STEPHANIE KITT, RN MSN
Formerly Clinical Specialist, Emergency Department
Northwestern Memorial Hospital
Chicago, Illinois

JUNE KAISER, RN MS
Clinical Research Associate
Curatek Pharmaceuticals
Elk Grove Village, Illinois

Formerly Practitioner/Teacher
Emergency Service
Rush-Presbyterian-St. Luke's Medical Center
Chicago, Illinois

EMERGENCY NURSING

A Physiologic and Clinical Perspective

W.B. SAUNDERS COMPANY
A Division of Harcourt Brace & Company
Philadelphia London Toronto
Montreal Sydney Tokyo

W.B. SAUNDERS COMPANY
A Division of
Harcourt Brace & Company

The Curtis Center
Independence Square West
Philadelphia, PA 19106

Library of Congress Cataloging-in-Publication Data

Emergency nursing.

   1. Emergency nursing I. Kitt, Stephanie.
II. Kaiser, June. [DNLM: 1. Emergencies—nursing.
WY 154 E52302]
RT120.E4E4744 1989   610.73′61   89-10164
ISBN 0-7216-2374-3

Editor: Michael Brown
Developmental Editor: Lisa Konoplisky
Designer: William Donnelly
Production Manager: Carolyn Naylor
Manuscript Editors: Lorraine Zawodny and Catherine Fix
Illustrators: Sharon Iwanczuk and Arlette Ramphal
Illustration Coordinator: Walt Verbitski
Indexer: Bernice Heller
Cover Designer: Terri Siegel

Emergency Nursing: A Physiologic and Clinical Perspective   ISBN 0-7216-2374-3

Last digit is the print number: 9 8 7 6 5 4

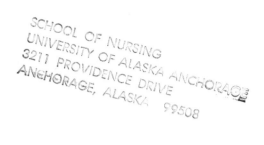
To our contemporaries who see emergency nursing as an art — an art that carves and paints the atmosphere in which we work, to effect the quality of the day.

Adapted from Henry David Thoreau

To Michael, who provided the greatest contribution of all — himself.

About the Authors

Stephanie Kitt began her career in emergency nursing as a staff nurse at Strong Memorial Hospital in Rochester, New York. Upon completion of a graduate degree in nursing from the University of Rochester, she became a clinical specialist in emergency nursing at Northwestern Memorial Hospital in Chicago. Ms. Kitt has a strong clinical background, has conducted numerous educational programs for emergency and critical care nurses, is a member of a clinical faculty for graduate programs in nursing, and lectures widely on trauma and other emergency-related topics. She is a member of the Special Committee on Trauma of the Emergency Nurses Association and the national faculty for the ENA trauma nursing core course.

June Kaiser gained a broad background in Emergency Nursing working as an emergency services staff nurse prior to accepting a faculty position as practitioner-teacher in emergency services at Rush-Presbyterian-St. Luke's Medical Center in Chicago. In this role, Ms. Kaiser was primarily responsible for clinical and classroom education of both nursing students and emergency services nursing staff. Ms. Kaiser is a member of ENA and has published, participated in, and coordinated seminars on a variety of topics related to emergency nursing. Currently, Ms. Kaiser is a clinical research associate for Curatek Pharmaceuticals in Elk Grove Village, Illinois, where she designs and monitors clinical trials for new drugs.

Contributors

Stephen L. Adams, MD FACP FACEP
Associate Chief, Section of Emergency
  Medicine
Department of Medicine, Northwestern
  University Medical School
Associate Medical Director, Emergency
  Medical Services
Northwestern Memorial Hospital
Chicago, IL
Neurologic Emergencies

Karen Smith Blesch, RN MS
Practitioner-Teacher
Department of Medical Nursing
Rush-Presbyterian-St. Luke's Medical
  Center
Chicago, IL
Oncologic Emergencies

Arlene Bonet, RN MS
Administrative Director
Emergency Services
Northwestern Memorial Hospital
Chicago, IL
Mass Casualty Management

Mary C. Brucker, CNM, DN Sc
Consultant, Women's Health
Dallas, TX
Obstetric and Gynecologic Emergencies

Janet Buckley, RN MSN
Practitioner-Teacher
Department of Medical Nursing
Rush-Presbyterian-St. Luke's Medical
  Center
Chicago, IL
Pulmonary Emergencies

Timothy Buckley, RRT
Regional Field Manager
Glasrock Home Health Care
Mount Prospect, IL
Pulmonary Emergencies

Michael F. Carter, MD
Associate Professor of Clinical Urology
Northwestern Memorial Hospital
Chicago, IL
Genitourinary Emergencies

Linda Clemmings, RN MA MS
Assistant Professor
Rush University College of Nursing
Practitioner-Teacher
Department of Community Health Nursing
Rush-Presbyterian-St. Luke's Medical
  Center
Chicago, IL
Gastrointestinal Emergencies

William Donnellan, MD PhD
Professor of Pediatrics
University of South Dakota
Sioux Falls, SD
Pediatric Trauma

Charles Drueck III, MD
Attending Surgeon
Director, Grainger Burn Center
Evanston Hospital Corporation
Evanston, IL
Burn Injuries

Jane Duda, RN MSN
Flight Nurse, University of Chicago
  Aeromedical Network
Pediatric Trauma Coordinator
University of Chicago Medical Center
Chicago, IL
Gastrointestinal Emergencies

Joan Duda, RN MS
Nurse Associate, Trauma Surgery
Cook County Hospital
Chicago, IL
Gastrointestinal Emergencies

Susan Fortin, RN MS
Unit Leader: Specialty Operating Rooms
Rush-Presbyterian-St. Luke's Medical
    Center
Chicago, IL
Ocular Emergencies

Marianne Genge, RN MS
Assistant Professor
Rush University College of Nursing
Practitioner-Teacher
Department of Surgical Nursing
Rush-Presbyterian-St. Luke's Medical
    Center
Chicago, IL
Musculoskeletal Emergencies

**Mary Beth Carrier Goldman, RN MS
    CCRN**
Practitioner-Teacher
Department of Maternal-Child Nursing
Rush-Presbyterian-St. Luke's Medical
    Center
Chicago, IL
Pediatric Medical Emergencies

Cheryl Jenkins, RN MS
Diabetes Clinical Specialist
Chicago Children's Diabetes Center
La Rabida Children's Hospital and
    Research Center
Chicago, IL
Endocrine Emergencies

Christine Jutzi-Kosmos, RN MS
Nurse Manager, Emergency Room
Former Trauma Coordinator
Michael Reese Hospital
Chicago, IL
*Assessment of Multiple Trauma and
    Thoracic Trauma*

Thomas Keeler, MD
Evanston Hospital
Evanston, IL
Genitourinary Emergencies

Rose Lach, RN MS
Practitioner-Teacher
Department of Medical Nursing
Rush-Presbyterian-St. Luke's Medical
    Center
Chicago, IL
*Quality Assurance in the Emergency
    Department*

James Mathews, MD FACEP
Associate Professor of Clinical Medicine
Chief, Section of Emergency Medicine
Northwestern University Medical School
Chicago, IL
Hypertension and Hypertensive Emergencies

Ruth E. Rea, RN PhD CEN
Lieutenant Colonel
Nurse Researcher
U.S. Army Nurse Corps
San Antonio, TX
Emergency Nursing Productivity Issues

Cheryl Ramler, RN MA
Gallstone Lithotripsy Project Coordinator
Northwestern Medical Faculty Foundation
Northwestern Memorial Hospital
Chicago, IL
Triage

Benita Reed, RN BSN MPH
Nurse Epidemiologist
Edward Hines, Jr., Veteran's Hospital
    Nursing Service
Hines, IL
Infectious Diseases

Nancy Jo Reedy, CNM MPH
Dallas, TX
Obstetric and Gynecologic Emergencies

Susan Santacaterina, RN
Staff Nurse, Emergency Department
Northwestern Memorial Hospital
Chicago, IL
Emergency Medical Services

**Michael K. Schroyer, RN MSN CCRN
    CNA**
Director of Organ and Tissue Bank
Rush-Presbyterian-St. Luke's Medical
    Center
Chicago, IL
Organ Donation

Elaine Scorza, RN MS
Staff Nurse, Level D
Department of Psychiatric Nursing
Rush-Presbyterian-St. Luke's Medical
    Center
Chicago, IL
Psychiatric Emergencies

Daniel J. Sheridan, RN MS
Coordinator, Family Violence Program
Rush-Presbyterian-St. Luke's Medical
    Center
Chicago, IL
Family Violence

Gary M. Sollars, MD FACEP
Emergency Physicians, Inc.
Phoenix, AZ
Thermoregulatory Emergencies

Leslee G. Stein-Spencer, RN MS
Chief, Division of Emergency Medical Ser-
    vices and Highway Safety
Illinois Department of Public Health
Springfield, IL
Emergency Medical Services

Rita Wickham, RN MS
Assistant Professor
Rush University College of Nursing
Oncology Clinical Nurse Specialist
Department of Medical Nursing
Rush-Presbyterian-St. Luke's Medical
    Center
Chicago, IL
Long-Term Venous Access Devices

James R. Wilson, MD
Assistant Professor of Medicine
Emergency Services
Rush-Presbyterian-St. Luke's Medical
    Center
Chicago, IL
*Maxillofacial Trauma and Ear, Nose, and
    Throat Emergencies*

Barbara G. White, RN MS
Vice President
Chesapeake General Hospital
Chesapeake, VA
*Fiscal Considerations in a Competitive
    Environment*

Mary Wlasowicz, RN MS
Nurse Consultant, Medicus Systems
    Corporation
Evanston, IL
Former Clinical Specialist/Supervisor
Midwest Regional Spinal Cord Injury Care
    System
Northwestern Memorial Hospital
Chicago, IL
Spinal Cord Injuries

Susan M. Woolley, RN
Burn Nursing Consultant
Evanston Hospital
Evanston, IL
Burn Injuries

Donna L. Young, RN MS
Vice President, Patient Care Services
Waterbury Hospital
Waterbury, CT
*Fiscal Considerations in a Competitive
    Environment*

Judith Zoellner-Hunter, RN MS
Clinical Nurse Manager
Division of Neurosciences Nursing
Northwestern Memorial Hospital
Chicago, IL
Shock; Head Trauma

David N. Zull, MD FACEP
Associate Chief of Medicine
Northwestern Memorial Hospital
Former Residency Director, Emergency
    Medicine
Northwestern Memorial Hospital
Assistant Professor of Clinical Medicine
Northwestern University Medical School
Chicago, IL
Anaphylaxis; Poisoning and Drug Overdose

Preface

The scope of Emergency Nursing practice is no longer viewed as providing episodic and crisis-oriented care. In an era characterized by exponential changes in health care and technology, the practice of professional nursing has expanded accordingly. Research and education, recognizing social, financial, and environmental influences in health care, are now incorporated into the expanded role of emergency nursing.

This text is based on a conceptual framework grounded in scientific, social, and psychologic sciences. It is divided into four content areas: core concepts, clinical systems, selected topics, and management issues. The core content chapters consist of broad-based topics covering all facets of emergency nursing practice. Clinical chapters are organized by physiologic systems and include a sound body of scientific knowledge relating to pathology of disease and trauma plus practical information that reflects optimal standards of care based on the nursing process. Throughout, the emphasis is on psychosocial integration. We believe incorporation of scientific principles enhances nursing care by enabling the nurse to anticipate physiologic and psychologic changes and act in accordance with the needs of the patient. Chapters in the selected topics section cover medical, surgical, and traumatic disorders that are not system-specific. Emergency department management issues are addressed in the final section of this text since we recognize that efficient management and fiscal responsibility promote better patient care. Specific topics are the economics of emergency care, quality assurance, and productivity planning.

Throughout this text, nursing diagnoses have been utilized within the nursing process. With few exceptions, we have used NANDA-approved nursing diagnoses. We believe much of emergency care is collaborative and health care professionals are interdependent. As such, treatment and nursing care discussed in relation to a particular nursing diagnosis include medical and nursing interventions. When a non-NANDA nursing diagnosis has been used, a footnote so indicates.

This text is intended as a comprehensive resource for emergency nurses, enhancing the delivery of holistic patient care in the emergency setting—a setting that is dynamic, broad-based, and in perpetual evolution to best serve millions of people in times of need.

Contents

Concepts Related to Emergency Nursing Practice

Susan Santacaterina, RN
Leslee Stein-Spencer, RN MS

Emergency Medical Services

Emergency Medical Services, or EMS, refers to an organized and coordinated system of prehospital providers, ambulance services, and, sometimes, hospital emergency department staff that respond to the needs of the acutely sick and injured. Like fire protection, Emergency Medical Services is a basic public service: that is, a service every citizen is entitled to.

Every emergency department in this country is currently involved in what is known as prehospital care. Any patient care rendered prior to arriving at an emergency facility can be defined as prehospital care. The concept of prehospital care is relatively new and has introduced health care roles such as the emergency medical technician, the EMS coordinator, and the mobile intensive care nurse. In addition, organized prehospital care has further expanded the role and responsibility of the emergency physician.

This chapter covers the evolution of EMS throughout this country and identifies current trends in this rapidly growing area of patient care.

HISTORICAL PERSPECTIVE

Military conflicts have served as training grounds for advancements in prehospital care. The concept of field resuscitation and emergency transportation of wounded soldiers proved effective in reducing battle casualties. In World War I mortality was 8%; it dropped to 4.5% in World War II, 2.5% in Korea, and less than 2% in Vietnam.

It became evident that rapid evacuation of the critically injured to facilities with highly trained personnel (Mobile Army Surgical Hospital units) saves lives.

The concept of reducing deaths from traffic accidents by prehospital care in the civilian sector first arose following the presidential campaign of 1960, during which John F. Kennedy stated that traffic accidents constituted one of the greatest, perhaps the greatest, of the nation's public health problems.

President Lyndon Johnson proposed a Traffic Safety Act, making him the first chief executive to give federal direction in this area. The Highway Safety Act of 1966 established guidelines and channeled funds to states for development of emergency medical services systems. The National Highway Traffic Safety Agency (NHTSA), which is part of the Federal Highway Administration of the Department of Transportation (DOT), is responsible for enforcing the Act. The Department of Transportation, in conjunction with the American Academy of Orthopedic Surgeons, was given responsibility for developing academic standards for training prehospital personnel. Curriculum development for prehospital education throughout the country continues to be a responsibility of the DOT.

Also in 1966, the National Academy of Sciences and the American Medical Association published a report that identified trauma as "the neglected disease of modern society," since little had been done for this problem in the civilian sector. This paper was the impetus for building emergency medical care programs in the United States.

In 1969, the first national conference on emergency medical services was held. Guidelines for organizing community-wide EMS councils were formulated as were standards for design and equipment of EMS vehicles. It was also suggested that hospital emergency departments be categorized according to the level of care offered.

Frank Pantridge, M.D. is credited with the first successful prehospital care system in the early 1960s in Belfast, Ireland. Although the Belfast system used physicians and nurses to staff emergency vehicles, which is not commonly done in this country, it was the first system to provide sophisticated prehospital care. Dr. William Grace, through St. Vincent's Hospital in New York, put the first mobile coronary care unit on the street in 1966. Dr. Eugene Nagel from Miami is credited with development of telemetry. These physicians were pioneers in developing EMS systems even before our country had legislation.

These early efforts and the NHTSA/DOT programs were aimed at improving care and transportation in the prehospital phase of EMS. In 1972, recognizing the need to further reduce death and disability from injury, President Nixon charged the Department of Health, Education and Welfare (HEW) with a new role in EMS. While NHTSA/DOT would continue to be responsible for prehospital transportation and communication, HEW would assume responsibility for the medical aspects of prehospital care and for upgrading services within hospitals.

In order to accomplish this task, HEW awarded five demonstration contracts totalling $16 million to test various approaches to providing emergency care in a systematic and comprehensive manner. The demonstration sites were Jacksonville, Florida; San Diego, California; Athens, Ohio; and the States of Arkansas and Illinois. Various models for regionalization and organization were tested.

Through the experiences of these EMS demonstration projects came the direction, guidelines, and models for the Emergency Medical Services Systems Act of 1973. This act provided funding and a way for communities across the United States to develop regional EMS Systems. Since the funding was federal, Congress mandated that a systems approach to emergency response and medical care be planned and implemented. The Act required that EMS systems provide training for EMS professionals and for public education in first aid techniques and in using the system. In addition, at least one hospital within every EMS system was to provide continuous physician coverage in the emergency department. Another important aspect of the act was that it forbade the withholding of emergency care to a victim because of inability to pay for the service. The EMS Systems Act started a major national effort in improving emergency care throughout the states. EMS programs developed in almost every community, regardless of size.

The Omnibus Budget Reconciliation Act of 1981 resulted in another major change in national EMS focus. The Federal EMS program with its "categorical" grants was integrated into the preventive Health and Health Services Block Grant. This action effectively ended federal leadership for EMS. The national office within the Department of Health and Human Services (formerly HEW) was closed, leaving NHTSA with its limited transportation and communications mandate in the only federal EMS role.

The responsibility for development, direction, and control of EMS Systems now lies with state and local governments. While the federal initiative certainly helped the early development of EMS across the country, the vast diversity of the nation ensured that each system would be implemented in a different way. Consequently, the recent return of decision making to the state and local level is appropriate.

In just over twenty years' time, EMS has grown from a concept unknown outside the military sector to a service taken for granted by the public.

THE EMS SYSTEMS

EMS systems join a number of resources in order to provide quality emergency care. Physicians and nurses must work with policemen, firemen, politicians, and government agencies in situations outside the familiar hospital environment. A cooperative effort between hospitals, municipalities, and health care givers is essential in establishing a successful EMS system.

In addition, advanced level EMS systems provide quality prehospital emergency care and emergency management through delegation of responsibility for assessment and the reporting of patient complaints by prehospital providers. The Project Medical Director or physician responsible for the system delegates this responsibility.

Access to the System

Each system has a mechanism by which ambulance service is provided. This is often accomplished through one of the municipal services such as fire, police, or health department personnel. In many cities the major ambulance provider is the local fire department. Since most police and fire departments are connected to an emergency access system such as 911, an ambulance response can easily be dispatched through this same emergency response network. Coverage by 911 systems, however, varies widely, ranging from three states with no 911 to six states with 100 percent coverage.

In some systems, the ambulances may be dispatched from the hospital itself and staffed with a physician, nurse, or emergency medical technician (EMT) from the emergency department. Most communities also have ambulance services that are privately owned. These ambulance companies usually provide the same type of care but are not necessarily dispatched through the 911 system as a first response. Private ambulances may be called by any consumer or institution seeking skilled transportation to a medical facility.

One current problem in the delivery of emergency medical services is lack of medical control at the basic life support (BLS) level. Medical control, in which physicians take direct responsibility (via radio or standing medical orders) for prehospital patient care, is commonly exercised only at the intermediate life support (ILS) and advanced life support (ALS) levels. However, most prehospital care is at the BLS level, and it is believed that adding physician involvement and accountability at this level could significantly improve patient care.

Medical Direction

Advanced level, in-field emergency care is carried out under directions from professionals employed by a hospital known as a resource hospital or base station. Each system sets up its own way of implementing this extension of emergency care. However implemented, the network must clearly define medical authority for the prehospital care rendered. In situations in which physicians do not provide prehospital care, the system must provide a mechanism to contact the resource hospital so that medical direction can be provided. This communication is usually accomplished by telemetry radio in which both voice and EKG strip can be transmitted from the field to the hospital.

The designation of a resource hospital is done on a statewide level through the local or state department of public health. Hospital designation is based on geographic location as well as ability to meet established criteria. The resource hospital or base station must provide personnel to staff the telemetry system at all times. Once treatment is initiated in the field, the resource hospital must have direct communication with the receiving or participating hospital; resource hospital personnel act as liaison between the prehospital team and the hospital staff receiving the patient. Although there are no studies to document the benefits of this liaison, it is thought that such communication is important in preparing for the patient, initiating treatment, and establishing estimated time of arrival. The resource hospital must be assured by agreement with participating hospitals that established minimum standards will be maintained once care is relinquished to them. The staff at the participating hospital is then in turn able to assess the care rendered in the field and to provide valuable feedback to the resource hospital and prehospital staff regarding appropriateness of treatment. Each link in this system is as important as the next. Without a full commitment from each component, EMS would be only a ride to the hospital.

Medical Director

In 1984, the American College of Emergency Physicians issued a position paper concerning medical control in EMS. It stated that prehospital emergency care provided by nonphysicians is considered to be an extension of the medical director, who is responsible for all clinical and patient care aspects of EMS. This philosophy places a great deal of responsibility on the medical director, which could not be assumed without a team approach to efforts in the field and at the resource hospital. The physician who is best suited to administer and coordinate medical control is the emergency – critical care physician who continues the care initiated by the prehospital care provider.

An important aspect of the team effort is development of protocols for care delivery. In most systems the medical director develops standing medical orders (SMOs) or protocols. In the event of radio communication failure, care can be given under specific standing orders. Standing medical orders must be designed to correlate with the needs and resources of a specific EMS system. Capabilities of the EMTs on the scene, rate of incidence, and transport times to the hospital are all important considerations in developing standing medical orders.

Developing protocols is a difficult task at best. However, most prehospital standing medical orders (SMOs) are designed to treat specific problems that can readily be identified and treated in the prehospital setting. The orders usually follow a logical algorithm similar in format to those developed by the American Heart Association for advanced cardiac life support.

Protocols should be designed to provide a standardized approach to patient management. However, the SMOs will be only as effective as the process by which they are implemented. This brings us to the issue of educational responsibilities. Philosophically, implementation of treatment by anyone other than the medical director is done by extending the use of that physician's medical license. Therefore, to reduce liability and ensure quality care, each system must establish internal educational requirements. Physicians have played a significant role in development of the national training curriculum for prehospital personnel through the DOT, which recommends

1. A physician should serve as the course medical director with responsibility for ensuring the medical accuracy of the course.

2. The in-hospital phase of training must be planned in conjunction with the course medical director and representatives of an emergency medical facility.

3. All EMT training must be arranged under the sponsorship of the local medical adviser to ensure medical accuracy and compliance with local treatment protocols.

Nursing Roles

In many resource hospital emergency departments, nurses have expanded their scope of practice to include telemetry communication. Since this responsibility has been designated by legislation to the medical director or qualified designee, only mobile intensive care nurses (MICNs) can qualify to provide on-line direction for prehospital care. The educational requirements for emergency department nurses to take on this responsibility vary from state to state and system to system. There currently are very few states that define MICN by legislation. Although there is not an established national curriculum for training, most systems require the minimum of a 40-hour course with documented proficiency in practical application.

The course must focus on prehospital care. Areas of specific concentration include the following:

1. Dysrhythmia recognition and management
2. Respiratory emergencies
3. Trauma management
4. Spinal cord immobilization and management
5. Medical and environmental emergencies
6. Obstetric/pediatric emergencies
7. Telemetry communications

The nurse has historically assumed the multidisciplinary tasks of patient advocate, educator, and facilitator. The MICN must likewise use similar skills in order to be a valuable member of the EMS team. It is important that MICNs as well as physicians involved in telemetry communication develop an appreciation for circumstances encountered in the prehospital setting. Staff education should include clinical experience in the field with the prehospital providers. There is a tendency for hospital staff to treat patients on telemetry as though they are in the hospital setting. Clinical experience in the field attunes the staff to conditions that can lead to unrealistic expectations. Telemetry orders such as starting an IV or recheck of vital signs may be simple enough in the sterile confines of the emergency department. At the scene, however, it may mean starting an IV in a bar or listening for lung sounds amid the noise of expressway traffic. Situational circumstances must always be considered.

Also, in-hospital EMT education is important. This experience may enhance the EMT's assessment skills with the advantage of follow-up information and the ability to spend more time with patients. The exchange of clinical experiences promotes working relationships and helps the EMT to understand difficulties such as a delay in answering telemetry in a busy emergency department.

EMS System Coordinator (Hospital-Based)

The EMS coordinator is a hospital staff person who integrates all aspects of emergency management by fostering the concept of emergency care starting "in the streets." Many of the resource hospital system coordinators have historically been nursing personnel. The EMS coordinator position in most systems is established to coordinate educational and on-line administrative functions of the EMS system. This position is usually held by a registered nurse who can integrate emergency skills, scientific knowledge, and education principles. The EMS coordinator is responsible for implementation of educational programs for both resource hospital/base station and prehospital personnel. In addition to educational responsibilities, the EMS coordinator must assume responsibility for quality assurance discussed within this chapter.

Prehospital Care Providers

Throughout the years, ambulance staffing has changed along with the changing focus of EMS. In the United States, ambulances are commonly staffed by EMTs. There are

TABLE 1-1
Required Areas of EMT-P Proficiency

Division 1: Prehospital Environment	**Division 4: Medical**
Section 1. Roles and responsibilities	Section 1. Respiratory
Section 2. EMS systems	Section 2. Cardiovascular
Section 3. Medical/legal considerations	Section 3. Endocrine emergencies
Section 4. EMS communications	Section 4. Nervous system
Section 5. Rescue	Section 5. Acute abdomen
Section 6. Major incident response	Section 6. Anaphylaxis
Section 7. Stress management	Section 7. Toxicology, alcoholism, and drug abuse
Division 2: Preparatory	Section 8. Infectious diseases
Section 1. Medical terminology	Section 9. Environmental injuries
Section 2. General patient assessment	Section 10. Geriatrics/gerontology
Section 3. Airways and ventilation	Section 11. Pediatrics
Section 4. Pathophysiology of shock	**Division 5: OB/GYN/Neonatal**
Section 5. General pharmacology	Section 1. OB/GYN/neonatal
Division 3: Trauma	**Division 6: Behavioral**
Section 1. Trauma	Section 1. Behavioral emergencies
Section 2. Burns	

a number of different levels of training for the EMT, and the type of training required depends on the level of service the system can afford to provide. Advanced life support (ALS) is the optimal level of prehospital emergency care. An ALS ambulance must be fully equipped with telemetry communication, cardiac monitor and defibrillator, and a full complement of emergency medications. It must be staffed by at least one EMT trained to the level of EMT-paramedic (EMT-P). The curriculum used for EMT-paramedic training has been established by the national DOT and is the accepted national standard; it supplies the didactic material, and the EMS system provides the clinical component. In order to provide prehospital advanced life support, the EMT-P must prove proficiency in the areas described in Table 1-1.

Although ALS paramedic-staffed ambulances provide a high level of care, these programs are expensive and lengthy and are not always available in all areas of a state, especially in rural and volunteer areas.

Some systems provide a BLS service that renders an advanced first aid type of care. The ambulances are staffed with two emergency medical technician attendants (EMT-As) and are equipped for basic supportive care. EMT-A training includes, as a minimum, a 106-hour course. The emergency care EMT-As are trained to provide includes the following: (1) airway management, (2) CPR, (3) control of shock and bleeding, and (4) splinting of fractures. The BLS provider is often used as a first response team. This means the BLS team may arrive at a scene and request ALS back-up and transport if the patient's condition warrants it.

Over the years, other levels of EMT training have been developed that fall in between that of the EMT-P and the EMT-A. For instance, there is a level called EMT-intermediate (EMT-I). This group may be trained to perform the following: (1) EMT-A skills, (2) intravenous therapy, (3) invasive airway management, (4) trauma care, and (5) defibrillation (optional). These skills vary from jurisdiction to jurisdiction. This level seems most useful in areas where transport times are lengthy and additional skills are beneficial, yet a full paramedic program would be too expensive.

Recent studies have focused on sudden fatal dysrhythmias and the importance of quick defibrillation. In response, some systems have developed a level of training called EMT-defibrillator (EMT-D). These technicians are EMT-As with additional training in recognition of ventricular fibrillation and defibrillation techniques. This level is also thought to be exceptionally useful in systems where long transport times might warrant the use of this skill in addition to basic life support care.

Continuing Education

Every EMS system must design programs to meet the continuing educational needs of its health care providers. EMTs must meet requirements for a specific number of continuing education hours as mandated by the local or state agency. Paramedic continuing educational programs are often provided by the resource hospital or training school (i.e., college). Programs may include telemetry review (in which telemetry recordings are reviewed and critiqued by paramedics, MICNs, and emergency department physicians) or clinical experience in the resource hospital. Emergency medical and nursing seminars now include topics relevant to prehospital care providers. Such continuing education experiences are extremely beneficial in promoting a team approach to patient care.

Along with meeting specific continuing educational requirements, EMTs must often go through rigid certification and recertification processes. Since most states certify EMTs for only two or three years, the process of recertifying must be included in system programs. National registry, for example, also mandates continuing education in order to be recertified, and this must also be taken into account.

EMS Quality Assurance

In the hospital setting nurses and physicians are often in a fishbowl atmosphere in which care is easily observed by peers or supervisors. Paramedics, on the other hand, practice in a setting that allows little scrutiny by supervisors or peers. Consequently, assuring quality care is difficult. The main connection between medical care rendered in the field and the physician responsible for that care is sometimes at best a radio. Although continuing education programs are designed to reinforce the potentially weak link, they are not enough. Establishing and monitoring standards of prehospital care is a burgeoning aspect of EMS systems today. There is a trend toward establishing programs that utilize paramedics, nurses, and physicians in a quality assurance capacity.

CONCLUSION

Prehospital care is here to stay. Studies have shown that prehospital care has had a significant impact on patient survival. For example, research from Seattle, ending in 1979, studied the impact of paramedic services on mortality from out-of-hospital cardiac arrest. The study showed higher rates of admission and discharge for patients treated by paramedics. Thirty-five percent of such patients lived to be admitted to the hospital, versus 18% of patients treated by nonparamedics.

For the future, there is a great need for public education. It has taken hospital personnel some time to understand what prehospital care providers are doing in the field; it is taking the public even longer. In Chicago, for example, 80% of persons requesting advanced life support by the Chicago Fire Department really require no medical intervention. Such inappropriate requests for care tie up ALS ambulances that may be needed elsewhere and add an intangible stress factor to the paramedic role in addition to increasing system costs. Public education that identifies paramedic roles and reasons for calling 911 will help promote EMS effectiveness as will call screening by EMT-Ps.

Recently two states, Pennsylvania and Illinois, have passed legislation allowing nurses to work in the prehospital care setting. Previously nurses had to become certified as EMTs in order to function in the field. This is an enormous step in expanding the role of a registered nurse. The field RN will be beneficial in areas where, although there are no paramedics, the patient still can be given ALS care in the field. In a recent article in the Journal of Emergency Nursing, the Emergency Nurses Association and the National Flight Nurses Association jointly endorsed the concept of specially prepared registered nurses working in the prehospital care setting.* These organizations feel that the nurse can provide care that is commensurate with his/her level of training and expertise. The "Field RN" would be looked upon as a leader in the prehospital care environment.

The work in managing in-field emergencies oftentimes goes unheralded. The development of prehospital care and its professionals have not been without growing pains. Work in the field can be physically demanding, emotionally stressful, and oftentimes unappreciated. The health care worker who chooses to work in a prehospital setting must indeed be an individual with high professional standards, and fortunately EMS systems are growing up with those standards.

REFERENCES

Boyd D. 1982. The conceptual development of EMS systems in the United States, Part I. Emerg Med Serv 11:19–23.

Boyd D. 1982. The conceptual development of EMS systems in the United States, Part II. Emerg Med Serv 11:26–35.

Department of Health, Education and Welfare, Public Health Service, Division of Emergency Medical Services. 1975, revised. Emergency Medical Services Systems Program Guidelines. Washington, DC, DHEW Publication No. HSA 75-2013.

Eleventh Annual EMS State and Province Survey. Emerg Med Serv 16:203–257.

ENA/NFNA. 1988. Role of the Registered Nurse in the Pre Hospital Environment. J Emerg Nurs 14:23A–24A.

Henry MC, Stapleton ER. 1985. EMTs and medical control. 1985 Almanac. Emerg Med Serv 10:32–34.

National Academy of Sciences-National Research Council. Division of Medical Sciences. 1966. Accidental Death and Disability—The Neglected Disease of Modern Society. Washington, DC.

Omnibus Budget Reconciliation Act of 1981. Public Law 97–35.

Turnock BJ. 1979. Illinois Comprehensive Plan for Emergency Medical Services, 1979–1983. 22–40.

USDOT/NHTSA. 1984. National Standard Curriculum, Instructor's Lesson Plans. Emergency Medical Technician—Ambulance. 3rd ed. Washington, DC.

USDOT/NHTSA. 1985. National Standard Curriculum, Instructor's Lesson Plans. Emergency Medical Technician—Paramedic.

---

* Developed jointly by Emergency Nurses Association and National Flight Nurses Association. Approved by ENA, August 2, 1987; approved by NFNA September 10, 1987.

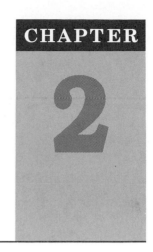
Stephanie Kitt, RN MSN

Interfacility Transfer

Transport of critically ill and injured patients has increased in both numbers and methods over the past two decades. Although most patients are able to receive comprehensive care in local hospitals, individuals with more serious illnesses and injuries may require specialized services beyond those locally available. An increasing number of centers provide advanced and comprehensive care to patients with complex problems. However, the volume of individuals with a particular problem (e.g., spinal cord injury) may not be large enough to enable development of expertise in management of these highly complex injuries. The physician should assess the institutional capabilities and limitations to ensure recognition of patients who could benefit from care available at specialty centers. Spinal cord and burn injury and neonatal care are a few examples of the kinds of specialty services provided primarily at tertiary health care facilities. As a patient advocate, the nurse should recognize the benefits of highly specialized and technologically advanced critical care and suggest transfer of appropriate patients to specialty centers.

METHODS OF TRANSFER

There are two primary methods, air and ground, by which an individual can be transferred from one facility to another. While both afford advantages and disadvantages, if criteria are applied according to well-considered guidelines, an optimum system for transfer can be attained. Ground transport is the more cost-effective method. Air transport should be reserved for patients requiring expeditious transfer between hospitals. Air transport may also be used by the first responder at the scene of rural accidents. The ideal system supports both methods of transport and utilizes each according to protocols to promote patient welfare. Coordinators for patient transport can be very effective in assuring proper use of regional resources.

MEDICOLEGAL RESPONSIBILITY

Individuals and agencies involved in patient transport bear responsibility that implies medicolegal liability. The sending institution is responsible for initial patient stabilization, notification of the receiving institution and transport service, obtaining a physician's order for transfer, maintaining medical responsibility for the patient until the receiving physician accepts responsibility, and informing family of the necessity for transport.

A physician from the receiving institution must accept the patient prior to transport. Transporting a patient without the consent of a receiving physician able to accept the patient is considered abandonment.

In most cases the transferring physician is liable for the patient until he has arrived at the receiving institution. In some situations a prearranged transfer agreement may specify when medical control exchanges hands.

PATIENT PREPARATION

Before transport the patient should be hemodynamically stable with pharmacologic support, adequate arterial blood gases, intubation, supplemental oxygen, and positive end-expiratory pressure as necessary. Certain routine diagnostic tests (ABGs, electrolytes, chest x-ray, CBC, and so forth) should be reported and repeated just before transfer to ensure that the patient's condition is stable.

Prior to transport the patient must be evaluated to detect any immediately or potentially life-threatening problems and to assure that appropriate actions are taken to prevent in-transport crises. The patient should have a secure and patent airway. Airway and breathing are evaluated for current as well as potential problems. Is the patient able to maintain a patent airway throughout transport or is there a possibility of airway compromise? The massively burned patient provides an excellent example of one whose status may change rapidly and who may therefore require prophylactic intubation to avoid airway compromise secondary to laryngeal edema. Unconscious patients must be intubated to aid in ventilation and to prevent aspiration. A patent airway is not enough to assure ongoing protection, since movement in an ambulance or aircraft may induce nausea and vomiting. The potential for aspiration and respiratory compromise is present.

Once the patient's airway is secured, adequate oxygenation and ventilation should be assured. Blood gas analysis is an essential part of assessment and stabilization of the patient. Because most patients require supplemental oxygen, it is the transport nurse's responsibility to assure that oxygen tanks are adequately filled to last during transport times.

Hemodynamic status can be determined by evaluation of the readily available physiologic parameters — blood pressure and pulse. A relatively new means of monitoring the patient's perfusion status is the transconjunctival oximeter. The oximeter is placed on the conjunctiva and senses changes in peripheral oxygen levels. In a hemodynamically stable patient, the concentration of conjunctival oxygen ($Pcjo_2$) is related to the Pao_2 (Abraham et al. 1984). In the hemodynamically unstable patient, the $Pcjo_2$ tracks the state of peripheral perfusion and oxygenation. The $Pcjo_2$ is more sensitive to changes in the oxygenation and circulatory status than heart rate, blood pressure, and clinical assessment of tidal volume (Lee 1987).

In critically ill individuals, an arterial line for purposes of invasive hemodynamic monitoring is in order. When the ABCs have been stabilized, one should assess all major systems, using a head-to-toe approach. Refer to Chapter 6 for more details. Individuals recently traumatized should have gone through a thorough examination with major diagnoses established prior to transfer.

Patients with actual or potential spinal cord injury must be maintained in full spinal immobilization with a hard collar, towel rolls laterally, and 2-inch tape across the forehead. In addition, the patient must be fully restrained to a full-length backboard with binders to prevent any movement of the body. The backboard can then be turned without moving the patient. Should vomiting occur, aspiration is less likely.

Psychologic support for the patient and family members or significant others is important in preparation for transport. Family members need to know exactly what the arrangements are. They must be directed to the appropriate facility by land maps, must be given an estimated time of arrival for the patient and transport team, and must be directed to appropriate individuals in the admitting hospital for overnight or long-term housing arrangements. It is also important for family members to know the admitting physician's name at the receiving hospital.

The patient who is being transported far from home requires special consideration. Patients fear unknown diagnostic procedures and treatments. In addition to the stress of the illness or injury, the patient experiences stress caused by removal from home and family, and often by transport to a large hospital in a strange city (Anderson 1987). Whatever the magnitude of anxiety, there is a consistent need for explanations regarding the many pretransfer preparations, what to expect en route, and the anticipated course of events during transfer.

TRANSPORT CONSIDERATIONS

Successful transport depends on proper equipment and supplies. Transport equipment is used primarily for monitoring and should be lightweight and compact and should have battery back-up modes of operation (Pearl 1987, 71). Basic equipment includes a cardiac monitor, transducers, defibrillator, portable suction unit, infusion pumps, pneumatic antishock garments, oximeter, oxygen cylinders, and a stretcher.

Vehicle limitations are a consideration whether transporting in ground ambulance or in fixed-wing or helicopter aircraft. Lighting and electrical power are limited, and patient access is more cumbersome than in hospital settings. The transfer must be carefully planned to ensure adequate supplies, equipment, and especially suction, oxygen, and battery-supported monitoring and defibrillation equipment. Refer to Table 2–1 for a sample adult transport equipment checklist.

Air transport is ideal in circumstances requiring rapid transport over relatively short periods of time. Although air transport decreases the amount of time the patient is not in a hospital setting, it does not necessarily decrease the overall transport time. Mobilizing the team and flying out to get the patient adds to overall transport time. Air transport may be utilized in congested areas for short transports during rush hours when traffic delays may significantly delay definitive care. Helicopters generally are neither the first nor the sole responders for on-scene care (Sroczynski 1985). However, rural communities lying long distances from any health care facility are increasingly using helicopters for first-line response and transport. This practice affords expeditious health care to communities previously exempt from immediate advanced level care.

PHYSIOLOGIC EFFECTS OF ALTITUDE

In preparation for air transport, whether fixed-wing or helicopter aircraft, one must anticipate the physiologic effects of altitude. The major effects of altitude reflect the change in atmospheric pressure (McNeil 1983). Increases in altitude are associated with decreases in atmospheric pressure. In an unpressurized aircraft, there is a lack of protection against the decreasing pressure as altitude is gained. The rate of decrease is relative to the rate of climb of the aircraft. The major physiologic effects of changing altitude relate to the expansion of gases. Boyle's law states that at constant temperature, the volume of a given mass of gas is inversely proportional to the pressure on it. It therefore follows that altitude and resultant drops in atmospheric pressure promote expansion of gases.

Expansion of Gases

The symptoms resulting from expansion of gases are most pronounced when gases expand in the gastrointestinal tract, middle ear, and sinuses (Saletta et al. 1984). When a cavity is closed or semiclosed, increased pressure can be harmful, painful, or both. Expansion of air in the inner ear is most painful when pressure equalization is not possible. When air in the gastrointestinal tract expands, there is potential for vomiting and aspiration. A nasogastric tube should be inserted prior to air transport. Any pneumothorax must be treated prior to transfer by air in order to prevent expansion of the trapped air. Even a small pneumothorax will expand in flight and in doing so may develop into a tension pneumothorax. A chest tube must always be inserted in the patient who has a pneumothorax. When the patient is transported with a chest tube in place, the tube must never be closed off as this allows no room for expansion of gases, and atelectasis may occur. A valve may be attached to the end of the chest tube to allow one-way flow of air.

TABLE 2–1
Adult Transport Equipment Checklist

Blue Box

Side A, Tier 1
- ☐ Redux paste × 1 tube
- ☐ Razor × 1
- ☐ #11 Scalpel × 1
- ☐ General all-purpose instrument tray × 1
- ☐ 25% albumin × 2, administration set × 1
- ☐ EKG paper × 1 roll
- ☐ 1 Each: rectal, oral thermometer

Side B, Tier 1
- ☐ Microdrippers × 4
- ☐ Macrodrippers × 1
- ☐ Nonvented tubing × 1
- ☐ Dial-A-Flow × 2

Side A, Tier 2
- ☐ EKG electrodes × 5
- ☐ Tycoe manometer × 1
- ☐ Screwdriver × 1
- ☐ Black Magic Marker × 1
- ☐ Tourniquet × 1
- ☐ Heparin lock adapter × 2

Tape:
- ☐ 1/2″ eye tape × 1
- ☐ 1/2″ pink tape × 1
- ☐ 1″ eye tape × 1

Plastic bag:
- ☐ 2″ pink tape × 1 roll
- ☐ 1″ adhesive tape × 1 roll
- ☐ 1″ paper tape × 1

Side B, Tier 2
- ☐ 12 ml Syringes × 4
- ☐ 5 ml Syringes × 5
- ☐ 3 ml Syringes × 3
- ☐ TB Syringes × 3
- ☐ 50 ml Regular Tip Syringe
- ☐ 50 ml Cath Tip Syringe
- ☐ 20 ml Syringes × 2

Side A, Tier 3
- ☐ Stopwatch
- ☐ 3-0 Nylon suture with straight needle × 4
- ☐ Assorted needles
- ☐ "D" batteries × 2

Side B, Tier 3
- ☐ Alcohol wipes
- ☐ 2 × 2 gauze sponges × 6
- ☐ Betadine swabsticks × 3

In small plastic bag:
- ☐ K-Y jelly
- ☐ Betadine ointment
- ☐ Benzoin ampules

Bottom

IV tubing bags:
- ☐ 4 ft. Cobe tubing × 3
- ☐ 1 ft. Cobe tubing × 2
- ☐ K-52 extension tube × 1
- ☐ K-51 extension tube × 2
- ☐ Holter pump tubing Size "B" × 2
- ☐ Holter pump tubing Size "C" × 2
- ☐ Holter pump tubing Size "D" × 2

Plastic bags:
- ☐ Bell & Howell transducer dome × 3
- ☐ Stopcocks × 10
- ☐ IV air filters × 4
- ☐ Male-male adapters × 3

IV catheter bag:
2 each: ☐ 18-gauge Quik Cath
- ☐ 20-gauge Quik Cath
- ☐ 14-gauge Jelco
- ☐ 16-gauge Jelco
- ☐ 18-gauge Jelco
- ☐ 20-gauge Jelco
- ☐ 18-gauge arterial needle

- ☐ 4 × 4 gauze sponges × 4
- ☐ Soluset × 1
- ☐ Blood set with pump
- ☐ Blood set Y-tube
- ☐ NS 1000cc × 3
- ☐ D5W 250cc × 4
- ☐ DS/.2NS 500cc × 1
- ☐ NS 250cc × 1

Black Bag

Side A
- ☐ Manifold × 2
- ☐ Guidewires #18, #25, #35 (1 ea)
- ☐ #14 Fr. suction catheters × 4
- ☐ Salem sump × 1
- ☐ Sterile gloves #7, #7 1/2, #8 (1 ea)

- ☐ Swan-Ganz 7 Fr. thermodilution × 1
- ☐ Arterial line tray × 1
- ☐ Cutdown tray × 1
- ☐ Transvenous pacing wire × 1 (disp. kit)
- ☐ External pacemaker with cable × 2

Center Section
- ☐ Flashlight × 1
- ☐ CVP manometer × 1
- ☐ Pressure bag × 1
- ☐ Blood pressure cuff × 1
- ☐ Chest tube 28 Fr. × 1
- ☐ Heimlich valve × 2

Side B
- ☐ CVP tray (Arrow disposable) × 1
- ☐ Swan tray (Arrow disposable) × 1
- ☐ CVP intrafusor × 2

Intubation Box

Top Shelf
- ☐ Magill forceps × 2
- ☐ Stylet × 1

Oral airways:
- ☐ #5 × 1
- ☐ #4 × 1
- ☐ #3 × 1
- ☐ #2 × 1

Nasal airways:
- ☐ 30 Fr.
- ☐ 28 Fr.

- ☐ Manometer for anesthesia bag

Tape:
- ☐ 1/2″ adhesive
- ☐ 1″ adhesive
- ☐ 1″ eye tape
- ☐ Extra bulbs
- ☐ Benzoin ampules
- ☐ 2% xylocaine jelly
- ☐ K-Y jelly
- ☐ Straight connector × 1
- ☐ "C" batteries × 2
- ☐ 9v batteries × 3

Second Shelf
- ☐ Laryngoscope handle × 2
- ☐ #2 Miller blade
- ☐ #3 Miller blade
- ☐ #4 Miller blade
- ☐ #3 Mac blade
- ☐ #4 Mac blade
- ☐ Q-tips × 3
- ☐ Tongue blades × 3
- ☐ Scissors
- ☐ Blue bite block

Bottom
- ☐ RT module
- ☐ ET tube #6, #7, #8 × 2
- ☐ 4% Xylocaine, topical
- ☐ #6 Shiley trach
- ☐ 14 Fr. suction catheters × 2
- ☐ Tonsil suction × 1

Source: Pearl RG, et al. 1987. Care of the adult patient during transport. Int Anesthesiol Clin 25:73.

Air expansion in equipment is a major consideration. Air splints, pneumatic antishock garments, blood pressure cuffs, and balloon cuffs on endotracheal tubes may present hazards to the in-flight patient if not properly attended. Care must be taken to reduce pressure in all pressure-filled equipment as indicated. Because balloons filled with air may expand and cause undue pressure on surrounding structures such as the trachea, one may consider substituting water for air to assure constant balloon pressures. Intravenous flow problems necessitate special regulation. Intravenous solutions in plastic bags are preferred to glass bottles since there is no risk of breakage. The air pressure that under normal atmospheric conditions allows intravenous fluid to flow is no longer sufficient at nonpressurized flight elevations.

Pressure cuffs applied around pliable intravenous solution bags are necessary to assure infusion. When IV glass bottles must be used, additional pressure above the fluid may be required to assure infusion. This can be accomplished by adding several milliliters of air to the bottle through the air vent in the IV tubing. In this case, the air above the fluid may be subject to expansive forces that are prevented from venting. This can cause air embolus if the intravenous solution is not changed prior to complete infusion. In addition, tape applied to completely cover glass bottles will provide a safety measure against glass shattering should the bottles break.

Temperature

Temperature decreases by approximately 2°C (3.5°F) for every 1000 feet above sea level (Dnenin 1978). Temperature changes generally pose no threat to the flight team or patient, since pressurized air ambulances have adequate temperature regulation. However, temperatures outside the cabin may fluctuate, and inside temperature controls, unable to respond immediately, may induce fluctuation in aircraft temperature. Blankets should be readily accessible for patient comfort in the event of a temperature fluctuation.

Humidity

Humidity also changes with altitude. As air is cooled, it loses moisture. Since helicopter and fixed-wing aircraft have decreased relative humidity, chapped lips, dry mucous membranes, sore throats, and hoarse voices may result. Adequate fluid intake and lip balm are means to avoid discomforts associated with long flights.

Orthopedic Considerations

Orthopedic patients present particular problems with respect to altitude. For patients with casted extremities and injuries less than 48 hours old, it may be wise to bivalve or split the cast in order to avoid constriction that may result as the extremity swells with increased altitude. The size of the aircraft may prohibit the use of hare traction splints. There are various alternative traction splints available that do not extend beyond the foot and are useful when space is limited.

Gravity

Gravitational effects or effects of acceleration are experienced with changes in speed during takeoff and landing and with changes in direction. A transient redistribution of body fluids can occur as a result of these forces. During takeoff, the acceleration forces act from the front to the back of the vehicle. If a patient is positioned in the head-aft position, he or she might experience a transient increase in venous return to the heart from a redistribution of blood from the lower extremities. Since most air ambulances exert only a small gravitational force during any type of flight maneuver, the potential for serious problems is minimal (Lachenmyer 1987, 30–31).

Turbulence

Turbulence, caused by rapid changes in wind speed and direction, may make patient monitoring more difficult. The aircraft movement may induce motion sickness in the patient as well as in the flight crew.

Vibration and Noise

Vibration and noise occur in varying degrees in both ground and air ambulances. The noise associated with medical transport makes auscultation impossible. Palpation of blood pressures and pulses is a good alternative means of monitoring hemodynamic status. Continuous airway assessment is extremely important, since sounds associated with airway compromise such as an endotracheal air leak or mucous congestion may be difficult or impossible to discern.

FLIGHT TEAM

Air transport requires a qualified flight team to ensure optimal care. Flight nursing has developed as a specialty over the past several years. The flight service has a responsibility to utilize professional standards in developing qualifications and performance guidelines needed to effectively employ professional nurses in the air ambulance setting (Sroczynski 1985, 267). The American Society of Hospital-Based Emergency Air Medical Services (ASHBEAMS) acknowledges in their national standards the need for nursing personnel who must be accepted for full recognition as members in that society (Sroczynski 1985). Flight team composition varies from program to program. While some flight programs favor the nurse, physician, and paramedic team, others prefer a flight nurse and paramedic combination, and still others advocate nurses as the sole healthcare personnel for air transport. The advantages and disadvantages of various combinations of flight-team members and of their various qualifications and specialty training are beyond the scope of this text.

TABLE 2–2
Objectives for Active Prevention of Injuries

1. Do not approach a helicopter until it has settled firmly onto the landing site. In the interim, stay at least 50 to 100 feet away from it.
2. Shield eyes or wear safety glasses while the helicopter is landing and while rotor blades are running. The highest winds and the greatest amount of flying debris are produced just before the helicopter touches the ground.
3. If two or more persons are at the landing site, they should be in one place, within the pilot's view. In general, if you can see the pilot, he can see you.
4. *Never* go to the rear of the helicopter. The tail rotor is at body height and may be very difficult to see when it is rotating.
5. *Never* raise your arms above shoulder level or stand on a stretcher. Do not place any part of your body higher than your body height, since the main rotor may dip low and cause lethal injuries. This is especially important with IV bags—do not raise them above your head until you have walked away from the helicopter.
6. Approach the helicopter at a 30- to 45-degree angle from the front of the helicopter. Because of the design of most helicopters, the main rotor dips lowest at the very front of the helicopter.
7. Secure loose objects such as long hair, hats, and stethoscopes. Remove mattresses and sheets from stretchers prior to entering the landing area.
8. Avoid running, especially when the surface is wet. Increased wind speeds under the main rotor can make surfaces very slippery.
9. When closing a door on the helicopter, make sure that it is securely closed and that no objects, such as straps or oxygen lines, are hanging out. Opened doors and/or loose objects can be safety hazards for people inside the helicopter when it takes off again.
10. Protect ears with earplugs or earmuffs. Sound levels from the jet engines and rotor blades may cause hearing loss.
11. Secure the patient onto the hospital stretcher carefully. If the patient is being transported *from* the hospital by helicopter, have the patient placed on a long board or in a Stokes basket and secure properly. Protect the patient's eyes from flying foreign bodies.
12. If you are at the landing site when the helicopter takes off, stay within view of the pilot and as far away from the helicopter as possible.
13. The pilot is ultimately in charge of the landing site while the helicopter is on the ground.
14. When a helicopter is expected to land, take time to clear the landing site of any loose debris that could become missiles. Wetting the landing area in advance of the landing in dusty conditions or on crude landing sites may reduce flying small debris.

Source: Adapted from CV Mosby Co. Taylor JE. Safety at the helicopter landing site: preventing injuries to emergency personnel and patients. J Emerg Nurs 11: 326–327, by permission of CV Mosby Co.

HELICOPTER SAFETY

Safety is a major consideration for all personnel involved with transportation of patients by rotary aircraft. There are certain guidelines that make patient transfer to and from the helicopter safer. Loading zone safety is particularly important for individuals who are involved in loading and unloading patients from the aircraft. Refer to Table 2–2 for guidelines and their associated rationale.

TRANSFER ARRANGEMENTS

Whether transporting by air or ground, arrangements between the transferring and receiving institutions require timely planning and communication. Transfer forms aid in assuring a methodic approach to communication as well as appropriate documentation for in-transit personnel.

CONCLUSION

Transfer of patients between institutions has become increasingly prevalent over the past two decades. The most commonly used modes of transfer are air and ground.

The nurse's responsibility includes care of the ill or injured at the sending or receiving institution or as transport nurse. Much planning and preparation provide for a smooth transfer. The overall theme of preparation is prophylaxis. The emergency nurse must ensure a smooth transition from one stable in-hospital situation to another. The two components of patient preparation are the physical/psychologic stabilization of the patient and the logistic organization of services. A thorough approach to assuring these components guarantees a safe and efficient transfer for the patient.

REFERENCES

Abraham E, Smith M, Silver L. 1984. Continuous monitoring of critically ill patients with transcutaneous oxygen and carbon dioxide and conjunctival oxygen sensors. Ann Emerg Med 13:1021–1026.

Anderson CA. 1987. Preparing patients for aeromedical transport. J Emerg Nurs 13:229–231.

Campbell PM. 1985. Transporting the critically ill and injured child. Crit Care Quarterly 8:1–12.

Committee on Trauma of the American College of Surgeons. 1986. Hospital versus prehospital resources for optimal care of the injured patient (Appendix C: Interhospital transfer of patients). Bull Am Coll Surg 71:19–22.

Dnenin G. 1978. Aviation Medicine: Physiology and Human Factors, London, Tri-Med, Ltd.

Lachenmyer J. 1987. Physiological Aspects of Transport. In Critical Care Transport, Int Anesthes Clin 25:15–41.

Lee G. 1987. Aeromedical transconjunctival oximeter hemodynamic monitoring in the trauma patient. J Emerg Nurs 13:241–243.

Lee G. 1986. Transport of the critically ill trauma patient. Nurs Clin North Am 21:741–749.

Lockwood BJ. 1982. Transport of multisystem trauma patients from rural and urban health care facilities. Crit Care Qu 15:22–37.

McNeil EL. 1983. Airborne Care of the Ill and Injured. New York, Springer-Verlag, 100, 106.

Pearl RG, Mihm FG, Rosenthal MH. 1987. Care of the adult patient during transport. Int Anesthesiol Clin 25:43–75.

Saletta AL, Behler DM, Chamings PA. 1984. Fit to fly. Am J Nurs 84:463.

Sroczynski M. 1985. Helicopter staffing regulations in Massachusetts. J Emerg Nurs 11:264–268.

Cheryl Ramler, RN MA

Triage

Triage is one of the most challenging responsibilities of the emergency nurse. The triage nurse is the first health care professional to interact with patients and families who are often anxious and upset. Consequently, this nurse must be capable of managing situations that evoke a variety of emotional responses.

The triage nurse must also possess excellent assessment skills. She or he is responsible for evaluating and documenting the chief complaint, determining acuity, and initiating diagnostic and first-aid procedures. All this must be accomplished while simultaneously establishing rapport with the patient. Brevity, thoroughness, and accuracy are key elements of the interviewing process. An expeditious interview helps to avoid delays in treatment that may jeopardize the health of critically ill individuals.

Obviously, the triage nurse works under stress and must be able to maintain his or her composure while making numerous decisions. Safe, effective patient care begins with the triage assessments, and interpersonal skills set the tone for the duration of the patient's stay.

HISTORY

The word *triage* is a French word that means *to sort*. The classification of patients for the purpose of determining treatment priorities originated on the battlefields of World War I. The intent of the military was to identify and treat those soldiers with minimal wounds who could be returned to battle. Performance of triage in this situation was guided by the maxim "the best for the most with the least by the fewest" (Simoneau 1985, 402). In other words, aggressive medical efforts were concentrated toward the many individuals with only minor wounds who were "most salvageable," as opposed to those with serious injuries who required extensive resources.

In addition to military situations, the concept of triage has been applied in two other settings, disasters and emergency departments. In large scale disasters, victims are subjected to triage and their dispositions are determined at the actual disaster site. This facilitates an even distribution of patients to surrounding emergency departments.

Implementation of the triage process in emergency departments was not initiated until the late 1950s or early 1960s. Impetus for its use came from two striking changes occurring in emergency departments throughout the country (Weinerman and Edwards 1964). First, there was a sharp rise in the number of cases being treated in emergency departments. Second, many of these patients were seeking treatment for nonurgent problems.

Weinerman and Edwards (1964) cite numerous circumstances contributing to these two trends. The public's changing perception of hospitals was one. Hospitals were no longer viewed as institutions established to treat only the seriously ill or injured. Instead, they were seen as community resources where medical treatment could be obtained for a variety of less urgent problems. A change in the role of the primary care provider was another factor that produced an increase in the number of cases being treated in emergency departments. As medical practice became more specialized, there was a decrease in the availability of office-based practitioners. Furthermore, these physicians no longer routinely managed acute problems that occurred during off-duty hours. They frequently directed patients to the emergency department on weekends, nights, and holidays.

Triage systems originated to deal with these increased numbers of nonacute cases that presented to emergency departments. The objectives of these systems were twofold: (1) prompt identification of patients requiring immediate medical treatment, and (2) determination of the appropriate area for treatment, i.e., outpatient clinic, medical or surgical area of the emergency department, and so forth.

URGENCY CATEGORIES

In many emergency departments, triage rating systems were implemented to classify the severity of an illness or injury. Most rating systems employ three categories: emergent, urgent, and nonurgent.

Emergent conditions are life-threatening disorders that require immediate medical attention. Examples of clinical problems that fall into this category are cardiopulmonary arrest, chest pain of cardiac origin, and pulmonary edema. Patients with such emergencies frequently arrive via ambulance and are sent immediately to the treatment area.

Urgent conditions include significant medical problems that require treatment as soon as possible. Sheehy and Barber (1985, 90) state that patients with illnesses or injuries in this category should receive medical attention within 20 minutes to 2 hours. However, these patients have stable vital signs and in some cases treatment may be delayed for several hours without impairment to the patient. Included in this category are simple lacerations, fever, and uncomplicated extremity fractures. Any patient in significant pain should also be classified as urgent (e.g., patients with renal calculi or sickle cell crises), as well as patients with chronic illnesses (diabetes, cancer, systemic lupus erythematosus). Patients in the last category warrant this acuity rating, regardless of their complaint, because of their increased potential for change in health status.

Nonurgent conditions include minor illnesses or injuries in which medical treatment can be delayed indefinitely. Sore throats, rashes, and chronic low-back pain fall into this category. Patients with such conditions often seek treatment in an emergency department because they do not have a primary physician.

Patients present to emergency departments with a wide range of symptomatology. Urgency ratings may be readily recognizable for patients with life-threatening disorders or those with low priority, nonurgent complaints. However, it is determining the urgency rating for less obvious problems that challenges the triage nurse's assessment skills and decision-making abilities.

Usually, the triage nurse makes a decision on the basis of a number of parameters evaluated during the initial assessment. These include the chief complaint, general appearance, vital signs, past medical history, current medications, and age of the patient. Rund and Rausch (1981) identify three methods used singly or in combination to determine an urgency rating:

1. Elicitation of symptoms or signs that by previous experience and training indicate to the triage nurse the rating and severity of the underlying disease or injury

2. Discovery of a symptom or sign that inherently warrants a particular urgency rating

3. Adherence to written protocols that outline a step-by-step approach to each problem until an urgency rating is determined

An example of the first method is found when the triage nurse identifies a set of symptoms that define a particular illness or injury. For example, the triage nurse would be concerned about a 28-year-old man who appears ill, complains of persistent vomiting for the past 24 hours, and has a history of insulin-dependent diabetes mellitus. A patient with this history would be categorized as emergent because of the seriousness of diabetic ketoacidosis. Although the purpose of triage is not to diagnose, experienced triage nurses are able to recognize clinical syndromes and use this knowledge when deciding on acuity.

Rund and Rausch (1981) identify a number of signs and symptoms that warrant a particular urgency rating. Patients with significantly abnormal vital signs, severe pain, excessive bleeding, or loss of function of a particular system all merit an emergent acuity rating. Also, signs and symptoms that occur acutely are usually more urgent than those chronic in nature.

A third method employed to determine acuities involves use of protocols or algorithms. Once the chief complaint has been determined, a series of questions directs the triage nurse to an appropriate acuity rating. Thompson and Dains (1982) have compiled an extensive collection of triage protocols organized on the basis of physiologic systems. The protocols outline the major subjective and objective data to be collected for each system and include 97 flow sheets that organize specific signs and symptoms into various urgency categories. Protocols promote consistency in acuity decisions. They are especially useful in teaching the triage process to new triage nurses, and experienced triage nurses can use them as references.

The significance of decisions regarding acuity cannot be overemphasized. The acuity rating determines in part the length of time the patient waits to see a physician, especially in busy emergency departments. Because access to medical treatment is controlled by the triage nurse, appraisal of the patient's condition and assignment to an urgency category must be accurate. When uncertainty exists with regard to a category decision, the patient should always be assigned to the higher priority category to prevent the possibility of serious error.

The acuity category also affects the schedule for reassessment of patients waiting at triage for assignment to an examination room. Because of the potential for change in the stability of these patients, they should be reassessed by triage personnel at periodic intervals. Thompson and Dains (1982, 37–38) recommend the following reassessment schedule in a four-category system: Category I patients are emergent and are sent directly to the treatment area; patients in category II should be reevaluated every 15 minutes; category III patients should be reassessed at 30-minute intervals; and category IV patients should be reevaluated every 60 minutes. This practice assures that any change in a patient's condition will be detected and the plan for care and the urgency rating modified accordingly. Observations made when patients are reassessed should also be documented.

TRIAGE SYSTEMS

Since its inception, the triage process has been conducted by individuals with widely varying qualifications (Slay and Riskin 1976). Receptionists, paramedics, laymen specifically trained for this purpose, and resident physicians have all performed this function. The responsibilities of the triage nurses vary according to the type of system. Thompson and Dains (1982) identify three major types: type I (traffic director), type II (spot check), and type III (comprehensive).

In the type I system nonprofessionals (i.e., receptionists, clerks, or allied health personnel) are the first persons to interact with the patient. Their assessment is cursory. They determine the chief complaint and classify the patient as "sick" or "not sick" on the basis of appearance. Patients are then directed to the acute care area of the emergency department or the waiting room. Documentation is sparse or absent, and no diagnostic procedures are initiated.

In the type II, or "spot check," system, assessment is done by an RN or a physician. Both subjective and objective data related to the chief complaint are evaluated and documented, and an urgency rating is assigned. Initiation of diagnostic procedures in this system may be inconsistent and varies with the institution. Patients may be directed to a specific care area, or they may even be treated and released by the triage physician. There is no plan for reevaluation of patients waiting for treatment in this system.

Type III, or comprehensive, triage is the most sophisticated system of triage. This system includes the major components of the type II system: assessment is performed by a professional, acuity ratings based on care priorities are assigned, and patients are directed to a specific care area or waiting room. The following characteristics distinguish the comprehensive system from other systems and improve the quality of care received by the patient:

1. Triage nurses (RNs) complete a triage education program that includes standards and protocols for basing assessments and decisions. This promotes quality and consistency in the care being provided.

2. The data base is expanded to include not only subjective and objective information about the chief complaint but also health care and learning needs of the patient.

3. Documentation is consistent and ongoing.

4. Ordering of diagnostic procedures is consistent and based on protocols.

5. Establishment of rapport with patients, families, and visitors is an expectation.

6. A schedule for periodic reassessment of patients waiting for treatment is provided.

In this system triage takes place in the lobby area near the entrance of the department. This enables the triage nurse to visually survey all persons entering the emergency department. Stationing the triage nurse in this location is beneficial to patients and visitors for several reasons. First, it affords patients immediate contact with a professional person. This reassures patients that they will receive appropriate treatment. The presence of a nurse in the lobby area is also comforting to visitors, who often feel isolated from their relative in the treatment area. They regard the nurse as a source of access to information about their loved one.

All patients are seen by the triage nurse before any registration procedures are initiated. Acutely ill (i.e., emergent) patients are sent immediately to the treatment area. Assessment of the chief complaint, along with documentation of the patient's subjective statements and the nurse's objective observations, is done on all other patients. This nurse is also responsible for evaluating the patient's vital signs. In certain cases a limited physical examination may be performed—e.g., orthopedic assessment in distal limb injuries. Other information that should be documented includes the patient's past medical history, current medications, and allergies.

On the basis of his or her assessment and the policies and procedures of the institution, the nurse may initiate first-aid measures, such as ice to an injured extremity or a dressing to a wound, and may also order certain diagnostic studies, such as distal limb radiographs and urinalyses. Completion of tests prior to the physician's examination often expedites the flow of patients through the department, thus decreasing the length of time spent in the emergency department and enhancing satisfaction with the service provided.

Once the triage assessment has been completed, the patient is assigned an urgency category—i.e., emergent, urgent, nonurgent. As indicated earlier, the emergent patient is sent to the treatment area immediately. Patients stable enough to wait in the lobby are sent to the registration area to complete that process. Reassessment at periodic intervals, depending on acuity classification, may be indicated.

A final responsibility of the triage nurse in this system is assignment of the patient to an examination room. A brief report is given to the nurse in the treatment area who assumes responsibility for the patient. There are a number of factors to consider when assigning a patient to a treatment room. The nurse must be aware of room availability and the urgency rating of each patient waiting to be seen. Additionally, she or he must consider the workload and capabilities of each staff member. If a patient with an emergent condition presents to a full emergency department, the triage nurse must notify staff in the treatment area that an examination room is needed immediately. In busy emergency departments, this may present a problem in that patients who are categorized as nonurgent may wait for hours as emergent and urgent cases receive priority treatment. The triage nurse must not lose track of nonurgent patients. Some emergency departments designate and staff an area where patients with nonurgent problems can be evaluated, treated, and discharged quickly. Such systems prevent unduly long waiting times for patients with nonurgent conditions.

The responsibilities of the triage nurse in a comprehensive system are numerous and diverse. The number of nurses required to staff such a system will vary, depending largely on the census of the department and its size and floor plan. If minimal requirements include two nurses, Thompson and Dains (1982, 34) recommend dividing their responsibilities so that the triage nurse assesses, documents, determines diagnostic tests/first aid, and assigns an urgency category. The patient then becomes the responsibility of the float nurse, whose duties include reassessment, assigning examination rooms, and reporting to the nurse in the treatment area.

Regardless of the staffing pattern, the skills required are constant. In addition to making accurate judgments about the patient's need for medical attention, triage nurses must have proficient organizational skills. They direct the flow of traffic through the department and have many factors to examine and judge in order to accomplish this aspect of their job in a safe and efficient manner.

TRIAGE INTERVIEW

The focus of the triage assessment is the chief complaint. Initially, open-ended questions may be used to obtain information. e.g., "Why did you come to the emergency department today?" Once the chief complaint has been determined, more details must be obtained before an acuity rating can be assigned. For example, if the patient stated, "I was in a car accident," the following information should be obtained:

1. When did the accident occur?
2. How fast was the car traveling?
3. Where were you sitting?
4. Were you wearing a seat belt?
5. Did your head hit the dash, or were you thrown against another part of the car?
6. Do you have head or neck pain?
7. Did you black out?
8. What hurts you now?

Guidelines and protocols may help the triage nurse obtain appropriate information. However, ability to interview skillfully is equally important in assuring that all relevant facts surrounding the chief complaint are elicited. In addition to knowing the right questions to ask, the triage nurse must be able to evaluate the patient's responses. Frequently, the nurse will have to clarify what the patient says in order to determine what is meant and must also know when to probe further. "Stomach pain" may actually be epigastric pain, and further questioning may elicit symptoms indicative of an acute myocardial infarction.

Evaluating the patient's description of his or her problem also involves knowing what semantics to use. The patient population in many emergency departments includes persons from various ethnic groups who use terms peculiar to their culture. In addition to questioning these patients about unfamiliar terms, the triage nurse should avoid using medical jargon that may not be understood. The nurse must evaluate the level of comprehension of all patients and adjust his or her vocabulary accordingly.

While collecting subjective data from the patient, the triage nurse must use observational skills to assess the overall appearance of the patient. Does he or she appear pale or diaphoretic, appear to be in pain, or display more anxiety than normally expected? This objective assessment actually begins the moment the triage nurse observes the patient, and in certain circumstances these observations become crucial factors in acuity determination. During peak periods in the department, when large numbers of patients arrive at once, the triage nurse relies on a visual survey to identify patients in obvious distress. These patients should receive immediate attention, even if assessment of another patient must be interrupted.

In certain circumstances, the triage nurse may have difficulty evaluating the exact nature of the patient's problem. Patients who speak little English may be unable to describe symptoms. The elderly patient may be forgetful and unable to give an accurate history. In such cases the triage nurse is forced to rely on observation and intuition to determine the acuity of the complaint. Expert practitioners are frequently able to identify acutely ill patients with only a superficial, cursory assessment. Their past experiences enable them to rapidly and instinctively determine when a patient is "sick." Although they may not be able to legitimize their decision, they are rarely wrong and should be taken seriously. Conversely, assessments should never be so cursory or instinctive that a truly ill patient who may not be vocal or who minimizes symptoms is overlooked.

Collecting subjective and objective data is only one aspect of triage interviews. Another purpose is to establish rapport with patients and their families. The interpersonal skills of the triage nurse are important in decreasing patient anxiety. She or he must be able to convey genuine concern, empathy, and a willingness to listen. Frequently patients with minor complaints, many of a nonurgent nature, believe that their problem is very serious. It is important to approach all patients with a nonjudgmental attitude and communicate that their complaints have been taken seriously. Psychosocial needs of some patients may be greater than their need for physical care. It is the responsibility of all emergency department nurses to respond to these needs. By communicating a desire to help, the triage nurse decreases the patient's anxiety, establishes rapport, and facilitates the patient's cooperation throughout the interview and stay in the department.

Consistency in approach is important with respect to all groups of patients. "Repeaters," substance abusers, and psychiatric patients should not be treated brusquely or made to wait an excessive amount of time. In addition to their overwhelming psychologic and emotional distress, they are often in poor physical condition, and even minor trauma can produce serious consequences. For example, an alcoholic is more susceptible to bleeding, and head trauma may precipitate an intracranial hemorrhage. As Turner (1981, 154) points out, "All psychoneurotic patients ultimately die of organic disease."

The purpose of the triage interview is to determine the acuity of the patient's condition by assessing the chief complaint. Analysis of both subjective and objective data is necessary. Broad knowledge of emergency health care is required because of the wide variety of chief complaints. The triage nurse must be able to determine what data are crucial in making an acuity decision and must possess highly developed interviewing skills in order to elicit this information. Finally, a nonjudgmental attitude and demonstrated concern are also needed to accomplish the second purpose of the interview, i.e., establishment of rapport with the patient and family.

SKILLS REQUIRED FOR TRIAGE

Triage can be a challenging position. Decisions regarding acuity of a complaint and the order in which patients will receive medical attention rest with the triage nurse. Frequently, responsibilities must be carried out in an environment which can be hectic and chaotic. There are times when a rush of clients can include acutely ill patients, agitated psychiatric patients, and distraught visitors. Such situations require the skills of an expert practitioner able to set priorities under stress.

In order to function effectively, the triage nurse must possess three critical qualities: (1) expert assessment skills, (2) demonstrated competence in interviewing and communicating with patients and families, and (3) well-developed organizational skills.

The triage nurse must be able to make rapid, accurate assessments, recognizing that the attitudes of other health care professionals along with the subsequent and timely care that patients receive are generated and guided by the appraisal of the chief complaint. Patients' conditions span a spectrum from seriously and acutely ill to minimally ill. Identifying patients in the extremes of the spectrum may not be difficult. However, many patients present with conditions that fall into the intermediate range, and a decision regarding how long they can wait before receiving medical attention is less clear.

The psychosocial skills of the triage nurse are as important as competence in assessing acuity of the complaint. A key role in triage involves providing psychologic support to patients and families. The triage nurse must possess an understanding of psychologic reactions to illness and injury as well as knowledge of behavioral responses to crises. The ability to empathize and communicate with patients and families is essential in establishing rapport, facilitating trust, and decreasing anxiety.

A final skill necessary for effective triage is the ability to organize. All patients presenting to the emergency department are screened by the triage nurse, who alone is responsible for determining the order in which they are treated and where they will be seen. Thus, the triage nurse regulates patient flow into the department and by organizing this flow of traffic assures that emergent cases are cared for immediately and urgent and nonurgent cases receive timely treatment. To function effectively the nurse must be able to organize the work load and have a thorough knowledge of the system and its setting.

CONCLUSION

Triage is a key position in the emergency department. The triage nurse plays a significant role in the delivery of optimal patient care. The responsibilities are numerous and include a number of important decisions. Because of this, the triage nurse must be proficient in several skills, including assessment, communication, and organization. The position is stressful, but many nurses find it both challenging and rewarding.

REFERENCES

Baldridge PB. 1966. The nurse in triage. Nurs Outlook 14:46–48.

Estrada EG. 1979. Advanced triage by a RN. J Emerg Nurs 5:15–18.

McLeod KA. 1975. Learning to take the trauma of triage. Part 1. RN 38:22–27.

Nelson D. 1983. Triage and assessment. In Warner CG, ed. Emergency care: Assessment and intervention. St. Louis, C.V. Mosby Co. 51–65.

Pool M. 1976. Triage nursing as problem solving. J Emerg Nurs 2:25–27.

Rund DA, Rausch TS. 1981. Triage. St. Louis, C.V. Mosby Co.

Sheehy SB, Barber J. 1985. Emergency Nursing: Principles and Practice, 2nd ed. St. Louis, C.V. Mosby Co.

Shields JE. 1976. Making triage work: the experience of an urban emergency department. J Emerg Nurs 2:37–41.

Simoneau JK. 1985. Disaster aspects in emergency nursing. In Budassi SA, Barber JM. Emergency Nursing: Principles and Practice, 2nd ed. St. Louis, C.V. Mosby Co., 390–425.

Slay LE, Riskin WG. 1976. Algorithm-directed triage in an emergency department. J Am Coll Emerg Physicians 5:869–875.

Thompson JD, Dains JE. 1982. Comprehensive Triage: A Manual for Developing and Implementing a Nursing Care System. Reston, Va., Reston Publishing Co.

Turner SR. 1981. Golden rules for accurate triage. J Emerg Nurs 7:153–155.

Weinerman ER, Edwards HR. 1964. "Triage" system shows promise in management of emergency department load. Hospitals 38:55–62.

Willis DT. 1979. A study of nursing triage. J Emerg Nurs 5:8–11.

Arlene Bonet, RN MS

Mass Casualty Management

The world today is at a greater risk for mass casualty disasters than ever before. The potential for catastrophic events will continue to increase as the population grows and people compete for resources. A densely populated area creates the potential for greater loss of life when a disaster does occur. The goal of this chapter is to assist the emergency nurse in recognizing the elements of management in disaster situations and in identifying methods that will help establish order out of chaos during a disaster.

The definition of a medical disaster has been stated in a variety of ways but most commonly in terms of an overtaxed emergency medical system. It is important to recognize that if any one component of the system is greatly compromised, a disaster may exist even though the remaining parts of the system are intact. Therefore, a medical disaster occurs when the number of victims exceeds the daily capabilities of an emergency medical services (EMS) system or any component of that system to deliver the customary standard of services. Disasters may be internal or external. Internal disasters occur within a medical facility and often are the result of fire, explosion, or chemical spill. If structural damage to the medical facility exists, functioning within it may still be possible. In external disasters the occurrence takes place outside the medical facility, thereby allowing the structure to remain sufficiently intact to prepare for incoming victims.

Disasters can be either manmade or natural. Manmade tragedies are caused by human error or technical failure and are not premeditated. Examples of a manmade tragedy include a train or jet crash, structure collapse, and radiation contamination from a nuclear accident. Wars and acts of terrorism are considered deliberate acts.

The responsibility society must accept is that most manmade disasters are predictable and in all cases are preventable. Natural disasters are events over which humans have little or no control. Although they are not preventable, predictability of occurrence may be possible. For example, earthquakes, hurricanes, floods, tornados, mud slides, volcanic eruptions, and avalanches typically occur in specific geographic locations. Evacuation may be possible in an effort to reduce fatalities.

CLASSIFICATION OF A DISASTER

For the purposes of this chapter, numbers of victims will be used as a guideline for classifying disasters. Numeric categorization alone may however not always accurately reflect the magnitude of a disaster. When assessing the ability of an emergency medical services system to provide the necessary resources to afford the most lifesaving potential, one must consider the following: number of victims, types and severity of injuries, and timing of the occurrences.

The term *minor disaster* usually conveys an upper limit of 25 persons injured or killed. The victims can be managed by the local EMS system; however, additional off-duty help from within the system may be required. Examples of these kinds of disasters include multiple-vehicle or bus accidents or something as unusual as the multiple shootings at the Bethesda IBM Building in May 1982. In such incidents the impact on the EMS system is short-term, lasting several hours.

A moderate disaster may include up to 100 persons injured or dead. This type usually occurs in a metropolitan area with a well-developed plan and ample resources. Most likely regional assistance would be necessary from surrounding municipalities. Whatever the cause, the number of victims alone would make this an unusual event. An example of such a tragedy occurred in Montreal in September 1972, when a cafe fire caused 54 injuries and 36 deaths.

If the number of victims exceeds 100, it is considered a major disaster. Local and regional EMS systems may require nearby military personnel to assist in rescue and evacuation. The 1981 Kansas City Hyatt incident is an example of a major disaster. Orr and Robinson (1982) report an initial count of 111 deaths and 188 injuries.

A fourth level is the catastrophic disaster. This is an event of such magnitude that numbers of injured and dead reach into the thousands. With the exception of a few wealthy and developed nations, this type of tragedy requires international assistance. The September 1985 earthquake in Mexico City, which affected thousands of people, constituted a catastrophic disaster. Although international assistance may be available, in these situations the aid may arrive some time after the initial impact. One can see that the immediate lifesaving efforts must be carried out by local and regional emergency medical systems. In a mass casualty event such as this, the EMS system may be involved for days or perhaps weeks until search for and rescue of victims terminate.

Timing refers to the spacing of injuries. Were all persons injured concurrently, or were injuries sustained over a period of time? Fourteen victims with multiple system injuries resulting from building collapse will tax an EMS system more than 14 victims of sniper shooting with wounds inflicted at various times over a 6-hour period.

The importance of a prepared approach to disaster cannot be underestimated. Preparation for disaster requires planning, practicing the plan with exercises, evaluating the exercises, identifying deficits, and then replanning. A good plan is periodically evaluated and updated. Drills demonstrate strengths and weaknesses at every level —regional, local, hospital, and departmental. Updating assures the changes necessary in accordance with system updates and alterations.

Preparation and practice are keys in the ongoing development of a disaster management system that will provide services to reduce morbidity and mortality. A moulage drill with enough victims to test the system is the preferred method of disaster preparation. This type of exercise better simulates the impact of victims on an EMS system than does use of mannequins, "pretend" injuries written on cards and strategically placed, or victims not "made up."

A good disaster plan is developed by adhering to specific principles. Preparedness by healthcare givers—i.e., nurses, physicians, paramedics—is one important component. Other aspects to consider include eight principles of disaster management as cited by Sanford (1984). They include preventing the occurrence of disaster, minimizing the number of casualties, preventing further casualties, rescuing, providing first aid, evacuating the injured, providing definitive care, and facilitating reconstruction-recovery.

COMMUNITY PLAN

Disaster preparedness according to Sanford's eight principles requires community cooperation. Since a comprehensive disaster system incorporates community, hospital emergency departments', national, and international plans, it is important that each sector collaboratively interface with the others. A variety of agencies both governmental and private must be involved in developing, implementing, and reviewing the community disaster plan. Plans may differ from region to region as each plan coordinates the resources available in a specific environment. A community plan should address the following issues: communication, activation of the plan, traffic control, criteria for designating participating hospitals, transportation, site teams, rescue and first aid, and evacuation.

Effective communication is critical. Ineffective or disrupted communication will have a deleterious effect on mass casualty management. Since disruption of normal communication modalities is quite possible in disastrous situations, practice exercises should simulate such breakdowns in traditional communication systems. Alternative methods for communication can be used. For example, walkie-talkies should be available in anticipation of disrupted phone activity, and consideration should also be given to the utilization of ham radio operators.

Just as cooperation is imperative between various systems involved in disaster preparedness, collaboration among disciplines is equally important. No discipline can function in isolation during a mass casualty incident. The planning committee must include representation from all community agencies involved, which may include the Department of Public Health, fire department/paramedics, police department, private ambulances, American Red Cross, hospitals, and the military.

Overall responsibility for coordinating the activities of an area-wide disaster program will depend upon the size and organizational structure of the community. Individuals in positions of recognized authority who can maintain objectivity in developing and overviewing the plan are best suited. Examples include a representative from the Department of Public Health or Public Safety. The coordinator or chairperson of the planning committee is not necessarily the prime decision maker during an actual disaster. The frontline leader should be decided by the community plan. The appointed individual is usually an official of the fire department, police department, public safety department, or the mayor.

HOSPITAL PLAN

The hospital disaster plan evolves around continued care or disposition of existing patients and simultaneous preparation for incoming casualties. The hospital master plan should address the following areas: identification of victims, notification of families, public relations, solicitation of additional staff, telecommunications, crisis intervention, and designated areas for family waiting. For realistic plans to be developed, subcommittees from various disciplines such as social service, security, environmental service, and food service should develop strategies that can be integrated into the master plan.

In addition, the master plan must include but is not limited to the following functions: triage at point of entry, designated treatment areas for patients in various categories, psychiatric management, and casualty discharge. In order to ensure an organized flow of patients during a disaster, the plan should designate an individual as the overall leader. This individual should be responsible for activating and terminating the disaster plan.

Calls coming into the hospital often congest the lines, making it impossible to complete outgoing calls for additional personnel. Consideration should be given to having rolls of coins available so that assigned staff can use public telephones to assist with outside communication or can use predesignated telephones that have private lines (such as in the office of administration). The internal telephone system may also be overtaxed; if possible, several walkie-talkie sets should be issued to key people so that staff members in vital areas can readily communicate. Hospitals can use intercommunication systems, and those with computers can also use these to augment standard communication.

EMERGENCY DEPARTMENT PLAN

The emergency department plays a predominant role in a hospital disaster plan. The department will be responsible for establishing procedures that provide for the most efficient management of incoming casualties.

Specific plans will vary considerably from hospital to hospital. Each emergency department must determine what will work best for them. All plans, however, must include the following elements: charge responsibility, disposition of patients currently in the department, preparation of triage site, patient flow, extent of initial treatment, alternate patient care areas, staffing, and supply needs. It is important that patients not be allowed to accumulate at the triage site. A backlog will affect the outcome of casualties waiting in ambulances and will eventually jeopardize the overall system.

CIVILIAN DISASTER MANAGEMENT

Civilian disaster management principles have evolved from military conflict. The military refers to echelons of care, whereas civilians refer to triage sites. The goal is the same—stabilization of victims. Triage during disaster serves to temporarily prioritize care at various stages or sites. There are three triage sites, and at each one the victim's category may be reassigned. Site I is prehospital, in the field. Site II is at the point of entry into the hospital and is based on categorization. Although they are located in different areas, the objectives of triage sites I and II are the same: examine rapidly, sort, move forward to resuscitation area, and evacuate.

The objective of field, or site I, triage is identification of injuries through a primary survey. An airway may be established if it can be accomplished manually. Initial assessment adheres to all the basic essentials of airway, breathing, and circulation. Initially, prehospital personnel will undertake the task of sorting, tagging, and moving to the designated areas victims tagged as hyperacute, serious, walking injured, or dead. When medical teams arrive, they will continue to assist with this task or begin initial stabilization or both, as directed by the disaster chief. The important point to remember in site I triage is not to attempt to treat victims to the extent that causes a bottleneck in the triage system.

Developed EMS systems use color coding as a means of identifying the level of emergency care and evacuation of victims. Universally recognized colors are red, yellow, green, and black. The tags are designed with perforations between colors so that all colors except the one that identifies the most recent priority assigned to a particular victim may be removed (Table 4–1).

Psychiatric manifestations are not uncommon during a disaster. The behavior of the victim will determine when it would be prudent to evacuate to the hospital. Although the patient may not be a first or second priority in terms of a life-threatening event, consideration must be given to disruptive behavior in an already chaotic situation.

Remembering the principles of disaster management, consideration must be given to minimizing and preventing further casualties. Crowd control and extinguishing spreading fires may be a higher priority than first aid to injured victims. Paramedics are usually the first upon the scene and are able to make initial surveys and advise central dispatch of the severity of the situation. Misdiagnosis in the chaos of the field is to be expected. The triage medical personnel do not stop to treat casualties but instead assign victims to one of the four categories listed above. Victims are transported to the hospital according to their triage categorization. Patients categorized as hyperacute are transported first and the dead last.

TABLE 4-1
Color Codes Used in Triage

Red Tag	Hyperacute, a first priority requiring immediate evacuation or care. Any injury producing 1. Life-threatening respiratory problem 2. Severe blood loss 3. Unconsciousness 4. Severe shock
Yellow Tag	Serious, a second priority in evacuation or care 1. Moderate blood loss 2. Head injuries (conscious) 3. Spinal cord injury 4. Extensive burns (uncomplicated respiratory status)
Green Tag	Walking injured, a third priority for evacuation or care 1. Minor lacerations 2. Minor fractures, minor injuries 3. Minor burns
Black Tag	Deceased, fourth priority

Site II triage occurs at the hospital point of entry. Each arriving casualty must have his or her field tag reviewed and physiologic status reevaluated. Because of the priorities of field triage, prehospital intervention may have been inadequate to maintain a seriously injured patient. It is possible the patient's status has changed, and if so, the category must therefore be reassigned.

Site III triage occurs in the designated hospital area. Here a thorough reevaluation occurs. The patient is completely undressed, and a head-to-toe survey is done. Assessment of injuries and immediate resuscitation are the primary activities in the initial care of the disaster victim. All efforts are geared toward determining injuries, stabilizing hemodynamic status, and planning for definitive care.

NATIONAL AND INTERNATIONAL PLANS

The National Disaster Medical System (NDMS) is a plan developed in response to a presidential mandate in December 1981. President Reagan appointed the Emergency Mobilization Preparedness Board (EMPB) to establish programs to improve emergency preparedness. The NDMS concept is based on the civilian-military contingency hospital system (CMCHS). CMCHS was developed in 1980 as a ready resource to the military in the event of great numbers of unexpected combat casualties. This was a program administered by the Department of Defense (DOD), the Veterans Administration (VA), and participating civilian hospitals. The local EMS system facilitates the triage and transport of the incoming casualties. Each community and hospital implements its own disaster plan. One major difference between NDMS and local disaster plans is that the former notifies hospitals that are to receive patients many hours in advance of the actual need to implement the plan. This advantage allows for an organized approach to freeing inpatient beds and preparing for casualties.

Until recently little attention has been given to how our nation would respond to a catastrophic incident involving an entire city or most of a state. Potential sites for a disaster of great magnitude include densely populated areas. Cities and states are not adequately prepared to deal with thousands of injured, dead, and homeless. Other problems can include interrupted communications, contaminated water supplies, loss of power or energy sources, and chaotic conditions that may leave a community without clear leadership.

Most of our EMS systems are decentralized and serve specific regions. There is a need for a plan at the national level to merge and coordinate these systems when regional resources are exhausted. The NDMS Implementation Task Force (1984) states

> NDMS Planners have scaled the system to deal with a great California earthquake. The system is therefore designed to accept up to 100,000 seriously injured patients requiring hospitalization. The system cannot handle more than this number and is thus not adaptable to nuclear war situations.

Mahoney and Brinley (1986) state that the system is designed to fulfill three objectives:

1. To assist a disaster-affected area by mobilizing medical assistance teams and medical supplies and equipment.

2. To evacuate victims who cannot be cared for in the affected area to designated centers in unaffected areas.

3. To provide hospital care in a network of participating hospitals throughout the nation.

NDMS is not intended to replace any regional EMS system. In order to activate the plan, a request must come from the governor of an affected state. There is still more planning and coordination required to fulfill the objectives of NDMS.

There are a number of world-wide organizations devoted to supplying resources during a disaster. International communication and collaboration make such actions possible. In 1976 The Club of Mainz for Improved Emergency and Disaster Medicine Worldwide was founded. One of the Club's objectives is to share scientific and social information relating to emergencies and disasters that may occur among a variety of populations. The Club of Mainz has established liaisons with the United Nations Disaster Relief Organization, the World Health Organization, the League of Red Cross Societies, the World Federation of Societies of Anesthesiologists, and the World Federation of Societies of Intensive and Critical Care Medicine.

RADIATION AND HAZARDOUS MATERIALS

In our society today, no disaster preparation is complete without a plan for victims of hazardous waste or radiation exposure. Past situations in the United States have usually been associated with the transport of hazardous material. Radiation victims have been limited to industrial accidents involving two or more people. A tragedy such as that at Chernobyl in April 1986 is dreaded by all nations with nuclear capabilities. Linnemann (1987) reports that of the 444 workers on site, 203 victims were hospitalized, and 30 eventually died. Skin damage caused by thermal injury was as much responsible for the deaths as radiation exposure.

As in any disaster, the number of victims, the geographic area involved, and the resources available determine how adequately a local EMS system will be able to respond. Distancing victims from the source of contamination will be a top priority. Two major principles underlying care of individuals in a radiation accident or one involving hazardous materials include preventing further exposure and providing appropriate treatment immediately. The emergency department should have references as well as a list of agencies such as the Environmental Protection Agency and the Department of Public Safety where they may call for guidance in the handling of victims exposed to specific hazardous material. Rescue personnel must be familiar with how to use protective clothing and appropriate techniques for removal of victims. This can only be accomplished by the development of a contingency plan for such a situation and implementation of the plan during practice exercises. The United States currently has two major agencies with dedicated 24-hour availability of emergency medical responses for nuclear accidents, the Radiation Emergency Assistance Center/Training Site (REAC/TS), located in Oak Ridge, Tennessee, and sponsored by the federal government, and Radiation Management Consultants (RMC), developed by the nuclear industry and located in Philadelphia, Pennsylvania. These two programs maintain teams that may be dispatched to the scene or to local hospitals to assist in radiologic evaluation and treatment of victims (Linnemann 1987).

Every hospital should have a plan for treatment of contaminated victims. Four principles to follow, in order of priority, are
1. Resuscitate and stabilize victims if injured
2. Decontaminate victims
3. Control contamination to specific area in hospital
4. Start radiation exposure evaluation

Assessment of contamination begins at the emergency door using a Geiger counter to scan the total body of the patient. Once recorded, the patient may be taken to a designated room for decontamination in a carefully defined, roped-off area. The floor area traversed should be covered with heavy plastic and taped to secure. The personnel resuscitating and decontaminating the patient should be gowned in total-body disposable suits, headgear, masks, and double latex gloves. They should also wear a rad meter, and should take readings before and after exposure to the radiation source.

Decontamination is achieved by washing the body with soap and water. It is important to dispose of the waste water in canisters or drums that allow for proper disposal and avoid main drain contamination. Specialized carts are available with drain boards that allow the water to empty into a proper receptacle.

Radiation exposure evaluation begins with history of the victim's exposure and of nausea, vomiting, or both; evidence of erythema; and baseline complete blood cell counts, including platelet counts.

NURSING CARE

The emergency nurse may assume a variety of roles during a disaster situation. There are basic characteristics of emergency nursing practice that make the emergency nurse one of the professionals best prepared to manage a mass casualty environment. These are

1. Crisis intervention skills
2. Flexibility in adapting to changing volume and acuity of patients
3. Daily use of triage assessment skills

These elements make the nurse a key component of the medical team that is dispatched to the disaster site. The nurse is autonomous in a field disaster setting. When the medical teams arrive at the disaster site they will assist with triage or begin initial stabilization as directed by the disaster chief.

In the hospital setting, there are a variety of roles the emergency nurse may be required to perform in a disaster situation. "Cheat sheets" stating responsibilities for each role provide quick reference. The emergency nurse becomes a key figure in all activities. It may be some time before additional medical staff arrives in the emergency area; therefore, the nurse plays a predominant role in the reevaluation and stabilization of casualties. The nurses will be required to assume responsibility for a detailed assessment of each victim and to respond with appropriate recategorization and intervention to achieve and maintain a stable patient.

Another important role is that of flow chief or disaster control officer. This is usually performed by the charge nurse. She or he should be clearly identified by wearing a colorful vest. The flow chief assures that every area has the supplies, equipment, and personnel necessary to keep the system moving. This nurse is constantly mobile and anticipates the needs of individuals assigned to various areas.

For base station hospitals, telemetry may also be a responsibility of the emergency nurse. The resource hospital command post is vital as the communication link between the field and participating hospitals. The past experience of the mobile intensive care nurse will help assure appropriate interpretation and transmission of field information. Other assignments may include the triage station, the hyperacute area, and ambulatory area. The respective responsibilities are listed in Table 4–2.

The ambulatory group of victims although not physiologically compromised

TABLE 4–2
Assignment Responsibilities in Disaster Relief

Triage
   Reassess quickly to establish current status
   Tag victim with hospital identification; registration information may not
      be available; use a pre-established numbering system and sex of
      patient as identification
   Briefly document injury on hospital disaster chart
   Assign victim to appropriate area

Hyperacute
   Reassess; completely undress victim
   Make thorough head-to-toe survey
   Use emergency interventions and resuscitation
   Monitor continuously
   Determine readiness for transport to appropriate area for definitive care

Ambulatory/Wheelchair
   Administer first aid
   Immobilize extremity(ies)
   Manage superficial wound
   Take tetanus history
   Intervene in crisis

---

may be emotionally distraught. Recognizing that they have survived a close brush with death may trigger a wide range of emotional responses. How each individual reacts is determined by past coping mechanisms, maturity, and perceptions of the situation. The psychologic support and intervention immediately available will be important in minimizing anxiety and establishing a basis for future psychosocial counseling. Individuals in crises will require much emotional support. In fact, psychologic management is often of higher priority than medical management. Emergency personnel should have an understanding of the effect of such a stressful event on victims and their families. Establishing a controlled environment will reduce anxiety and provide a better milieu for treatment.

There is another aspect to the psychologic impact of a critical incident: the potentially damaging effects of stress following the event. This phenomenon is not limited to victims and their families but may also include members of the rescue team and health care providers involved in a catastrophic occurrence of any nature. It is important to recognize this stress as a normal response to an overwhelmingly powerful event. Since emergency personnel devote so much of their physical and emotional energy to others, the fact that they, too, may require special interventions during and after a crisis is sometimes overlooked. Critical incident stress debriefings have been developed by some agencies to assist with diffusing the psychologic effects of a devastating event.

The nurse is too often overlooked as a participant in regional disaster planning. Hospitals and other agencies tend to appoint administrative personnel as representatives for planning disaster preparedness. However, the emergency nurse, experienced in the EMS system and the realities of caring for patients in an uncontrolled environment, is apt to provide insight on many aspects of disaster preparedness. Most emergency departments have experienced an event in which they have been responsible for several patients involved in one incident. As such, this exposure to handling multiple victims, although on a smaller scale, establishes the emergency nurse as a reliable resource. Every hospital participating in the development of a disaster plan should include emergency nurse representatives.

CONCLUSION

Disaster preparedness requires planning, practice, critiques, and revision. Nothing should be overlooked that will help bring organization from chaos; therefore, elements of management should be universal. Because of their background, clinical expertise, and crisis intervention skills, emergency nurses provide continuity and stability in the development and implementation of mass casualty preparedness systems.

REFERENCES

Burkle SM Jr, Sanner PH, Wolcott BW, eds. 1984. Disaster Medicine. New York, Medical Examination Publishing Co.

Butman AM. 1983. The challenge of casualties en masse. Emerg Med 15:110–151.

Campbell PM, Pribyl CA. 1982. The Hyatt disaster: two nurses' perspectives. J Emerg Nurs 8:12–16.

In the shadow of radiation. 1987. Emerg Med 19:68–84.

Herman RE. 1983. Disaster preparation: developing a plan. Emergency 15:28–29.

Jacobs LM Jr, Goody MM, Sinclair A. 1983. The role of a trauma center in disaster management. J Trauma 23:697–701.

Linnemann RE. 1987. Soviet medical response to the Chernobyl nuclear accident. JAMA 258:637–643.

Mahoney LE, Brinley FJ. 1986. The national disaster medical system. Top Emerg Med 7:75–85.

Nash JR. 1977. Darkest Hours. New York, Pocket Books.

Facts on the National Disaster Medical System. 1984. National Disaster Medical Systems Implementation Task Force, Rockville, MD.

Orr SM, Robinson WA. 1982. The Hyatt disaster: two physicians' perspectives. J Emerg Nurs 8:6–11.

Parker JG. 1984. Disaster planning. In Parker JG, ed. Emergency Nursing: A Guide to Comprehensive Care. New York, John Wiley & Sons, 585–595.

Richtsmeier JL, Miller JR. 1985. Psychological aspects to disaster situations. In Garcia LM, ed. Disaster Nursing, Planning, Assessments, and Intervention. Rockville, Md, Aspen Systems Corporation, 185–202.

Sanford JP. 1984. Civilian disasters and disaster planning. In Burkle SM Jr, Sanner PH, Wolcott BW, eds. Disaster Medicine. New York, Medical Examination Publishing Co.

Emergency Nursing Care: A Systems Approach

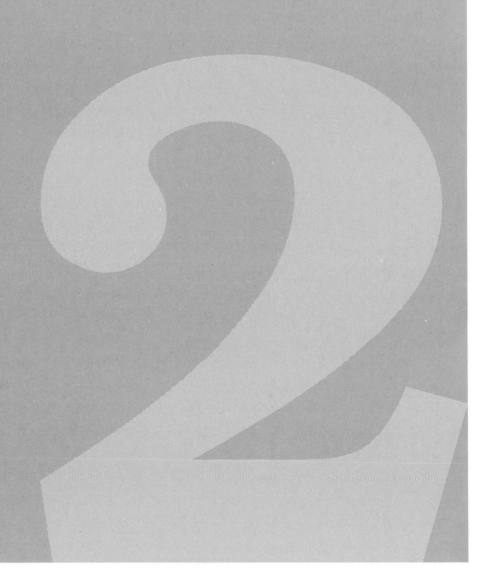

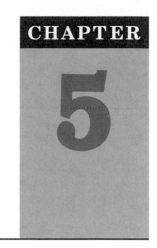

CHAPTER

5

Judith Zoellner-Hunter, RN MSN

Shock

Any definition of shock must focus on the cell, since cellular death is central to all forms of shock. Shock is a syndrome that produces failure of perfusion at the cellular level, which may or may not be flow related. Shock in all its forms is accelerated entropy. If patients are to survive shock, it must be recognized early by health care practitioners. Recognizing the early changes in shock demands a skilled and comprehensive approach. The purpose of this chapter is to provide a comprehensive review of the pathophysiology, assessment, clinical manifestations, and interventions for the patient in shock.

PATHOPHYSIOLOGY OF SHOCK: CELLULAR MECHANISMS

Normal homeostatic mechanisms that maintain the human body in hemodynamic equilibrium are balanced among three separate components: cardiac pumping action, blood volume, and vascular capacity (Fig. 5–1). Normally, the body adapts to changes in any one of these components through compensatory adjustments in the others. Should the compensatory mechanism fail, an imbalance will occur and produce decreased cellular perfusion. If cellular perfusion is decreased to the point of cellular death, then shock has occurred.

In shock, the cell has been deprived of perfusion and therefore has received insufficient glucose and oxygen, the substrates that cells require in order to function

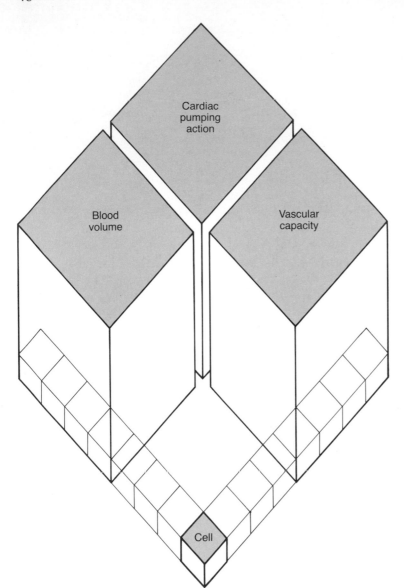

FIGURE 5-1. Critical components affecting cellular perfusion: blood volume, cardiac pumping action, and vascular capacity.

at peak efficiency. Aerobic metabolism (with oxygen) is far more efficient than anaerobic metabolism (without oxygen). One mole of glucose in aerobic metabolism produces 36 mol adenosine triphosphate (ATP) (Ayres, Gianelli, and Mueller 1974). ATP is the "coin of the cellular realm" and allows energy to be released in a slow, step-wise fashion. Alternatively, 1 mol glucose in anaerobic metabolism produces only 2 mol ATP (Fig. 5-2). One can readily see how much more efficient aerobic metabolism is. Some cells, mostly in skeletal muscle, function primarily in the anaerobic state with its obligatory build-up of lactic acid. However, many body cells, particularly those of the vital organs (heart, brain, kidney, liver), which must produce energy more efficiently than the skeletal muscles, need more ATP and do not tolerate

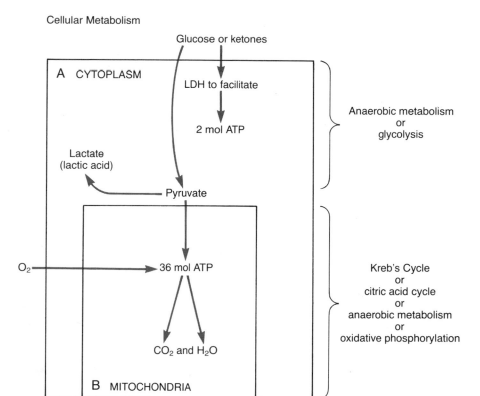

Cellular Metabolism

FIGURE 5-2. *A*, Anaerobic metabolism occurring within the cytoplasm, facilitated by lactate and producing 2 mol adenosine triphosphate (ATP). *B*, Aerobic metabolism occurring within the mitochondria, facilitated by pyruvate (an enzymatic breakdown product of glucose) and oxygen and producing 36 mol ATP.

an accumulation of lactic acid. They depend on aerobic metabolism for adequate energy production, and when deprived of oxygen, their mitochondria become dysfunctional and produce much less energy in the form of ATP.

With the failure of perfusion at the cellular level, many changes take place within the cell. Lactic acid builds up within the cell and eventually leaks into the circulation. Weil and associates (1975) discuss the implications of lactic acid measurements for determining the severity of shock states. As the cell pH falls as a result of accumulating lactic acid, several other destructive phenomena occur. Cell wall integrity and the osmotic gradient between the cell and the serum is maintained by the sodium-potassium pump, which is fueled by ATP. Trump and colleagues (1971) discuss the events in the cell as the sodium-potassium pump fails. Sodium begins to enter the cell and with it, water. The cell in shock becomes waterlogged and develops blebs as it swells. Potassium leaks from the cell into the serum, producing cardiac dysrhythmias. The energy deficit continues as ATP production falls and sodium and water begin to enter the mitochondria. As a terminal event, calcium, which is normally an extracellular cation, enters the mitochondria. The contents of the mitochondria coalesce, and the cell literally falls apart (Fig. 5–3).

Lysosomes, which are cytoplasmic organelles, are very much involved in shock. As sodium and water enter the cell, they also enter the lysosomes. As the lysosomes swell, their membranes rupture, and the intralysosomal contents spill into the cell. This is disastrous for the cell, because the lysosome's proteolytic enzymes function well in an acidic medium and the cellular acidity from lactic acid now provides the

CELL DEATH

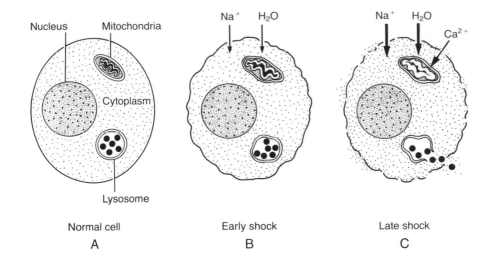

FIGURE 5-3. *A*, Sodium and water move from extracellular space to intracellular space during early shock; mitochondria are intact. *B*, Massive amounts of water and sodium enter the cytoplasm, causing blebs to develop; calcium enters the mitochondria and causes destruction; the cell wall loses integrity.

perfect environment. Just as the contents of the lysosomes enter the cell and contribute to its destruction, they also enter the circulation, contributing to cell damage elsewhere.

In summary, the process that leads to death from shock is cumulative. When enough cells die, the organ system to which they belong also dies. When major organ systems fail, the individual dies. Cell death is the beginning of shock and also the cause of death from shock.

EFFECTS OF SHOCK ON MAJOR ORGAN SYSTEMS

Measuring shock as it occurs at the cellular level is difficult. Instead, clinical assessment is based on the effects of shock on the major organ systems. The first major organ to be affected by shock is the sympathetic nervous system (SNS). Many shock symptoms represent the effects of the SNS as it acts to rescue the organism under duress: vasoconstriction, tachycardia, tachypnea, and anxiety. Many of the effects of the SNS stimulation, although initially lifesaving, contribute to the overall pathology in shock. The alpha-adrenergic effects, primarily caused by norepinephrine, produce vasoconstriction. This maintains systolic blood pressure and elevates the diastolic blood pressure. Therefore, a narrowed pulse pressure is usually evident early in shock. Although stimulation of alpha receptor sites improves circulation to the heart and the brain, there is a dramatic decrease in perfusion to other organs of the body. This is costly over time, because the cells of these deprived organs die as the supply of oxygenated blood is reduced. Beta-stimulating effects, primarily due to epinephrine, cause increased cardiac output through an increased heart rate, increased contractility, and increased stroke volume; this produces an inevitable increase in myocardial

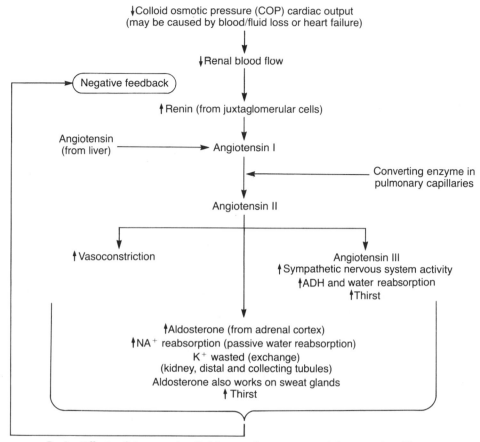

FIGURE 5–4. Effects of decreased colloid osmotic pressure and decreased cardiac output on the renin-angiotensin-aldosterone system in the body's effort to maintain vascular volume. ADH = antidiuretic hormone.

oxygen demands. Beta stimulation also causes bronchodilation and postcapillary vasodilation. The renin-angiotensin-aldosterone system is activated early in an effort to maintain volume (Fig. 5–4).

As shock progresses, acidosis, the effects of histamine and bradykinin, and the rupture of lysosomes cause the capillaries to dilate. Fluid leaks out of the capillaries into the tissues, and perfusion continues to deteriorate. This fluid shift into the tissues contributes to a diminished preload, producing a fall in stroke volume and a compensatory tachycardia in an attempt to sustain cardiac output. As a terminal event, blood pressure plummets, and the patient's skin becomes mottled, cold, and clammy.

Metabolic acidosis occurs as a result of anaerobic metabolism and the consequent build-up of lactic acid. Acidosis can precipitate serum electrolyte abnormalities. Hyperkalemia is often present in conjunction with acidosis. Potassium, a positive intracellular ion, moves from its intracellular habitat to the extracellular serum and changes places with the hydrogen ion (H^+). As the pH is corrected, potassium reenters the cell (Guyton 1986, 331), correcting the hyperkalemia.

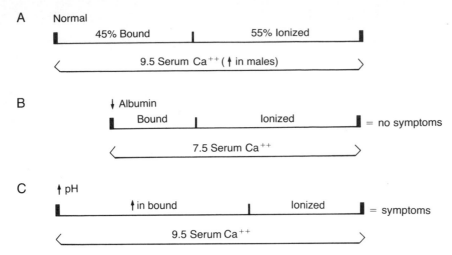

FIGURE 5–5. *A*, Normal percentage of calcium that is bound and ionized in blood serum and normal serum values. *B*, Effects of a decreased albumin on bound and ionized calcium. *C*, Effects of alkalosis on bound and ionized portions of calcium.

Ionized calcium levels may be altered in shock if the patient is hyperventilating as a result of hypoxemia or if the patient is receiving multiple blood transfusions. Calcium binds to citrate (the anticoagulant used in banked blood). This leads to a decrease in available or ionized calcium within the circulating blood. The total serum calcium in an average male is about 10 mEq/L. Of that amount, approximately 4.5 mEq is bound and thus is inactive. Approximately 5.5 mEq is available for use and is termed *ionized*. Although the serum calcium may not change in the face of pH shifts, the amount of calcium that is ionized decreases as the bound portion increases (Fig. 5–5). This occurs in alkalosis, when more calcium is bound to the serum proteins and is therefore unavailable for use. Whenever the amount of calcium available to the tissues decreases, symptoms of hypocalcemia such as tetany, laryngospasm, and seizures can appear.

Sodium abnormalities are common in the shock patient. Antidiuretic hormone, released from the posterior pituitary during the shock state, causes retention of water and dilutional hyponatremia. A low serum sodium, whether it is due to absolute loss (true hyponatremia) or to an increase in water (which produces a relative decrease in sodium), produces a decreased level of consciousness and if uncorrected can lead to seizures or coma (Fig. 5–6).

Blood gases measure oxygenation and ventilation. Early in shock, a reasonable Po_2 is likely because of the compensatory tachypnea and hyperventilation. As shock progresses, the skeletal respiratory muscles fatigue as a result of the work of breathing and become increasingly inefficient. The Po_2 falls as the Pco_2 normalizes and then rises. These changes lead to the release of autoregulating prostaglandins, causing the pulmonary vasculature to vasoconstrict, and pulmonary function deteriorates further. If a patient loses the ability to protect his or her airway, aspiration may occur, and the stage may be set for adult respiratory distress syndrome (ARDS).

As perfusion to the kidney is reduced, urine volume falls. Refer to renin angiotensin (see Fig. 5–4). The systemic blood urea nitrogen (BUN) rises as a result of increased protein breakdown and increased time for reabsorption in the renal tubules. Potassium fails to be excreted. Red blood cells, white blood cells, and albumin

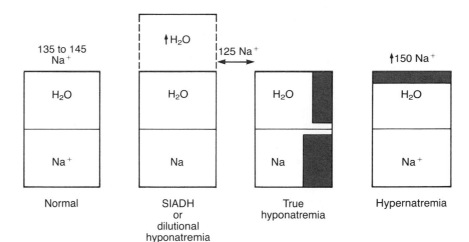

FIGURE 5-6. Effects of ratios of sodium to water on serum sodium levels.

appear in the urine, since they squeeze through the compromised glomerular capillaries in Bowman's capsule. Casts appear in the urine as the linings of the tubules slough. This signals the death of nephron units.

The remaining effects of shock on the splanchnic bed are due to the profound vasoconstriction that alpha stimulation has engendered throughout the system. The mucosa of the stomach is affected as the mucin cells, which require ATP for their production, fail. Mucin, which protects the stomach from hydrochloric acid (HCl), is no longer present in sufficient amounts, and the HCl attacks the stomach unimpeded. Additionally, the pyloric sphincter becomes incompetent as the blood supply is decreased, allowing a backwash of duodenal contents—sodium bicarbonate, proteolytic enzymes, and bile. This seems to be an important mechanism in hastening the formation of stress ulcers.

In shock the pancreas is affected as proteolytic, lipolytic, and digestive enzymes produced in the pancreas leak out of their channels and consume the pancreas itself. An elevated serum amylase is common in shock.

The liver in shock is increasingly unable to clear bacteria, glucose, and ammonia from the blood. In addition, the inability of the liver to inactivate lactic acid accelerates the progressive acidosis the individual is suffering. Most significant for the patient's ultimate survival is the inability to destroy the gram-negative organisms from the gut. As shock is prolonged, sepsis is likely.

It should be remembered that prevention or early treatment is the optimal treatment to avoid cellular death and all the events that follow.

ASSESSMENT

The initial priorities in the assessment of a patient at risk for shock are airway, breathing, and circulation. Is the airway open? Is the patient breathing? What is the level of peripheral perfusion as evidenced by blood pressure, pulse quality, and capillary refill? When available, a history from the patient or significant others can be helpful, but identification of the patient at risk for shock is vitally important, and demands a skilled emergency department clinician.

Most of us were taught that the patient in shock has a thready pulse and low blood pressure and is cold and clammy. These traditional assessment parameters reflect shock in the late stages, when maximal therapy is sometimes to little avail, and can be recognized by any lay person. Emergency department clinicians need to recognize impending shock early, when therapy will be most efficacious. Some texts divide shock into early, middle, and late. Others discuss shock, particularly hemorrhagic shock, as occurring in stages I, II, III, and IV. These somewhat artificial categories are rather clumsy and difficult to use in an emergency clinical setting. A more useful approach uses the following assessment criteria, which rely not on technology but on "hands on" assessment by the clinicians caring for the patient: level of consciousness, arterial blood pressure, pulse quality, urinary output, and capillary perfusion. Ongoing assessment and integrating these parameters into a holistic approach will help to identify the patient in impending shock and track the success of ongoing therapy.

Level of Consciousness

The level of consciousness is an important measurement of shock because it directly reflects cerebral perfusion. Early in shock states, blood is passively shunted to the brain and heart. This protective mechanism assures perfusion of these vital organs in preference to viscera and other less vital organs. A decreasing level of consciousness in the patient who has no obvious neurologic problems indicates a decrease in brain perfusion. When the well-protected brain shows signs of decreased cellular perfusion, it is indicative of a deterioration in the patient's overall status. Many of the early signs of decreased cerebral perfusion are mediated by the sympathetic nervous system. Symptoms such as anxiety, agitation, and inability to concentrate should provoke suspicion of diminished blood flow to the brain. As shock progresses, the patient becomes increasingly lethargic and apathetic, progressing to obtundation and coma. One should remember that hearing is the last sense lost. Many patients have reported conversations that took place in the emergency department when all concerned were quite sure the patient was not conscious.

Arterial Blood Pressure

Early in shock the diastolic pressure is elevated by vasoconstricting catecholamines produced by the SNS. This often occurs prior to any significant fall in systolic blood pressure and reflects an attempt by the body to compensate for decreased volume by tightening up the vascular bed. There are a few points concerning blood pressure that must be kept in mind. There is no absolute value in blood pressure that signifies a shock state; rather, it is the deviation from normal that is important. For a patient in shock with significant vasoconstriction, cuff pressure is often quite inaccurate. Measurement of arterial pressure via an arterial line allows for precise monitoring of the blood pressure. Pressure taken with a Doppler device is more reflective of actual pressure than is cuff pressure.

Pulse Quality

Pulse quality is an important assessment parameter. Quality is far more important than rate alone. The patient with a strong pulse, no matter what the pulse rate is, is probably not in shock, whereas a weak and thready pulse reflects a diminished cardiac output. Tachycardia is common in most shock states as a result of the SNS-mediated response to tissue hypoxia. It must be remembered, however, that a slow and bounding pulse is typical for the patient in spinal cord shock (discussed further in Chap. 19). Also patients in cardiogenic shock secondary to an inferior wall myocardial infarction often present with bradycardia. Early in distributive shock the patient may have an increased cardiac output.

Urinary Output

Urine output and quality are important measurements in the shock state. An indwelling catheter with an attached urometer should be inserted. Generally, a minimum of 30 ml urinary output per hour should be seen, although 20 ml/hour may be acceptable for a short period of time. Children should maintain an output of 0.5 ml/kg/hour. Urine should be measured for specific gravity: a low, fixed, specific gravity of 1.01 implies a dilute urine, most likely related to a deterioration in tubular function. A high specific gravity may indicate dehydration, the effect of renal compensatory mechanisms, or the presence of radiologic contrast dyes. Urine should be tested for red blood cells, white blood cells, casts, and albumin, the presence of which indicates renal dysfunction.

Capillary Perfusion

Finally, skin color, temperature, moisture, and capillary refill reflect important information regarding the patient's peripheral perfusion. Cold, moist, and pale or ashen skin indicates potent vasoconstriction and compensatory sympathetic activity to shift blood to the brain and heart. Capillary refill is tested by compressing the patient's nailbed, releasing pressure and mentally saying, "capillary refill." The color in the nailbed of the patient with adequate peripheral perfusion will return within two seconds or the time it takes to say "capillary refill."

TREATMENT AND NURSING CARE

General treatment and nursing care for patients in shock are discussed in this section. Since all forms of shock carry the same pathology, death of the cell, resuscitation at the cellular level is mandatory. All patients in shock will need to be returned to a reasonable homeostatic state by oxygenation, fluid resuscitation, and restoration of acceptable electrolyte and pH status.

Altered Tissue Perfusion: (Cerebral, Cardiopulmonary, Peripheral), Related to

- **Fluid Volume Deficit (Serum or Blood)**
- **Myocardial Pump Failure**
- **Massive Vasodilation**

Patients in shock universally have a decreased ability to supply oxygen to the tissues. Since oxygenation is essential, all shock patients will require oxygen therapy. Initially, a 10-L non-rebreather face mask or Venturi mask should be used as a means of providing high-flow oxygen supplementation. The patient who is unable to manage secretions or is ventilating poorly will require endotracheal intubation. The patient's oxygenation should be assessed on a continuum in order to provide appropriate therapy. Arterial blood gases are monitored for gas exchange—Pco_2 and bicarbonate as well as Po_2. A rising Pco_2 indicates hypoventilation and potential respiratory failure. A falling bicarbonate level often reflects metabolic acidosis caused by rising lactate levels.

Hemorrhage and its accompanying decrease in red blood cell mass will necessitate early O_2 support. Soft tissue injury to the face may mandate intubation or tracheostomy. In caring for the trauma patient, a high level of suspicion must be maintained for injury to the chest or lungs that may demand ventilatory support.

Fluid Volume Deficit, Actual or Relative, Related to

- **Volume Loss (Blood or Plasma)**
- **Volume Shifts (to Cells or Interstitium)**
- **Alterations in Vascular Capacity**

Fluid resuscitation is a difficult problem and the most controversial area of shock resuscitation. All patients in shock will need fluids owing to intracellular, intracapillary, and interstitial fluid losses and shifts. *How much, when,* and *what kind* are questions that must be answered for each situation rather than by applying a standardized formula. The patient with fluid volume deficit related to dehydration or hemorrhage should have at least two large-bore (16-gauge, 1½–inch long) catheters inserted to aid in rapid fluid administration. Maintenance of urine volume at 30 ml/hour is desirable.

In the last 10 years, there has been ongoing discussion in the literature of crystalloid versus colloid therapy. The crystalloid school believes that crystalloids (lactated Ringer's solution, normal saline) resuscitate individuals from shock quite nicely, and the cost is significantly less than for colloids. The colloid supporters claim that although the colloids (blood products, albumin, dextran, hetastarch) are more expensive, it takes far fewer fluids to resuscitate an individual with colloids, and the chances of producing pulmonary edema and significant peripheral edema are much less. If the individual has a leaky cell – leaky capillary syndrome, both types of fluids will leak into the interstitial space. This can produce marked edema of the face and extremities. The crystalloid school thinks that a leaky capillary membrane, which allows the large colloid particles to leak into the interstitial space, will produce more significant problems by pulling water into the interstitial space. Certainly, both sides have valid arguments, and most clinicians agree there is room for both approaches in shock resuscitation.

The best guide to volume resuscitation is a right-side heart balloon flow-directed catheter, an option not available in most emergency settings. A central venous pressure catheter (CVP) is a reasonable alternative and is helpful in assessing fluid status. An initial reading must be taken at the time of insertion of the catheter. This baseline reading provides a comparison point for further readings taken as volume resuscitation is underway. A maintenance of baseline may suggest that the patient is dehydrated, whereas increases may warn of fluid volume overload.

In the absence of a CVP, volume resuscitation must be guided by clinical signs and symptoms. Crackles on auscultation of lung fields or an S_3 murmur heard on assessment of heart sounds may imply fluid overload. Tachycardia is not particularly helpful as a guideline for fluid resuscitation since it can occur in hypovolemia as well as hypervolemia. In addition, patients with some cardiac pathologies (heart block, nodal disease, inferior wall myocardial infarctions (MIs), increased vagal tone or a combination of these) may manifest a low cardiac rate with little ability to adjust through cardioacceleration. Blood gases may indicate deterioration of pulmonary function related to fluid overload. If the Pco_2 is falling, the patient may be hyperventilating in response to hypoxemia. Urine output provides a useful means of monitoring fluid volume status. Thirty ml/hour is considered adequate.

Fluid volume resuscitation should be monitored carefully and correlated with changes in the patient's clinical condition. Collaboration with the physician is necessary in order to meticulously adjust fluids according to the patient's response to therapy.

Acid-Base Disturbance, Related to

• **Shock**

Once oxygenation and fluid resuscitation are underway, acid-base homeostasis needs to be addressed. If the patient has respiratory acidosis, evidenced by an elevated Pco_2, he or she should be treated with ventilatory support. If the patient has metabolic acidosis, alleviation of the hypoxic state as the cause of a lactic acidosis must be considered. Sodium bicarbonate may be appropriate. However, care must be taken not to overtreat the acidosis, as metabolic alkalosis is as deleterious to the patient as metabolic acidosis. Compensating for metabolic alkalosis is difficult, since the kidneys are slow to clear bicarbonate from the serum. Blood gases should be used as a guide to replacement. Patients are better off in a slightly acidemic state, since oxygen is more readily dissociated from hemoglobin at lower pH levels. In acidemia the oxyhemoglobin dissociation curve is shifted to the right, and more oxygen is efficaciously delivered to the tissues: an ideal effect in the shock state (Ayres 1974, 14) (Fig. 5 – 7).

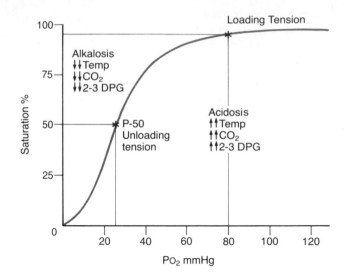

FIGURE 5-7. Oxyhemoglobin dissociation curve. P-50 is oxygen tension corresponding to 50% oxyhemoglobin saturation. Factors shown on the right shift the curve to the right; factors shown on the left shift the curve to the left. (Adapted from Ayres SM. 1972. Respir Care 17:291, by permission.)

Correction of electrolyte abnormalities should not be attempted until the pH is stabilized. This will allow endogenous electrolyte stabilization and help clinicians to make appropriate adjustments.

SPECIFIC FORMS OF SHOCK AND RELATED THERAPIES

Shock can be classified into three major categories and is derived from the three major mechanisms responsible for tissue perfusion. The first classification, distributive shock, occurs when the primary problem is maldistribution of blood volume: in other words, there is a mismatch between blood volume and vascular space. The subtypes are neurogenic shock, septic shock, and anaphylaxis. The second classification is hypovolemic shock, typified by a loss of circulating volume. Blood losses from hemorrhage and fluid loss seen in the victims of burns typify this form of shock. The third major category is cardiogenic shock, in which the cause of the shock state is myocardial pump failure. The commonality shared by all three major categories of shock is decreased perfusion to the cells. Anaphylactic shock is covered in Chapter 27.

Neurogenic Shock

Neurogenic shock is due to profound vasodilation which results in an increase in total vascular capacity and a subsequent decrease in blood volume to vascular space ratio. Inadequate tissue perfusion results.

Fainting and spinal cord injury both produce this syndrome. The person who faints has a massive vasodilation secondary to vagal stimulation and loss of sympathetic tone. For some, the sight of blood or a vagal maneuver such as bearing down with a bowel movement may cause this syndrome. The patient with a spinal cord injury at the cervical level also suffers loss of sympathetic tone and increased parasympathetic control that results in vasodilation below the level of the injury.

Neurogenic shock can also result from drugs that cause significant vasodilation. Lidocaine in excessive doses causes vasodilation and a drop in blood pressure. Barbiturates, alcohol, and narcotics alone or in combination cause vasodilation. In addition, barbiturates produce a significant negative inotropic effect (decreased strength of myocardial contractility) and therefore contribute to a decreased cardiac output.

Clinical Manifestations

Patients in neurogenic shock are hypotensive and bradycardic and have a slow and bounding pulse. The skin is generally pale, warm, and dry. In patients with spinal cord lesions, reflexes are absent and there is loss of sensation and motor function below the level of the lesion. For details of spinal cord shock refer to Chapter 19.

Treatment and Nursing Care

Tissue Perfusion, Altered (Cerebral), Related to

- **Increased Vascular Capacity Secondary to Spinal Cord Injury or**
- **Vasodilating Drugs**

Patients in neurogenic shock should be maintained in the supine position for maximum cerebral perfusion. If the patient shows signs of compromised cardiac output, such as change in mental status, drop in blood pressure, cold clammy skin, diaphoresis, decreased urine volume, or chest pain, fluid replacement will usually be necessary. If the patient is not ventilating, oxygenating, or protecting his or her airway, ventilatory support may be necessary.

Septic Shock

Septic shock is generally caused by endotoxins released by gram-negative organisms — e.g., *Escherichia coli, Serratia.* However, in recent years, gram-positive organisms have been implicated in septic shock. Toxic shock syndrome, caused by *Staphylococcus,* and pneumococcal shock syndrome, caused by pneumococcus, have been seen with increasing frequency.

Septic shock has a high mortality rate, as it is more common in patients with a damaged or incompetent immune system. Patients on chemotherapy or radiation therapy are susceptible as are those on steroids. Diabetics and individuals who have undergone invasive procedures such as cystoscopy may also develop sepsis. The progression of sepsis from its early stages marked by a hyperdynamic state to late septic shock with depressed myocardial contractility is a continuum with unmarked borders. Progression may be very rapid or may occur over days. The mechanism of sepsis and septic shock involves the cell wall of the invading organism and its interaction with the cell walls of the individual. The complement cascade, a complex sequential event, is precipitated and a number of what Guyton (1986) and others call noxious polypeptides are released. Some of these include bradykinin, which causes powerful arteriolar dilation and increased capillary permeability, and histamine, which acts in much the same way. Shunting is enhanced around the area of the capillaries, and perfusion is decreased (Shoemaker 1984, 54–56).

Clinical Manifestations

An early sign of sepsis is usually an elevated temperature. However, patients who are immunosuppressed, neonates, and the elderly may be unable to mount an adequate immune response, and their temperature may fall as a result of vasodilation and loss of core temperature. The more usual presentation, however, is the patient who is flushed and warm. Early septic shock is called "warm shock," or high-output shock because of this. The patient appears pink owing to a combination of endotoxins, high cardiac output, fever, and vasodilation. This robs the brain of perfusion, and a change in the patient's affect is often marked. The endotoxins affect the carotid bodies and cause tachypnea and hyperventilation; therefore, these patients often have a marked decrease in their Pco_2. Septic patients may have a metabolic alkalosis although the mechanism for this is not clearly understood. As septic shock progresses, the patient goes into "cold shock," or low-output shock, and is vasoconstricted.

The patient in sepsis may have an altered white blood cell count. Initially, there will be a slight fall in total white blood cell count, particularly in the polymorphonuclear neutrophils (Fig. 5–8).

Treatment and Nursing Care

Infection, Potential for, Related to

- **High Risk History**

Patients at risk for sepsis should be identified quickly. As with all patients in shock, oxygen therapy will be necessary. The vasodilation produced by the endo-

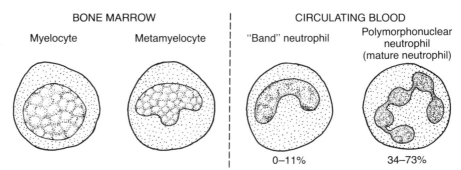

FIGURE 5–8. The immature neutrophils: "Band" neutrophil metamyelocytes and metamyelocytes are released from the bone marrow as the mature (polymorphonuclear) neutrophils are consumed in antimicrobial defense. This is called a shift to the left (left shift). As the infection or sepsis "matures" and the body responds, the total white blood count rises. With a chronic infection or with viral infections, the macrophages (lymphocytes, monocytes) become more numerous.

toxins usually requires large volumes of fluid to maintain homeostasis. Antibiotic therapy is necessary. Generally, antibiotics are selected for both gram-negative and gram-positive organisms: aminoglycosides and cephalosporins.

Meticulous blood cultures should be done on patients in whom there is a probability of or who are exhibiting signs and symptoms of sepsis. Sputum and urine cultures should be obtained in addition to cultures from other potential sites of infection (abscesses, indwelling lines, and so forth). Some consideration may be given to performing a spinal tap if meningitis is suspected.

Noncardiogenic pulmonary edema, adult respiratory distress syndrome, acute tubular necrosis, and disseminated intravascular coagulation often follow sepsis and septic shock, owing at least in part to the "leaky capillary syndrome" produced by the endotoxins and the complement cascade they release.

The patient will need frequent arterial blood gas analyses, an indwelling urinary catheter to monitor urine output, and a central line to measure fluid volume status. A cardiac monitor is helpful. If massive vasodilation is present and large volumes of fluid present a problem to the heart, some consideration may be given to the use of dopamine at alpha levels (over 10 μg/kg/minute) or norepinephrine to produce vasoconstriction. If the shock is severe, the patient may have passed through the early part of the spectrum (high output/warm shock) to the late spectrum (low output/cold shock). This would be shown by markedly diminished urine output and cold, mottled skin. These patients usually need positive inotropic support—i.e., dopamine at midrange dosage (5 to 10 μg/kg/minute). (See Chap. 9 or refer to Cardiogenic Shock, in this section.)

The role of steroids in increasing cell wall and capillary integrity is debatable. However, they are used in some settings with the thought that stabilization of lysosomal membranes occurs and prevents cell dysfunction. If instituted, they should be started early, used in large doses, and continued only a few days.

Hypovolemic Shock

Hypovolemic shock is divided into two subtypes; hemorrhagic shock and fluid loss. Hemorrhagic shock, the most familiar to emergency department nurses, is most easily understood and has the best prognosis. Hemorrhagic shock has been studied since the seventeenth century, when Harvey in England correctly ascertained that the heart circulated blood. Hemorrhagic shock was further studied in England during the eighteenth and nineteenth centuries when condemned prisoners were given a choice of being bled to death privately or hung publicly. It was determined at that point that 40% blood loss caused death. Demling (1986) states that this determination is still valid.

Survival statistics for hemorrhagic shock are relatively good. This most likely relates to the fact that trauma victims, many of whom have hemorrhagic shock, tend to be a younger and healthier population than those who develop other forms of shock. The point that blood often galvanizes the clinicians caring for these patients into early and appropriate actions should not be minimized.

Hypovolemic shock caused by fluid losses has a more dismal outlook than hemorrhagic shock. Fluid losses can be due to a variety of causes, and because the fluid losses are often subtle, the patient may be quite sick before the diagnosis is made and interventions are initiated. Often these patients are elderly with underlying illnesses, which make their survival more questionable. Examples of patients with potential for fluid deficits include those with prolonged vomiting or diarrhea, burns, and diabetic ketoacidosis. Patients with significant peritoneal fluid accumulations, or patients with an ileus that promotes stagnation of fluids within a distended loop of bowel (dead space fluids) may also suffer profound intravascular fluid volume deficits.

The effects of plasma and other fluid losses are more serious with smaller percentage losses than in whole blood loss. This is because plasma and other fluid losses produce an increase in hemoglobin and hematocrit concentration within the blood. This causes increased blood viscosity, sequestration in the capillaries, clotting, and decreased blood flow.

Clinical Manifestations

Individuals presenting to the emergency department in hypovolemic shock may have a history of trauma and external bleeding (e.g., vaginal bleeding or epistaxis) or recurrent nausea, vomiting, and diarrhea or a combination of these plus burns and diuresis. Early in shock the patient may appear anxious, may have cool and pale skin, may appear dehydrated, may have tachycardia, and may demonstrate a decreased pulse pressure. As shock progresses, the capillary refill time will be delayed, heart rate will increase above 130 beats per minute, pulse will become thready, and systolic blood pressure will fall to less than 60. Skin will be cool, clammy, and diaphoretic. Respirations may be rapid, shallow, or agonal.

Although the complete blood count may be altered in a patient suffering from hemorrhagic shock, changes occur slowly. Since the patient is losing serum as well as blood cells, the ratio for iron (hemoglobin) to serum and red blood cells to serum (hematocrit) may remain unchanged initially. The initial hemoglobin and hematocrit values reflect the patient's baseline, not the losses (Fig. 5–9). After 24 hours or when the patient's fluid volume is replaced, the true state of the hemoglobin and hematocrit can be determined. In fluid loss, serum has been lost, and the ratio of red blood cells to serum is increased, so that the hemoglobin and hematocrit will increase.

Treatment and Nursing Care

Fluid Volume Deficit, Actual or Relative; Related to

- **Hemorrhage**
- **Fluid Shifts**

When a patient covered with blood enters an emergency department most clinicians feel relatively comfortable because they know what to do and know the outcome is likely to be relatively good. When the bleeding source is not obvious, copious irrigation often reveals the source of the bleeding. Pressure points seldom seem useful, but a sterile dressing with firm direct pressure over the bleeding site will

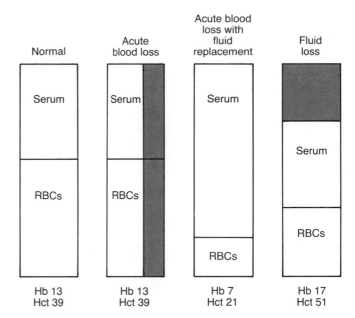

FIGURE 5–9. Effects of blood loss, blood loss with fluid replacement, and serum loss on hemoglobin and hematocrit levels. Hgb = hemoglobin; Hct = hematocrit.

usually control and often stop the bleeding. A tamponading object should be left in place until a physician can remove it under controlled circumstances. A blood specimen should be obtained for type and cross match. A high-flow O_2 mask should be placed, and fluids, usually lactated Ringer's solution, should be started with a 16- or 18-gauge IV catheter (refer to the section on fluid resuscitation). Tourniquets are not necessary and should not be used. A vigorous search should be made for the source of suspected internal bleeding and may involve peritoneal lavage, the use of radiology and contrast agents, or surgery.

Cardiogenic Shock

Cardiogenic shock represents an anatomic disaster. Rackley (1985) discusses this problem. Patients who develop cardiogenic shock have lost 45% to 50% of their left ventricle, either with one massive myocardial infarction (MI) or several smaller events. Approximately 12% of patients suffering an MI will develop some degree of cardiogenic shock. Until recently, the mortality rate approached 90%. Even with the assistance of positive inotropic agents, preload and afterload manipulation, and the use of counterpulsation assistive devices, the mortality rate is still approximately 60%. Of those patients who do survive, few survive longer than one year. The crippled myocardium cannot pump the required blood to the system and, more critically, cannot generate enough pressure to perfuse the atherosclerotic coronary arteries. The only real hope for this fixed anatomic problem is prevention. Angioplasty, thrombolytic therapy (streptokinase or tissue plasminogen activator), or both performed in the early stages of MI may allow revascularization to occur. Failing early presentation, in the best case, cardiogenic shock would be treated by a donor heart.

Clinical Manifestations

Individuals with cardiac failure severe enough to cause cardiogenic shock will appear acutely ill and may have altered mentation. They may be anxious, restless, confused, or lethargic. Hypotension reflects a diminished cardiac output, and poor peripheral perfusion will be evidenced by cool and clammy skin, weak peripheral pulses, prolonged capillary refill, and cynanosis. Cardiac dysrhythmias and evidence of massive myocardial infarction are common. Tachypnea and orthopnea may be present and crackles may be heard on auscultation of lung fields. Hypoxemia and metabolic acidosis may occur as a result of decreased cardiac output and poor peripheral perfusion.

Treatment and Nursing Care

Decreased Cardiac Output, Related to

- **Decreased Myocardial Contractility**
- **Altered Preload or Afterload**

The patient with alteration in cardiac output related to a decrease in myocardial contractility will require drug therapy to increase cardiac output. Drugs that increase cardiac contractility are positive inotropic agents. Most are beta stimulators, which cause an increase in heart rate and contractility, vasodilation of the postcapillary sphincters, and bronchodilation in the lungs.

Epinephrine stimulates both alpha and beta receptor sites, and it is primarily used to promote beta stimulation. Isuprel is a synthetic drug that produces pure beta stimulation. Dopamine has a wide range of effects related to the dose given. In the low range (2 to 5 μg/kg/minute), it produces a dopaminergic effect, increasing renal blood flow with minimal effects on blood pressure. In the midrange (5 to 10 μg/kg/minute), the dominant effect is beta stimulation. In the high range (over 10 μg/kg/minute), dopamine produces alpha effects, or vasoconstriction.

Beta stimulation usually results in a modest increase in blood pressure caused by the increase in cardiac output. Cardiac output is a product of rate times stroke volume. The physiologic price for increased output is an increased demand for oxygen, which can be costly to the patient with a decrease in myocardial oxygen reserves. Tachydysrhythmias and premature ventricular contractions (PVCs) often occur in these patients. All patients on inotropic drug therapy require close monitoring of their response to therapy.

Most patients in shock, with the exception of those in neurogenic, anaphylactic, and early septic shock, will have an increased afterload caused by peripheral vasoconstriction. Volume loss through hemorrhagic fluid loss and intracellular and interstitial losses will decrease preload. Both an increase in afterload and a decrease in preload decrease cellular perfusion and produce misleadingly low blood pressure cuff readings.

Vasoconstrictive drugs — high-dose dopamine, norepinephrine, phenylephrine, and aramine — increase blood pressure through vasoconstriction, but decrease perfusion, particularly in the gut, kidneys, and skin. Vasodilator drugs, or afterload reducers, have now become a component of therapy for many patients in shock. Sodium nitroprusside is often the drug of choice, as it vasodilates peripheral vessels and augments perfusion. Refer to Chapter 29 for more discussion on nitroprusside therapy.

Nitroglycerin, another vasodilator, primarily causes venous vasodilation and therefore is a preload reducer for both the left and the right heart. Its efficacy in angina therapy may be related to its preload reduction effect in decreasing the amount of blood presented to the heart. The decrease in the stretch on the myocardium decreases oxygen demands. The same effects may be desirable in cardiogenic shock. Morphine is also a vasodilator, and its central calming and analgesic effects make it a useful drug for cardiogenic shock.

All vasoactive drugs need to be titrated carefully to changes in the patient's condition. The patient in shock with decreased tissue perfusion related to capillary sludging will need fluid resuscitation to complement vasodilator therapy. Patients in cardiogenic shock should be transferred to the intensive care or coronary care unit as soon as possible.

CONCLUSION

Shock is a syndrome and represents failure in perfusion at the cellular level. The cells must be rescued from their decreased perfusion if the patient is to survive. An integrated, thoughtful approach to assessment, knowledge of pathophysiology and of clinical manifestations (both early and late), and appropriate interventions can make a profound difference in the patient's stabilization and recovery.

REFERENCES

Ayres SM, Gianelli S, Mueller H, Buehler M. 1974. Care of the Critically Ill. New York, Appleton-Century-Crofts, 8, 14.

Ayres SM, Schlightig T, Sterling MJ. 1988. Care of the Critically Ill, 3rd ed. Chicago, Year Book Medical Publishers, Inc.

Bremer C. 1987. Shock emergencies. In Rea R, Bourg P, Parker JG, Rushing D, eds. Emergency Nursing Core Curriculum. Philadelphia, WB Saunders, 674–687.

Demling RH. 1986. Shock and fluids. In Chernow B, Shoemaker WC, eds. Critical Care: State of the Art, Vol 7, 318. Society of Critical Care Medicine. Fullerton, California.

Guyton AC. 1986. Textbook of Medical Physiology, 7th ed. Philadelphia, WB Saunders.

Rackley CE. 1985. Treatment of acute myocardial infarction. In Chernow B, Shoemaker WC, ed. Critical Care: State of the Art, Vol 6. Society of Critical Care Medicine. Fullerton, California.

Rodman GH. 1984. Bleeding and clotting disorders. In Shoemaker WC, Thompson WL, Holbrook PR, eds. The Society of Critical Care Medicine: Textbook of Critical Care. Philadelphia, WB Saunders, 722–732.

Schiffer CA. 1984. Transfusion Therapy in Critical Care. In Shoemaker WC, Thompson WL, Holbrook PR, eds. The Society of Critical Care Medicine: Textbook of Critical Care. Philadelphia, WB Saunders, 752–768.

Shoemaker WC, Thompson WL, Holbrook PR. 1984. The Society of Critical Care Medicine: Textbook of Critical Care. Philadelphia, WB Saunders, 505–580.

Trump BF, Croker BP, Mergner WJ. 1971. In Richter GW, Scarpelli DG, eds. Cell Membranes: Biological and Pathological Aspects. Baltimore, Williams & Wilkins, 84.

Weil HM, Shubin H, Carlon RW. 1975. Treatment of circulatory shock, use of sympathomemetic and related vasoactive agents. JAMA, 231:1280–1286.

Christine Jutzi-Kosmos, RN MS

Assessment of Multiple Trauma and Thoracic Trauma

Trauma is the leading cause of death for Americans between the ages of 1 and 44 years and the fourth leading cause of death overall. A 15-year-old white male has a 1 : 110 risk of dying from a motor vehicle accident by the time he is 30. A 20-year-old black male has 1 : 50 chance of dying from homicide by the time he is 35 (Trunkey 1987a). Annually, more than 4 million potential years of life are lost owing to traumatic deaths. In 1984, the cost of trauma to our nation was almost $97 billion. This figure amounts to over $265 million per day (Trunkey 1987a).

Trauma is an unexpected, unplanned, yet often preventable event that affects not only the victim and his or her family but society as well. It is one of the major health and social problems facing the United States today.

The expanded role of the nurse includes a responsibility to educate patients on issues such as trauma prevention. Programs such as "First Time Feet First" (developed after a rash of spinal cord injuries occurred over one holiday weekend owing to people diving into shallow water) are excellent examples. Additionally, trauma nurses may choose to become involved in legislative issues that directly affect trauma nursing. Drunk driving, seat belt usage, and child car seat laws are examples.

Health care professionals need to address these issues in a direct, aggressive manner. The nursing profession has a responsibility to itself and to the public for educating members of their profession to become specialists in trauma and the prevention of trauma. In effect, the only true "cure" for trauma is its prevention.

This chapter is intended not to make the reader an expert in trauma (for this takes many years of hard work) but to provide a solid framework from which sound nursing diagnoses can be formulated and subsequent interventions planned. Trauma nursing can be a challenging and rewarding specialty. For those who choose to pursue trauma nursing, welcome to our group. We need your special talents and skills!

EVOLUTION OF PRESENT-DAY TRAUMA MANAGEMENT

Over the past four decades, three key factors have been recognized as having positively influenced the administration of care to trauma patients. They are military conflict, the Emergency Medical Services (EMS) systems, and designation of area trauma centers.

Military Conflict

Military conflict creates high demands for greater efficacy in the treatment of injured military personnel and civilians. Past and current methods of trauma care delivery are frequently re-evaluated. Subsequent changes in treatment protocols, surgical techniques, and trauma care principles are made (e.g., training of field medical personnel in triage and life-saving maneuvers, shorter intervals between the time of injury and definitive treatment) that are transferable to the care of trauma victims during peacetime. These changes, in addition to medical advances, have resulted in a consistent decline in mortality of battlefield casualties reaching medical facilities between World War I and the Vietnam conflict.

The EMS System

The Vietnam conflict has resulted in improvements in management of trauma victims. We learned, for example, that placing properly trained personnel in the field to perform life-saving procedures for victims of trauma without sacrificing rapid transport will ultimately result in an improved outcome for those individuals. This principle is a basic component in our present-day (EMS) systems.

Designation of Area Trauma Centers

The goal of designated area trauma centers is to see that the right patient gets to the right hospital at the right time. (A primary strategy utilized to effect this goal is trauma scoring, which is discussed in the following section.) Hospitals that are designated as area trauma centers are responsible for maintaining 24-hour coverage by a specialty trained trauma team and for providing for all of the possible needs of multiply injured patients. The trauma nurse is a very important member of this team. His or her role is expanding and growing more complex. Primary responsibilities include assessment of trauma patients utilizing the nursing process, anticipating the needs of the physician team leader (as well as patients' and their families' needs), and efficiently and skillfully performing life-saving interventions for multiply injured individuals.

TRAUMA SCORING

Great strides have been made since the late 1960s in development of indices of injury. The two major incentives for index development include triage of patients from the field to appropriate trauma centers and the need for the development of a common language for comparative studies. Although no one index has been universally accepted, it is agreed that the criteria by which these indices should be judged include practicality, ease of use, validity, and reliability (Thompson and Dains 1986). Current research is directed toward the Trauma Score and the Injury Severity Score, which are indices (tools) utilized during field triage to enhance the effectiveness of trauma regionalization by attempting to identify which patients should be brought to a trauma center.

Two commonly used trauma scoring scales are the Champion and the CRAMS. The Champion trauma score consists of the rating (or measurement) of four physiologic parameters plus the Glasgow coma score. Respiratory rate, respiratory effort, systolic blood pressure, and capillary refill are each given a value that reflects the patient's cardiopulmonary function. High scores indicate normal function and low scores indicate impaired function. The Glasgow coma score is obtained and then converted into a number that equals one third of the raw score. This allows a more balanced grading system considering both cardiopulmonary and craniocerebral compromise. Severity of injury is then estimated by summing the five numbers. The lowest score is 1 and the highest score is 16 (Table 6–1). The projected estimate of survival for each value of the trauma score is listed in Table 6–2. It is suggested that patients with a trauma score of 12 or less be candidates for level I trauma care. Survival declines precipitously with scores below 12.

The trauma score has recently been revised and is believed to be easier to use and more accurate than the version discussed previously. The revised trauma score (RTS) consists of Glasgow coma scale, systolic blood pressure, and respiratory rate with coded values from zero to four (Table 6–3). The coded values are based on data from more than 26,000 major trauma patients. The survival probability for the sum of coded RTS variable values is listed in Table 6–4. The triage guideline, which sends patients whose sum of RTS coded variable values is 11 or less to the trauma center, has demonstrated a substantial gain in sensitivity, with only a modest loss in specificity (Committee on Trauma of the American College of Surgeons 1987, 44).

Because rating trauma severity is not in and of itself precise as a predictor of which patients will require care at a level I trauma center, other readily available information should be considered in triage of trauma patients. It is thought that more accurate predictions could be made if decisions were based on information such as

TABLE 6–1.
Trauma Score*

	Value	Points	Score
A. Respiratory rate			
Number of respirations in 15 seconds, multiply by four	10–24	4	
	25–35	3	
	>35	2	
	<10	1	
	0	0	A. _____
B. Respiratory effort			
Shallow: markedly decreased chest movement or air exchange	Normal	1	
Retractive: use of accessory muscles or intercostal retraction	Shallow or retractive	0	B. _____
C. Systolic blood pressure			
Systolic cuff pressure: either arm; auscultate or palpate	>90	4	
	70–90	3	
	50–69	2	
	<50	1	
No carotid pulse	0	0	C. _____
D. Capillary refill			
Normal: forehead, lip mucosa, or nail bed color refill in 2 seconds	Normal	2	
Delayed: more than 2 seconds for capillary refill	Delayed	1	
None: no capillary refill	None	0	D. _____

E. Glasgow Coma Scale		GSC Points	Score
1. Eye opening			
Spontaneous _____ 4		14–15	5
To voice _____ 3		11–13	4
To pain _____ 2		8–10	3
None _____ 1		5–7	2
		3–4	1 E. _____
2. Verbal response (arouse patient with voice or painful stimulus)			
Oriented _____ 5			
Confused _____ 4			
Inappropriate words _____ 3			
Incomprehensible words _____ 2			
None _____ 1			
3. Motor response (response to command or painful stimulus)			
Obeys commands _____ 6			
Purposeful movement (pain) _____ 5			
Withdraw (pain) _____ 4			
Flexion (pain) _____ 3			
Extension (pain) _____ 2			
None _____ 1			

Total GCS points (1 + 2 + 3) _____

Trauma Score _____
(Total points A + B + C + D + E)

Source: From Champion HR, Sacco WJ, Carnazzo AJ, et al. Crit Care Med 9:673. Copyright by Williams & Wilkins Co., 1981. Reprinted by permission.

* Patients with trauma scores of less than 12 should be considered candidates for level I trauma centers.

TABLE 6–2.
Estimated Survival Rates as
They Relate to Trauma Score*

Trauma Score	Percentage Survival
16	99
15	98
14	96
13	93
12	87
11	76
10	60
9	42
8	26
7	15
6	8
5	4
4	2
3	1
2	0
1	0

Source: From Champion HR. Sacco WJ, Carnazzo AJ, et al. Crit Care Med 9:673. Copyright by Williams & Wilkins Co., 1981. Reprinted by permission.

* Projected estimate of survival for each value of the Trauma Score based on results from 1509 patients with blunt or penetrating injury.

mechanism of injury and co-morbid factors (whether or not others were killed in the accident). In any case, problems to be avoided during field triage are undertriage and overtriage to level I trauma centers. Undertriage is the incorrect identification of a patient as not having an injury when in fact one is present. Overtriage consists of incorrectly identifying patients as trauma center candidates when they are not. The increasing numbers of trauma centers being designated and the regionalization of trauma care make development of an accurate, easy to use, and reliable method of

TABLE 6–3.
Revised Trauma Score Variable Breakpoints

Glasgow Coma Scale	Systolic Blood Pressure	Respiratory Rate	Coded Value
13–15	<89	10–29	4
9–12	76–89	>29	3
6–8	50–75	6–9	2
4–5	1–49	1–5	1
3	0	0	0

Source: Committee on Trauma of the American College of Surgeons. 1987. Hospital and Prehospital Resources for Optimal Care of the Injured Patient. Quality Assurance in Trauma Care, 44.

TABLE 6–4.
RTS Scores and Probability of Survival

Sum of coded RTS variable values	12	11	10	9	8	7	6	5	4	3	2	1	0
Survival probability	.995	.969	.879	.766	.667	.636	.630	.455	.333	.333	.286	.259	.037

Source: Committee on Trauma of the American College of Surgeons. 1987. Hospital and Prehospital Resources for Optimal Care of the Injured Patient. Quality Assurance in Trauma Care, 44.

rating the severity of injury critical in the assessment and management of trauma patients.

The CRAMS scale is another tool utilized to determine which patients should be brought to a trauma center. Five components, as the acronym suggests, are measured: C, circulation, R, respiration, A, abdomen, M, motor, and S, speech. Each parameter is assigned a value from 0 to 2. Lower scores indicate more severe injuries (Table 6–5).

The injury severity score (ISS) was developed by Baker and coworkers in 1974 in an effort to quantify the effect of the severity of injury and the number of body areas involved in multiply injured individuals (Baker et al. 1974). The ISS is scored from 0 to 75, with higher scores indicating increased injury severity and mortality. The ISS is generally reserved for scoring trauma patients in the hospital setting. Although it more closely correlates with morbidity and mortality than the previously discussed trauma scoring scales, it takes more time and requires more information to complete.

TABLE 6–5.
CRAMS Scale

Components	Score
C Circulation	
Normal capillary refill and BP > 100	2
Delayed capillary refill or BP > 85 < 100	1
No capillary refill or BP < 85	0
R Respirations	
Normal	2
Abnormal (labored or shallow)	1
Absent	0
A Abdomen	
Abdomen and thorax nontender	2
Abdomen or thorax tender	1
Abdomen rigid or flail chest*	0
M Motor	
Normal	2
Responds only to pain (other than decerebrate)	1
No response (or decerebrate)	0
S Speech	
Normal	2
Confused	1
No intelligible words	0
Score ≤ 8: Major trauma	
Score ≥ 9: Minor trauma	

Source: From Gormican SP. 1982. CRAMS scale: Field triage of trauma victims. Ann Emerg Med 11:133.
* "Penetrating wounds to the abdomen or thorax" was added after the study was published.

ASSESSMENT AND MANAGEMENT OF THE MULTIPLE TRAUMA PATIENT

The most comprehensive and continuous form of assessment utilized to identify and prioritize patient problems can be broken down into two separate phases according to priorities in patient management: the primary assessment (or survey) and the secondary assessment (or survey). The primary survey provides vital information to the trauma nurse regarding a patient's airway, pulmonary, and cardiac function as well as a brief neurologic evaluation. The ultimate goal of this survey is to perform rapid and simultaneous evaluation and intervention for life-threatening injuries. The secondary survey does not begin until the primary survey is completed and resuscitation for life-threatening conditions has begun. The secondary survey is a systematic head-to-toe evaluation of the trauma patient (American College of Surgeons, Committee on Trauma 1984, 6.) If at any time during the secondary survey a patient's condition deteriorates, returning to the primary survey with institution (or reinstitution) of resuscitative measures is in order.

The primary and secondary approach to assessment quickly identifies actual or potential life-threatening problems early, before they progress and become more difficult to manage, and it provides a baseline from which all future nursing assessments can be evaluated. Utilizing the primary and secondary survey approach to assessment for all trauma victims will ultimately enhance the Emergency Department (ED) nurse's skill and proficiency in performing such an assessment.

Primary Survey (ABCDE)

During the primary survey, life-threatening conditions are identified and simultaneous management is begun. An experienced trauma nurse can complete this survey within 30 seconds. The primary survey assesses or performs the following:
1. *A*irway maintenance with cervical spine control
2. *B*reathing
3. *C*irculation with hemorrhage control
4. *D*isability (neurologic status) and
5. *E*xposes the patient so that all injuries can be readily identified

Any life-threatening problems identified through this survey must be dealt with immediately rather than after completion of this survey.

Specific Problems Identified During Primary Survey: Airway Obstruction

Airway obstruction is the partial or total occlusion of a person's airway by various means. This is the most rapidly fatal problem seen in EDs. If not treated properly, the patient will die within a few minutes. Usually patients develop airway obstruction within the first few minutes following onset of trauma. Because of this, assessment of the airway is given top priority. In most cases, airway obstruction can be relieved quickly and easily.

Etiology

Airway obstruction is most commonly seen in unconscious patients. This is because unconscious individuals lack the ability and instincts necessary to protect their own airways. The most common reason for airway obstruction in the unconscious victim is partial or complete occlusion of the oropharynx by the tongue. The posterior portion of the tongue simply relaxes into the oropharynx. Saliva, vomitus, bloody secretions, and blood clots may exacerbate the problem. Foreign bodies from maxillofacial trauma may obstruct the upper airways and may even occlude the right or left main stem bronchus. Conscious victims of trauma are not exempt from these previously mentioned causes of airway obstruction; however, their instincts to protect their airways are intact. Airway obstruction may also be due to direct trauma to the larynx. Clinical history is extremely important when diagnosing trauma of the larynx. Typically the history will reveal a direct blow to the anterior neck on a steering wheel or dashboard, or it may be suggestive of a clothesline injury to the neck (Wilson 1986).

Facial trauma and facial fractures (especially midfacial and mandibular fractures) increase the patient's risk for developing airway obstruction. The bony construction of the face is disrupted and may allow the tongue to fall back into the oropharynx.

Soft tissue swelling of the tongue and neck may cause disruption of the normal anatomy of the airway and lead to eventual airway obstruction.

Pathophysiology

Airway obstruction is really a descriptive term for a variety of occurrences that result in partial or complete occlusion of the airway. The physiologic result of this obstruction is hypoxia. The patient is unable to get enough oxygen to the red blood cells or tissues. Therefore, arterial blood gases (ABGs) will reveal a clinical status of hypoxia with respiratory acidosis. Owing to the decrease in available oxygen, the patient reverts to anaerobic metabolism and produces lactic acid, adding to the existing acidosis. Lactic acid levels will continue to rise as long as there is anaerobic metabolism and will eventually reach a point that cannot be reversed. Very high lactic acid levels are associated with very low survival rates. The end result of airway obstruction is hypoxia of the brain and myocardium.

Clinical Manifestations

The signs and symptoms of airway obstruction depend somewhat on the amount of air exchange taking place. With partial airway obstruction and good air exchange, the patient should be able to cough forcefully; however, most likely he or she will be wheezing between coughing. As air exchange diminishes, symptoms of a partial airway obstruction become much like those of complete airway obstruction. Victims cannot speak and commonly are clutching at their throats if they are still conscious. Coughing is ineffective and respiratory distress worsens. Tachypnea, stridor, intercostal retractions, cyanosis, agonal breathing, use of accessory muscles, and anxiety become evident (Buschiazzo et al. 1986). Clinical manifestations of laryngeal damage include local tenderness, subcutaneous emphysema with crepitus over the neck, voice changes, and inspiratory stridor (Wilson 1986).

Treatment and Nursing Care

The patient who is experiencing airway obstruction has a true emergency and requires immediate stage I care. The obstruction must be alleviated immediately.

Airway Clearance, Ineffective, Related to

- **Airway Obstruction**

As stated previously, airway obstruction may be the result of a multitude of causes; swelling of the airway, displacement of the tongue, secretions (blood, vomitus), foreign bodies, and direct laryngeal trauma are examples. Regardless of cause, the oropharynx should be cleared with suction or by the nurse's fingers. The back of the tongue can be brought forward in a variety of ways. The jaw thrust can be used to open the airway and keep the tongue forward (Fig. 6–1). An oral or nasal airway can assist in opening the airway and preventing the tongue from falling back into the oropharynx. Keep in mind, however, that an oral airway improperly placed may actually push the tongue back into the airway, thereby exacerbating the problem. Also, oral airways are not well tolerated by the conscious patient owing to the gag reflex. Other methods for pulling the tongue forward include wrapping a 4 × 4–inch

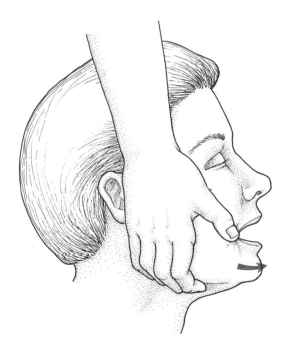

FIGURE 6–1. Jaw thrust. Place fingers of both hands behind the angles of the patient's lower jaw and forcefully bring it forward. If cervical spine injury is suspected, this maneuver should be modified to maintain the head in a neutral position. (Redrawn from American Academy of Orthopaedic Surgeons. 1987. Emergency Care and Transportation, 80.)

gauze square around the tip or inserting a suture through the tip of the tongue and pulling forward.

All patients who are unconscious are at risk for airway occlusion because, as stated previously, they are unable to protect the airway. Therefore, all unconscious victims of trauma should be intubated. A conscious patient who is not at risk of cervical spine injury may have the head of the bed elevated or may be rolled onto his or her side in an attempt to eliminate airway obstruction associated with secretions or tongue displacement.

Injury (Possible), Related to

* **Cervical Spine Fracture Secondary to Trauma**

Patients with airway problems and possible concurrent cervical spine fractures present a difficult dilemma. Any patient with a history of blunt head trauma, neck trauma, or gunshot wound to the neck, or with any injury above the clavicle, in addition to significant decelerative injuries, is at potential risk for cervical spine fracture. These patients need to have the neck immobilized with a hard collar and should be placed on a back board with sandbags or towel rolls on either side of the neck. The forehead should also be taped to the board. The question always arises on whether to intubate the patient in respiratory distress who may have a cervical spine injury. Patients who are having difficulty maintaining a patent airway need to be intubated immediately before waiting for cervical spine radiographs to rule out a fracture. Intubation in these patients can be accomplished in several ways. One option is nasal intubation. This does not require hyperextension of the neck but does require spontaneous respirations and takes time. Spontaneous respirations are required because the tube is advanced with inspiration to assist with placement. Nasal intubation may be contraindicated in the patient suspected of having a basilar skull fracture because of the danger that the tube may enter the anterior cranial fossa through a fractured cribriform plate. Signs and symptoms of basilar fractures are discussed further in the secondary assessment. A second option (and one that is used if the patient is suspected of having a basilar skull fracture) is oral intubation. This can be done safely if a second person maintains in-line manual immobilization of the head and cervical spine while another person proceeds with oral intubation, as in Figure 6–2 (Rice and Enderson 1987).

If oral or nasal intubation fails to secure an airway in the patient with obstruction within 60 seconds and the patient cannot be ventilated with an Ambu bag and mask owing to facial fractures, the trauma nurse should prepare for emergency cricothyrotomy. This is accomplished by cutting down to the cricoid membrane with a No. 11 blade scalpel and inserting the handle of the scalpel or a curved clamp into the trachea and twisting it to enlarge the opening. The opening should be large enough to insert a No. 5 or No. 6 cuffed endotracheal tube (Trunkey 1982, 2). Cricothyrotomy is contraindicated in the patient with a history of laryngeal trauma. Complete tracheolaryngeal separation would defeat the purpose of endotracheal intubation or cricothyrotomy. In cases such as these, tracheostomy is the preferred method of access to the airway. Tracheostomy, however, requires extension of the neck and needs to be considered carefully if a cervical spine injury is suspected. Tracheostomy, along with

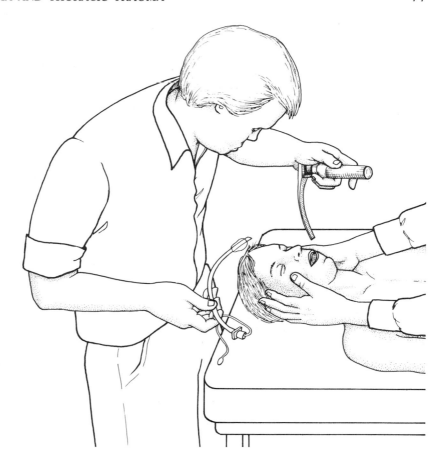

FIGURE 6-2. Cervical spine immobilization during oral intubation. One person straddles patient, holding his or her neck in a neutral position, while another inserts the tube. (Redrawn from American Academy of Orthopaedic Surgeons. 1987. Emergency Care and Transportation, 566.)

the predominant method of oral intubation, requires extension of the neck for optimal visualization. The question often arises whether these methods of securing an airway should be utilized in the unconscious patient when a cervical spine injury is possible and cervical spine films have not yet been obtained. In these circumstances that which poses the greater threat to the patient—the obstructed airway or the possible cervical spine fracture—must be determined. If the airway does not require immediate intervention, it is wise to obtain cervical spine films to rule out a fracture as soon as possible.

Potential airway problems are significantly diminished following successful intubation or cricothyrotomy. It is the conscious patient with the potential for development of airway problems who is not intubated or who does not have a cricothyrotomy that needs constant evaluation. Many conscious patients are able to maintain their own airways. Attempts to intubate aggressively and suction these patients may only lead to vomiting and aspiration. In some cases, however, restlessness and agitation may be a sign of hypoxia and airway obstruction. These patients need immediate intubation. Knowledge of the signs and symptoms of airway obstruction will assist the trauma nurse in differentiating between the patient who is simply restless and the patient who is experiencing hypoxia as a result of airway obstruction. The patient with possible cervical spine fracture and concomitant airway obstruction needs immediate intervention.

The *B* of the primary survey stands for *breathing,* or ventilation. Airway patency does not ensure adequate ventilation. Adequate air exchange along with a patent airway is required for sufficient ventilation and oxygenation. Three life-threatening traumatic conditions that often compromise ventilation are tension pneumothorax, open pneumothorax, and large flail chest.

Tension Pneumothorax

Tension pneumothorax is a potentially lethal problem that results from a continuous increase in pressure in the pleural space. This occurs when air enters the pleural space on inspiration and cannot escape during expiration.

Etiology

Tension pneumothorax is frequently the result of a closed (simple) pneumothorax and commonly occurs in patients who are being ventilated with an endotracheal tube and an Ambu bag or ventilator. A spontaneous pneumothorax (e.g., a ruptured bleb) can also develop into a tension pneumothorax if the leak from the injured lung fails to seal. Penetrating trauma may also cause a tension pneumothorax.

Pathophysiology

The continuous increase in positive pressure on the affected side of a tension pneumothorax causes the lung on that side to collapse, resulting in mediastinal displacement toward the unaffected side. Collapse of the affected lung and mediastinal displacement both contribute to respiratory embarrassment, the latter because it eventually compresses the unaffected lung. Diminished lung expansion occurs bilaterally. Compression of the heart and great vessels (e.g., inferior and superior vena cava) as the result of mediastinal displacement causes a decreased venous return to the heart and shock-like symptoms (Fig. 6–3). The mediastinal shift may eventually become so severe it causes a kink or closes off the abdominal aorta, resulting in cardiac arrest (Knezevich 1986, 91).

Clinical Manifestations

Patients with tension pneumothorax will have increasing dyspnea, hypoxia, and shock-like symptoms: a decrease in blood pressure, increase in heart rate, anxiety, and cool, clammy skin. Physical examination will reveal a trachea deviated toward the unaffected side. Breath sounds may be diminished or absent on the affected side, and there will be hyperresonance to percussion. Heart sounds are distant. Distended neck veins (in the absence of hypovolemia) and cyanosis may also be present. Chest radiograph confirms diagnosis.

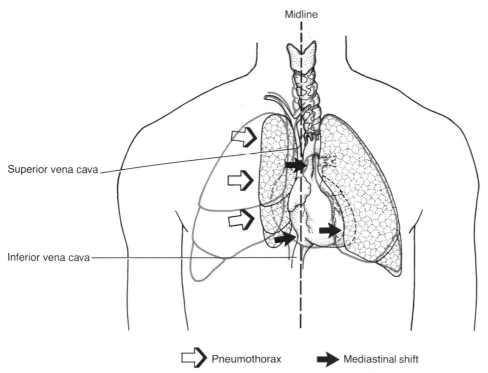

FIGURE 6-3. Tension pneumothorax. As pleural pressure on the affected side increases, mediastinal displacement ensues with resultant respiratory and cardiovascular compromise. Gray line indicates normal anatomic position.

Treatment and Nursing Care

Tension pneumothorax is a true medical emergency. Immediate stage I care is required. Therapeutic measures to relieve the tension pneumothorax should be undertaken prior to obtaining the chest radiograph. Delaying treatment to obtain a chest radiograph may prove detrimental to the patient.

Impaired Gas Exchange, Related to

- **Tension Pneumothorax**

Respiratory embarrassment in a patient with a tension pneumothorax is evident. Relieving the tension through chest tube insertion or needle thoracentesis should provide immediate relief to the patient. Trauma nurses should prepare for a chest tube insertion of a large-bore (36 to 40 F caliber) chest tube on the affected side, at the fifth intercostal space anterior to the mid-axillary line. Once inserted, suction drainage should be established. If a delay is anticipated before the insertion of a chest tube, a large-gauge needle (14 to 18) can be inserted into the second intercostal space in the mid-clavicular line of the affected side. This relieves some of the pressure and converts the tension pneumothorax into a simple pneumothorax (American College of Surgeons, Committee on Trauma 1984, 75). Supplemental oxygen in the form of a non-rebreather mask should also be available.

Decreased Cardiac Output, Related to

- **Decreased Venous Return Secondary to Compression of Great Vessels Resulting from Tension Pneumothorax**

A decrease in cardiac output as the result of a tension pneumothorax is not uncommon. Treatment of the tension pneumothorax should immediately improve venous return to the heart and alleviate shock-like symptoms.

Evaluation

Patients with tension pneumothorax need constant respiratory evaluation to identify signs and symptoms of hypoxia, such as agitation or tachypnea. Patients with advanced tension pneumothorax need to be evaluated continually for signs and symptoms of shock due to decreased venous return. Therefore, vital signs must be closely monitored and life-saving interventions initiated expediently. Once treatment has been initiated, significant improvement in the patient's respiratory and hemodynamic status should be evident.

Open Pneumothorax

Open pneumothorax (also called sucking chest wound) occurs when there is significant penetration of the chest wall that results in free communication between the pleural space and the atmosphere (Lewis 1986).

Etiology

All penetrating wounds to the chest can be considered open pneumothoraces. Most penetrating chest wounds, however, are sealed off by the tissue of the chest and do not communicate with the atmosphere. True open pneumothoraces are associated with close-range shotgun blasts and high velocity missiles (for example, a .44 Magnum).

Pathophysiology

Because of the open communication between the pleural space and the environment, equilibration of intrathoracic and atmospheric pressures occurs. The negative intrathoracic pressure required to generate adequate ventilation is no longer present. As

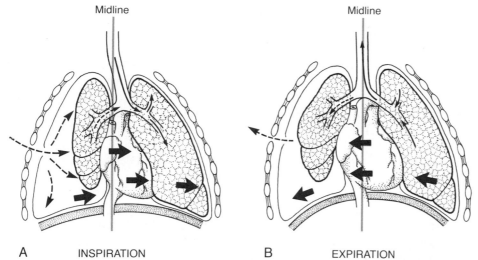

FIGURE 6–4. Open pneumothorax. *A*, Inspiration. As air enters the pleural space, intrapleural pressure increases, causing the affected lung to collapse and shift the mediastinum toward the unaffected side. *B*, Expiration. As air escapes, intrapleural pressure decreases and the mediastinum returns to midline. Large arrows indicate normal air movement; dashed arrows indicate abnormal air movement; small arrows indicate structural movement.

the person inspires, atmospheric air is sucked into the intrapleural space, increasing intrapleural pressure. This increase in intrapleural pressure collapses the lung on the affected side and shifts the mediastinum toward the unaffected side, resulting in compromised lung expansion bilaterally. During expiration intrapleural air escapes, decreasing intrapleural pressure, and allowing the mediastinum to swing back toward the midline (Fig. 6–4). A "to-and-fro" movement of the mediastinum occurs.

Clinical Manifestations

Diagnosis of open pneumothorax should be obvious. History reveals penetrating chest trauma. There is a large gaping wound to the chest. It is usually associated with frothy blood at the wound site. Air can be heard moving back and forth through the wound with respiration. The patient generally experiences anxiety, air hunger, and pain.

Treatment and Nursing Care

Immediate stage I interventions are required for patients with open pneumothorax. Care must be taken to prevent the development of tension pneumothorax while treating an open pneumothorax.

Impaired Gas Exchange, Related to

- **Loss of Negative Intrapleural Pressure Secondary to Open Pneumothorax**

The loss of negative intrapleural pressure impairs gas exchange, leading to inadequate ventilation. Stage I care is required for any patient with open pneumothorax. The open wound must be sealed immediately with an occlusive dressing or nonporous material (e.g., petrolatum gauze, plastic wrap) and taped on three sides. In this way a flutter valve effect occurs; on inspiration the occlusive dressing is sucked onto the open wound, not allowing air to enter the pleural space, and on expiration the opened end of the dressing allows air to escape. (If, however, a flap forms, allowing air to enter into the pleural space on inspiration but not to escape on expiration, intrapleural pressure continues to increase and a tension pneumothorax may develop.) In this case the dressing should be removed immediately. If a foreign object is lodged in the chest wall it should never be removed until the patient is in a controlled medical setting. Removal of the object may convert a closed pneumothorax to an open pneumothorax and also induce bleeding.

The trauma nurse should immediately set up for insertion of a large-bore (36 to 40) French chest tube in the affected hemithorax. This chest tube will be placed in the affected hemithorax away from the open wound. Surgical closure of the wound may then follow. Supplemental high flow oxygen should be administered. ABGs will need to be determined at frequent intervals to assess respiratory status. Also, a chest radiograph will be needed following chest tube insertion to check placement and also to assess for related thoracic injuries. Antibiotics and tetanus prophylaxis may also be indicated.

Evaluation

The patient with open pneumothorax will need close monitoring to assess for the development of tension pneumothorax. Any shock-like symptoms should alert the ED nurse to this possibility. The patient's respiratory status will also require careful observation for indications of increasing respiratory embarrassment.

Large Flail Chest

A flail chest occurs when a segment of the chest wall (usually three or four ribs) does not have bony continuity with the rest of the thoracic rib cage. The loss of bony continuity of a segment of the chest wall with the remainder of the thoracic cage results when fractures occur in more than one place in the same plane (anterior or posterior plane) in two or more adjacent ribs.

Etiology

Flail chest is with few exceptions the result of blunt trauma, such as motor vehicle accidents, falls, and crushing injuries. It is usually associated with high-force injuries, and, although this is not common, can include fractures of the first and second ribs.

Fractures of the first or second rib, or both, may be associated with contained rupture of the descending thoracic aorta or rupture of the subclavian artery or vein.

Pathophysiology

Flail chest is responsible for varying degrees of respiratory and cardiovascular compromise. Respiratory compromise occurs because the bellows function, which is required for normal ventilation, is no longer present. The flail segment of the chest wall and its underlying lung tissue respond to intrapleural pressure changes and no longer move in continuity with the remainder of the chest wall. During inspiration, when intrapleural pressure becomes increasingly negative, the flail segment and its underlying lung tissue are sucked inward when they should normally be expanding outward. This causes the affected lung and mediastinum to be shifted toward the unaffected side, compromising the amount of air inspired in both the affected and the unaffected lung. On expiration, when intrapleural pressure is less negative, the flail segment and underlying lung tissue are pushed outward when they should normally be collapsing inward. This causes the mediastinum to be shifted toward the affected side. This opposing movement between the flail segment and its underlying lung tissue and the remainder of the chest wall is referred to as paradoxical chest movement.

Paradoxical chest movements impair gas exchange not only by compromising the amount of inspired air on inspiration, as already described, but also by shunting air between the lungs instead of its passing through the trachea and upper airway (Fig. 6–5). Paradoxical chest movements, in addition to the pain associated with flail chest, diminish lung expansion, resulting in atelectasis, hypoxia, and hypercapnea. Pulmonary contusions also are frequently associated with flail chest and contribute to impaired gas exchange.

Cardiovascular compromise as the result of flail chest occurs in response to the "mediastinal swing." Venous return to the right heart may be impeded with a resultant drop in arterial pressure and eventually in cardiac output. Venous pressure remains high initially.

Clinical Manifestations

Patients with flail chest usually complain of severe chest pain during inspiration and dyspnea. History reveals blunt or crushing chest trauma.

Physical examination reveals asymmetry and uncoordinated movement of the thorax with respiration. Palpation of this area may reveal crepitus. Respirations are usually rapid and shallow. The patient may be cyanotic. Arterial blood gases will reveal varying degrees of hypoxia, hypercapnea, and respiratory acidosis.

Treatment and Nursing Care

Medical and nursing interventions that are required for patients with flail chest focus primarily on ensuring adequate oxygenation and cardiac output, promoting comfort, and alleviating anxiety.

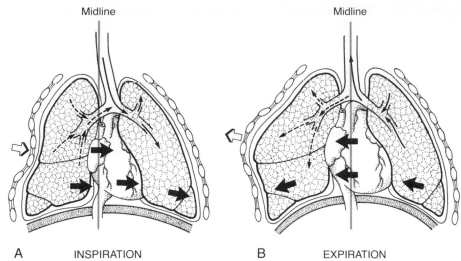

FIGURE 6-5. Flail chest. *A*, Inspiration. As intrapleural pressure becomes increasingly negative, the flail segment and its underlying lung tissue are sucked inward, collapsing the lung on the affected side and causing the mediastinum to shift toward the unaffected side. *B*, Expiration. As intrapleural pressure becomes less negative, the flail segment and underlying tissue are pushed outward and the mediastinum shifts to the affected side. Some air moves between lungs instead of passing through upper airways. Large arrows indicate normal air movement; dashed arrows indicate abnormal air movement; open arrows indicate structural movement.

Impaired Gas Exchange, Related to

- **Pulmonary Contusion(s)**
- **Paradoxical Chest Movements Secondary to Flail Chest**
- **Pain Secondary to Flail Chest**

Paradoxical chest movements, concurrent pulmonary contusions, and pain all contribute to ventilation-perfusion abnormalities and impaired gas exchange in the person with flail chest. It used to be thought that stabilization of the flail segment was necessary to regain normal ventilation. This was achieved by placing a 2-pound sandbag over the flail segment or by placing firm pressure with one's hand on the flail segment. Currently, however, it is realized that splinting restricts chest wall movement altogether and does not promote normal ventilation or oxygenation. Intubation and mechanical ventilation will provide adequate ventilation without restricting chest wall movement. However, if this is not contraindicated because of possible cervical spine fracture, the patient may be rolled over to the affected side in order to splint the flail segment. This temporary measure can be utilized to provide some immediate relief of pain. The patient should also have a diagnostic chest radiograph and ABG determinations to assess for hypoxia.

Decreased Cardiac Output, Potential, Related to

- **Pulmonary Contusion(s)**
- **Ruptured Aorta**
- **Mediastinal Swing Secondary to Flail Chest**

Pulmonary contusions with associated interstitial and intra-alveolar hemorrhage, a ruptured aorta, and mediastinal displacement all may contribute to altered hemodynamics and a decrease in cardiac output. Vital signs must be closely monitored. Intravenous access must be initiated for the possible administration of blood, blood components, or intravenous fluids. Overhydration of the patient with a pulmonary contusion must be avoided, however, as this may worsen the clinical condition of the patient.

Pain, Related to

- **Flail Chest**

As mentioned previously, stabilizing the fracture site may decrease the patient's pain. The most effective method of pain control has been the administration of bupivacaine (Marcaine) intercostal nerve blocks. This provides immediate relief and breaks the pain cycle. Allowing the patient to breathe with normal respiratory excursions will reduce the incidence of atelectasis.

Infection, Potential for, Related to

- **Pulmonary Contusion**

Many patients with flail chest have associated pulmonary contusions. These persons are at risk of developing pulmonary sepsis due to extravasation of blood into the tissue of the lung. This blood is an excellent culture medium and may become contaminated. Although this is largely a concern in in-patient nursing care, the ED nurse may need to administer antibiotics as prescribed. The patient's white blood cell (WBC) count and temperature should also be closely monitored.

Evaluation

Evaluation of the patient who has a flail chest includes continuous assessment for signs and symptoms of increasing respiratory or cardiovascular difficulty, or both. Agitation, confusion, and tachycardia are all symptoms that should be watched for and may indicate that more aggressive management is in order.

The *C* of the primary survey denotes *circulation* with hemorrhage control. Patients who have uncontrolled bleeding greater than 15 ml/minute are at risk for developing hypovolemic shock if the bleeding is not managed aggressively. The primary survey should identify conditions associated with alterations in circulation that can lead to loss of life if aggressive intervention is not undertaken.* These conditions include pericardial tamponade, traumatic aortic dissection (or other injuries to the great vessels), massive hemothorax, and uncontrolled external hemorrhage. (For a discussion on uncontrolled internal hemorrhage, see Chap. 5.)

Pericardial Tamponade

Pericardial tamponade is the filling of the pericardium with blood from the heart or great vessels.

Etiology

Pericardial tamponade may be caused by blunt trauma but is more commonly the result of penetrating injuries to the heart.

Pathophysiology

The pericardial sac is a fibrous structure that surrounds the heart. Leaking of blood into the sac raises the intrapericardial pressure, restricting venous blood flow into the heart. Ventricular filling is decreased and cardiac output falls. Eventually, if it is allowed to continue, the patient will go into cardiogenic shock.

Clinical Manifestations

The signs and symptoms of pericardial tamponade may be subtle at first. Patients will usually reveal a history of blunt or penetrating chest trauma and may complain of dyspnea. Objective symptoms are the result of impaired right-sided ventricular filling, a distended pericardial sac, and a diminished cardiac output. An elevated central venous pressure (CVP) with jugular vein distention (JVD), muffled heart tones, and hypotension* constitute Beck's triad—a cluster of symptoms that are seen in approximately 40% of all patients with cardiac tamponade. Pulsus paradoxus, a narrowed pulse pressure, cyanosis, tachycardia, and restlessness may also be present. Chest radiograph will reveal an enlarged heart and mediastinum, and electrocardiographic (EKG) voltage is usually decreased.

---

* Blood pressure should not be relied on for early detection of an alteration in circulatory status. Compensatory mechanisms maintain normal adequate systemic systolic and diastolic pressures until the later stages of shock. Because it is an unreliable indicator, blood pressure is not included in the primary survey. The pulse, however, can give the nurse an estimate of the systolic blood pressure. Generally, if the radial pulse is palpable, the systolic blood pressure will be above 80 mmHg. If the femoral pulse is palpable, the systolic pressure will be above 70 mmHg. If the carotid pulse is palpable, the systolic pressure will be above 60 mmHg.

Treatment and Nursing Care

Pericardial tamponade may be quickly fatal if immediate stage I care does not rapidly ensue once the diagnosis is made.

Decreased Cardiac Output, Related to

- **Decreased Ventricular Filling Secondary to Pericardial Tamponade**

A decrease in ventricular filling ultimately leads to a decrease in cardiac output. The nurse must prepare for immediate pericardiocentesis (and possible thoracotomy) so that intrapericardial pressure can be decreased, allowing for increased ventricular filling.

Pericardiocentesis is performed using sterile technique by inserting a 16- or 18-gauge spinal needle or 6-inch angiocatheter into the pericardial sac, thereby relieving some of the pressure. To perform pericardiocentesis, the patient should be placed in a semi-Fowler's position, if not contraindicated, to allow for pooling of blood in the apex of the heart. The patient is placed on a 12-lead EKG. The needle should be attached to a 50-ml syringe with a three-way stopcock. A sterile alligator clamp should be attached from the hub of the needle to the V lead of the EKG machine. The xyphoid and subxyphoid areas are prepared with an iodine solution and a complete explanation of the procedure is given to the patient if possible.

The needle is inserted subxyphoid at a 45-degree angle, toward the left shoulder (Fig. 6–6). If the needle is advanced too far and enters the epicardium, the monitor will show extreme ST-T wave changes, widened QRS complexes, or premature ventricular contractions (PVCs). If this should occur, the needle should be withdrawn until baseline rhythm returns. As much blood as possible is withdrawn. It is thought that blood that clots in the syringe after several minutes is ventricular blood

FIGURE 6–6. Pericardiocentesis.

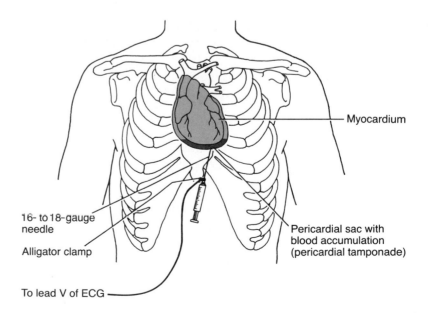

Myocardium

16- to 18-gauge needle

Alligator clamp

Pericardial sac with blood accumulation (pericardial tamponade)

To lead V of ECG

and nonclotting blood is pericardial in origin. It is not uncommon for pericardial taps to aspirate only small amounts (15 to 25 ml) of blood. Aspiration of small amounts of blood, however, may be enough to save the patient's life. Observe the patient for a drop in CVP and an increase in blood pressure after aspiration. After completion of the aspiration, remove the syringe and leave the needle in place with the stopcock closed. Secure the needle to the chest by taping it securely to prevent displacement. This procedure then can be repeated if necessary by simply placing a syringe on the stopcock, opening it, and aspirating.

Impaired Gas Exchange, Related to

- **Hypoxia Secondary to Decreased Cardiac Output Resulting from Pericardial Tamponade**

Patients with pericardial tamponade may also have respiratory distress owing to a decreased cardiac output with resultant hypoxia. High-flow oxygen should be administered. If the patient is unconscious or is in severe respiratory distress, intubation should be considered.

Fluid Volume Deficit, Related to

- **Fluid Accumulation in Pericardial Sac**
- **Decrease in Cardiac Output Secondary to Pericardial Tamponade**

All patients with significant trauma including pericardial tamponade should have two large-bore (No. 14 to 18) intravenous (IV) lines inserted. The rate of the IV infusion can be adjusted according to the patient's individual needs. Patients who have severe hypovolemia and are not responsive to initial IV therapy may need more than two peripheral IV lines. An indwelling Foley catheter should be placed to monitor urine output every 15 minutes. Urine output is the best indicator of the adequacy of volume resuscitation.

Anxiety, Related to

- **Fear of Dying**

The trauma nurse needs to maintain a calm and reassuring manner. The patient is understandably upset and confused over the circumstances, the strange surroundings, and fear of the unknown. The patient's family is also experiencing similar emotions. The trauma nurse needs to be open, direct, honest, and compassionate when attempting to allay the fears of the patient and his or her family.

Evaluation

The trauma nurse needs to monitor the patient post pericardiocentesis for signs of improvement or worsening of his or her status. A decrease in blood pressure will indicate continued filling of the pericardial sac. The trauma nurse also needs to evaluate fluid volume status closely for indications of hypovolemic shock.

Injuries to Great Vessels

Injuries to the great vessels, whether from blunt or penetrating trauma or from acceleration-deceleration injuries, are associated with very high mortality rates. Injuries to these vessels result in rapid exsanguination into the chest. The vast majority of these patients die at the scene of the accident. Our discussion of injuries to the great vessels will focus on traumatic aortic dissection.

Traumatic Aortic Dissection

A common cause of sudden death following blunt chest trauma and acceleration-deceleration injuries is aortic rupture or dissection. According to Greendyke (1966), one in every six fatality victims of motor vehicle accidents has sustained an aortic rupture. High vehicular speeds, substance abuse, and failure to use seat belts were factors that contributed to this type of injury.

Etiology and Pathophysiology

Traumatic aortic dissection occurs commonly in sudden horizontal or vertical acceleration-deceleration injuries (e.g., falls, motor vehicle accidents). The most common site of disruption involves the thoracic aorta just distal to the left subclavian artery (Piano and Turney 1988) (Fig. 6–7). The aorta is relatively mobile within the chest cavity, secured only by its attachment to the other great vessels and the ligamentum arteriosum (ductus arteriosus in the fetus). Sudden impacts producing deceleration forces cause shearing of the aorta away from its attachment. Another common site of disruption occurs at the take-off of the innominate artery. Less commonly, when the heart is displaced laterally from blunt force, the ascending aorta may rotate and shear away from the heart, causing disruption at the aortic valve. Rapid exsanguination into the chest is responsible for the high mortality rates associated with aortic dissection.

Clinical Manifestations

The patient in whom aortic dissection is suspected will have a history of blunt trauma to the chest or an acceleration-deceleration type of injury. Major deceleration injuries should always raise a high index of suspicion of aortic dissection even in the absence of obvious trauma. If the patient is awake on arrival, he or she may complain of chest pain or back pain between the scapulae. Severe shortness of breath, hemoptysis, and a loud systolic murmur may signal loss of aortic valvular integrity. Shock-like symptoms will most likely be present. There may be a difference in blood pressure from right to left sides depending on where the dissection is and how blood flow is altered. Reflex hypertension occurs in a small percentage of patients. Sympathetic fibers located in the aorta respond to the stretching stimulus from a hematoma or a torn intimal flap. This is referred to as the acute coarctation syndrome and is evident by

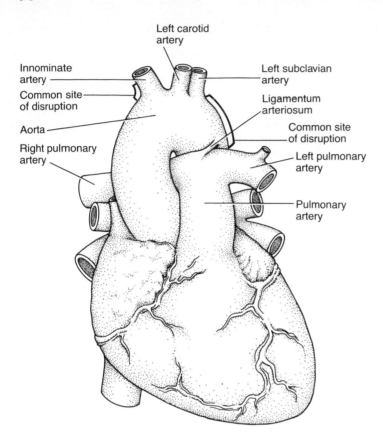

FIGURE 6–7. Common sites of aortic dissection.

elevated upper extremity blood pressure and decreased or absent lower extremity blood pressure.

The chest radiograph may show a widened mediastinum, a depressed left main stem bronchus, displacement of the nasogastric tube or trachea to the right, or loss of the aortic knob shadow (Stiles et al. 1985). Patients with any of these signs, a history of acceleration-deceleration injuries, or evidence of blunt chest trauma should have further radiographic studies of the aorta. Some authors believe that a true erect chest radiograph, rather than the commonly performed supine film, depicts the anatomy of the chest more accurately and should be performed whenever feasible to avoid unnecessary follow-up studies (Mirvis 1988).

Treatment and Nursing Care

Because the majority of patients with aortic disruption have multisystem injuries, the initial management focuses on stabilization of the cardiovascular system and identification of injuries through diagnostic testing and ongoing monitoring. Stage I treatment is required immediately.

Fluid Volume Deficit, Related to

• *Traumatic aortic dissection*

Surgical repair is nearly always indicated in the treatment of traumatic aortic dissection or rupture. Immediately upon arrival in the ED intravenous access with large-bore needles should be established if traumatic aortic dissection or rupture is suspected. The patient's blood should be typed and cross-matched for 6 to 10 units and the patient rapidly prepared for surgery. He or she may require an arch angiogram or injection of contrast dye into the aorta via a catheter threaded through the femoral artery to diagnose the injury. Explanations to the patient regarding the procedure are necessary.

Medical therapeutic interventions may include measures to decrease the hemodynamic stresses on the aorta and prevent rupture of the intact layers of the aorta (Hammond 1986, 681). Beta-adrenergic blocking agents or vasodilators may be used to maintain a systolic blood pressure between 100 and 120 mmHg.

Evaluation

Continuous monitoring of blood pressure, pulse, and respiratory status is necessary while the patient is in the ED. Postoperatively, the patient is closely monitored for complications, and associated injuries are managed.

Massive Hemothorax

Massive hemothorax is the accumulation of large amounts of blood in the pleural space (Fig. 6–8). It is associated with about a 50 to 75% mortality rate upon arrival in the ED (Trunkey 1987b).

Etiology

Massive hemothorax usually results from penetrating injuries to the aortic arch, hilum of the lung, or intercostal or internal mammary arteries. Rupture of these large vessels may cause the patient to have blood loss into the hemithorax of 500 to 1000 ml/hour.

FIGURE 6–8. Massive hemothorax.

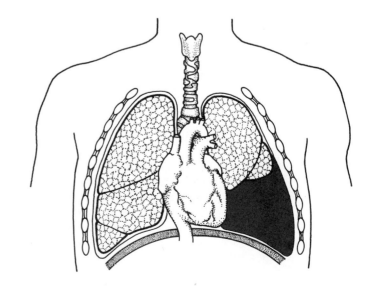

Pathophysiology

Patients with massive hemothorax have high-volume blood loss because their injuries involve the arteries in the chest. The arteries within the chest are at systemic pressure and therefore the amount of the exsanguination depends on the pressure within the systemic system. It is obvious that exsanguination can occur rapidly.

Clinical Manifestations

The patient, if not dead on arrival in the ED, exhibits signs of respiratory distress, shock, and mediastinal shift. A chest radiograph will confirm a diagnosis of massive hemothorax, but definitive treatment should not depend on or be delayed for confirmation.

Treatment and Nursing Care

Fluid Volume Deficit, Related to

- *Hypovolemia secondary to massive hemothorax*

The nurse should prepare for immediate placement of a 36- to 40-French chest tube on the affected side. In many cases, a gush of blood is obtained immediately on insertion of the chest tube.

Patients will also require aggressive fluid resuscitation in an attempt to replace lost blood volume and reverse hypovolemic shock. The patient will need at least two or more large-bore peripheral IV lines. Blood should be sent for immediate typing and cross-matching. Administration of type-specific blood may be indicated in patients who cannot wait for cross-matched blood. If there are no associated abdominal injuries to cause contamination of the blood, autotransfusion should be considered.

Autotransfusion, a procedure described in the early 19th century and perfected in the 1960s and 1970s, is designed to collect blood and prepare it to reinfuse through an IV line. In the emergency setting autotransfusion is used most often for patients with massive hemothorax.

Blood can be easily collected from a hemothorax through a chest tube attached to a collection bag. Once 1 liter of blood is collected, it can be reinfused into the patient. Although blood from a hemothorax is essentially incoagulable, most centers add citrate phosphate dextrose (CPD), an anticoagulant, to the blood prior to reinfusion. The ratio of CPD to blood is $1:10$. A 20-μm filter should be utilized to provide ultrafiltration.

The major benefits of autotransfusion are the immediate availability of blood, the diminished incidence of transfusion reactions, and the lower cost as compared with use of banked blood. The potential risks of autotransfusion include air embolism, sepsis, coagulopathies, and electrolyte abnormalities.

The risk of air embolism can be reduced by carefully removing all air from the blood bag prior to reinfusion. Because sepsis is likely when the patient is transfused with contaminated blood, autotransfusion should not be performed whenever the possibility of thoracoabdominal communication is present.

Massive autotransfusion has been found to contribute to the development of significant coagulopathies. Autotransfusion from a hemothorax of 25 per cent estimated blood volume has been associated with a mild reduction of platelets, fibrinogen, and clotting factors but did not significantly compromise the adequacy of the clotting system (Napoli et al. 1987). Replacement therapy of hemostatic components should be considered when autotransfusion exceeds 25 per cent of estimated blood volume (Napoli et al. 1987).

Hyperkalemia may result from red blood cell destruction during autotransfusion. Red blood cell hemolysis occurs secondary to mechanical forces during collection and reinfusion and prolonged exposure to serosal linings of the body cavities.

Impaired Gas Exchange, Related to

- *Massive hemothorax*

As blood accumulates in the pleural space, the negative pressure that is usually present to allow for lung expansion on inspiration is diminished. As lung expansion is diminished, gas exchange becomes impaired, and respiratory distress ensues. High-flow oxygen or intubation is required to relieve hypoxia.

Essentially all patients with massive hemothorax will require thoracostomy and chest tube insertion. Consent should be obtained from the family if possible because these patients usually are not in any condition to consent for themselves. Usual operating room (OR) preparation will depend on policies of the specific institution.

Evaluation

Trauma nurses must closely monitor and record drainage from the chest tube. This volume in general will need to be replaced times three with IV fluids and blood when available. The patient also needs to be evaluated continuously for signs of hypovolemic shock and respiratory distress.

Uncontrolled External Hemorrhage

Uncontrolled external hemorrhage can be caused by any major injury, blunt or penetrating. Hemorrhage may be due to a variety of injuries and results in the acute loss of circulatory blood volume. Exsanguination accounts for 30% to 40% of all traumatic deaths (Lewis 1984). External hemorrhage is usually due to penetrating trauma to a major vessel—for example, a stab wound to a femoral artery. The physiologic effects and clinical manifestations of uncontrolled external bleeding are the same as for those discussed for hypovolemic shock (see Chap. 5).

Treatment and Nursing Care

External hemorrhage must be controlled as quickly as possible or hypovolemic shock may develop rapidly.

Fluid Volume Deficit, Related to

- *Uncontrolled external hemorrhage*

Rapid external blood loss can be managed by constant direct pressure to the wound. Sterile 4 × 4 gauze squares applied with firm hand pressure or an elastic wrap may be helpful in decreasing blood loss. Pneumatic splints may also be used to tamponade bleeding sites. In general, hemostats should not be used because they may cause further damage to the blood vessels and cause nerve deficits. Tourniquets cause anaerobic metabolism and therefore should not be used. Abdominal or lower extremity hemorrhage can be controlled or decreased with the use of the pneumatic anti-shock garment (PASG) or military anti-shock trousers (MAST suit). Much controversy has evolved over the last few years regarding the use of the MAST or PASG. Initially, it was thought that the PASG increased blood pressure by causing an autotransfusion effect of 1.0 to 1.5 liters of blood from the lower extremities back to the systemic circulation. Recent evidence indicates that only about 200 ml of blood is actually shunted back into the circulation. The rise in blood pressure is more likely the result of an increase in peripheral vascular resistance in the lower extremities.

PASGs also cause anaerobic metabolism to occur in the lower extremities, resulting in the production of lactic acid. When the PASG is deflated rapidly, this lactic acid is released into the systemic circulation, causing pH imbalance and metabolic acidosis. In addition, there is a profound hypotensive effect on rapid deflation, which may lead to cardiac arrest. Deflation of the PASG is done in an orderly fashion starting with the abdominal section. The nurse should take a baseline blood pressure before deflation and immediately afterward. The abdominal compartment is slowly deflated until a 5-mm decrease in blood pressure is noted. At this point, deflation is discontinued and IV fluids are increased until the blood pressure returns to baseline. Deflation is resumed in the same manner while checking blood pressure until the abdomen is completely deflated. Once the abdomen is deflated, each leg is individually deflated while constantly monitoring the blood pressure (Carter and Smith 1982). If the patient's injuries require an OR procedure for stabilization of blood loss, the PASG or MAST suit should not be deflated until the patient is safely in the OR.

In some instances, inflation of the PASG will exacerbate bleeding from injury sources above the level of the garment and may complicate ventilation owing to elevation of the diaphragm. In addition, examination of the abdomen and legs is difficult when the PASG is on.

In summary, the advantages and disadvantages of applying the PASG need to be weighed for each individual patient. In addition to the above measures, all patients with uncontrolled external hemorrhage need to have at least two large-bore IV lines inserted peripherally. Blood samples should be drawn for typing and cross-matching as well as the usual blood chemistry tests. Hematocrit should be obtained on an ongoing basis until the patient's condition is stable and hemorrhage is controlled.

Evaluation

Patients need constant monitoring by the nurse for any increase in bleeding from the source of injury. Successful volume resuscitation will be indicated by warm dry skin, urine volume greater than 0.5 ml/kg/hr, capillary refill within 2 seconds, normal pulse rate and blood pressure, and absence of deteriorating mental status.

The *D* of the primary survey stands for *disability*. This consists of a brief neurologic examination that is undertaken at the end of the primary survey. The examination should take no longer than 20 seconds and should establish the patient's level of consciousness and pupil size and reactivity. A mnemonic using the acronym AVPU is utilized to evaluate the patient's level of consciousness (American College of

Surgeons, Committee on Trauma 1984, 8):

A = alert
V = response to verbal stimuli
P = response to painful stimuli
U = unresponsive

The patient's extremities are checked for spontaneous movement, movement in response to pain, or absence of movement. This survey is done to establish a baseline from which future assessments can be evaluated.

The *E* in the primary survey stands for *exposure*. All trauma patients need to be completely undressed before an adequate examination can be completed.

The Resuscitation Phase

The resuscitation phase is composed of ongoing patient assessment and continued management of all previously identified life-threatening conditions. In essence, the primary survey is reviewed during the resuscitation phase. Additionally, therapeutic interventions that may not have been done during the primary survey may be initiated during this phase.

Supplemental oxygen is given to all trauma victims to reduce further strain on the heart, and a minimum of two large-bore peripheral IV lines should be placed (16- or larger gauge, if possible), if needed. Aggressive IV therapy should be initiated with a balanced salt solution, such as lactated Ringer's solution or normal saline. The controversy continues over whether to initiate fluid resuscitation with a crystalloid (lactated Ringer's solution or normal saline) solution or a colloid solution (albumin and plasma). According to Virgilio (1979) no significant advantage was found for albumin over crystalloids. Remember that 3 ml of crystalloid per 1 ml of estimated blood volume lost is to be replaced. Remember also that the rate of the IV infusion is determined not by the size of the vein but by the internal diameter of the catheter and is inversely affected by its length. Initially two peripheral IV lines should be placed in the upper extremities if not contraindicated. IV lines should not be started in injured extremities. If additional IV lines are needed, one or more cut-downs should be started. In general, central percutaneous subclavian and internal jugular veins should be avoided in hypovolemic patients because of a danger of producing a pneumothorax. Blood must be drawn for typing and cross-matching, basic chemistry tests, and spun hematocrit determination. Remember that massive fluid resuscitation can result in hemodilution and in a falsely lowered hematocrit value. A MAST suit (or PASG) may be applied if hypotension persists and its use is not contraindicated. The patient's EKG should be monitored for dysrhythmias and ST wave changes. Whole blood may be given to those patients who do not respond to 3 liters of lactated Ringer's solution infused over 10 to 15 minutes. The optimum method for transfusing trauma patients is to use blood that has been typed and cross-matched. Unfortunately, there is usually a delay in obtaining typed and cross-matched blood. Type-specific blood can be used in those cases in which it would be detrimental to wait for blood that has been cross-matched. The risk of transfusion reactions is low with type-specific blood and such blood generally is tolerated as well as cross-matched blood. Low-titer type O negative blood may be used in extreme cases when type-specific blood is not available. All emergency rooms should have one to two units of type O negative blood available and in stock for immediate use. In some cases however, the use of type O negative blood may cause transfusion reactions and difficulties with future typing and cross-matching.

A nasogastric (NG) tube should be inserted to decrease gastric dilation caused by either an ileus or air in the stomach owing to ventilation assistance with an Ambu mask device. Gastric contents should be checked for the presence of blood. NG tubes should not be inserted through the nose in patients suspected of having skull fractures. Signs and symptoms of skull fractures are discussed further in the section on secondary assessment. An NG tube inserted nasally into the patient with a skull fracture may inadvertently be inserted into the intracranial cavity. If necessary, the NG tube may be inserted orally.

A Foley catheter should be inserted to monitor output and evaluate effectiveness of fluid resuscitation. Foley catheters should not be inserted in patients suspected of having a urethral tear. Men with urethral tears will have blood at the meatus, a high-riding prostate on rectal examination, or blood in the scrotum. Women are less likely to have urethral tears owing to intraabdominal protection of the urethra. Women with blood at the meatus should be suspected of having a urethral tear. Insertion of a Foley catheter in the presence of these signs may cause a complete tearing of the urethra. A urethrogram should be obtained prior to insertion of a Foley catheter to rule out urethral tear if one is suspected. If catheterization is possible, a urine sample should be obtained and tested for the presence of blood.

Secondary Survey

Once the primary survey is completed and life-threatening injuries are treated surgically, stabilized, or ruled out and the resuscitation phase is completed, a secondary survey is performed. The secondary survey consists of a history and a rapid complete head-to-toe examination to identify problems that may not have been identified as immediately life-threatening during the primary survey and other potentially debilitating conditions. The secondary survey does not begin until the primary survey has been completed and the resuscitation phase has been initiated. If at any time during the secondary survey the patient's condition deteriorates, returning to the primary survey with implementation of life-saving interventions is indicated.

The secondary survey begins with completion of the subjective history of the patient. This history really began in the primary survey and is continued throughout the secondary survey; it should include the patient's past and present medical history, drug and allergy history, and specific details of the traumatic event (e.g., mechanism and velocity of injury, precipitating events). The secondary survey ends with an objective head-to-toe physical examination.

Medical History

Pertinent past and present medical conditions of the patient need to be elicited. Any history of cardiac, respiratory, neurologic, endocrine, or hematologic disorders is

TABLE 6-6.
Guide to Tetanus Prophylaxis in Routine Wound Management

History of Adsorbed Tetanus Toxoid (Doses)	Clean, Minor Wounds		All Other Wounds*	
	Td†	*TIG*	*Td*†	*TIG*
Unknown or < three	Yes	No	Yes	Yes
Three‡	No§	No	No‖	No

Source: From Immunization Practices Advisory Committee. 1985. Diphtheria, tetanus, and pertussis: Guidelines for vaccine prophylaxis and other preventive measures. MMWR 34:422.

* Such as, but not limited to, wounds contaminated with dirt, feces, soil, saliva, etc.; puncture wounds; avulsions; and wounds resulting from missiles, crushing, burns, and frostbite.

† For children under 7 years old, DTP (DT, if pertussis vaccine is contraindicated) is preferred to tetanus toxoid alone. For persons 7 years old and older, Td is preferred to tetanus toxoid alone.

‡ If only three doses of fluid toxoid have been received, a fourth dose of toxoid, preferably an adsorbed toxoid, should be given.

§ Yes, if more than 10 years have elapsed since last dose.

‖ Yes, if more than 5 years have elapsed since last dose. More frequent boosters are not needed and can accentuate side effects.

Td = tetanus diphtheria; TIG = Tetanus immune globulin (Hypertet).

especially important to note. Additionally, any history of alcohol or substance abuse should also be sought out. When the patient last ate is important if surgery is required, and whether or not women are pregnant should also be determined.

Drug and Allergy History

Current medications which the patient is taking (or should be taking) not only are important features in a patient's medical history but may also be relevant in assessing the cause of an accident or injury. In the face of any alterations in skin integrity, a tetanus immunization history must be obtained. If indicated, tetanus prophylaxis should be administered (Table 6–6).

Details of Incident

Eliciting details related to the mechanism of an accident (e.g., blunt versus penetrating trauma, force of impact) may assist the ED nurse in assessing likely related injuries. Automobile accidents account for the majority of cases of severe blunt trauma. The severity of blunt trauma is dependent on the amount of energy transferred from the object to the body (American College of Surgeons, Committee Trauma 1984, 12). Table 6–7 lists some examples of questions that should be asked for a variety of traumatic injuries.

TABLE 6–7.
Questions to Be Asked of Patients with Various Traumatic Injuries

Motor vehicle accidents
- Were you the driver or passenger?
- Were you wearing a seatbelt or shoulder harness (or both)?
- Did you hit the steering wheel or the dashboard? If so, with what part of your body?
- Did you lose consciousness? If so, for how long?
- How fast was the vehicle going?
- What did the vehicle hit?
- Did the vehicle hit a moving object or a nonmoving object? (Paramedics may assist by describing the condition of the car.)
- Where is your pain?
- How far were you thrown?
- What is the condition of the other passengers?

Blunt trauma from falls
- How far did you fall?
- What precipitated the fall?
- What did you land on?
- Where is your pain?
- Did you lose consciousness?

Gunshot wounds
- How long ago did the incident occur?
- How many shots did you hear?
- What type of gun was it?
- From what direction do you think the bullet entered you?
- Where is your pain?

Penetrating wounds or stab wounds
- How long ago did it happen?
- How many times were you stabbed?
- How long was the knife?
- How far did it go?
- From what direction were you stabbed?
- Where is your pain?

Note: The severity of penetrating trauma will depend on two factors: 1. Anatomic location of the injury. 2. The amount of energy transferred to the body. (This is determined by the force of the penetrating object at the time of impact. In general, stab wounds have less force than gunshot wounds and therefore are associated with a comparatively better prognosis when occurring in the same anatomic location.)

Physical Assessment

In beginning physical assessment during the secondary survey, the patient's general appearance (even though noted in the primary survey) should be closely assessed. Whether or not the patient is favoring a particular position or is guarding should be noted. Skin should be checked for color and temperature. The presence or absence of cuts, bruises, ecchymoses, bony deformities, and impaled objects must also be noted, along with the patient's general state of orientation and level of consciousness. A brief but thorough head-to-toe examination and neurologic evaluation then follows.

Assessment of Scalp and Face

The scalp is inspected and palpated for evidence of lacerations, bony or soft tissue deformity, pain, tenderness, or bleeding. All facial bones should be inspected and palpated for pain, deformity, and swelling. Palpation includes the orbital rims, nose, zygomatic arch, mandible, and maxilla. Fractures of the maxilla may be identified by grasping the upper incisors and attempting to rock the upper jaw back and forth.

Assessment of Eyes, Ears, Nose, Throat, and Neck

Eyes should be checked for extraocular movements by having the patient look as far up, down, to the left and right, and diagonally as he or she can. Limitation of upward gaze suggests a blowout fracture of the orbit. Disconjugate gaze suggests neurologic damage. Raccoon eyes or periorbital ecchymoses may be indicative of a basilar skull fracture. Pupils are also checked for size, symmetry, and reaction. Vision can be evaluated grossly by having the patient read the printing on an IV bag. The doll's eye maneuver should be checked in the unconscious patient once cervical spine injury is ruled out. The presence of doll's eye response indicates an intact brain stem (Fig. 6–9).

Blood in the external ear canal or behind the tympanic membrane is a presumptive sign of basilar skull fracture until ruled out. A halo test can be performed on blood or other drainage from the external nose, mouth, or ears to help determine basilar skull fracture. This is done by placing a drop of blood or drainage on a sheet or towel. Blood within cerebrospinal fluid will disperse from the center of the drop and become progressively lighter as it moves away from the center. There will be gradation of color from dark red in the center to pink-tinged away from the center. Battle's sign or mastoid ecchymosis is also indicative of a basilar skull fracture.

The nose should also be inspected and palpated for signs of fracture. Uncontrolled bleeding from the nose can be tamponaded by inserting a 20 French Foley catheter with a 30-cc balloon through the nostril into the nasopharynx. The balloon is then inflated and traction is applied to ensure proper placement. Clear fluid from the nose may also suggest basilar skull fracture. To differentiate between rhinorrhea and cerebrospinal fluid, the glucose concentration of the blood and exudate from the nose can be checked with a Dextro stick. Glucose content of the cerebrospinal fluid, when present, will closely approximate a blood glucose level.

The throat is inspected to examine the airway. Brisk bleeding from the nose or

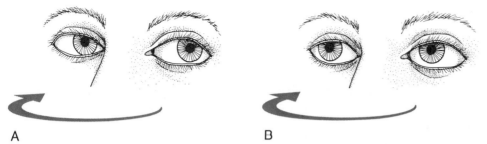

A   B

FIGURE 6–9. Doll's eye maneuver. *A*, Normal reflex: as head is rotated to one side, eyes move opposite to the direction of the head turning (i.e., contraversion). *B*, Abnormal or absent reflex: as head is rotated to one side, eyes remain fixed. (Redrawn by permission from Emergency Nursing: Principles and Practice, Sheehy SB, Barber J, St. Louis: 1985, The CV Mosby Co.)

mouth can cause clot formation in the airway of the supine patient, leading to obstruction and respiratory distress. Frequent suctioning with a Yankauer suction may be all the intervention needed to prevent this problem. At this time fractured or avulsed teeth may also be noted.

Inspection of the neck includes evaluation of swelling due to hematoma formation. This swelling may eventually displace the trachea and make it difficult to intubate the patient. Intubation in cases such as this should be performed before the patient develops respiratory distress.

Palpation of the neck may reveal a shift in the trachea away from the midline, suggesting tension pneumothorax. Subcutaneous emphysema may be indicative of a laryngotracheal disruption, esophageal tear, or injury to the tracheobronchial tree. Tenderness of the cervical spine is highly suggestive of cervical spine fracture, and these patients should have the neck immobilized with a hard collar and sandbags or towel rolls placed on either side of the neck and tape placed across the forehead and to the spine board bilaterally to secure the patient's head.

Assessment of Chest

Visual examination of the chest will identify paradoxical chest movements associated with flail chest and large sucking chest wounds. Palpation of the chest should include the sternum, each rib, and both clavicles. Point tenderness is usually indicative of rib fracture(s). Pressure placed on the sternum with the palm of the hand will be painful if rib fractures are present.

Auscultation is utilized to identify pneumothorax and hemothorax. Decreased breath sounds at the apex of the affected lung or along the anterior chest at the second or third intercostal space may indicate a pneumothorax. A hemothorax or pulmonary contusion can be identified by decreased breath sounds at the base of the affected lung. Distant heart sounds, venous distention, and narrow pulse pressure are the three components of Beck's triad for identifying cardiac tamponade. Injuries that may be identified through examination of the chest (which have not been discussed previously) include rib fracture(s), pulmonary contusion, myocardial contusion, and simple pneumothorax.

Rib Fractures

Ribs form a bony protection for all of the structures within the chest. Rib fractures are a disruption of this bony structure and are one of the non–life-threatening injuries that can be identified while evaluating the chest.

Etiology

Rib fractures are usually caused by blunt force to the chest but may also be caused by a gunshot wound in the rib itself.

Pathophysiology

Rib fractures may be single or multiple. Most commonly seen are fractures of the fourth through tenth ribs because these are most exposed. Although rib fractures are not life-threatening in and of themselves, concomitant injuries associated with rib fractures must be ruled out. Injuries to the first and second ribs may be associated with vascular injury because they overlie subclavian arteries and veins. Injuries to the lower six ribs are more likely to be associated with abdominal injuries; right-sided lower rib fractures may involve liver injury and left-sided lower rib fractures may involve splenic injury. Fractures of the ribs are painful. The effect that this pain has on the patient may result in major complications. Pain associated with rib fractures causes splinting and hypoventilation. The patient may be unwilling to cough and breathe deeply, thereby limiting his or her ability to clear secretions. Eventually, this splinting and hypoventilation may result in atelectasis. Patients who develop atelectasis and are not forced to clear out their secretions are good candidates for developing pneumonia.

Clinical Manifestations

Point tenderness upon palpation of the ribs and pain with sternal pressure are probable indications of rib fractures. Patients with rib fractures have pain with ventilation. Ventilations will be rapid and shallow. Chest radiograph will confirm the diagnosis.

Treatment and Nursing Care

Patients with rib fractures in the absence of other concomitant injuries will usually be discharged home from the ED. Goals in the management of rib fractures are aimed at ensuring effective ventilation for the patient and minimizing discomfort. Stage II care for these individuals usually is adequate.

Breathing Pattern, Ineffective (Potential), Related to

• Pain Secondary to Rib Fracture

Patients with rib fractures should be instructed to splint their chest with a pillow for coughing and deep breathing. This should be done every hour while awake. An incentive spirometer practiced 10 times per hour will help prevent hypoventilation.

Pain, Related to

• Rib Fractures

Analgesia with opiates may allow for pain relief but also may depress normal respiration. Therefore, opiates should be used judiciously. Intercostal nerve blocks with bupivacaine (Marcaine) provide immediate relief from the pain of rib fractures without depressing respirations.

Evaluation

Ventilation should be adequate if the patient carries out instructions on splinting, deep breathing, and the use of incentive spirometry. Pain should be minimized by splinting and the use of a prescribed analgesia.

Pulmonary Contusion

Pulmonary contusion refers to bruising of the lung. It occurs most often following blunt trauma to the chest and is often associated with rib fractures and flail chest.

Pathophysiology

Pulmonary contusion results in damage to lung parenchyma. There is hemorrhage and edema within the lung resulting in an increase in pulmonary vascular resistance, a decrease in pulmonary blood flow, and subsequent ventilation-perfusion abnormalities.

Clinical Manifestations

History will reveal significant penetrating or blunt chest trauma. The patient will usually complain of chest pain and dyspnea. There may be evidence of chest contusions or abrasions. Hypoxia is usually evident from ABG values. Crackles over the affected area may be auscultated. Not all patients with pulmonary contusion will have clinical findings on admission chest radiograph, as it may take 4 to 6 hours for edema to develop.

Treatment and Nursing Care

Treatment is supportive and directed primarily at maintaining adequate ventilation and preventing atelectasis through coughing and deep breathing. Intercostal nerve blocks, as stated before, may provide significant relief of pain.

Patients with pulmonary contusions must be adequately hydrated (as must all trauma patients), but care must be taken not to cause fluid overload. Fluid overloading will back up into the lung and extend the contusion, exacerbating the problem. Tracheobronchial suctioning can be utilized to stimulate coughing and sputum production. Supplemental oxygen should also be given by nasal cannula or Venti-mask.

Infection, Potential for, Related to

- **Pulmonary Contusion**

Patients with pulmonary contusions are susceptible to pneumonia because a contused lung does not clear bacteria at a normal rate (Hart, 1986). These patients therefore should receive antibiotic therapy, especially if mechanical ventilation is required.

Evaluation

Proper and aggressive management of patients with pulmonary contusions will be reflected in ABG values and vital signs. Arterial blood gases will reveal a Pao_2 greater than 55 mmHg, and a Pco_2 less than 50 mmHg. The patient's respiratory rate should be less than 30 breaths per minute. He or she should have a patent airway and minimal pain.

Myocardial Contusion

Myocardial contusion is the bruising of the myocardial muscle of the heart. It is most commonly associated with blunt chest trauma, especially after a motor vehicle accident. Typical history would include a blunt injury to the chest from a steering wheel. The right ventricle is most often involved.

Pathophysiology

Myocardial contusion is similar to a myocardial infarction (MI) in that both are characterized by an injury to an area of the myocardial muscle. A contused myocardial muscle has diminished contractile ability and compliance. As a result, cardiac output drops. In addition to direct muscle damage, perfusion abnormalities of the coronary microcirculation have also been implicated in myocardial contusion (Hammond 1986).

Clinical Manifestations

Patients with myocardial contusions may experience chest pain similar to that experienced during myocardial ischemia. Diagnosis is based mainly on a high index of suspicion. EKG changes may be nonspecific. Myocardial enzymes, if absent from the serum, do not definitely rule out myocardial contusion. Patients with myocardial contusions may develop ventricular dysrhythmias.

Treatment and Nursing Care

Management of persons with myocardial contusions is somewhat similar to that of patients with suspected MI. Patients should be placed in a monitored unit for 24 hours post injury to watch them continuously for dysrhythmias. If ventricular dysrhythmias do occur, the drug of choice is lidocaine. Patients can be discharged from the unit when they are free of dysrhythmias for 24 hours. Serial EKGs and myocardial enzyme determinations should be obtained over a 48-hour period. Both, however, are nonspecific in the diagnosis of myocardial contusion. Although ST-T wave changes are common in myocardial contusion, they also commonly occur in the absence of cardiac trauma. Likewise, an elevated creatine kinase (CK) with a positive MB fraction, although suggestive of a cardiac contusion, may also be present in the absence of cardiac trauma. Supplemental oxygen should be administered to decrease cardiac workload.

Evaluation

Patients suspected of having myocardial contusions are treated as if they had an MI. Close monitoring of vital signs, EKG rhythm, and cardiac enzyme levels helps ensure a stable clinical status.

Simple or Closed Pneumothorax

Simple pneumothorax or closed pneumothorax results from a tear or puncture of an internal respiratory structure, causing air to enter the pleural space (Luckman and Sorensen 1987, 806). Partial or total collapse of the lung on the affected side occurs.

Etiology

Any rupture or tear of internal respiratory structures (e.g., bronchioles, bronchus, alveoli) may cause a closed pneumothorax. Damage of internal respiratory structures may be the result of blunt or penetrating chest trauma; however, more commonly it results from mechanical ventilation or a ruptured bleb in a patient with chronic obstructive pulmonary disease (COPD).

Pathophysiology

In simple pneumothorax, air enters the pleural space, causing a decrease in the negative pressure necessary for ventilation. This loss of negative pressure causes a total or partial collapse of the affected lung. Lung expansion during inspiration is impaired, and ventilation is subsequently diminished.

Clinical Manifestations

As mentioned previously, decreased breath sounds at the apex of the affected side or along the anterior chest at the second or third intercostal space may indicate a pneumothorax. The patient may also experience tachypnea, shortness of breath, chest pain, and hyperresonance with percussion. Confirmation of the diagnosis can be made by chest radiograph.

Treatment and Nursing Care

Therapeutic intervention may range from simple observation if the pneumothorax is small and the patient is asymptomatic to chest tube placement in the affected side. Insertion of the chest tube (as with all procedures) must be explained to the patient and consent obtained. Consent may usually be obtained from the patient because this is a non–life-threatening condition and usually does not require immediate intervention. Patients with pneumothorax should also be given supplemental oxygen to ease respiratory distress and facilitate lung re-expansion.

Evaluation

Evaluation of the patient without a chest tube will focus on monitoring for signs and symptoms of increasing respiratory distress. The trauma nurse will evaluate and document any increase in respiratory rate or worsening dyspnea. If this should occur, insertion of a chest tube will then become necessary.

In patients with chest tubes, a chest radiograph should be obtained after insertion to ensure proper placement. Patients should begin to express relief from respiratory distress soon after chest tube placement.

The most common forms of trauma identified during the chest examination of the secondary survey have been reviewed. In addition to all specific measures discussed with each entity, a chest radiograph should be obtained in all trauma patients. The major purpose of this radiograph is simply to identify or eliminate the chest as a major source of blood loss and to rule out any pneumothoraces or hemothoraces. If the chest radiograph reveals no hemothorax, blood loss most likely is occurring in the abdomen or, less commonly, comes from a long-bone fracture.

Assessment of Abdomen

Missed abdominal injuries are an all too frequent cause of preventable death following blunt trauma (Moore 1985). Abdominal injuries are often overshadowed by more obvious injuries, such as fractures, or masked by alcohol influence or head trauma.

Patients with suspected intraabdominal injuries need to be evaluated frequently to detect subtle changes in the abdominal examination. Abdominal injuries are usually due to blunt trauma and are most often sustained from motor vehicle accidents (MVAs). In penetrating injuries the degree of tissue damage is usually related to those structures in the path of the injuring agent. The major concern with penetrating trauma is the specific organs injured, the number of organs injured, the degree of organ obstruction, and the amount of hemorrhage.

Inspection of the abdomen is of prime importance. The presence of ecchymoses and abrasions suggests underlying organ injury. Inspect the contour of the abdomen for symmetry, distention, old scars, and obvious trauma. Document all physical findings.

Auscultation of the abdomen in all four quadrants for bowel sounds should be performed and documented. A decrease in bowel sounds may not be significant in all trauma patients and may represent a temporary ileus. This temporary ileus often occurs in patients with extraabdominal trauma and usually resolves within 48 hours.

Percussion of the abdomen can detect gastric distention and abdominal peritoneal irritation. Palpation is also useful in the determination of peritoneal tenderness and hematomas. An abdomen that is dull to percussion suggests intraabdominal fluid, most often blood. The pelvis is evaluated by pushing down with the hand on the pubis and compressing the iliac wings toward the midline. Pain with palpation may be due to a pelvic fracture. A rectal examination must also be done to assess for blood in the rectal vault, a high-riding prostate, and loss of sphincter tone.

Assessment of Extremities: Musculoskeletal System

The musculoskeletal system is next evaluated in the secondary survey. The upper and lower extremities are inspected for gross bony deformities, ecchymoses, abrasions, lacerations, and swelling. Motor ability of all extremities should be assessed.

Patients with suspected fractures should have the extremity splinted and immobilized from above to below the injury. Splinting stabilizes and decreases the movement of the extremity. Splinting helps prevent further soft tissue and neurovascular damage, and reduces pain. Grossly deformed limbs should be gently straightened and splinted. Palpation will elicit tenderness, crepitance, and abnormal movements of the fracture site. All extremity pulses should be palpated and documented as present or absent. The fingers and toes of the extremity with suspected fracture should be evaluated for warmth, color, capillary refill, and neurovascular status. Fracture sites in addition to splinting should be elevated and iced. Open fractures need to have cultures performed and to be covered with a sterile saline dressing. Patients with fractures are usually experiencing pain, and analgesics should be used if they are not contraindicated.

Neurologic Evaluation

In the primary assessment, the AVPU method was utilized to determine level of consciousness. This method is continued in the secondary survey along with the Glascow coma scale. The Glascow coma scale is a more detailed evaluation of neurologic status. It evaluates three criteria (responses), utilizing a numerical scale: eye opening, verbal response, and motor response (see Table 6–1). A total Glascow coma scale score of 14 to 15 is within normal limits.

Assessment of the 12 cranial nerves along with sensory and motor nerves is also performed in the neurologic evaluation of the secondary survey.

It is important to note that hypotension generally does not occur because of head injury. The exceptions to this include loss of brain stem function, spinal shock, or profusely bleeding scalp lacerations. In general, however, if hypotension is the problem, the nurse needs to look at sources other than head trauma for its cause.

Neurologic evaluations should continue every 15 to 30 minutes with patients displaying any changes in mental status. Patients who have mental status changes owing to alcohol or drug use should improve over time. Neurologic deterioration of these patients indicates that organic disease also is present, and the patient's condition can no longer be dismissed as solely alcohol- or drug-related.

CONCLUSION

Trauma patients are, for the most part, young, heretofore healthy persons who have experienced an unplanned noxious event. At best, it is a frightening occurrence with no long-term effects. At worst, it is a life-taking, life-threatening, or permanently disabling occurrence. This segment of the patient population has a great need for nursing support throughout the time of psychologic and physical crisis. Top-notch trauma nursing requires that the nurse be observant, systematic, assertive, supportive, and quick-thinking. It is hoped that this chapter has aided in accomplishing that goal.

REFERENCES

American College of Surgeons, Committee on Trauma. 1984. Advanced Trauma Life Support. Chicago, American College of Surgeons.

Baker SP, O'Neill B, Haddon W Jr, et al. 1974. The injury severity score: A method for describing patients with multiple injuries and evaluating emergency care. J Trauma 14:187–196.

Buschiazzo L, Possanza C, LeDent M. 1986. Coordinating your efforts to manage multiple trauma. Nurs Life 6(5):34–39.

Carter JL, Smith BL. 1982. Use of military antishock trousers: Nursing implications. Heart Lung 11:422–425.

Champion HR, Sacco WJ, Carnazzo AJ, et al. 1981. Trauma score. Crit Care Med 9:672–676.

Committee on Trauma of the American College of Surgeons. 1987. Hospital and Prehospital Resources for Optimal Care of the Injured Patient. Quality Assurance in Trauma Care. 44–45.

Eastman AB, Lewis FR, Mattox KL. 1987. Regional trauma system design. Am J Surg 154:79–87.

Gormican SP. 1982. CRAMS scale: Field triage of trauma victims. Ann Emerg Med 11:132–135.

Greendyke RM. 1966. Traumatic rupture of the aorta: Special reference to automobile accidents. JAMA 195:527–530.

Hammond BB. 1986. Nursing assessment of blunt cardiac trauma. Nurs Clin North Am 21:677–684.

Hart LH. 1986. Hidden chest trauma in the head-injured patient. Crit Care Nurse 6:51–55.

Immunization Practices Advisory Committee. 1985. Diphtheria, tetanus, and pertussis: Guidelines for vaccine prophylaxis and other preventive measures. MMWR 34:405–414, 419–426.

Knezevich BA. 1986. Trauma Nursing: Principles and Practice. East Norwalk, CT: Appleton-Century-Crofts.

Lewis FR. 1984. Prehospital trauma care. In Trunkey D, Lewis FR eds. Current Therapy of Trauma. Toronto, BC Decker, 1–6.

Luckman J, Sorensen KC. 1987. Medical-Surgical Nursing: A Psychophysiologic Approach. Philadelphia, WB Saunders.

Mirvis SE. 1988. Traumatic disruption of the thoracic aorta: Imaging diagnosis. Trauma Q 4(2):49–60.

Moore E. 1985. Resuscitation and evaluation of the injured patient. In Zuidema GD, Rutherford RD, Ballinger WI eds. The Management of Trauma. Philadelphia, WB Saunders, 1–22.

Napoli VM, Symbas PJ, Vroon DH, et al. 1987. Autotransfusion from experimental hemothorax: Levels of coagulation factors. J Trauma 27:296–300.

Piano G, Turney SZ. 1988. Traumatic rupture of the thoracic aorta: Surgical management. Trauma Q 4(2):61–65.

Rice CL, Enderson BL. 1987. Hemorrhagic shock/resuscitation. In Hurst JM ed. Common Problems in Trauma. Chicago, Year Book Medical Publishers, 10–15.

Stiles OR, Cohlmia, GS, Smith JH. 1985. Management of injuries of the thoracic and abdominal aorta. Am J Surg 150:132–140.

Thompson J, Dains J. 1986. Indices of injury development and status. Nurs Clin North Am 21:655–672.

Trunkey DD. 1987a. Foreword. In Hurst JM ed. Common Problems in Trauma. Chicago, Year Book Medical Publishers.

Trunkey DD. 1987b. Torso trauma. Curr Prob Surg 24:215–264.

Trunkey DD. 1982. Surgical Profiles (pamphlet). West Point, PA, Merck, Sharp, and Dohme.

Virgilio RW. 1979. Balanced electrolyte solutions: Experimental and clinical studies. Crit Care Med 7:90–106.

Wilson RF. 1986. Larynx, trachea, bronchi, and lungs. In Trunkey DD, Lewis FR eds. Current Therapy of Trauma 2. Toronto, BC Decker, 243–248.

James Wilson, MD

Maxillofacial Trauma and Ear, Nose, and Throat Emergencies

The anatomy and physiology of the head and neck are quite complex. Housed within the facial architecture are most of the major senses with which patients experience the world around them. Traumas to the face vary in severity, from minor soft tissue injuries sustained in an altercation, to major distortions caused by the impact of the victim's head against a windshield during a high-speed motor accident. As shocking as maxillofacial trauma may appear to emergency personnel, it is not commonly an immediate threat to life.

Infections involving the head and neck similarly vary in severity, from self-limiting viral pharyngitis to extremely serious retropharyngeal abscesses. A systematic approach to the patient with a head and neck injury or complaint is vital to accurately assess the extent of the injury or condition. This chapter discusses most of the common problems seen by emergency department (ED) personnel relating to emergencies of the head and neck. The first half of the chapter addresses maxillofacial trauma, with focus on facial fractures and soft tissue injuries. The second half of the chapter addresses other ear, nose, and throat (ENT) emergencies of infectious and noninfectious origin.

MAXILLOFACIAL TRAUMA

Persons who arrive at EDs with maxillofacial trauma often have multiple injuries. Assessment of these patients must proceed in a fashion similar to that described for multiple trauma victims in Chapter 6. Rarely are maxillofacial injuries life-threatening; however, they may be if airway compromise or hemorrhage is present. Therefore, treatment must oftentimes be delayed as more urgent life- or limb-threatening emergencies take precedence. Depending on the nature and severity of concomitant injuries, treatment of maxillofacial injuries may be delayed as long as hours to days after the accident.

Assessment

Assessment of the patient with maxillofacial trauma must include a detailed description of the nature (e.g., how and when the accident or injury occurred) and mechanism (e.g., speed, force, direction) of the trauma. Questions such as "How fast were you or the object or vehicle(s) traveling on impact?" and "From which direction did the object or vehicle hit you?" are appropriate. Additionally, information surrounding and immediately following the traumatic event regarding the patient's vital signs and mental status at the scene of the accident, and the condition of the objects or vehicles involved (e.g., shattered windows, bent steering columns, other casualties, position in the car in which the patient sat, whether or not a seat belt was used) are all critical in assisting the emergency nurse to determine not only the type of facial injury(ies) most likely sustained, but also the likelihood of central nervous system involvement. (Specific facial injuries that most commonly result from specific types of trauma are discussed in appropriate subsequent sections of this chapter.) If the patient is unable to relate an accurate history of the trauma sustained, information should be sought from bystanders, paramedical personnel, or people accompanying the patient.

If the patient's condition is stable, a careful and orderly examination of the head and neck can be performed (Schultz and Oldham 1977). Objective evaluation should begin with inspection of the face. Alterations in skin integrity often are readily observable, and their size, location, amount of associated bleeding, and surrounding swelling should be described. Sometimes spreading the hair is required to discover a scalp abrasion indicating head trauma. Asymmetry of facial structures also is frequently evident (e.g., downward displacement of the globe of the eye, depression of the lateral canthus, asymmetry of nasolabial folds) and should be noted in addition to the presence or absence of malocclusion, epistaxis, and cerebrospinal fluid (CSF) rhinorrhea. The mastoid and ear are inspected next for ecchymosis, lacerations, or discharge (i.e., blood or CSF otorrhea). Perforation of the eardrum, CSF drainage, blood behind the tympanic membrane, and hearing loss are important findings. Next the zygomas and bony orbits are palpated for deformity. Visual acuity and extraocular movements (to detect extraocular muscle entrapment) are assessed. The presence of diplopia usually means an orbital floor blow-out fracture is present. The orbit itself is best evaluated at this point. The nose is next examined for alignment, swelling, septal deformity, and hematoma. Maxillary fractures are discovered by palpating a deformity or demonstrating midface mobility while pulling on the upper incisors.

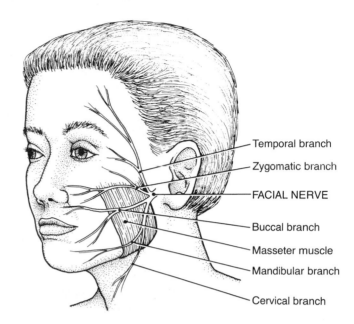

Temporal branch
Zygomatic branch
FACIAL NERVE
Buccal branch
Masseter muscle
Mandibular branch
Cervical branch

FIGURE 7-1. Anatomy of the facial nerve.

Next, all teeth should be examined with a gloved finger for fractures and avulsions. Lacerations in the mouth are found with a tongue blade and light source. Finally, the mandible is palpated with a gloved finger, jaw occlusion is assessed, and pain with range of motion is evaluated.

Owing to the facial anatomy and location of the seventh cranial nerve (facial nerve), motor and sensory function reflective of this nerve should be assessed in cases of maxillofacial trauma before analgesics or anesthetics are administered (Fig. 7-1). Facial nerve assessment includes the assessment of facial muscle strength and taste sensation in the anterior two thirds of the tongue.

If the foregoing examination sequence is followed, it is unlikely that significant facial injuries will be overlooked. Assessment findings can be further evaluated by plain radiographs or craniofacial computed tomographic (CT) scanning.

FACIAL FRACTURES

As specific facial fractures are discussed, their causes, pathophysiologies, and clinical manifestations are presented in more detail. Principles of nursing care common to all types of facial fractures are then discussed. The specific treatment for each type of facial fracture also is covered and integrated as appropriate.

Nasal Fractures

Because the nose is the most prominent facial feature, it is the most vulnerable and therefore is the most commonly fractured facial bone. In addition, it requires the least amount of force to fracture.

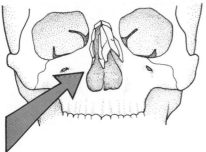

LATERAL TRAUMA

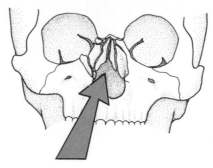

POSTERIOR DIRECTED TRAUMA

FIGURE 7–2. Nasal fractures as they relate to the mechanism of trauma. (Redrawn from Zook EG. 1980. The Primary Care of Facial Injuries. PSG Publishing Co, 90.)

Etiology and Pathophysiology

Blunt blows to the face are the most common cause of nasal fracture. Motor vehicle accidents, sports injuries, and interpersonal altercations are most commonly responsible. The direction and force of trauma causing the fracture will most likely reveal the type of fracture sustained and whether or not there will be displacement (Fig. 7–2). Laterally directed trauma displaces the nasal bones laterally (Zook 1980), whereas posteriorly directed trauma often results in comminuted fractures of the nasal bones with inward displacement.

Clinical Manifestations

Patients who come to the ED with a nasal fracture most often report a history of facial or nasal trauma in addition to some degree of pain at the site of injury. Epistaxis may or may not be present.

Inspection often reveals swelling, edema, and ecchymosis. Gross deformity, however, is not always observable. Palpation usually reveals tenderness, pain, and some degree of crepitus. Radiographs confirm the presence of a nasal fracture but help little in deciding on management. They are most useful in ruling out associated injury to surrounding structures. The inside of the nose should be examined for the presence or absence of septal hematoma.

Zygomatic Fractures

The zygoma is composed of the malar eminence (or body of the zygoma) and the zygomatic arch and is most commonly associated with two types of fractures. The first is a trimalar or tripod fracture, which involves depression of the malar eminence along with fractures at the zygomatic-frontal, zygomatic-temporal, and zygomatic-maxillary interfaces (Fig. 7–3). The second is depression of the zygomatic arch (which results from a central fracture in addition to fractures at both ends of the zygomatic arch) (Fig. 7–4).

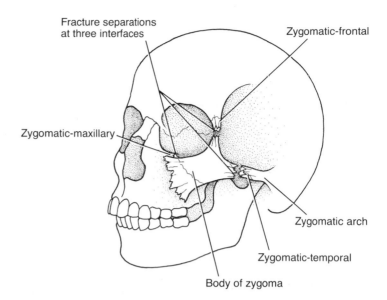

FIGURE 7–3. Tripod (trimalar) fracture.

Etiology and Pathophysiology

There are many causes of zygomatic fractures; however, in nearly every case, some type of blunt trauma is involved. The types of trauma most likely to be associated with zygomatic fractures include direct blows to the zygoma and falling on the side of

FIGURE 7–4. Depressed fracture of the zygomatic arch.

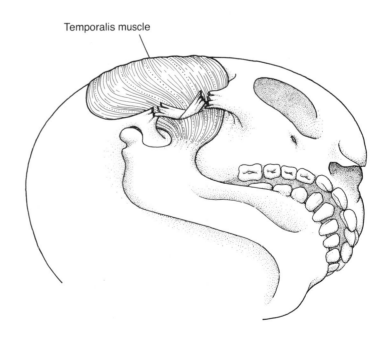

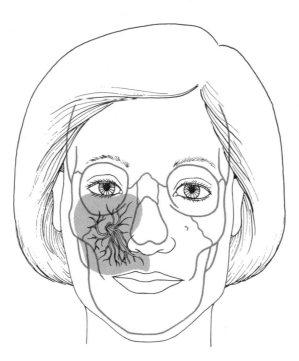

FIGURE 7–5. Sensory area of the infraorbital nerve and its anatomic exit from the skull.

the face. Sports injuries and interpersonal altercations are most commonly responsible.

Clinical Manifestations

Persons who come to the ED with zygomatic fractures will have some history of facial trauma. They most likely have some degree of pain (especially with jaw movement), tenderness, and swelling at the site of the injury. Because the zygomatic bone forms a portion of the lateral and inferior orbital rim, the patient may also complain of visual disturbances (e.g., diplopia).

On physical examination, visual evidence of trauma will usually be present. In addition to obvious alterations in skin integrity surrounding the injury site, periorbital ecchymosis and subconjunctival hemorrhage are usually present. Point tenderness, flatness of the affected cheek, and a palpable deformity also will be found. Additionally, there may be depression of the lateral canthus of the eye with downward displacement of the globe (as a result of inferior rectus muscle entrapment) and infraorbital nerve anesthesia manifested as paresthesias of the cheek, nose, and upper lip of the affected side (Fig. 7–5). Owing to the close proximity of the temporalis muscle (a major muscle of mastication) and the zygomatic arch, trismus often is associated with depression of the zygomatic arch.

Because many combinations of zygomatic fractures may occur, history and clinical examination (although critical) often are not enough. Radiographs, specifi-

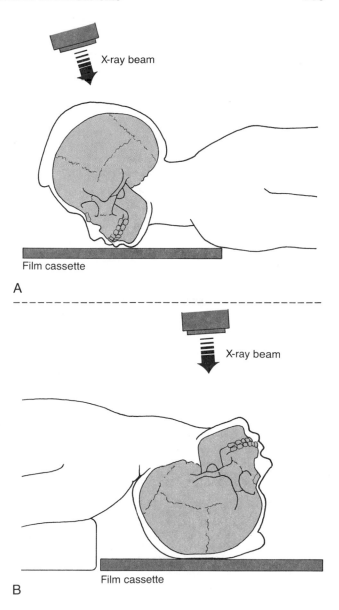

FIGURE 7–6. Radiographic positioning and the structures outlined. *A,* Waters view outlines the orbital floors and facial bones. *B,* Submental-vertex view outlines the zygomatic arches. (Redrawn from Zook EG. 1980. The Primary Care of Facial Injuries. Littleton, MA, PSG Publishing Co, 109.)

cally the Waters view and the submental-vertex view, are most helpful in diagnosing zygomatic fractures definitively (Fig. 7–6).

Maxillary Fractures

Maxillary fractures represent severe facial trauma and are frequently associated with multisystem injuries. They are classified by the LeFort system, named after the French surgeon LeFort who devised the system in the nineteenth century.

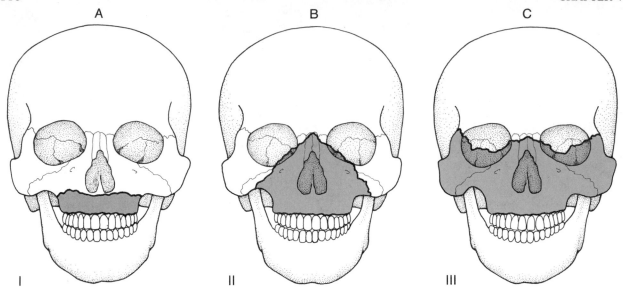

FIGURE 7–7. LeFort Fractures. *A*, LeFort I. *B*, LeFort II. *C*, LeFort III.

Etiology and Pathophysiology

Maxillary fractures result from high-velocity trauma. Gunshot wounds to the face, high-speed deceleration motor vehicle accidents, and blunt blows to the face are commonly responsible. LeFort I fractures are low and transverse and give mobility to the upper teeth and lower maxilla. The fracture site is just above the apices of the teeth and below the floor of the nose (Zook 1980). LeFort II fractures or pyramidal fractures involve the nasomaxillary segment with fractures of the medial orbital rims, orbital floors, and nose. A complete separation of the facial skeleton from the cranial skeleton, or craniofacial disjunction, is found in LeFort III fractures (Fig. 7–7).

Clinical Manifestations

As the force required to cause a person to sustain a LeFort fracture is quite significant, patients with LeFort fractures have a history of severe facial trauma. Although symptoms may vary somewhat depending on the type of the LeFort fracture sustained, midface mobility, periorbital swelling and ecchymosis, pain, asymmetry, elongation of the mid-face, and malocclusion are common findings. CSF rhinorrhea may also be present with LeFort II and LeFort III fractures. The Waters view is the most informative radiograph in the diagnosis of maxillary fractures.

Mandibular Fractures

Mandibular fractures result from blunt trauma of significant force directed at the mandible. They are classified according to the region in which they occur and

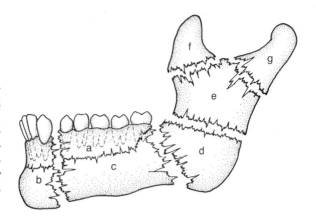

FIGURE 7-8. Common mandibular fracture sites: *a,* alveolar process; *b,* symphysis; *c,* body; *d,* angle; *e,* ascending ramus; *f,* coronoid process; *g,* condyle. (Modified with permission from Schultz RC: Facial Injuries. Copyright © 1977 by Year Book Medical Publishers, Inc., Chicago.)

whether or not they are open or closed. Mandibular fractures are considered open whenever there is communication with either the oral cavity or the skin surface (Gerlock et al 1981).

Etiology and Pathophysiology

Catapulting forward on impact during vehicular accidents, interpersonal altercations, and falling forward on the chin are common causes of mandibular fractures. Owing to the horseshoe shape of the mandible, fractures can occur at a point opposite the point of impact, or multiple fractures may occur. Common mandibular fracture sites are identified in Figure 7-8.

Clinical Manifestations

Clinical manifestations of mandibular fractures may vary somewhat depending on the locations of fractures; however, assessment of patients with such fractures usually reveals malocclusion, pain, decreased range of motion in the jaw, or a palpable, bony deformity. Patients with only mild pain but full range of motion (including right and left lateral motion), normal bite, and normal strength are unlikely to have mandibular fractures. A patient is considered to have normal jaw strength if he or she can bite with both sides of the mouth on a tongue blade such that the examiner is unable to withdraw the instrument. Trismus and ecchymosis of the floor of the mouth also are common findings of mandibular fractures. CSF otorrhea may be present with mandibular fractures at the condyle, and paresthesias of the lip and chin are usually evidence of alveolar nerve damage and diagnostic of mandibular fractures of the alveolar process. A mandibular series and panoramic radiographs (Panorex) are both adequate studies in evaluating these fractures.

Treatment and Nursing Care: Facial Fractures

Stage I care for patients with facial fractures usually is not required. As stated previously, only in cases of airway compromise or hemorrhage are maxillofacial injuries an immediate priority in the trauma patient (Manson 1984). Many of the patients have other, more urgent injuries that cannot be overlooked. The importance of following the usual approach to the trauma victim as outlined in Chapter 6 cannot be overemphasized.

Definitive care of facial fractures can be given early in the course of treatment or delayed several days, depending on the extent of concomitant injuries. If life- or limb-threatening emergencies are present, immediate interventions must center on establishment and maintenance of airway, breathing, and circulation. Cervical spine injury in the multiply injured accident victim with facial trauma, and in persons with isolated maxillofacial trauma, should always be assumed unless proved otherwise.

The airway can be cleared by using a jaw thrust or chin lift, by removing foreign material from the mouth (such as fractured teeth and blood clots) using Yankauer suction, and using oropharyngeal or nasopharyngeal airways. Nasotracheal or oro-tracheal intubation using a two-person technique is the procedure of choice in securing an airway except in apneic patients with central facial trauma. In the latter cases immediate needle or surgical cricothyroidotomy is indicated. Shock, which is treated by rapid fluid administration through large-bore intravenous lines, does not commonly occur with facial injury, and if present, another bleeding site should be sought. Facial hemorrhage is best controlled by direct pressure, not by blind clamping, which risks injury to branches of the facial nerve or other important structures. The head and neck must be immobilized using sandbags and a hard cervical collar.

Once life- or limb-threatening emergencies are ruled out or treated, stage II care for persons with facial fractures relates to three primary nursing diagnoses: anxiety related to possible permanent alteration in facial appearance, alteration in comfort, and knowledge deficits related to the care, treatment, and sequelae of sustained injuries.

Anxiety, Related to

- **Possible Permanent Alteration in Facial Appearance Secondary to Facial Fractures**

There is almost no injury that creates as much emotional stress as injury to the face. People who sustain these injuries are unaware of how they are treated, how long they take to heal, and whether or not they can expect permanent physical deformity as a result. The answers to these questions are not always absolute and often depend on the type of fractures sustained and whether or not malalignment is present. The patient can be reassured, however, that although at the present time his or her facial appearance seems grossly altered, most likely the alterations noted are temporary and correctable. Additionally, the patient is preoccupied with possible disfigurement and scars that may alter his or her acceptability to society, friends, and loved ones. It is very important to reassure the patient, lend support, and understand his or her concerns. Explanations regarding procedures to be done and what the patient can expect should be provided throughout the ED stay. Keeping significant others informed as well about procedures is critical in helping to allay their fears and anxieties. In addition, explanations can diminish the likelihood that significant others will display shock, fear, or disgust when seeing the patient for the first time in the ED. As many of these cases will eventually result in litigation, meticulous documentation, drawings, and even photographs are important and should be part of the patient's medical record.

Pain, Related to

- **Facial Fracture(s)**

Persons who sustain facial fractures commonly experience an alteration in comfort that is usually localized to the fracture site. Ice applications to the fracture site, positioning the patient for comfort, and elevating the head of the bed (unless contraindicated) assist in reducing pain and edema. A local anesthetic (especially when there is concurrent soft tissue injury) often is effective in reducing pain. Systemic analgesics (given orally or intramuscularly) also may be administered if needed; however, special attention must be paid to the patient's respiratory status.

Knowledge Deficit, Related to

- **Care, Treatment, and Sequelae of Facial Fractures**

As stated previously, persons who sustain facial fractures usually have knowledge deficits related to their care, treatment, and sequelae. This section discusses knowledge deficit with respect to specific facial fractures.

Nasal Fractures

When a nasal fracture with displacement is sustained, reduction is indicated early and may be done in the ED if edema is minimal or if there is obvious malalignment. Otherwise the patient is re-evaluated in 4 to 7 days, after swelling has subsided.

Prior to reduction, the nasal mucosa is anesthetized with a 5% cocaine solution. Occasionally, local injections of procaine (Novocain) are also given. Reduction is then accomplished with manual manipulation. Following reduction, an external splint and nasal packing with bismuth tribromophenate (Xeroform) or petrolatum gauze may be required to maintain the fracture segments in good alignment. Ice applications and analgesics are recommended to control swelling and pain. All children with nasal fractures, however, should be referred to appropriate specialists because minor deformities may yield major deformities in adulthood.

Epistaxis associated with nasal fractures is usually self-limited. When present, it can be controlled by direct pressure or, less commonly, it will require nasal packing (see discussion of epistaxis). If, however, septal hematomas are present, they will need to be incised and drained to prevent septal perforation. Most commonly this is done by an otolaryngologist. Following evacuation of the hematoma, bilateral nasal packs should be placed and antibiotics prescribed.

Prior to discharge, the patient with a nasal fracture must be instructed on follow-up care. Medication and prescriptions should be thoroughly explained. Ice should be applied to the fracture site over the next 24 hours. If epistaxis becomes severe, the patient should be instructed to return to the ED.

Zygomatic Fractures

Treatment of zygomatic fractures depend on the nature and severity of the fractures. If a zygomatic fracture is minimally displaced, without cosmetic deformity or extra-ocular muscle involvement, treatment may not be required. In such instances, the patient may be discharged home with instructions to apply ice to the fracture site for the next 24 hours and to keep his or her head elevated (if cervical spine injury is ruled out) to reduce facial edema. Referral to a plastic surgeon for the following day should also be arranged. Most zygomatic fractures, however, do require open reduction with internal wire fixation. Stabilization is then required for 4 to 6 weeks.

LeFort Fractures

Although treatment depends on the type of LeFort fracture sustained, nearly all require some degree of intermaxillary (maxillomandibular) fixation with open re-duction to reduce fracture fragments (Fig. 7–9). Although admission to the hospital is required for this, rarely is emergency surgery necessary. Emergency care for these individuals must center on the identification and treatment of concurrent injuries, promotion of comfort, and maintenance of an adequate airway.

Considering that significant force is required to fracture the maxilla, it is not unlikely that the bone has become displaced and has obstructed the airway. Should this occur, a tracheostomy and mechanical ventilation will be required as an endo-tracheal tube is difficult to pass in such cases. Suctioning may be required frequently if clots, vomitus, teeth, or other materials are compromising the patient's airway. In the absence of cervical spine injury, a semi-Fowler's or Fowler's position not only assists the patient in maintaining an open airway but probably also is more comfort-able.

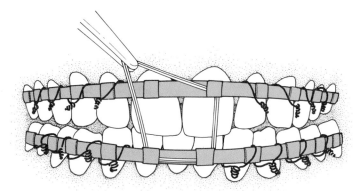

FIGURE 7–9. Intermaxillary fixation. (Redrawn from Zook EG. 1980. The Primary Care of Facial Injuries. PSG Publishing Co, 139.)

Mandibular Fractures

As with other facial fractures, treatment of mandibular fractures may often be delayed until stabilization of the patient's condition is ensured. Although they are not life-threatening in and of themselves, mandibular fractures may pose a significant threat to life by directly or indirectly occluding the patient's airway. Therefore stage I nursing assessment and care may be required to either prevent or treat airway obstruction.

Fractured mandibles may cause a loss of support for the tongue, allowing it to be displaced posteriorly, obstructing the patient's airway. Additionally, fractured or misplaced teeth from mandibular trauma may also cause airway obstruction. Emergency personnel must be cognizant of these possibilities and make every effort to prevent airway obstruction. Suctioning may need to be done frequently, and bleeding may be controlled by direct pressure. If the patient's neurologic condition is stable, he or she should be in a sitting position with the head tilted forward. Intubation and emergency equipment should be readily available in case of complete airway obstruction.

In the absence of airway obstruction, treatment depends on the type and severity of the fracture(s). Asymptomatic, nondisplaced mandibular fractures may not require treatment. Patients may be sent home with instructions to eat a blenderized diet and to make a follow-up visit to a plastic surgeon. Most mandibular fractures, however, will require some sort of jaw immobilization for 6 weeks to promote both healing and comfort. Open reduction with some form of interdental or intermaxillary fixation usually is required. Most mandibular fractures are considered to be open fractures, and prophylactic antibiotics (penicillin or erythromycin) should be given.

Dental Fractures

Dental fractures and avulsions are best handled by a dentist, but ED personnel often must treat such injuries when they occur in the setting of multiple trauma, or in the evening hours when most dentists are unavailable. Tooth fractures not involving the dental pulp can be protected with a zinc oxide splint and the patient referred for follow-up visit to a dentist. Pulp is identified by its red vascular appearance. If the pulp is showing, a pulpectomy will need to be done because of the risk of infection and associated pain (Medford and Curtis 1983). A loose tooth may be teased back into position and splinted (Medford 1982). An avulsed tooth may be reimplanted after thorough cleaning if the time outside the oral cavity is less than 30 minutes. Otherwise reimplantation should be done by a dentist within 6 hours.

SOFT TISSUE INJURIES

Soft tissue injuries of the face may occur alone or concomitantly with underlying facial fractures. Consequently, facial fractures should be ruled out in any individuals with facial soft tissue injuries.

Etiology

Like facial fractures, soft tissue injuries of the face are commonly the result of motor vehicle accidents, sports injuries, and interpersonal altercations. Human and animal bites also are common causes.

Clinical Manifestations

Soft tissue injuries of the face may range from isolated simple lacerations or puncture wounds to massive facial trauma accompanied by edema, airway obstruction, fractures, and multisystem injuries (Kaiser 1987). As a result, the presence or absence of symptoms reflective of concurrent (and potential) injuries or problems must be sought out. The importance of the usual approach to trauma victims, as discussed in Chapter 6, again cannot be overemphasized.

Treatment and Nursing Care

Stage I care for maxillofacial soft tissue injuries is usually not required unless airway compromise or blood loss is significant (see Treatment and Nursing Care: Facial Fractures). In the absence of life- or limb-threatening emergencies, stage II care for individuals with maxillofacial soft tissue injuries usually is all that is required. This nursing care relates to four primary nursing diagnoses: anxiety related to the possible permanent alteration in facial appearance, pain, alteration in skin integrity, and knowledge deficits related to the care, treatment, and sequelae of sustained injuries.

Anxiety, Related to

- *Possible Permanent Alteration in Facial Appearance Secondary to Facial Soft Tissue Injuries*

See the discussion of anxiety, related to possible permanent alteration in facial appearance secondary to facial fractures.

Pain, Related to

- *Facial Soft Tissue Injuries*

See the discussion of pain, related to facial fractures.

Skin Integrity, Impaired, Related to

- *Facial Soft Tissue Injuries*

The usual principles of wound management, including tetanus prophylaxis, apply to maxillofacial soft tissue injuries with few exceptions. Because of the vascularity of the face, facial lacerations may primarily be closed up to 24 hours after an injury is sustained. The skin should be cleaned and painted with a 10% povidone-iodine solution, and the wound itself irrigated copiously with a sterile saline solution. Human or animal bites and soil-engrained lacerations are highly contaminated and need special attention to débridement and high-pressure irrigation if they are to be closed primarily. Débridement of road abrasions needs to be done with care to avoid future "tattooing" of the face. Shaving of eyebrows prior to the repair of surrounding lacerations should be avoided as this removes a facial landmark and makes symmetric closure difficult; also, regrowth is often irregular.

Prior to closing a laceration on the face, care must be taken in evaluating injury to underlying structures such as the facial nerve and Stensen's duct. Movement of the muscles of the face must be fully assessed for symmetry. Stensen's duct may need to be cannulated to demonstrate that no transection exists. Lacerations anterior to a vertical line from the lateral canthus of the eye are rarely associated with damage to Stensen's duct or with irreparable facial nerve injury (Fig. 7–10).

Local anesthesia is best obtained with 1% or 2% lidocaine with 1:100,000 epinephrine. The only sites where epinephrine should be avoided are the very tip of the nose and (questionably) the ear. A solution of 4% lidocaine on a gauze sponge may be used to anesthetize abrasions. Marking the vermilion border prior to anesthetizing the lip allows for more accurate approximation during suturing because swelling usually accompanies local lidocaine injection.

FIGURE 7–10. Anatomy of the parotid gland, parotid duct, facial nerve branches, and masseter muscle. (Lacerations anterior to line A are rarely associated with damage to the parotid duct.)

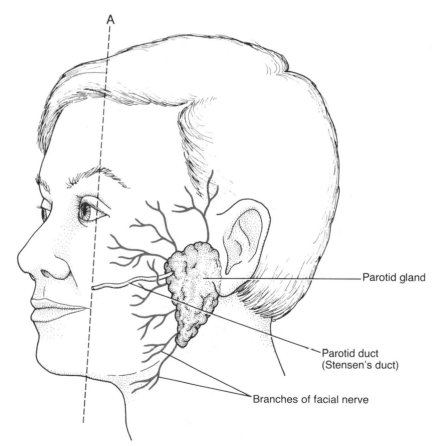

Parotid gland

Parotid duct
(Stensen's duct)

Branches of facial nerve

Foreign bodies such as glass are best removed using a gloved finger and forceps, and with a lot of patience. Rarely is a radiograph helpful.

Suture material for deep stitches is usually 4-0 or 5-0 synthetic absorbable with 5-0 or 6-0 nylon monofilament for the skin. Silk is best for lip lacerations. Silk or chromic catgut is used for intraoral lacerations. Skin sutures are usually left in place for three to five days, and then Steri-strips are applied using tincture of benzoin.

Ear lacerations, as well as many other facial lacerations, should be closed in layers. If the cartilage of the ear was repaired, the ear should be splinted with dry or petrolatum-soaked gauze in and around the pinna, and then wrapped with a circumferential dressing about the ear and head. A subperichondrial hematoma is usually produced by blunt injury to the ear (often seen in boxers). Because this is sometimes a prelude to a cauliflower ear, the hematoma should be aspirated with an 18-gauge needle or incised surgically. A compression dressing is then used for the ensuing five to seven days.

Knowledge Deficit, Related to

• *Care, Treatment, and Sequelae of Soft Tissue Injuries*

Patients discharged from the ED following repair of soft tissue injuries must be instructed on follow-up care. Sutures are usually removed three to five days later. Medication prescriptions must be explained to the patient thoroughly. Instructions about the method and frequency of dressing changes, and information on signs and symptoms indicative of infection, should also be given to the patient.

Summary: Maxillofacial Trauma

Traumatic injuries to the face may be isolated, or they may occur concomitantly with other injuries. In either instance severity may be highly variable and so is treatment. Some facial fractures (in the absence of concomitant injuries) may be treated on an outpatient basis, whereas others may require surgical repair. Likewise, some facial lacerations may be sutured in the ED and the patient sent home, whereas others require extensive evaluation and repair by a specialist. Identification and stabilization of all concurrent life-threatening injuries, however, is always the priority of the ED personnel.

EAR, NOSE, AND THROAT (ENT) EMERGENCIES: INFECTIONS OF THE HEAD AND NECK

Pharyngitis

Pharyngitis, or sore throat, is one of the more common problems seen in EDs. Pharyngitis causes more than 200,000,000 lost workdays per year in the United

States. The great majority of cases are caused by viruses and do not represent serious illness, but caution should be exercised before assigning the patient to a nonurgent status on triage. The key is to recognize those cases in which more serious disease could be present, including severe streptococcal infection, peritonsillar abscess, diphtheria, epiglottitis, and deep fascial infections of the head and neck.

Clinical Manifestations

The primary goal of the ED practitioner in the assessment of persons with pharyngitis is to identify those with serious or potentially serious illness. Certain signs and symptoms are clues to the identification of these persons. Stridor is one. In adults, stridor can be caused by epiglottitis, deep fascial infections, and diphtheria. In children, croup and bacterial tracheitis are additional causes of stridor. Patients with high fevers, dehydration, and difficulty in swallowing oral secretions are also more seriously ill.

Diphtheria should be considered in patients with marked swelling of lymph glands in the neck, fever, pharyngitis with a gray-green membrane, shortness of breath, profound weakness, and an irregular pulse. Patients with facial swelling, trismus (inability to open the mouth), fever, poor dental hygiene, airway obstruction, drooling, or neck pain may have a deep fascial infection of the head or neck. Systemic antibiotics and surgical consultation will be necessary (Patterson et al 1982). A prolonged illness, associated with exudative tonsillitis, numerous swollen lymph nodes, and an enlarged spleen indicates mononucleosis. Patients with exudate or pus over the tonsils may have "strep throat" (streptococcal pharyngitis) which can result in peritonsillar abscess, otitis media, rheumatic fever, or acute glomerulonephritis. Streptococcal pharyngitis occurs most commonly in late winter and early spring. Its clinical presentation varies. Even with the classic findings of severe sore throat, exudative pharyngitis, tender anterior cervical lymphadenopathy, fever, and headache, only about half of such cases will be due to group A beta-hemolytic streptococci (Gwaltney 1985). The diffuse red, blanching rash of scarlet fever is the most suggestive finding of streptococcal infection, but it is uncommonly present. Throat culture is quite reliable in making the diagnosis.

Patients with peritonsillar abscesses have sore throat, drooling, fever, a strained "hot-potato" voice, and variable trismus. The key physical finding here is unilateral midline displacement of the tonsil with distortion of the soft palate.

Treatment and Nursing Care

Treatment for patients coming to the ED with pharyngitis obviously depends on the cause. Once serious illness is ruled out, most of the time treatment is symptomatic.

Fluid Volume Deficit, Actual or Potential, Related to

• **Dehydration Secondary to Pharyngitis, Dysphagia, or Fever**

Patients with significant pharyngitis should be encouraged to drink large amounts of fluid to prevent dehydration. Symptomatic relief is best obtained with over-the-counter sore throat lozenges. Occasionally, combinations of viscous lido-caine, kaolin and pectin (Kaopectate), diphenhydramine hydrochloride (Benadryl) elixir, and antacids may be prescribed as a gargle. Liquids are more easily consumed right after gargling with these preparations.

Antibiotic therapy is necessary for those persons with suspected or known group A beta-hemolytic streptococcal pharyngitis. Although it will not hasten resolution of the sore throat, the administration of antibiotics will help prevent suppurative complications. In adults over the age of 30 years antibiotics are of questionable benefit in preventing acute rheumatic fever.

Treatment of individuals with peritonsillar abscess involves intravenous antibiotics along with incision and drainage or needle aspiration of the abscess. These patients usually require hospital admission and an ENT consultation should be obtained.

Sinusitis

Sinusitis is an inflammatory condition of the mucous membranes lining the paranasal sinuses. Acute sinusitis is usually a bacterial complication of a viral upper respiratory tract infection. Other predisposing factors for acute infection include dental abscess, allergic rhinitis, nasal foreign bodies in children, nasogastric tubes, and altered ciliary function produced by smoking, air pollution, and cocaine use. *Streptococcus pneumoniae* and *Haemophilus influenzae* are the most common bacteria involved.

Clinical Manifestations

The clinical presentation of sinusitis can be quite variable, from no symptoms to symptoms of a prolonged upper respiratory tract infection, to classic facial or retro-ocular pain, purulent nasal discharge, headache, fever, and marked sinus tenderness to palpation. Transillumination of the maxillary sinus is done by shining a penlight percutaneously over the maxillary sinus and looking for light transmission in the mouth through the hard palate. Similarly, the light can be directed in a superior and medial direction through the bony rim of the orbit, and transillumination is looked for over the frontal sinus. Normal light transmission is good evidence that no infection is present. X-ray examination showing opacity, air-fluid levels, or mucosal thickening of more than 5 mm is the most sensitive test for sinusitis (Reiter 1983).

Treatment and Nursing Care

Treatment of acute sinusitis involves antibiotics (especially amoxicillin, trimethoprim-sulfamethoxazole, or cefaclor), 0.25% to 0.5% phenylephrine hydrochloride (Neo-Synephrine) nose drops to reduce swelling around the sinus ostia in the nose, humidification of the home environment, and isotonic saline nose drops. Sinus drainage usually is not required.

Chronic sinusitis is largely not an infectious problem. Normal mucociliary columnar cells are replaced by stratified squamous epithelial cells, with a resulting loss of sinus sterility. With acute exacerbations, symptoms and signs similar to those of acute sinusitis appear. Antibiotics are indicated, especially those directed against anaerobic organisms (e.g., clindamycin). Occasionally the underlying cause of chronic sinusitis will be neoplasm or vasculitis.

NONINFECTIOUS, NONTRAUMATIC ENT EMERGENCIES

Epistaxis

Epistaxis, or bleeding from the nose, is a common presenting complaint in EDs. Some patients may have spontaneous resolution of their bleeding, but many will need some intervention, such as nasal packing, to control blood loss (Juselius 1974). An occasional patient may even have life-threatening bleeding, requiring aggressive support and blood transfusions. In either case, a systematic and comprehensive approach to the assessment and management of persons experiencing epistaxis will help to ensure successful resolution of the problem.

Etiology and Pathophysiology

Epistaxis may be anterior or posterior. In younger patients, it is often anterior and originates at Kesselbach's plexus (Fig. 7–11). This area is richly supplied by several anastomosing arteries. Bleeding from this area may result from trauma, allergies, environmental irritants, low humidity, nose picking, and foreign body insertion or obstruction of the nares. The majority of these nose bleeds will either stop spontaneously or cease with firm pressure applied by pinching the soft portion of the nose.

Unfortunately, however, the majority of patients seen in EDs for this problem are elderly and often have underlying cardiovascular disease. In this group of pa-

FIGURE 7–11. Vasculature of the nasal cavity.

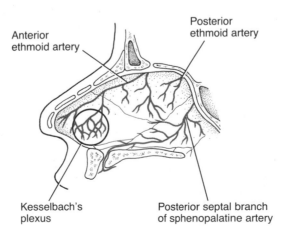

Anterior ethmoid artery

Posterior ethmoid artery

Kesselbach's plexus

Posterior septal branch of sphenopalatine artery

tients, bleeding is not from Kesselbach's plexus but from sites more posterior in the nose, behind the inferior and middle turbinates. Some common causes of posterior epistaxis include atherosclerosis of nasal vasculature, hypertension, and anticoagulant drug therapy. Hematologic disorders as well as hepatic pathology may also be responsible for posterior epistaxis.

Clinical Manifestations

When the patient arrives in the ED, active epistaxis will be readily apparent. Even if bleeding has diminished or ceased, most likely the patient will be holding blood-stained tissues, handkerchiefs, or cloths. His or her clothing is also usually blood stained. Initial assessment of these patients must focus on evaluation of airway, breathing, and circulation. Vital signs, including orthostatic changes, should be checked quickly to assist in the evaluation of the extent of blood loss. Patients with active bleeding, airway obstruction, orthostatic changes, underlying heart disease, trauma with associated injuries, or known bleeding diathesis (e.g., those taking anticoagulants) should have their status judged urgent on triage and brought to the treatment area as soon as possible.

Subsequent history, if not already obtained at triage, should include the duration and amount of bleeding, the side on which bleeding began, any past history of epistaxis and methods of control, any current medications being taken (e.g., aspirin, coumadin, quinidine), and any known bleeding disorders. A history of trauma, hypertension, recent respiratory tract infection, and nose picking should also be ascertained. Past medical history is important not only because certain diseases predispose the patient to abnormalities in hemostasis (e.g., leukemia, liver disease, multiple myeloma) but also because advanced atherosclerotic heart disease makes the patient less able to withstand mild hypovolemia, tachycardia, and excess autonomic stimulation to the heart.

Treatment and Nursing Care

The nature and severity of blood loss will determine the priorities of treatment for patients experiencing epistaxis. If blood loss is significant or the patient is experiencing respiratory distress, stage I medical and nursing care will need to be initiated. Airway management and circulatory support must be arranged for.

Fluid Volume Deficit, Actual or Potential, Related to

- **Epistaxis**

When a fluid volume deficit exists in the face of epistaxis, aggressive management for the treatment of hypovolemic shock must be instituted. An intravenous (IV) infusion of Ringer's lactate or 0.9% normal saline via a large-bore IV catheter should be begun. Blood should be obtained for typing and crossmatching, complete

TABLE 7–1
Equipment Used in the Control of Epistaxis

Nasal speculum
Bayonet forceps
Petrolatum gauze ($\frac{1}{2}''$ wide, 72″ long)
Silver nitrate sticks
Head mirror and bright light
ENT chair
Emesis basin
Tissues
Point suction
Cotton
Vasoconstrictor and anesthetic
    4% lidocaine (Xylocaine) and 1 : 100,000 epinephrine
    5% cocaine solution
    2% procaine (Novocain)
Antibiotic ointment
14 French (Red Robinson) catheter
4″ × 4″ gauze pads
2-0 silk sutures
14 French Foley catheter with 30-ml balloon

blood count (CBC), platelet count, and coagulation studies. Application of a pneumatic antishock garment (PASG) and cardiac monitoring may be required. (See Chapter 5.)

Fortunately, the majority of patients with epistaxis do not experience hypovolemic shock. Treatment for active nose bleeding often begins by having the patient sit up and blow the nose gently once or twice to remove excess clots. The anterior portion of the nose is then firmly pinched for 10 to 15 minutes. If this is not effective (as often it is not in the elderly) preparation should be made for more aggressive evaluation and intervention. Equipment listed in Table 7–1 should be readily available.

Medical interventions to control epistaxis include cautery, anterior packing, posterior packing, and, rarely, arterial ligation. Good local anesthesia is important in difficult cases and can best be obtained by using a 10% cocaine solution. The main side effects of this drug are tachycardia, hypertension, and increased contractility of the heart. Nurses should be especially alert for problems associated with these side effects, especially in the elderly patient. Patients with coronary artery disease may even experience angina when cocaine is given.

Once local anesthesia is obtained, chemical cautery with silver nitrate sticks can be utilized if the bleeding site is identified. Anterior packing using 72 inches of ¼-inch petrolatum gauze may be necessary if the bleeding site is not identified. Because anterior packing obstructs sinus drainage, antibiotics may be given prophylactically to prevent sinusitis. After bleeding is controlled, the patient should be observed for another one half to 1 hour before discharge. Patient discharge instructions can be given during this time (Table 7–2). Any blood sent to the laboratory (e.g., for CBC, platelet count, coagulation studies) must be checked before sending the patient home.

When bleeding continues in spite of anterior packing, posterior packing be-

TABLE 7–2
Discharge Instructions for
Patients Presenting with Epistaxis

Prevention
  Humidify the home
  Avoid straining (lifting, exercise, stooping)
  Avoid nasal trauma (fingers, cotton-tipped applicators)
  Avoid forceful nose-blowing
  Open mouth when sneezing
  Avoid hot liquids
  Avoid high altitude
Recurrent Bleeding
  Sit upright, be calm
  Squeeze lower (soft) half of the nose between thumb and index
    finger for 15 minutes by the clock
  If the above is unsuccessful, return to the emergency department

comes necessary (Fig. 7–12). In this case, a gauze pack or Foley balloon is used as a posterior buttress against which an anterior pack can be firmly placed (Cook et al. 1985). Posterior packing is considered an invasive procedure, which carries with it the risk of airway obstruction if the pack becomes displaced. All patients who have posterior packs should be admitted to the hospital, placed on humidified oxygen, and have serial arterial blood gas (ABG) determinations obtained.

Anxiety, Related to

*   **Epistaxis**

    Anxiety and fear are common responses to epistaxis, especially when there has been significant blood staining of the patient's clothes or handkerchiefs. In addition,

FIGURE 7–12. Nasal packing for severe epistaxis.

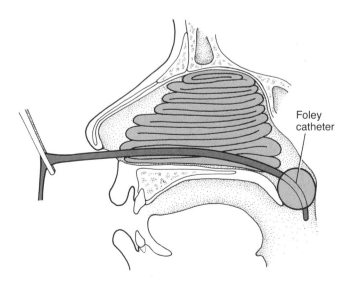

Foley
catheter

the discomfort of the nasal examination and packing contribute to the patient's apprehension and anxiety. For these reasons, explanations surrounding procedures to be done, along with a calm, reassuring attitude throughout all phases of patient's ED stay, are important.

Vertigo

Dizziness is a common complaint in EDs. Vertigo is a feeling of unsteadiness, of the room spinning, or of the patient's turning in space. Vertigo needs to be differentiated from a lightheaded or floating feeling, in which the patient sometimes feels as if he or she is about to lose consciousness. The latter often implies circulatory compromise with inadequate blood flow to the brain from dehydration, blood loss, or cardiac dysrhythmia. A true spinning feeling, on the other hand, implies a problem in the labyrinth of the inner ear, or less commonly a primary problem in the central nervous system. True ataxia or balance problems without lightheadedness or a sensation of spinning indicates a primary cerebellar problem.

Etiology and Pathophysiology

There are many causes of labyrinthine dysfunction. Drugs such as cimetidine, neuroleptics, antihypertensives, antihistamines, aminoglycosides, furosemide, and high-dose aspirin are commonly implicated (Baldwin 1984). A history of recent head trauma is important because the second most common complaint in the postconcussion syndrome is dizziness. New eyeglasses and hysterical personality are two other causes to be considered. Otitis media and other disorders of the middle ear can frequently affect the inner ear.

Central causes of vertigo arise mostly from lesions involving the brain stem. Cerebrovascular disease, neoplasms, and multiple sclerosis are examples.

Clinical Manifestations

The physical assessment of the patient with vertigo starts with the determination of vital signs, in particular identifying any orthostatic changes. The ear should be examined for any abnormalities or hearing loss. Hearing loss can be assessed grossly by determining the patient's ability to hear a watch tick, fingers being rubbed together, and a soft spoken voice. Any abnormality in neurologic assessment, especially the inability to walk, is important. The presence of nystagmus or jerking eye movements should be documented.

Nystagmus seen mostly with upward gaze is usually due to a central cause, whereas rotatory nystagmus almost always indicates a peripheral inner ear problem. The presence of tinnitus or ringing in the ears and hearing loss usually implicates inner ear pathology.

Treatment and Nursing Care

There are two major reasons to admit a patient with vertigo to the hospital. The first is because of severe vertigo with nausea, vomiting, and dehydration; the second is suspicion of central nervous system disease. A central nervous system cause should be suspected when there is an abnormal neurologic finding or when the patient is unable to ambulate even with encouragement. Recurrent and discrete episodes occurring in any position, lasting 10 to 15 minutes, can be transient ischemic attacks.

Patients who can be sent home often may benefit from meclizine hydrochloride (Antivert), which has been found to be effective in the management of dizziness. Patients should increase their activity only as tolerated. Depending on the cause, some patients may have symptoms for 4 to 6 weeks, although severe symptoms rarely last more than 1 to 2 days.

Rupture of the Tympanic Membrane

Trauma to the external ear can result in tympanic membrane perforation. Often this trauma is self-induced through the insertion of hairpins, cotton-tipped applicators, and similar objects into the ear. Perforation may also occur as a complication of otitis media. Occlusion of the eustachian tube from mucosal inflammation and swelling may create positive or negative pressure within the middle ear, leading to perforation of the ear drum. Significant changes in barometric pressure experienced during underwater diving or in air travel also predispose to tympanic membrane rupture.

Perforation from trauma does result in some hearing loss; however, significant hearing loss or the presence of vertigo should alert the nurse to more serious damage to the inner ear. Pain and discharge from the ear are variable findings with ruptured tympanic membrane. Fortunately, even in the presence of infection, most tympanic membrane ruptures will heal in days to months. The ear should be kept dry, and topical or systemic antibiotics are indicated only when infection is evident on examination.

Temporomandibular Joint Dislocation

Temporomandibular joint dislocations typically occur after yawning (Stair 1986). The dislocation usually is bilateral, with both mandibular condyles slipping anteriorly out of the glenoid fossae (Fig. 7–13). A persistent open bite and inability to move the jaw or close the mouth is characteristic. Radiographs usually are not necessary. Treatment involves downward pressure over the molar teeth on both sides, while pivoting the mandibular symphysis up and around a central axis defined by the condyles (Stair 1986). Reassurance and encouragement, as well as use of parenteral muscle relaxants (e.g., diazepam), often are needed to accomplish reduction. After joint relocation, the patient should have minimal pain and full range of motion. The patient should be cautioned against yawning, and should be instructed to adhere to a blenderized diet for several weeks. Follow-up by an otolaryngologist is preferable because many of these patients can have subsequent temporomandibular joint dysfunction.

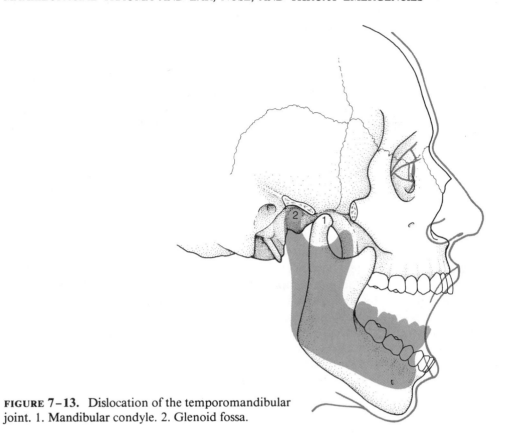

FIGURE 7–13. Dislocation of the temporomandibular joint. 1. Mandibular condyle. 2. Glenoid fossa.

Foreign Bodies in the Ear

Children may place a variety of objects into the ear canal. In adults, parts of instruments used to clean or scratch the ear frequently are broken off and become lodged in the canal. Insects not infrequently wander into this space and cannot exit, a situation that is quite distressing to the patient. Removal of these objects can be difficult. The adult external auditory canal is 24 mm long, with the narrowest portion about 7 mm lateral to the tympanic membrane. Round plastic or metal objects caught behind this narrowest part create the most problems.

If perforation of the tympanic membrane is not suspected, irrigation of the external canal with tap water at body temperature is a reasonable first step. One very effective method uses a Teflon IV catheter (with the needle removed) and a 30- ml syringe. The water is directed in superiorly and anteriorly. It may take 200 to 300 ml of water to remove the object. Other useful equipment includes large ear speculums, a head mirror with a good light source, an ear curette, a right-angled hook, ear suction equipment, and alligator forceps. Insects will occasionally leave the ear canal in response to bright light or cigarette smoke, but most will need to be killed first with mineral oil or topical lidocaine and then removed manually (Stair 1986).

Foreign Bodies of the Pharynx and Airway

Foreign bodies of the hypopharynx are usually seen in adults following a choking episode precipitated by the inadvertent swallowing of a chicken or fish bone. In children, any one of a number of objects can cause a similar presentation. Larger objects may pass into the upper one third of the esophagus, becoming lodged especially at the level of C6 or C7. Sharp objects may pass through the esophagus, leaving a mucosal scratch whose presentation mimics a foreign body sensation.

In addition to a foreign body sensation, patients complain of pain on swallowing. The patient often is accurate in localizing the level and side on which the foreign object is trapped. Xeroradiograms, which give better edge enhancement than regular soft tissue radiographs, are preferred, but objects may still not be visualized. Indirect laryngoscopy or fiberoptic laryngoscopy is of prime importance in fully assessing the patient with a foreign body sensation. Failure to diagnose the condition correctly may lead to perforation of the hypopharynx or esophagus with abscess formation or mediastinitis. If no object is found, and a scratch of the mucosal surface is suspected, the patient can expect dramatic improvement in one to three days. The importance of close follow-up by an otolaryngologist should be stressed to the patient.

Foreign bodies of the airway may be manifested by signs of upper airway obstruction, especially stridor, hoarseness, inability to talk, drooling, and inability to swallow. If the object is aspirated into more distal airways in a pediatric patient, history of the aspiration may not be obtained. The majority of children with aspirated foreign bodies are less than 2 years old (Kim et al 1973). The offending foreign matter frequently is a peanut or like vegetable matter. These children may have localized wheezing and recurrent pneumonias, and the diagnosis frequently is missed or delayed. On chest radiographs, atelectasis, mediastinal shift, or obstructive emphysema may not be evident (Blazer et al 1980).

Treatment of total upper airway obstruction from aspiration includes back blows, chest thrusts, and (in adults) abdominal thrusts. As long as the patient can breath or cough forcefully on his or her own, none of these maneuvers should be employed. A laryngoscope with Magill forceps or Kelly clamps may be quite useful in retrieving the object. If none of these attempts is successful in relieving the obstruction, needle or surgical cricothyroidotomy is indicated. Pediatric patients who have aspirated objects into more distal airways need general anesthesia and bronchosopy.

CONCLUSION: ENT EMERGENCIES

The existence of a multitude of ENT emergencies, along with their associated and potentially life-threatening complications, necessitates that the ED nurse be astute in his or her assessment skills. Additionally, he or she should have a sound scientific knowledge base so that both immediate care and appropriate anticipatory planning may be accomplished.

The nature and degree of severity of maxillofacial trauma and other ENT emergencies are highly variable. A patent airway, adequate ventilation, and circulatory stability with attention to actual or potential cervical spine injury remain priorities of care for patients experiencing such emergencies.

REFERENCES

Baldwin RL. 1984. The dizzy patient. Hosp Pract 19:151–162.

Blazer S, Naveh Y, Friedman A. 1980. Foreign body in the airway: A review of 200 cases. Am J Dis Child 134:68–71.

Cook PR, Renner G, Williams F. 1985. A comparison of nasal balloons and posterior gauze packs for posterior epistaxis. ENT J 64:446–449.

Gerlock AJ, Sinn DP, McBride KL. 1981. Clinical and Radiographic Interpretation of Facial Fractures. Boston, Little, Brown.

Gwaltney JM. 1985. Pharyngitis. In Mandell GL, Douglas RG, Bennett JE, eds. Principles and Practice of Infectious Diseases, 2nd ed. New York, John Wiley, 355–359.

Juselius H. 1974. Epistaxis: A clinical study of 1,724 patients. J Laryngol Otol 88:317–327.

Kaiser, J. 1987. Facial emergencies. In Rea RR, Bourg PW, Parker JG, et al, eds. Emergency nursing core curriculum, 3rd ed. Philadelphia, WB Saunders, 254–282.

Kim IG, Brummitt WM, Humphry A, et al. 1973. Foreign body in the airway: a review of 202 cases. Laryngoscope 83:347–354.

Manson PN. 1984. Maxillofacial injuries. Emerg Med Clin North Am 2:761–782.

Medford HM. 1982. Temporary stabilization of avulsed or luxated teeth. Ann Emerg Med 11:490–492.

Medford HM, Curtis JW. 1983. Acute care of severe tooth fractures. Ann Emerg Med 12:364–366.

Patterson HC, Kelly JH, Strome M. 1982. Ludwig's angina: an update. Laryngoscope 92:370–378.

Reiter D. 1983. A primer of ENT emergencies. Emerg Med 15:120–178.

Schultz RC. 1977. Facial Injuries, 2nd ed. Chicago, Year Book Medical Publishers.

Schultz RC, Oldham RJ. 1977. An overview of facial injuries. Surg Clin North Am 57:987–1010.

Stair TO. 1986. Practical Management of Eye, Ear, Nose, Mouth, and Throat Emergencies. Rockville, MD, Aspen Systems.

Zook EG. 1980. The Primary Care of Facial Injuries. Littleton, MA, PSG Publishing Company.

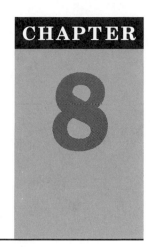
Susan Fortin, RN MS

Ocular Emergencies

Each year nurses see over 2 million cases of ocular trauma. These injuries may have a wide variety of causes, as unusual as jellyfish stings and gunpowder burns or as common as corneal foreign bodies or BB gun injuries. Half of the patients will be under 15 years of age and 65 per cent under age 31 (Keeney, 1974).

Patients with eye injuries will be anxious about a permanent vision loss. Even nontraumatic ocular conditions that are not emergencies will be of significant concern to patients who experience them.

This chapter begins with a review of ocular anatomy and physiology, followed by guidelines for history-taking and physical examination of the eye. Various ocular emergencies (traumatic and nontraumatic) are then discussed in relation to their causes, clinical manifestations, and treatments. The chapter closes with a discussion of eye donation.

OCULAR ANATOMY AND PHYSIOLOGY

To be able to assess abnormal conditions in a patient's eye, the nurse must first be familiar with the basic anatomy and physiology of the globe and orbit (Fig. 8–1).

The globe rests in the bony orbit surrounded by fat and connective tissue. Only the anterior portion of the globe is exposed and it is protected by the orbital rim and eyelids. Six extraocular muscles are attached to the globe, which allow for eye movements in all directions.

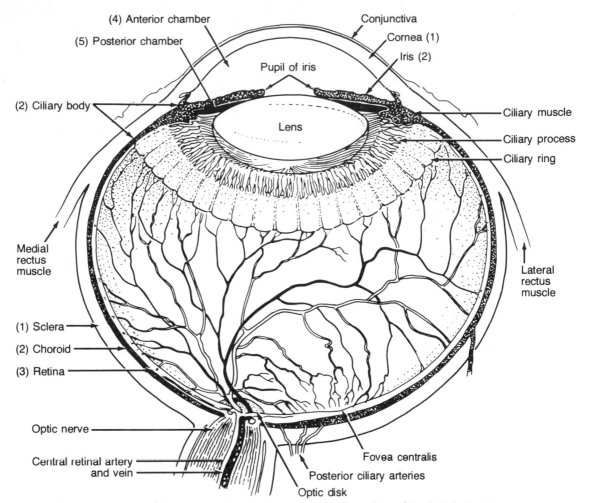

FIGURE 8–1. Anatomy of the eye. (Reprinted with permission from Care of the Ophthalmology Patient, by Elaine Thomson-Keith, 1986. Copyright © AORN, Inc, 10170-East Mississippi Avenue, Denver, CO, 8.)

The eye has three layers. The anterior portion of the outer layer is the curved, clear cornea, which is responsible for the refraction of light rays that enter the eye. The corneal epithelium is continuous with the conjunctiva, which covers the white sclera on the anterior portion of the eye (bulbar conjunctiva) and also lines the inside of the eyelids (palpebral conjunctiva). The conjunctiva forms a fornix, which prevents objects, such as contact lenses, from getting behind the eye.

The middle layer, or uvea, is a vascular, pigmented layer made up of the iris, ciliary body, and choroid. The iris, with its constrictor and dilator muscles, controls the amount of light that enters the eye by varying the size of the pupil. The ciliary body produces aqueous humor, the clear, watery liquid that fills the anterior and posterior chambers of the eye. In addition, the ciliary body contains muscles, which through their attachment to the lens via fine fibers called zonules, affect the shape and

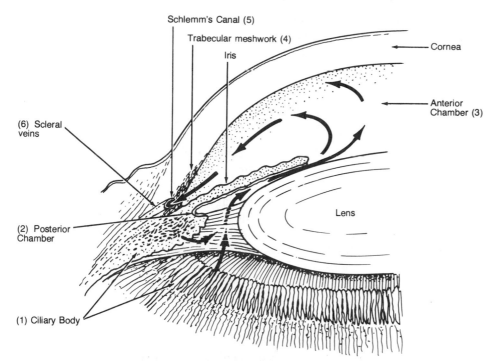

FIGURE 8–2. Aqueous fluid flow. (Reprinted with permission from Care of the Ophthalmology Patient, by Elaine Thomson-Keith, 1986. Copyright © AORN, Inc, 10170-East Mississippi Avenue, Denver, CO, 12.)

focusing power of the lens in the process known as accommodation. The choroid, along with the central retinal artery, supplies oxygen and other nutrients to the inner layer, the retina. The retina consists of sensory cells that are stimulated by light and send impulses to the brain via the optic nerve.

The eye has three chambers, which are filled with two different kinds of fluids, aqueous humor and vitreous humor.

Both the anterior chamber (behind the cornea and in front of the iris) and the posterior chamber (behind the iris and including the area occupied by the lens) are filled with aqueous humor. The lens is bathed in aqueous humor and provides some of the refractive power of the eye. The space the lens occupies is replaced by aqueous humor when the lens is removed, as in cataract extraction, but the focusing power must be replaced with an intraocular lens, contact lens, or glasses.

Aqueous humor enters the anterior chamber from the posterior chamber through the pupil and exits the eye into the venous system through the trabecular meshwork and Schlemm's canal, located in the angle between the iris and the cornea (Fig. 8–2). The amount of fluid in the eye determines the intraocular pressure, which is normally between 11 and 20 mm Hg. Increased intraocular pressure is termed glaucoma and may be acute or chronic.

Vitreous humor is the substance found in the space posterior to the lens. Vitreous humor is a clear, jelly-like substance present at birth and not synthesized postnatally as is aqueous humor.

Light rays enter through the clear cornea, pass through the pupil, lens, and vitreous space, and are focused on the retina. Swelling of the cornea, an opacity in the lens, or inflammation or bleeding in the anterior chamber or vitreous space may interrupt these light rays and decrease visual acuity.

OCULAR ASSESSMENT

The importance of a thorough ocular assessment in patients with ocular complaints cannot be overemphasized. With an accurate history and a sound knowledge base, many ocular problems will be easy to diagnose. Questions that should be included in every history taken from a patient with ocular complaints are listed in Table 8–1.

   Physical assessment of the patient with an ocular complaint includes the following examinations: visual acuity, visual fields, ocular motility, pupillary reactivity, and direct ophthalmoscopy. Proper completion of the physical examination depends on the ability of the examiner to perform the aforementioned tasks.

Visual Acuity

Emergency department (ED) nurses are accustomed to determining vital signs. The main vital sign in ophthalmic nursing is visual acuity. For legal reasons the determi-

---

TABLE 8–1
Questions to Be Asked While Obtaining
an Ophthalmic History

What are your symptoms (pain, loss of vision, diplopia, tearing, photophobia, discharge)?

When did this problem or injury begin or occur?

Has this problem or injury been treated in the past? If so, by whom, how, and what was the response?

Have you experienced any loss of vision or vision changes? If yes, ask the patient the following related questions:
- Is this the first time you have experienced a loss of vision?
- When did your loss of vision occur?
- Has your vision been decreasing gradually, or was this a sudden loss?
- What were you doing at the time of vision loss?

Do you have any history of eye problems (e.g., glaucoma, previous trauma, or surgery)?

Do you have an ophthalmologist?

Do you have any significant medical problems (e.g., atherosclerotic heart disease, diabetes)?

Do you wear glasses or contact lenses, or do you have a false eye?

When was your last tetanus shot?

Do you have any allergies?

Are you currently taking any medication?

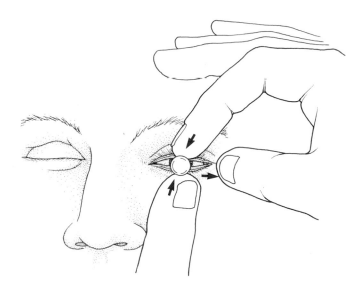

FIGURE 8–3. Removal of hard contact lenses.

nation of the patient's visual acuity must be done before any further treatment or examination is undertaken. The only exception to this rule involves chemical burns, for which immediate irrigation of the eye should precede any diagnostic maneuvers.

Prior to testing the visual acuity, determine whether or not there was any pre-existing visual deficit. If a patient wears glasses the vision should be tested both with and without correction. Patients who wear contact lenses may be tested with correction if their lenses are already in place or without if the eye is injured or has an abrasion.

When removing any type of contact lens it is important for the eye to be well lubricated in the area between the cornea and the contact lens to prevent corneal damage. If the eye appears dry, instill several drops of saline solution before attempting to remove the lens. It is best to have the patient in a supine position or reclining in a chair to prevent the lens from "popping" out onto the floor.

To remove hard contact lenses stretch the skin of the eyelid taut at the lateral canthus with your thumb and use one finger from each hand (one on the upper lid and one on the lower) to push the lids toward each other (Fig. 8–3). The lid margin should catch the edge of the contact lens and break its suction to the cornea. If a suction cup especially designed for removing contact lenses is available, it may be used by pressing it onto the contact lens until suction occurs and then pulling the contact lens straight away from the eye.

Soft contact lenses are removed by having the patient look upward, retracting the eyelids, and pinching the contact lens to break its suction to the cornea (Fig. 8–4).

Contact lenses should be stored in saline solution in separate containers labeled "left" and "right" that include the patient's name.

Whenever possible, test vision using a Snellen chart at a distance of 20 feet. Test one eye at a time, making sure that the eye not being tested is completely occluded. It may be necessary to lightly tape an eye patch over that eye to prevent "cheating." Record the lowest line the patient can read with each eye — for example, OD (oculus

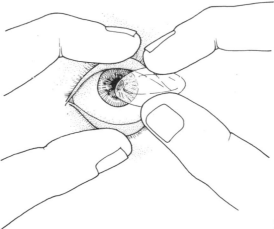

FIGURE 8–4. Removal of soft contact lenses.

dexter, or right eye) 20/30; OS (oculus sinister, or left eye) 20/40. Also record the number of mistakes made on that line (e.g., 20/30 − 2).

If the patient cannot read the top line on the chart his or her vision may be determined in the following manner. Standing 10 feet from the patient, hold up some fingers and see if the patient can count them. If not, continue to move toward the patient until he or she can tell how many fingers you are holding up. Record this as "Counts fingers (CF) at X feet." If when you are within a foot or two, the patient still cannot identify the number of fingers step back and try waving your hand around to see if the patient can see hand motion. This is recorded "Hand motion (HM) at X feet." If the patient has only light perception (LP), use a penlight or transilluminator to see if he or she can tell which direction the light is coming from and record the perception of light in all four quadrants if present. The visual acuity of a patient unable to perceive light is recorded as "no light perception" (NLP).

If the equipment to test distance vision is unavailable, near vision can be tested using a hand-held Rosenbaum vision chart (Fig. 8–5). Patients who wear reading glasses should be tested with corrective lenses in place. Record the lowest line the patient can read along with the distance at which the patient holds the card from the eye. If no "near card" is available, use a newspaper or book.

Attempt to determine the patient's best potential vision by using a pinhole. Pinholes are helpful when examining patients with refractive errors who have lost or broken their glasses or can't wear their contact lenses. Use the pinhole to test vision any time the visual acuity is 20/30 or less.

The concept of a pinhole is very simple. Normally the cornea bends light rays as they enter the eye and converges them to a point of focus on the retina. In persons with a refractive error, this point may be in front of or behind the retina owing to an unusual curve of the cornea (astigmatism) or a long or short eyeball. Using a pinhole blocks those light rays entering from the periphery and lets the patient concentrate on those rays that enter the central cornea and are not bent to be focused. If there is no improvement in vision when a pinhole is used it is unlikely that a refractive error is the cause of visual loss.

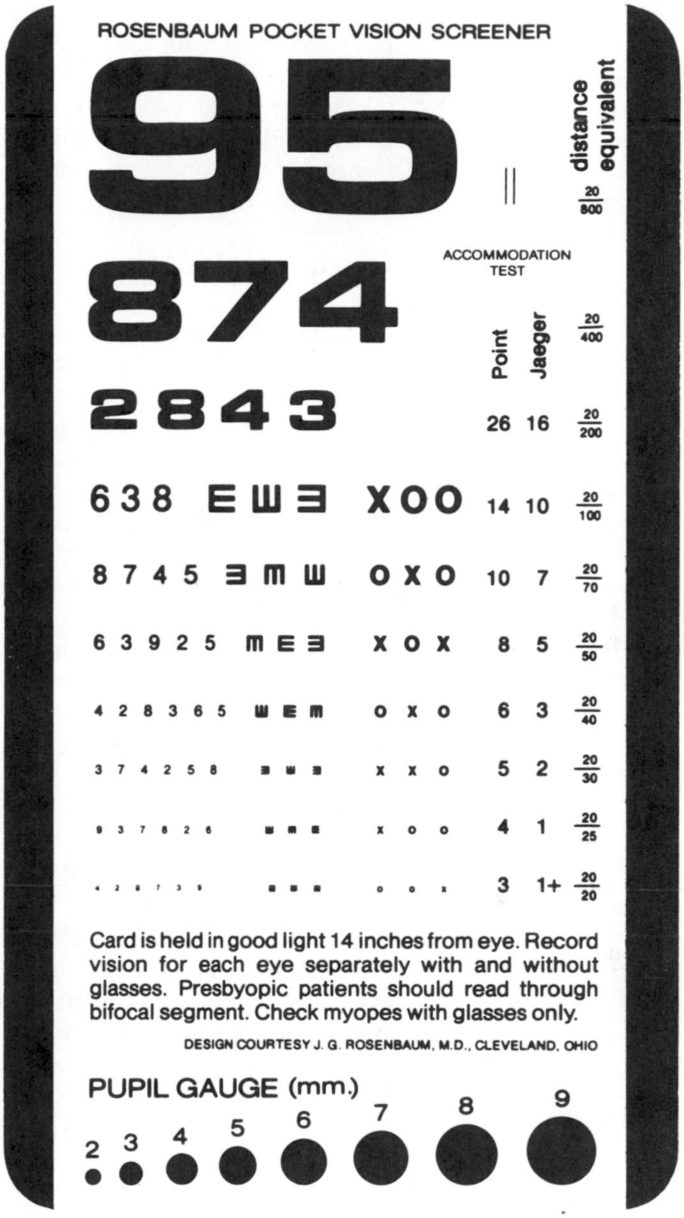

ROSENBAUM POCKET VISION SCREENER

distance equivalent

95 ‖ $\frac{20}{800}$

ACCOMMODATION TEST

874

	Point	Jaeger	
			$\frac{20}{400}$
2843	26	16	$\frac{20}{200}$
638 E Ш Ǝ X O O	14	10	$\frac{20}{100}$
8 7 4 5 Ǝ M Ш O X O	10	7	$\frac{20}{70}$
6 3 9 2 5 M E Ǝ X O X	8	5	$\frac{20}{50}$
4 2 8 3 6 5 Ш E M O X O	6	3	$\frac{20}{40}$
3 7 4 2 5 8 Ǝ Ш Ǝ X X O	5	2	$\frac{20}{30}$
9 3 7 8 2 6 Ш M Ǝ X O O	4	1	$\frac{20}{25}$
4 2 8 7 3 6 M M Ш O O X	3	1+	$\frac{20}{20}$

Card is held in good light 14 inches from eye. Record vision for each eye separately with and without glasses. Presbyopic patients should read through bifocal segment. Check myopes with glasses only.

DESIGN COURTESY J. G. ROSENBAUM, M.D., CLEVELAND, OHIO

PUPIL GAUGE (mm.)

2 3 4 5 6 7 8 9

FIGURE 8–5. Rosenbaum pocket vision screener. Reproduced by permission.

Visual Fields

The simplest method of assessing the patient's field of vision is by confrontation. As with visual acuity the eyes are examined separately, with the eye not being tested completely occluded.

The patient and the examiner should face each other about three feet apart. The examiner occludes his or her own eye opposite that of the occluded eye of the patient and while moving his or her fingers on the opposite hand slowly, brings the hand into the visual field from the periphery. The patient should indicate when he or she can first see the examiner's hand, which should be at the same time the examiner sees it, provided that the examiner has normal visual fields. All four quadrants should be tested, and absence of vision in any quadrant should be recorded as it may be indicative of retinal detachment.

Ocular Motility

The ability of the patient to move the eyes in all directions should be evaluated. While facing the examiner, the patient should follow an object up and down, to both sides, and diagonally. This is also the time to ask the patient if he or she is experiencing double vision (diplopia). Diplopia and an inability to move the eye up and down may indicate a blow-out fracture and entrapment of the inferior rectus muscle following blunt trauma.

To assess the reactivity of the pupil the anterior chamber must be clear, and the patient should not have received any dilating drops. Try to assess the depth of the anterior chamber and look for a crescent of whitish-yellow cells (hypopyon) or blood (hyphema) within the eye. A hypopyon occurs as the result of infection, whereas a hyphema appears as a dark layer and results most commonly from trauma.

If blood or white cells are present in the anterior chamber be sure to draw a picture of the eye in your nursing notes documenting the level observed. Hyphema may also be documented according to the grading system listed in Table 8–2.

Pupillary Reactivity

If the anterior chamber is clear, continue your assessment by checking pupil size, symmetry, and reactivity to light. The pupil should constrict both directly and consensually. Failure to constrict from a mid-dilated position may indicate acute, narrow-angle glaucoma.

TABLE 8–2
Grading System for Traumatic Hyphema

Grade I: Layered blood occupies less than one third of the anterior chamber
Grade II: One third to one half of the anterior chamber is filled with blood
Grade III: At least one half but not the entire total anterior chamber is filled with blood
Grade IV: The anterior chamber is completely filled with clotted blood; this is referred to as an eight-ball or blackball hyphema

Source: From Read JE, Crouch ER. 1984. Trauma: Ruptures and Bleeding. In Duane TD, ed. Clinical Ophthalmology, vol. 4. Harper & Row, 6.

Direct Ophthalmoscopy

Each eye should be examined, noting the appearance of the retina in all four quadrants. The optic nerve cup-to-disc ratio should be estimated and the macula examined for hemorrhages.

With practice, the use of a direct ophthalmoscope will become a routine part of your physical examination. Many books provide in-depth instruction on the proper use of the instrument, a discussion of which is beyond the scope of this.

The remainder of this chapter discusses specific ocular emergencies. Those of traumatic origin are discussed first, followed by those of nontraumatic origin.

TRAUMATIC OCULAR EMERGENCIES

Chemical Burns

Chemical burns of the eye, whether from acid or alkali, require immediate attention and generally do not have a good prognosis.

Etiology and Pathophysiology

Alkali burns are most often caused by ammonia, plaster, and products containing lye, such as oven cleaner. Alkalis combine with lipids of cell membranes and soften the tissue. Thus, alkalis easily penetrate the cornea and anterior chamber, resulting in a rising intraocular pH with subsequent damage to intraocular structures.

Acids tend to bind with tissue proteins and set up barriers to tissue penetration. Although acid burns are generally considered to be less serious than alkali burns, certain acids, such as hydrofluoric acid and those containing heavy metals, can also cause extensive damage. Acid burns of the eye are often associated with car battery explosions.

Clinical Manifestations

Patients who come to the ED with chemical burns of the eye(s) will have a history of a caustic substance being splashed onto the face and into the eye(s). They will complain of eye pain and decreased vision. Physical examination will most likely reveal burns of varying degrees. The cornea will appear white and opaque and the conjunctiva pale (Fig. 8–6).

Treatment and Nursing Care

Stage I care is not often required for patients who have eye problems alone because ocular injuries or diseases are not usually life-threatening. A chemical burn, however,

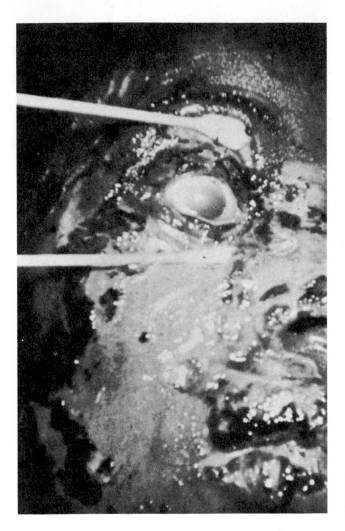

FIGURE 8-6. Chemical burn of the face and eye. (From Deutsch TA, Feller DB. 1985. Paton and Goldberg's Management of Ocular Injuries. WB Saunders, 95.)

is a true emergency, and treatment of patients with such burns should be instituted within *minutes* of their arrival in the ED.

Injury, Ocular, Related to

• Chemical Burn of the Eye

No matter what the agent, the first course of action in treating a patient with a chemical burn is copious irrigation of the eye and fornices with water or normal saline solution. Irrigation should be from the inner to the outer canthus to prevent contamination of the other eye. An irrigating contact lens called a Morgan therapeutic lens may be used to aid in flushing the eye over an extended period of time. This flushing will not reach all areas of the eye, and the eyelids should be everted and the conjunctival fornices swept with wet cotton-tipped applicators to remove debris. Periodically the tear film should be tested with a pH indicator, such as litmus paper. Irrigation should continue until the pH returns to the normal range of 7.2 to 7.4.

Once the pH has returned to a normal level, the patient is treated with a broad-spectrum topical antibiotic to prevent corneal infection and ulceration. Additionally, cycloplegics are used to ease discomfort by relieving iris and ciliary body spasm. Dilation of the pupil will help prevent the formation of lens-iris adhesions and secondary glaucoma.

Intraocular pressure should be measured, if possible, or at least estimated by palpation. If the intraocular pressure is elevated, acetazolamide (Diamox), given orally, and timolol (Timoptic), given topically, may be used to lower the pressure.

Impaired Gas Exchange, Potential, Related to

- **Chemical Burns of the Face**

Toxic chemicals that strike the eye may also enter the mouth and nose and may be aspirated or swallowed. An assessment of the patient's ability to breathe and to swallow should be made promptly. Emergency resuscitation equipment should be close at hand in case intubation is required.

Anxiety, Related to

- **Possible Loss of Vision Secondary to Ocular Injury**

The loss of vision, no matter how minor or temporary, is anxiety provoking. Patients with chemical burns of the eye are justified in fearing a permanent visual loss because the prognosis is poor in most cases. Nursing care for these patients and their families centers on providing a supportive but truthful environment and allowing the patient to express his or her frustrations and fears.

Injury, Physical (Potential), Related to

- **Sensory Perceptual Alteration Secondary to Ocular Injury**

Although a patient's eye may not be patched, he or she may still have difficulty in opening it or in keeping it open. The inability to see must be compensated for by giving the patient detailed, verbal information about procedures or examinations that will be performed.

The patient will be in unfamiliar surroundings and may require assistance in ambulating. It may be helpful to have a friend or relative stay with the patient to aid in any necessary relocation.

Blunt Trauma

Patients may suffer blunt ocular trauma from a variety of sources. Blunt ocular trauma may appear as an isolated injury or as part of multisystem trauma (Joondeph 1988). Some common offenders are baseballs, snowballs, toys, and fists.

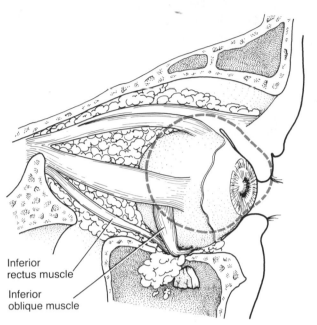

**Inferior
rectus muscle**

**Inferior
oblique muscle**

FIGURE 8–7. Blow-out fracture of the orbital floor. Dashed
line indicates the normal position of the globe. (Redrawn from
Deutsch TA, Feller DB. 1985.
Paton and Goldberg's Management of Ocular Injuries. WB
Saunders, 40.)

Blow-out Fractures

Blunt trauma to the eye and orbit may cause a fracture of the orbital wall. The most
well known of these fractures is a blow-out fracture of the ethmoid bone.

Etiology and Pathophysiology • Although an orbital fracture can occur in any part of
the orbit, the most common fracture site is the ethmoid bone on the orbital floor. The
ethmoid is the weakest bone in the orbit and therefore the most likely to give way
when the intraorbital pressure is increased by the force of a blow to the eye. Often the
orbital contents, including fat, the inferior rectus and oblique muscles, the infraorbital nerve, and — in rare cases — the globe itself, may herniate through this hole into
the maxillary sinus (Fig. 8 – 7). Radiographs will help to confirm this diagnosis.

Clinical Manifestations • The patient will complain of double vision (diplopia) and a
loss of sensation of the skin along the inferior orbital rim of the involved eye. The eye
may have a sunken appearance (enophthalmos) from prolapse of orbital contents.
Additionally, there will be limited vertical movement because of inferior rectus
muscle entrapment.

Treatment and Nursing Care • Blow-out fractures are never considered an emergency. Many times diplopia will resolve over a two-week period, making surgery
unnecessary. In those cases in which diplopia or enophthalmos persists, corrective
surgery may be performed up to 14 days after the insult with minimal risk.

Anxiety, Related to

• *Fear of permanent loss of vision secondary to ocular trauma*

Patients who have blow-out fractures and are experiencing double vision will expect
some kind of treatment or surgery to relieve their symptoms. These patients need to

be reassured that blow-out fractures often resolve without intervention and that no additional damage to the eye will occur by waiting. The role of the nurse is largely educational and supportive for these patients.

Hyphema

A second serious injury that may occur as a result of blunt trauma is bleeding in the anterior chamber of the eye, or hyphema.

Etiology and Pathophysiology • The iris and ciliary body of the eye are highly vascular. As a result of blunt trauma, hemorrhage from the aforementioned structures may fill all or part of the anterior chamber. Blood may clot and block the outflow of aqueous humor from the eye, resulting in a secondary glaucoma. Prolonged high pressure can cause permanent damage to the optic nerve and may also force blood into the corneal epithelium, resulting in permanent rusty-brown staining. Some hyphemas are nontraumatic in origin; patients with sickle cell anemia or other hemoglobinopathies are at higher risk for hyphemas and their complications.

Clinical Manifestations • The patient with a hyphema will usually, although not always, arrive in the ED after a recent incident of blunt trauma. He or she may complain of some degree of eye pain, seeing a reddish tint, and overall decreased visual acuity. The patient may also complain of extreme drowsiness. This somnolence is common among hyphema patients, although its cause is unknown. On examination with a penlight or ophthalmoscope, a level of blood will be visible in the anterior chamber (Fig. 8–8). This hyphema should be documented in the progress notes according to the grading system described in Table 8–2 or by drawing a picture of the eye.

Treatment and Nursing Care • Any patient who comes to the ED with a hyphema should be seen by an ophthalmologist. Until the doctor arrives, the patient should sit

FIGURE 8–8.   Hyphema, grade I. (From Deutsch TA, Feller DB. 1985. Paton and Goldberg's Management of Ocular Injuries. WB Saunders, 188.)

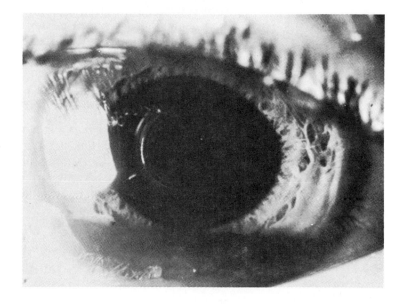

in a quiet, low-traffic area with the affected eye covered with a metal shield to avoid further trauma.

Pain, Related to

- *Ocular trauma*

The patient may be experiencing ocular or head pain following trauma and may request medication for pain relief. Because patients with hyphema have a tendency to rebleed, the patient should not be given any aspirin or aspirin-containing compound as aspirin is known to affect blood clotting.

The patient will probably be admitted to the hospital for observation by the ophthalmologist. Rebleeding occurs in up to one third of all hyphema patients, usually three to five days after the initial insult, when the clot begins to retract.

Retinal Detachment

The retina has two layers, an outer retinal pigment epithelium and an inner sensory retina. A retinal detachment occurs when the sensory retina is separated from the pigment epithelium. Trauma accounts for about 15 per cent of these detachments (Deutsch and Feller 1985).

Etiology and Pathophysiology • Retinal detachments may occur as a result of trauma, traction on the retina from membranes in the posterior segment, or retinal degeneration. When the sensory retina is separated from the pigment epithelium, it loses its source of blood supply and nourishment. Retinal detachments occur in men more often than in women, in patients with degenerative myopia, and in elderly patients. Those patients who are aphakic are 100 times more likely to develop a retinal detachment than those patients who have not had the lens removed (Newell 1986).

Clinical Manifestations • A retinal detachment should be suspected when the patient reports seeing flashes of light (even with the eyes closed), a shower of black dots in the peripheral vision, or a decrease in vision with a "curtain" blocking part of the visual field. On ophthalmoscopy, the detached retina appears gray or translucent and lacks the normal choroidal pattern. The retina may be folded, and it may move as the eye changes position. There is a bright red choroidal color shining through the opaque veil of detached retina. Performance of visual field testing will show lack of vision in a quadrant of the eye, indicative of the area of detachment.

Treatment and Nursing Care • Patients with suspected retinal detachments should be referred to an ophthalmologist immediately for confirmation of the diagnosis and surgical intervention. Bilateral eye patches and bed rest with minimal activity to limit eye movements and prevent further damage are indicated while waiting for an ophthalmic consultation (Joondeph 1988).

Anxiety, Related to

- *Fear of permanent loss of vision or impending surgical procedure or both*

As with any loss of vision, the patient will be fearful of a permanent visual deficit. The patient can be reassured that retinal detachments are often treated successfully with a surgical procedure. This operation consists of a scleral buckling with an encircling band or sponge to appose the sensory and pigment retinal layers and drainage of any retinal fluid that may have seeped between the layers.

The thought of a surgical procedure may also make the patient anxious, and the nurse should provide reassurance as the patient is prepared for surgery.

Lid Ecchymosis, Subconjunctival Hemorrhage, and Orbital Hematomas

Not all blunt traumas to the eye result in blow-out fractures, hyphemas, and retinal detachments. Lesser injuries include lid ecchymosis, subconjunctival hemorrhage, and orbital hematomas.

The eyelids have a plentiful blood supply and bruise easily. In the days following the injury, blood may seep to the other side of the face, making the patient appear to have two "black eyes." If no other injury is found, treatment for simple blunt trauma consists of cold compresses for 24 hours to reduce swelling. Thereafter warm compresses may be used to promote resorption of blood from subcutaneous tissues.

A subconjunctival hemorrhage appears as a patch of erythema under the conjunctiva. This should not be confused with conditions in which the conjunctiva itself is inflamed. No medications are known to aid in the resorption of this blood, which usually occurs within a few weeks.

Not uncommon after blunt trauma are orbital hematomas. These hemorrhages may not be visible unless blood seeps anteriorly along the extraocular muscle sheath. Hematomas may limit extraocular muscle mobility and in severe cases may be the cause of a central retinal artery occlusion.

Lacerations and Perforating Injuries

A laceration of the eyelid may be superficial, requiring only a few stitches for its repair in the ED. Other lacerations, however, may be associated with and hide perforations (injuries that traverse the full thickness of the sclera or cornea and disrupt the intraocular cavity).

Etiology and Pathophysiology

Lacerations and perforations of the eyelids and globe may have a wide variety of causes, ranging from animal or human bites to knife cuts or gunshot wounds. These injuries, depending on their severity, may have an effect on numerous portions of the visual system.

Clinical Manifestations

Patients with lacerations or perforating ocular injuries, or both, will manifest a wide variety of clinical signs and symptoms depending on the cause and severity of the

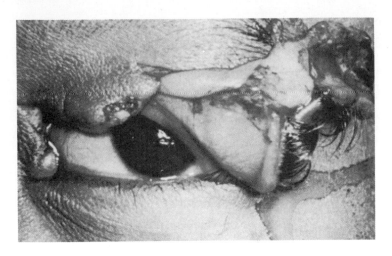

FIGURE 8–9. Upper eyelid injury following a dog bite. (From Deutsch TA, Feller DB. 1985. Paton and Goldberg's Management of Ocular Injuries. WB Saunders, 24.)

injury. Some lid lacerations may be superficial, whereas others may extend through the full thickness of the eyelid. In the case of animal bites, a large amount of tissue may be avulsed from the lid (Fig. 8–9). If available, this tissue should be saved and kept moist with saline as it makes the best material for repair. Varying degrees of pain, redness, irritation, or foreign body sensations, along with an altered visual acuity, will usually be present with lid lacerations. Nearly complete loss of vision, pain, bleeding, and occasionally leakage of intraocular contents onto the cheek or lid will occur with large lid lacerations and penetrating injuries (Lubeck 1988).

If the lids are uninjured, they should be retracted gently against the bones of the orbit to inspect the globe. It is important not to put pressure on the globe because a perforation may have occurred, and the contents of the eye may be expelled through the wound. Check the globe for abrasions, corneal foreign bodies or edema, or visible wounds of the cornea and sclera. Anterior chamber depth should be assessed and documented. If a foreign body such as a knife is sticking out of or embedded in the eye or orbit, do not attempt to remove it.

Treatment and Nursing Care

Superficial lacerations of the eyelids with no other ocular injury may be repaired by the ED physician. If the lacerations involve the eyelid margin, the medial portion of the eyelid (and therefore the lacrimal drainage system), the levator muscle, or the full thickness of the eyelid with or without tissue avulsion, the injury should be repaired by an ophthalmologist familiar with the anatomy and functioning of the eyelid.

A perforation of the globe of any size must be treated by an ophthalmologist. Aqueous fluid may leak from the eye, decreasing the intraocular pressure below acceptable levels. In addition, tissues may be extruded through the perforation, thus damaging delicate intraocular structures. Protruding objects should be immobilized and the injured eye should be protected with a metal eye shield until the patient can be examined by an ophthalmologist. The patient should be given nothing by mouth as surgery is likely.

Pain, Related to

- *Laceration of the eyelid*
- *Perforation of the globe*

If the repair of a lid laceration is to be done in the ED, the nurse should position the patient supine for maximum safety and comfort as well as accessibility by the physician who will perform the repair. An intravenous (IV) line may be started at a keep-open rate or a heparin lock placed to allow for ease of sedation or emergency drugs should the patient require them. A drop of topical anesthetic in each eye will ease any discomfort that may be caused by the entrance of soap and allows for the placement of protective contact lenses worn by the patient during the repair. Cotton placed in the patient's ear on the affected side will prevent the entrance of blood or irrigating solutions. Most repairs will be done using local anesthetics, which are administered by the physician in the form of a nerve block.

Patients with perforations of the globe will require surgery in the main operating room and should be positioned supine with the injured eye protected until the time of surgery. If a perforation is suspected, no topical anesthetics should be administered.

Infection, Potential, Related to

- *Laceration of the eyelid*
- *Perforation of the globe*

Before the repair of any ocular laceration in the ED, the skin around the patient's eye should be washed with a surgical soap and rinsed with normal saline solution. The eye should be irrigated to remove foreign bodies, and iodine compounds may be used on the skin to help prevent infection. If a perforation of the globe is suspected, the eye should not be irrigated, nor should any eyedrops be given. Antibiotics, if required, should be administered systemically. Depending on the nature of the injury, it is also wise to consider giving the patient a tetanus shot or rabies vaccine.

Injury, Ongoing (Potential), Related to

- *Foreign body in the eye or orbit*

Patients who present to the ED with obvious foreign bodies embedded in the eye, such as knives or hooks, have the potential for further injury if the object is bumped or removed improperly. The nurse should carefully protect the eye with a metal shield or—if the foreign body is too large—by covering it with a cup or other protector. The patient's uninjured eye may also be patched to decrease ocular movement.

NONTRAUMATIC OCULAR EMERGENCIES

Central Retinal Artery Occlusion

Artery occlusions in the eye, especially those of the central retinal artery, are an ominous sign for the patient's vision. Recovery of vision following an occlusion is minimal, and investigation of the cause of the occlusion may lead to the discovery of other arterial disease.

Etiology and Pathophysiology

Occlusion of the central retinal artery is often associated with vascular disease and may be caused by emboli from carotid artery atherosclerotic plaques in older patients, valvular heart disease in younger patients, and thrombosis from arteriosclerosis (Newell 1986). Additionally, artery occlusions may be associated with orbital hematomas or acute angle closure glaucomas, which cause increased intraocular pressure.

Clinical Manifestations

The only symptom a patient may report on presentation to the ED with central retinal artery occlusion is a sudden, painless loss of vision. On further questioning, however, there may have been transient visual loss in the weeks or months preceding the onset of blindness.

Using ophthalmoscopy, the examiner will usually find the following characteristic funduscopic appearance: pale optic nerve and narrowed arteries throughout the fundus, which may show segmentation or "box car" effect. There will also be diffuse retinal whitening from ganglion cell edema and a cherry red spot on the macula where the absence of ganglion cells allows the normal choroidal coloration to show through (Fig. 8–10). The cherry red spot may begin to appear within 20 minutes of the occlusion.

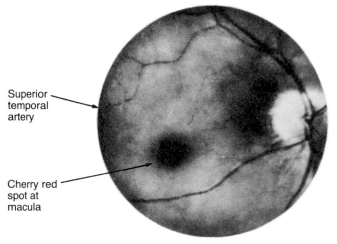

Superior temporal artery

Cherry red spot at macula

FIGURE 8-10. Central retinal artery occlusion. Note "box-car" effect in superior temporal artery and the cherry-red spot on the macula. (Reproduced by permission from Newell FW, Ophthalmology, Principles and Concepts, St. Louis, 1986, The CV Mosby Co.)

Treatment and Nursing Care

Central retinal artery occlusion is another true ophthalmic emergency that requires immediate initiation of treatment.

Tissue Perfusion, Altered, Ocular, Related to

- *Central retinal artery occlusion*

Treatment is directed toward lowering the intraocular pressure in order to raise, relatively, the arterial pressure and possibly move the block, restoring blood flow to the previously occluded areas. Methods of lowering the intraocular pressure include vigorous massage of the eye, administration of 250 mg of intravenous acetazolamide (Diamox), 300 ml of 20% mannitol (Osmitrol) over 10 minutes, or 0.5% timolol (Timoptic), one drop in the affected eye.

An ophthalmologist may perform immediate paracentesis, removing some of the aqueous humor from the anterior chamber with a tuberculin syringe in an attempt to decrease the intraocular pressure further and dilate the central retinal artery.

If the occlusion occurs as a result of an orbital hemorrhage or mass, the pressure may be relieved by performing a lateral canthotomy. After a small amount of lidocaine (Xylocaine) is injected near the lateral canthus, a straight clamp is used to clamp about 4 mm of the canthus. This area is then cut with a straight scissors. This allows the contents of the orbit to push forward slightly and relieves some of the pressure on the arteries.

As already noted, the prognosis for return of vision in central retinal artery occlusion is not good, with 75% of patients retaining vision only for "count fingers" and "hand motion" in the affected eye (Brown 1985). If the occlusion has been caused by emboli, it is important to refer the patient to an internist or cardiologist for further evaluation. By the time the patient arrives in the ED, it may be too late to save the eye, but you may save a life with an appropriate referral.

Anxiety, Related to

- *Possible permanent loss of vision secondary to central retinal artery occlusion*

Loss of vision due to central retinal artery occlusion usually occurs suddenly and without warning, and this lack of obvious explanation for the vision loss provokes anxiety in the patient. Patients need to be comforted and to have honest explanations about their condition, but the nurse should avoid false reassurances, as the return of vision is uncommon.

Fluid Volume Deficit, Potential, Related to

- *Use of carbonic anhydrase inhibitors*

Acetazolamide (Diamox) is a carbonic anhydrase inhibitor; carbonic anhydrase is an enzyme responsible for the production of aqueous humor. As the production of aqueous humor is slowed, intraocular pressure decreases. Carbonic anhydrase inhibitors also have a slight diuretic effect, and when they are used in conjunction with

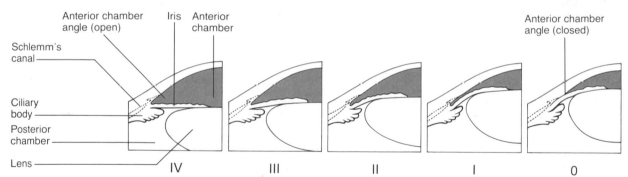

FIGURE 8–11. Grades of anterior chamber angle width. IV shows the lens touching the iris, blocking the flow of aqueous humor to the anterior chamber with the angle open and Schlemm's canal still accessible. The increasing pressure in the posterior chamber pushes the lens forward (III–I), until the lens pushes the iris into the angle, completely blocking drainage through the canal (0). (Redrawn from Peyman GA, Sanders DR, Goldberg MF. 1980. Principles and Practice of Ophthalmology. WB Saunders, 679.)

mannitol (Osmitrol), rapid fluid loss may affect the patient's fluid and electrolyte balance. The patient's intake and output should be monitored and signs of hypokalemia noted.

Acute, Narrow-Angle Glaucoma

Narrow angle glaucoma accounts for about 5% of all cases of glaucoma and occurs only in patients whose eyes provide a narrowed access to the trabecular meshwork and Schlemm's canal for drainage of aqueous humor.

Etiology and Pathophysiology

An attack of narrow-angle glaucoma may occur when the pupil is dilated midway by either pharmaceutical or natural means. When the pupil is dilated midway (such as in a darkened movie theater), the iris is thicker and may partially occlude the outflow of aqueous humor as it bunches up in the angle of the eye. In some patients the thickened iris may touch the lens, blocking the flow of aqueous humor from the posterior to the anterior chamber. The pressure in the posterior chamber rises quickly and forces the already thickened iris into the angle, possibly completely occluding flow out of the eye (Fig. 8–11).

Clinical Manifestations

Patients who come to the ED with acute, narrow-angle glaucoma may complain of an intense headache located in the brow on the affected side. They may also state that they see halos around lights and have a marked decrease in vision. Nausea and vomiting are common.

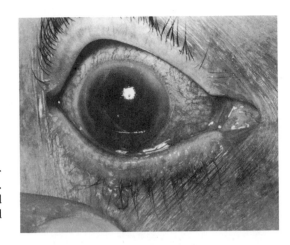

FIGURE 8–12. Narrow-angle glaucoma as viewed through a slit lamp. Note the hazy cornea and mid-dilated pupil. (From Haas J. Invest Opthalmol Vis Sci 7:140, 1968, with permission.)

Examination of the eye will reveal a pupil fixed in a midway-dilated position and unreactive to light. The cornea may be hazy and blood vessels may be prominent at the corneoscleral limbus (Fig. 8–12). Intraocular pressure may be as high as 60 mmHg, and the eye will feel rock-hard. Angle closure often occurs in only one eye, and the other eye may be used to compare the intraocular pressure by palpation.

Treatment and Nursing Care

Although it is not considered a true ocular emergency that requires treatment within minutes, acute, narrow-angle glaucoma poses a serious threat to the patient's long-term visual prognosis if not treated within a few hours.

Tissue Perfusion, Altered, Ocular, Related to

- *Altered flow of aqueous fluid*

Once again treatment is directed toward lowering the intraocular pressure. Interventions described previously for lowering the intraocular pressure in central retinal artery occlusion are also utilized for the treatment of acute, narrow-angle glaucoma. Application of eyedrops, such as 4% pilocarpine (one to two drops every 5 minutes three times) to constrict the pupil will help pull the iris away from the cornea and out of the angle. Effects are usually noted in 20 to 60 minutes.

Fluid Volume Deficit, Potential, Related to

- *Administration of carbonic anhydrase inhibitors*
- *Vomiting*

As with patients experiencing a central retinal artery occlusion, the use of carbonic anhydrase inhibitors in the patient with acute, narrow-angle glaucoma may lead to fluid and electrolyte imbalance. This state of imbalance may be compounded by the patient's vomiting prior to treatment. Watch the patient carefully for signs of hypovolemia and electrolyte imbalance. Nausea may be increased if oral glycerol (Osmoglyn) is given. Oral glycerol is administered by mouth over cracked ice with fruit juice, and in this form it is very sweet. Patients already nauseous may have trouble retaining the fluid. It may be necessary to administer antiemetics on doctor's order.

When the attack is broken the patient should be referred to an ophthalmologist, if he or she has not already seen one, for a peripheral iridectomy. A small opening is made at the periphery of the iris using a laser beam, which provides an alternative path for aqueous flow from the posterior to anterior chamber in the event of future pupillary block.

NONTRAUMATIC AND NONEMERGENT OCULAR CONDITIONS

A number of patients will arrive in the ED suffering from what they believe to be emergent conditions, characterized by redness, itching, burning, tearing, and "sticking" of the eye. These patients do not require emergency treatment to save their vision but do require an examination to rule out hidden pathology.

Etiology and Pathophysiology

Common nontraumatic and nonemergent conditions for which patients request emergency services are blepharitis, conjunctivitis, chalazions, and styes.

Blepharitis is an inflammation of the lid margins and may be related to seborrhea or staphylococcal antigen reaction. Conjunctivitis is an inflammation of the conjunctiva, which may be of bacterial, viral, or allergic causation. A stye results from an infection of one of the small glands located at the lid margin, and a chalazion is an inflamed meibomian gland.

Clinical Manifestations

Blepharitis causes burning and itching of the eye and occasional tearing. A close look at the lid margin reveals crusting on the lid and on the lashes.

Bacterial conjunctivitis is characterized by redness, irritation, crusting, and sticking together of the eyelids. Viral conjunctivitis causes irritation and tearing of the eyes accompanied by redness. The patient will also have a palpable preauricular lymph node on the affected side, which helps to distinguish it from allergic conjunctivitis, which has a similar presentation without a palpable node.

A stye is a small bump at the lid margin resulting from an infection of one of the small glands located there. A chalazion appears as a bump some distance from the lid margin and is an inflamed meibomian gland.

Whenever you are examining a patient who you believe may have an infection or conjunctivitis of some kind, it is important to remember how easily the infection can be transmitted to another eye. Human tears have been known to harbor chlamydia, bacteria, herpes simplex virus, and the AIDS virus. A patient's tears on your hand, examination instrument, tissue, or eyedrop bottle can infect the patient's other eye, your own eye, or the eye of another patient. Gloves should be worn. Handwashing is an important step in the prevention of this transmission.

Treatment and Nursing Care

Although this group of patients has no threat to vision they should have the diagnosis confirmed and the course of treatment determined by an ophthalmologist. Patients should be referred to and seen by an ophthalmologist within a few days. Treatment includes warm compresses four times daily, antibiotic ophthalmic ointment, and sometimes topical steroids.

Infection Transmission, Potential, Related to

- ### *Infectious Ocular Conditions*

Although some ocular conditions may not be contagious patients should always be instructed in proper hygiene to prevent cross infection of the other eye or the eyes of other family members. Patients should not touch or rub one eye and then the other; they should wash their hands immediately after touching the eye, and should use separate washcloths and towels from those of everyone else in the family to help contain the infection.

CORNEAL ABRASIONS AND FOREIGN BODIES

The cornea, richly supplied with nerve endings, is the most sensitive part of the eye. A corneal abrasion from any cause is an extremely painful ocular condition for which a patient will demand immediate attention and relief.

Etiology and Pathophysiology

Corneal abrasions can occur as a result of blunt trauma, a foreign body under the eyelid, overwearing of or poorly fitted contact lenses, or overexposure to ultraviolet light (suntanning lamps). When an abrasion occurs, there is damage to the corneal epithelium, which exposes the sensitive corneal nerves.

Clinical Manifestations

Patients will have sharp, stabbing pain, photophobia, and increased tearing in the affected eye. They may also complain of a feeling of something in the eye. Patients

CHAPTER 8

with corneal abrasions are in extreme pain, and a drop of topical anesthetic in the affected eye will relieve the pain temporarily and allow you to examine the patient.

To examine the patient, use fluorescein dye to stain the cornea and abrasion. A blue cover on the end of a flashlight will make the abrasion appear as a yellow-greenish area brighter than the rest of the cornea. Draw a picture of the abrasion in the chart. If the abrasion has a vertical, linear pattern suspect a foreign body under the eyelid.

Treatment and Nursing Care

No matter what the patient tells you, always suspect that there may be a foreign body in the fornix or under the eyelid. A corneal abrasion alone, and a foreign body and a corneal abrasion combined, feel exactly alike to the patient and cannot be differentiated without a thorough examination.

Pain, Related to

• *Corneal Abrasion Secondary to Ocular Injury*

The cornea is the most sensitive part of the eye, and corneal abrasions are extremely painful for the patient. Topical anesthetics are helpful in relieving pain but have only a short-term effect. Patients may request a bottle of the drops that made the pain go away, but *never,* under any circumstances, should any patient be sent home with a bottle of topical anesthetic or a prescription for such an eyedrop. Topical anesthetics impair corneal healing, and the patient who continues to use them may reinjure the eye without knowing it because of a lack of sensation. Patients who repeatedly use topical anesthetics often develop corneal ulcers.

An antibiotic ointment may be used to help lubricate the eye, and the eye should be double-patched. One eye pad is folded in half and placed on the eye and covered with another single eye pad, both of which are taped securely in place. Taping should be done from the area above the nose to the lateral cheek on the affected side. The patient should be referred to an ophthalmologist for further evaluation. He or she should be cautioned that depth perception is altered when one eye is patched, and safety precautions should be taken.

EYE DONATION

Cornea transplant surgery is one of the oldest and most successful types of transplant surgery performed. Thousands of patients in the United States and around the world are on waiting lists to receive a transplant to restore their vision. Patients who die in the ED are potential donors of this valuable tissue, and federal law requires that families be approached regarding tissue donation.

Cornea donors may be of any age and are not limited by a previous need for glasses. The requirement for brain death is not a factor in cornea donation as in other types of organ donation.

To help preserve the cornea, the eyelids should be gently closed and light ice-packs placed over the closed lids to cool the cornea and slow tissue breakdown. Some states require the permission of the next of kin before the eyes are removed; others assume consent unless otherwise previously indicated by the decedent or family member. Local eyebanks can provide information on the laws in each state and the appropriate methods to retrieve donated eyes.

CONCLUSION

Despite federal law requiring safety glasses in the workplace and public education programs on eye safety, ocular injuries continue to occur to the unprotected eye. A systematic approach will aid in the diagnosis and treatment of patients coming to the ED with ocular conditions of various causes. Although chemical burns and central retinal artery occlusion remain the most serious of ocular injuries, any ocular condition will be serious to the patient and requires prompt attention.

REFERENCES

Brown G. 1985. Retina vascular obstruction signals systemic disease. J Ophthal Nurs Technol 4:20–25.

Deutsch TA, Feller DB. 1985. Paton and Goldberg's Management of Ocular Injuries, 2nd ed. Philadelphia, WB Saunders Co.

Joondeph BG. 1988. Blunt ocular trauma. Emerg Med Clin North Am 6:147–167.

Keeney A. 1974. Prevention of ocular injuries. Int Ophthalmol Clin 14:1–10.

Lubeck D. 1988. Penetrating ocular injuries. Emerg Med Clin North Am 6:127–146.

Newell FW. 1986. Ophthalmology, Principles and Concepts, 6th ed. St. Louis, CV Mosby Co.

Peyman GA, Sanders DR, Goldberg MF. 1980. Principles and Practice of Ophthalmology. Philadelphia, WB Saunders Co.

Read JE, Crouch ER. 1984. Trauma: Ruptures and bleeding. In Duane TD, ed. Clinical Ophthalmology, vol 4. Hagerstown, MD, Harper & Row, 1–17.

Sheehy SB, Barber J. 1985. Emergency Nursing: Principles and Practice. St. Louis, CV Mosby Co.

Thomson-Keith E. 1986. Care of the Ophthalmology Patient. Denver, Association of Operating Room Nurses, Inc.

Stephanie Kitt, RN MSN

Cardiac Emergencies

Cardiovascular diseases affect 40 million people in the United States. It is estimated that more than one million individuals in the United States suffer myocardial infarction annually (Missri et al. 1984). Although mortality from coronary artery disease has declined over the past decade, it still remains the number one cause of death in this country. Health prevention and education focused on the reduction of risk factors along with early identification and intervention is paramount in reducing the morbidity and mortality associated with the disease. Emergency health care providers can significantly affect the incidence, morbidity, mortality, and severity of coronary artery disease and its sequelae.

CARDIOVASCULAR ASSESSMENT

Individuals who present to the emergency department with symptoms of myocardial insult must be identified immediately. The triage nurse is usually the first person with whom these individuals come in contact; therefore astute assessment skills become critical. The differentiation of symptomatology of cardiac origin from that which is not and determining the individual's acuity status are critical responsibilities of the triage nurse. Therefore stability of the individual's cardiovascular system must quickly be ascertained during the initial patient assessment.

    The chief complaint, the patient's reason for seeking health care, is a subjective statement by the individual to the triage nurse. Although patients with cardiovascular

163

disorders may present with a myriad of complaints, chest discomfort or pain is by far the most common. Other chief complaints that may also indicate cardiovascular pathology include palpitations, lightheadedness, dizziness, and loss of consciousness. Additionally, dyspnea on exertion (DOE), paroxysmal nocturnal dyspnea (PND), orthopnea, or fluid accumulation (e.g., weight gain, leg swelling, frothy sputum, and so forth) also suggests cardiovascular pathology.

When individuals present with any of the listed symptoms, additional information is necessary to determine the etiology of the complaint. Chest discomfort or pain (when present) should be described in terms of character (i.e., sharp, dull, stabbing, and so forth), intensity (i.e., rating on a scale of 1 to 10), location (including whether or not the discomfort or pain is localized or diffuse), and radiation. Additionally, the timing of all symptoms should be ascertained: when it began, how long it has lasted, whether it is continuous or intermittent. The presence of aggravating or alleviating factors or both and any associated symptoms such as nausea, vomiting, diaphoresis, and shortness of breath (SOB) should be sought.

Objective assessment at this time should include vital signs and a cursory physical assessment focused on level of consciousness and the integumentary and respiratory systems. When obtaining vital signs, the rate and regularity of the patient's pulse and respirations should be noted. The skin, often reflective of an individual's cardiovascular status, should be assessed for its color, temperature, and moisture. Is pallor or cyanosis present? Is the skin cool or warm? Is it clammy and diaphoretic, or is it dry? Signs of respiratory distress should also be noted: Are the patient's respirations deep or shallow? Are intercostal retractions, pursed lip breathing, or nasal flaring evident? Is the patient assuming a compromised breathing posture?

In addition to the presence or absence of previous cardiovascular pathology, other data that the triage nurse should attempt to obtain include the patient's medication and allergy history.

The triage history for an individual presenting with suspected cardiovascular disease should only take a few moments to obtain. If at any time during the triage assessment it however becomes apparent that significant cardiac or respiratory embarrassment, or both is present, the patient should be taken immediately to the treatment area. Details of the chief complaint (CC), and the history of present illness (HPI) can then be obtained either from the patient or a relative concurrently with the initiation of treatment.

When severe respiratory or cardiovascular compromise or both is overt, the triage nurse should have little difficulty in determining an acuity rating. Any individual with a presenting history compatible with cardiovascular insult (whether accompanied by a past medical history of cardiovascular disease or not) or with unstable vital signs (whether resultant of cardiovascular origin or not) should be taken to the treatment area without delay.

When individuals present with symptoms that are less overt, are somewhat vague, and are not clear in origin, the triage nurse may have more difficulty in the assignment of an acuity rating. The following paragraphs may assist in this determination and should also guide more detailed questioning later in the individual's emergency stay.

The chest discomfort or pain of cardiac origin may be experienced and described in various ways by different individuals. A variety of adjectives such as squeezing, choking, stabbing, pressing, or sticking may be used to describe the sensation. A feeling of tightness, heaviness, or indigestion may also be described. It is important to let individuals describe their symptomatology in their own words.

Chest discomfort or pain of cardiac origin results from an imbalance between myocardial oxygen supply and demand. Typically, its location is substernal and over the left anterior chest. It may radiate across the patient's entire chest, or to the shoulder(s), arm(s), back, neck, or jaw, or to any combination of these. The pain is not localized and is not altered by musculoskeletal movements. Anything that increases the oxygen requirements of the heart as in exercise, hypertension, and tachycardia may induce or aggravate pain of myocardial origin. Rest, which tends to decrease myocardial oxygen requirements, usually alleviates the pain. The longer and steadier the pain, the greater the likelihood of cardiac etiology. Pain specific to coronary atherosclerotic heart disease (CAHD) usually cannot be reproduced by palpation of the chest wall and is not usually associated with movement.

The most common noncardiac causes of chest discomfort or pain can be categorized by three systems: gastrointestinal, respiratory, and musculoskeletal (see Table 9–1).

Associated signs and symptoms are crucial in determining the etiology of chest discomfort or pain. Pain stemming from gastrointestinal distress is generally described as burning in the epigastric area. It may be associated with certain foods and may be relieved by an antacid. Chest pain originating in the lungs, surrounding pleura, or both is generally associated with chest wall movement and may be exacerbated by a deep breath. Additionally, respiratory assessment reveals areas of diminished ventilation indicating a number of potential pulmonary etiologies. Musculoskeletal pain is generally suspected if there is point tenderness on palpation of the chest wall. Sharp pain that can be elicited on palpation is also most likely of musculoskeletal origin. Questions related to unusual physical activity can elicit information as to whether the discomfort is secondary to trauma.

Although these descriptions may help the reader identify origins of symptomatology, they should be used only as general guidelines. The patient who is clinically unstable or reports a feeling of impending danger should be taken to the treatment area immediately. Although there are atypical presentations for various disorders, a patient with an acute MI can present without chest discomfort or pain and possibly with only referred pain. In these instances, "an ounce of prevention is worth a pound of cure."

Once inside the treatment area, further details of the patient's present illness, past medical history, and family history should be queried. Any details not yet obtained regarding the location, radiation, duration, intensity and quality, relation to movement, associated symptoms, and aggravating and alleviating factors of chest discomfort or pain (if present) and other symptomatology should be sought. Reasons for hospitalizations, diagnostic findings, and responses to treatments should be ascertained. Additionally, the past medical history is explored to determine the presence of hypertension, angina, previous MI, rheumatic heart disease (RHD), congenital anomalies or peripheral vascular disease (e.g., intermittent claudication, deep venous thrombosis [DVT], varicose veins, and the like).

Unfortunately, not all patients are accurate historians. Often, current medications can lend insight into past medical history for those who cannot recall specific problems. When obtaining a medication history, questions such as "Do you take any heart pills or water pills?" may be appropriate. Women of childbearing age should

TABLE 9–1
Characteristics of Chest Pain of Cardiac and Noncardiac Origins

Category	Characteristics	Makes Pain Worse	Makes Pain Better
Cardiac origin			
Acute myocardial infarction	Pressure, burning tightness, squeezing	Activity/exertion Hypertension Tachycardia	Morphine sulfate
	Epigastric area, substernal, between shoulder blades, radiation to arms and jaw or neck/back—lasts over 30 minutes		
Angina	Same as above but usually has history of angina and/or pain stops in a few minutes	Activity Eating Smoking Stress Anger	Rest Nitroglycerin
Gastrointestinal origin			
Indigestion	Heartburn or burning sensation in epigastric area, nonradiating and not associated with activity	Heavy meals	Antacids Walking Bland diet
Peptic ulcer	Burning epigastric pain	Empty stomach	Food Antacids
Hiatal hernia	Sharp epigastric pain	Heavy meal, bending Lying down	Small meals
Musculoskeletal pain			
Costochondritis	Sharp pain with point tenderness around the ribs on palpation May have cold with cough	Cough and palpation	Rest
Traumatic	Tenderness on palpation and with movement in addition to a history of trauma		
Pulmonary origin			
Pleuritic	Localized, sharp, gradual onset	Cough and deep breath	
Parenchymal (as with pneumonia)	Described as dull discomfort, patient may feel short of breath		
Pneumothorax	Sharp, sudden onset		Splinting
Pulmonary embolus	Crushing, sudden onset, associated with difficulty breathing	Deep breath	

also be asked specifically if they are on birth control pills. Information to be noted regarding medications includes name, date ordered, dosage schedule, and the patient's compliance with the schedule. Occasionally, the chief complaint is secondary to a problem with medications such as a depleted supply or taking out-dated and ineffective stock. A past medical record or call to the patient's health care provider may also clarify important information.

Last, subjective data collection should include a review of all body systems to ensure that subtle symptoms of other organ system pathology are not overlooked. The presence or absence of constitutional symptoms, such as fatigue, weight loss, anorexia, activity intolerance, fever, and even mental status changes must be documented.

Objective assessment usually includes a physical examination, electrocardiogram (EKG), chest radiography (CXR), and laboratory analysis. Indications for specific laboratory tests are discussed under specific disorders.

The most important aspect of physical assessment is the ABCs: airway, breathing, and circulation. Airway assessment should include visual observation of the patient's ability to move air in and out of the lungs. Airway patency and respiratory rate, depth, and effort are all parameters to be monitored. Supraclavicular retractions during inspiration usually indicate acute ventilatory difficulty. A patient who is severely dyspneic may be using accessory muscles to aid in ventilation. This is evidenced by intercostal retractions during inspiration and usually indicates a more pronounced inspiratory effort than normal.

An individual in respiratory distress has rapid, shallow, and sometimes noisy ventilations. Nasal flaring and pursed-lip breathing may be evident. Breath sounds may be decreased secondary to decreased movement of air. A prolonged expiratory phase may be noted. Crackles, wheezes, or both on auscultation are evidence of fluid or mucus in the small and large airways, respectively.

Once an effective airway is assured and adequate breathing patterns are established, circulatory status can be assessed. Blood pressure, pulse, and cardiac rhythm reflect the patient's hemodynamic status, which may vary on initial presentation. Autonomic disturbance and a host of reflex responses in an effort to maintain cardiovascular stability may be evident and are commonly seen at the onset of acute MI (Pantridge and Geddes, 1967). It is not unusual for patients to present with hypertension. They may have a history of chronic hypertension, or sympathetic stimulation can result from fear, anxiety, pain, or hypoxemia. This occurs in response to stimulation of the chemoreceptor sites on the carotid bodies and the arch of the aorta. These receptors cause the release of catecholamines (epinephrine and norepinephrine) from storage sites in response to hypoxemia, fear, anxiety, and pain. Heart rate is increased, and force of contractions is strengthened. Tachycardia increases myocardial oxygen consumption and consequently is detrimental to the individual with an imbalance between myocardial oxygen supply and demand. In addition, vasoconstriction of the blood vessels peripherally leads to elevated blood pressure. Similarly, stimulation of the sympathetic nervous system may be responsible for cool and diaphoretic skin. The patient experiencing hypotension secondary to pump failure will present with tachycardia as a result of baroreceptor response (Fig. 9–1).

FIGURE 9–1. Physiologic response to pain, fear, hypoxemia, and hypotension.

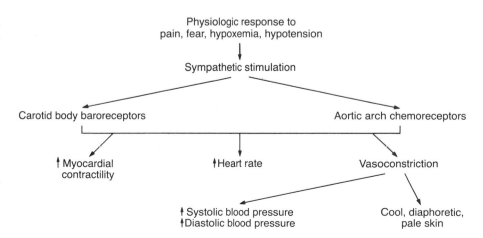

Patients experiencing cardiovascular compromise may also present with brady-cardiac rhythms, as may individuals taking medications that slow heart rate, such as digoxin and propranolol. Individuals who have been vomiting may experience bradycardia as a result of vagal stimulation from the Valsalva maneuver. Additionally, ischemic damage to the conduction system may induce a bradycardiac rhythm.

Data regarding organ and tissue perfusion can be obtained through assessment of the pulses, skin temperature and moisture, and level of consciousness. Weak pulses, cool and clammy mottled skin, and a diminished sensorium suggest compromised tissue perfusion.

Individuals presenting to the emergency department with actual or suspected cardiovascular insult also exhibit a host of emotional and psychologic responses. Apprehension, fear, and anxiety are the most notable. Patients may fear their very existence is threatened. They may be anxious because of a perceived (and often real) loss of control. The stark realization that one cannot eliminate or decrease symptoms can escalate the sense of helplessness.

There are also individuals who deny their vulnerability. Denial may be observed through their delay in seeking medical attention, refusal to cooperate in diagnostic work-ups, and inability to identify their cardiac status as a higher priority than work, family, or social responsibilities. These patients may eventually attempt to leave the emergency department against medical advice.

CORONARY ARTERY DISEASE

Coronary artery disease is a generic term for a variety of conditions that affect the coronary arteries. The most common of these conditions is coronary atherosclerotic heart disease (CAHD), which is characterized by local accumulation of lipids and fibrous tissue in the coronary arteries. These accumulations lead to arterial narrowing. The vascular changes result in diminished functional ability of the arteries to dilate and the characteristic manifestations of myocardial ischemia.

Etiology

Although the exact cause of CAHD is unknown, a number of risk factors have been shown to contribute to its existence. Some of these risk factors can be modified and others cannot. Hypertension, cigarette smoking, and elevated serum cholesterol have been consistently linked with coronary artery disease. Diabetes, obesity, lack of exercise, and type A personality traits have been correlated with an increased risk for development of coronary artery disease. The factors that cannot of course be modified include age, sex, race, and family history.

Susceptibility to CAHD steadily increases in men with age. The incidence sharply increases in females following menopause. This increase is thought to be related to loss of the protective effect of estrogen. Blacks have a greater incidence of hypertension than whites and therefore have a greater likelihood of developing CAHD. Last, although a strong family history of cardiovascular disease is suggestive in predicting the occurrence of CAHD, whether it causes any particular predisposition independent of other known risk factors remains to be seen.

Studies remain inconclusive concerning the importance of serum triglycerides as a coronary risk factor. Other factors, however, that may be associated with the development of CAHD include the use of oral contraceptives, high alcohol and coffee consumption, and gout. The role of alcohol is an area of considerable debate. Recent studies report that regular alcohol intake of up to two drinks a day in fact is protective against CAHD. The mechanism is thought to be peripheral vasodilation and increase in serum HDL (high-density lipoprotein) levels. Other reports indicate no protective influence as a result of alcohol consumption (Alpert 1984).

It is generally accepted that the greater the number of risk factors which an individual has, the greater his or her chances of acquiring CAHD. However, not all persons with significant risk factors acquire CAHD, and not all patients with CAHD have significant risk factors.

Pathophysiology

With atherosclerosis and progressive CAHD, the lumina of arterial vessels narrow. When this process occurs within the coronary arteries, there is a reduction of blood flow to the myocardium. This reduction in blood flow manifests itself symptomatically when the supply is inadequate to meet the demand for oxygen in the myocardium. Myocardial ischemia, with its characteristic manifestations of angina, myocardial infarction, and perhaps sudden death, results.

The ischemic process may be transient and may produce signs and symptoms that are reversible when the underlying cause is eliminated. Alternatively, severe or prolonged ischemia may result in myocardial infarction with cellular necrosis.

MYOCARDIAL ISCHEMIA

Myocardial ischemia results when there is a temporary imbalance between oxygen supply and demand in the myocardium. Therefore, ischemia follows when there is either a sudden decrease in coronary perfusion without a change in demand or an acceleration of myocardial oxygen demand without an adequate increase in supply.

Etiology

To understand the causes of myocardial oxygen supply and demand imbalances, one must consider the factors that determine myocardial oxygen supply and demand. Although numerous conditions affect myocardial oxygen supply, the most critical determinant is coronary blood flow. In the resting state, the myocardium extracts approximately 65% to 70% of the oxygen from the blood that flows through the coronary arteries. Therefore, when oxygen demands of the myocardium increase, there is very little "extra" oxygen to extract from the same amount of coronary blood flow. In order to prevent ischemia, increased oxygen demands must be met by increased coronary perfusion. In CAHD, this function becomes increasingly difficult.

As stated previously, although compromised coronary artery perfusion most often occurs as a result of CAHD, there are many other causes which should be considered: acute aortic dissection, hypovolemia, anaphylaxis, coronary artery spasm, tachydysrhythmias, and valvular disease. All can contribute to a reduced cardiac output and a subsequent fall in coronary artery perfusion and myocardial oxygen supply.

There are three major determinants of myocardial oxygen demand: heart rate, myocardial contractility, and myocardial wall tension. As each of these increases, so, too, does the myocardial oxygen demand. Myocardial wall tension is a direct function of intraventricular pressure and radius, and is inversely related to ventricular wall thickness.

$$T \text{ (tension)} = \frac{P \text{ (pressure)} \times r \text{ (radius)}}{h \text{ (wall thickness)}}$$

Therefore hypertension and ventricular dilation result in a greater demand for oxygen by the myocardium. Conversely, increased ventricular wall thickness, as in ventricular hypertrophy, decreases the wall tension necessary to achieve a given ventricular pressure. The result is a reduction in the amount of oxygen required. However, with a larger ventricular mass, the diffusion distance for oxygen to travel from the capillaries to myocardial cells is increased, and there is a greater amount of tissue requiring oxygenation. Although ventricular hypertrophy may initially be beneficial as a compensatory mechanism, it is not ultimately effective in decreasing myocardial oxygen demands.

The central mechanism all etiologies share is a fall in cardiac output and a subsequent decrease in myocardial oxygen supply. In descending aortic dissection and hypovolemia there is simply a reduced amount of blood in the central circulation. Tachydysrhythmias result in a fall in cardiac output as a result of diminished diastolic filling time. In anaphylaxis, massive histamine release causes vasodilation and promotes venous pooling, thus decreasing blood return to the heart. Aortic stenosis may disturb blood flow through the heart by causing a dilated and inefficient left ventricle. Ventricular hypertrophy results from repeated attempts to overcome the resistance to blood flow produced by the stenotic valve.

Pathophysiology

A number of metabolic alterations occur in myocardial cells during periods of ischemia. Under normal circumstances myocardial cells produce high-energy phosphate compounds by oxidative metabolic reactions. Within 15 seconds of the onset of ischemia, myocardial contractile function becomes depressed. Intracellular levels of high-energy phosphate compounds decline as anaerobic metabolic reactions are activated to produce ATP; lactate is a by-product of this anaerobic metabolism. The net result is an alteration in electrical conduction, a reduction in pumping ability, and elevated left ventricular diastolic pressures. The increased ventricular pressure occurs

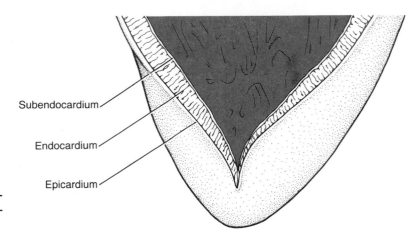

FIGURE 9-2.   Endocardial, subendocardial, and epicardial zones of the myocardium.

since relaxation of myocardial cells is energy-dependent. Oxygen-deprived cells cannot produce the high-energy phosphates necessary for diastolic activity (Alpert 1984).

Under normal circumstances coronary blood flow is uniform throughout the entire myocardium. If coronary blood flow declines, the subendocardial regions experience ischemic conditions before the epicardial zones (Fig. 9-2). Vessels in the subendocardial zone are more susceptible to ischemia, since they suffer greater compressive forces from overlying myocardial contractile activity. These subendocardial vessels are already vasodilated and have little reserve capacity to further dilate and increase blood flow (Alpert 1984).

Prolonged ischemia can result in myocardial infarction with cellular necrosis. Within hours after the onset of myocardial infarction, decreased contractile function in and around the necrotic myocardium results in ventricular dilation. Left ventricular filling pressures become elevated. This elevated pressure is transmitted to the left atrium and pulmonary veins, and finally, pulmonary capillaries. Increased pulmonary capillary pressure results in increased transudation of fluid into the pulmonary parenchyma, producing abnormal pulmonary compliance and blood gas exchange. The patient senses dyspnea (Alpert 1984).

A number of compensatory mechanisms attempt to oppose the deleterious effect of a myocardial infarction. Activation of the sympathetic nervous system increases circulating norepinephrine, which results in increases in myocardial contractile force, heart rate, and cardiac output. Unfortunately, these compensatory mechanisms may exaggerate myocardial ischemia by increasing myocardial oxygen consumption.

Clinical Manifestations

Angina pectoris is a term used to describe a cluster of symptoms characterizing myocardial ischemia. These characteristic symptoms may be likened to those of acute myocardial infarction. The pain is generally substernal in location and radiates to the shoulder and subsequently down the left arm or more rarely to the neck or abdomen. There may be associated dyspnea, diaphoresis, dizziness, nausea, and palpitations. Generally, episodes of angina are paroxysmal, lasting from a few seconds to several minutes as opposed to the longer duration of pain usually associated with infarction. Additionally, angina pain is usually brought on by exertion and relieved by rest and sublingual nitroglycerin. Individuals will often be able to tell if their pain is similar to their "usual" angina. If a difference is noted, myocardial damage should be suspected. Although the EKG may show signs of ischemia in conjunction with episodes of pain, there is no evidence of myocardial necrosis. Ischemia can be seen as T-wave alteration on the EKG. Cardiac enzymes remain within normal limits.

Prinzmetal's angina is caused by spasm of the coronary arteries as a result of increased neurogenic tone. This form of angina varies from classical angina in that the pain is not brought on by activity and is not relieved by rest. Prinzmetal's angina is usually more severe and of longer duration than classic angina. It waxes and wanes in cyclic fashion and often occurs at about the same time each day. This type of angina has been associated with sudden death.

Myocardial infarction occurs when ischemia is present for prolonged periods of time. If blood flow in an ischemic area is not reestablished within 3 to 4 hours, the destruction of myocardial cells is irreversible. Myocardial necrosis spreads from the subendocardial tissue through the myocardium toward the epicardium over a period of 4 to 6 hours (Bullas 1983).

Cardiac enzymes and a 12-lead EKG are mainstays of diagnostic testing for individuals with suspected myocardial insult. Creatine kinase (CK) and lactic acid dehydrogenase (LDH) are the enzymes reflective of myocardial damage. CK can be fractionated into isoenzymes according to catalytic rates as well as according to predominant tissue concentrations. The CK-BB isoenzyme found in brain tissue is slow acting, CK-MB found in myocardial cells is intermediate acting, and CK-MM found in skeletal muscle is fast acting.

CK-MB is the enzyme that rises first in acute MI (Fig. 9–3). Because of CK's early peak, the blood should be drawn when the patient first arrives in the emergency

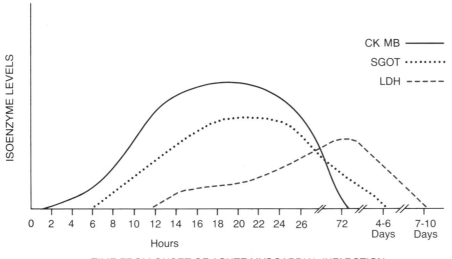

FIGURE 9–3. Isoenzyme alterations in acute myocardial infarction. CK MB = creatine kinase myocardial band; SGOT = serum glutamic oxaloacetic transaminase; LDH = lactic acid dehydrogenase.

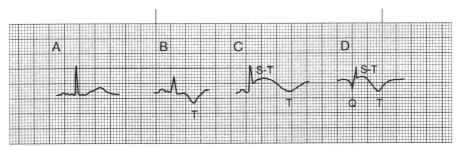

FIGURE 9-4. Electrocardiographic (EKG) wave changes indicative of ischemia, injury, and necrosis of the myocardium. *A,* Normal left ventricular wave pattern; *B,* ischemia indicated by inversion of the T wave. *C,* Ischemia and current of injury indicated by T wave inversion and S-T segment elevation. The S-T segment may be elevated above or depressed below the baseline, depending on whether or not the tracing is from a lead facing toward or away from the infarcted area and depending on whether epicardial or endocardial injury occurs. Epicardial injury causes S-T segment elevation in leads facing the epicardium. *D,* Ischemia, injury, and myocardial necrosis. The Q wave indicates necrosis of the myocardium. (Reproduced by permission from: Zipes DP, Andreoli KG. Introduction to electrocardiography. In Andreoli KG, Zipes DP, Wallace AG, et al., eds. Comprehensive Cardiac Care, 6th ed. St. Louis, 1987, The C.V. Mosby Co., 96.)

department. Many people do not seek care with the initial onset of symptoms preceding an acute MI. In this group of patients, the CK may have already peaked and leveled off by the time professional care is sought. For this reason, additional enzyme determinations are necessary.

LDH is abundant in kidney, cardiac, liver, and muscle tissues, as well as in blood, and is therefore elevated in many disorders. Since erythrocytes in blood contain LDH, hemolysis will cause an elevation of the enzyme. To avoid hemolysis when drawing blood samples, gently rotate the tube of blood after drawing and take care not to shake it vigorously.

The onset of LDH elevation occurs 12 to 24 hours after tissue damage, and levels do not usually return to normal until 7 to 10 days post infarction. LDH determinations are particularly helpful in instances where patients present several days after initial symptom onset.

Although serum glutamic-oxalacetic transaminase (SGOT) is the enzyme least specific to myocardial damage, it is still used in some institutions. SGOT is found in liver, red cells, skeletal muscle, and renal tissue. Consequently, damage to cells in any of these organs or systems will precipitate a rise in serum SGOT (Hudak 1986, 112).

The standard 12-lead EKG, although not definitive, is critical as an aid in the determination of the presence or absence of myocardial damage. EKG changes can be related to the evolution of an acute MI. If patients seek medical care early, the most prominent sign on EKG may be S-T segment elevation greater than 2 mm. Often Q waves do not develop for many hours. T wave inversion may not be seen for several days.

S-T segment alteration usually indicates myocardial tissue injury. Q waves are viewed as the most specific in identifying infarction (Fig. 9-4). Because Q waves may be normal, major importance is placed on the development of new Q waves in EKG leads where they previously were not present. Comparison of past and current EKGs

TABLE 9–2
Location of Myocardial Infarction

Area of Infarction	Leads Showing Wave Changes
Anterior	V1, V2, V3
Diaphragmatic (inferior)	II, III, aVF
Lateral	I, aV1, V5, V6
Posterior (pure)	V1 and V2: tall broad initial R wave, S-T segment depression, and tall upright T wave

Source: Reproduced by permission from: Zipes DP, Andreoli KG: Introduction to electrocardiography. In Andreoli KG, Zipes DP, Wallace AG, et al, eds. Comprehensive Cardiac Care, 6th ed. St. Louis, 1987, The C.V. Mosby Co., 104.

is compulsory. Significant Q waves have the following features: (1) 0.04 second or longer in duration, (2) greater than 4 mm in depth, and (3) appear in leads that do not normally have deep, wide Q waves (i.e., leads other than aVR/V1). In addition, pathologic Q waves are usually present in several leads that reflect the area of infarction (Andreoli et al. 1987, 103). While EKG changes may occur with an acute MI, a normal EKG in no way rules out myocardial ischemia or infarction. History is of major importance.

Characteristic patterns of EKG changes from normal may indicate damage in specific areas of the myocardium as shown in Table 9–2.

The anterior region of the heart is the most common location for MI (Sommers 1984). Occlusion of the left anterior descending coronary artery limits blood flow to the large anterior wall of the left ventricle (Smith 1984) (Fig. 9–5). Because a large amount of muscle mass is often involved, these infarctions may be complicated by hemodynamic compromise resulting from pump failure, heart block, and ventricular aneurysms. The EKG leads most reflective of anterior infarctions are V1, V2, and V3 (Fig. 9–6 *A*).

Occlusion of the right coronary artery limits blood flow to the upper portion of the conduction system and to the inferior (diaphragmatic) portion of the left ventricle (see Fig. 9–5). Occlusion of this coronary artery is particularly dangerous because it supplies the SA and AV nodes in most people. Heart block may appear and often progresses gradually from first or second to third degree. Rupture of papillary muscles, resulting in mitral insufficiency, is not uncommon. When this occurs, a systolic murmur heard best at the apex during systole is present. The EKG leads most reflective of inferior wall MIs are II, III, and aVF (Fig. 9–6 *B*).

Occlusion of the left circumflex coronary artery limits blood flow to the lateral wall of the left ventricle (see Fig. 9–7). A lateral wall MI may manifest as ventricular hypertrophy and heart failure secondary to a bulging ventricular aneurysm. Stasis of blood in the "outpouching" of the aneurysm forms mural thrombi termed *emboli* once they break free and enter the systemic circulation. The nurse should assess peripheral pulses and mental status and should be alert to any patient complaints of numbness or tingling or visual disturbance, as these symptoms may signify microemboli release. The EKG leads most reflective of lateral wall myocardial infarctions are I and AVL (Fig. 9–6 *C*).

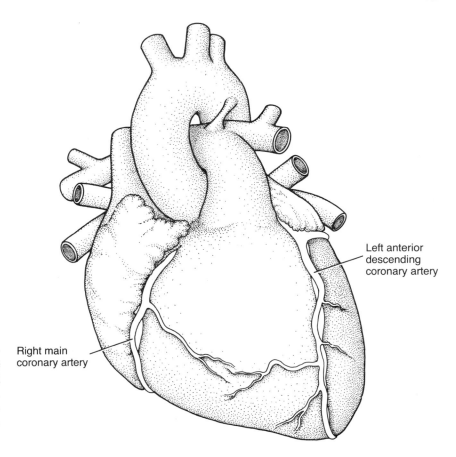

Left anterior
descending
coronary artery

Right main
coronary artery

FIGURE 9–5. *A,* Schematic drawing of the anterior heart showing the left anterior descending and the right main coronary arteries. (Redrawn from Abeloff D. Medical Art: Graphics for Use, Vol. 4, p. 5. © by Williams & Wilkins, 1982.)

Finally, a chest radiogram is likely to be obtained for any patient presenting with chest pain. Although it does not confirm or negate the possibility of a cardiac event, it is of value in reflecting cardiomegaly and congestive heart failure. It is also helpful in the differential diagnosis of chest pain of questionable cause. Cases in point include acute pulmonary embolism, acute pericarditis, and dissecting aneurysms (Rosen et al. 1988, 1367). Portable x-ray machines, although not ideal in terms of visualization, often are necessary in order to avoid catastrophe during radiography.

In summary, the clinical manifestations of myocardial ischemia or infarction are best sorted out by combining history, clinical status, and EKG findings. Further evaluation on an inpatient basis, for those admitted to the hospital, will confirm or negate myocardial damage. Initial myocardial enzyme levels and EKG findings on admission are important as they provide a baseline for comparison with subsequent diagnostic studies.

Treatment and Nursing Care

The focus for patients presenting to the emergency department with signs and symptoms indicative of myocardial ischemia or infarction is twofold: physical and psycho-

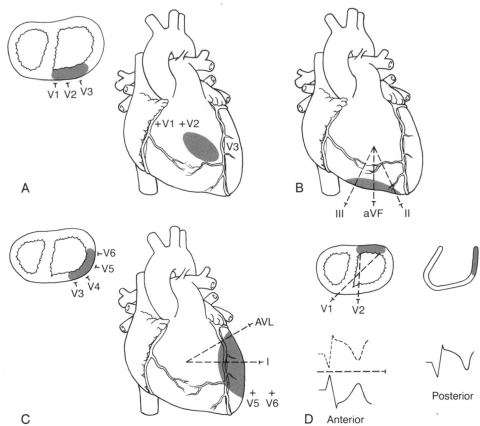

FIGURE 9–6. *A,* Leads demonstrating an anterior MI. *B,* Leads demonstrating an inferior MI. *C,* Leads demonstrating a lateral MI. *D,* Posterior surface shows a Q wave, elevated S-T, and inverted T wave. Leads on the anterior surface demonstrate reciprocal changes of a tall R wave, depressed S-T segment, and tall T wave (mirror image). (Redrawn from Lewis VG. 1987. Nurs Clin North Am 111:24–27.)

logic stabilization. As the clinical presentations of patients with potential cardiac problems is variable, so may be the proportion of nursing time spent on stage I and stage II care. Many people have myocardial infarctions without experiencing any complications. Others develop complications ranging from asymptomatic ventricular ectopy to cardiogenic shock (Sommers 1984).

Stage I nursing care will need to be initiated when individuals with suspected myocardial ischemia, infarction, or both present to the emergency department with life-threatening complications such as dysrhythmias, hypotension, pulmonary edema, or heart failure or a combination of these. Immediate interventions include the support of airway, breathing, and circulation (if needed), the establishment of intravenous access, and EKG monitoring.

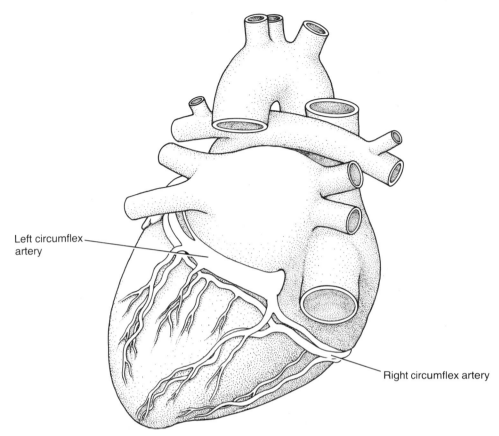

Left circumflex artery

Right circumflex artery

FIGURE 9–7. Schematic drawing of the posterior heart showing the left circumflex coronary artery. (Redrawn from Abeloff D. Medical Art: Graphics for Use, Vol. 4, p. 6. © by Williams & Wilkins, 1982.)

Breathing Pattern, Ineffective, Related to Decreased Cardiac Output Secondary to

• *Imbalance Between Myocardial Oxygen Supply and Demand*

Ensuring a patent airway and effective breathing pattern must be a priority when caring for individuals with alterations in breathing patterns related to compromised cardiac output. Positioning the patient in a sitting or semi-Fowler's position aids in ventilation by reducing pressure on the diaphragm. This position also promotes venous pooling and a decreased cardiac preload. Supplemental oxygen should be started. There is evidence suggesting that an elevation of arterial oxygen tension may reduce infarct size (Maroko 1975; Madias 1976). Oxygen should not be withheld while awaiting an arterial blood gas sample. The age-old concern of interrupting a CO_2 retainer's intrinsic drive for breathing (low Po_2) is not a sound consideration when treating a person in respiratory distress.

TABLE 9–3
Guidelines for Estimating Fio_2 with
Low-Flow Oxygen Devices

100% O_2 Flow Rate (L)*	Fio_2
Nasal cannula	
1	0.24
2	0.28
3	0.32
4	0.36
5	0.40
6	0.44
Oxygen mask	
5–6	0.40
6–7	0.50
7–8	0.60
Mask with Reservoir Bag	
6	0.60
7	0.70
8	0.80
9	0.80+
10	0.80+

Source: Reproduced with permission from Shapiro BA, Harrison
RA, Kacmarek RM, Cane RD: Clinical Application of Respiratory
Care, 3rd ed. Copyright © 1985 by Year Book Medical Publishers,
Inc., Chicago.
* Normal ventilatory pattern is assumed.
Fio_2 = fraction of inspired oxygen.

When oxygen is used prophylactically or in the mildly dyspneic patient, it should be administered by mask or nasal cannula at a flow rate of 4 to 6 l/minute (Andreoli 1983). For patients who are in respiratory distress, as evidenced by the use of accessory muscles, abnormal or worsening ABGs, and the like, a more aggressive means of assisting respiration and ventilation will be necessary. In this situation intubation will provide adequate ventilation and increase the concentration of inspired oxygen (FIo_2) available for exchange in the alveoli. Refer to Table 9–3 as a guideline in estimating FIo_2.

Suctioning is an integral part of airway management and should be done periodically to free the airways of mucus and secretions that interrupt proper ventilation and gas exchange. Caution is necessary to avoid hypoxia and dysrhythmias. Suction should be limited to 5-second periods.

Anxiety, Related to

- *Breathing Pattern Secondary to Compromised Cardiac Output*
- *Alteration in Health Status and Inability to Control, Diminish, or Change Symptom Complex*
- *Fear of Death*

Ongoing explanations, reassurance, and support are necessary to assist patients and their significant others in allaying fear and anxiety. Basic explanations regarding the rationale for diagnostic and therapeutic procedures should be given. Additionally, patients should not be left alone for prolonged periods of time, as they may fear their inability to summon help. Attempts to de-escalate anxiety are extremely important in reducing the sympathetic stimulation that increases heart rate and contractility and oxygen consumption and that contributes to an imbalance between myocardial oxygen supply and demand.

Decreased Cardiac Output, Related to

- *Conduction Disturbances Secondary to Imbalance Between Myocardial Oxygen Supply and Demand*
- *Hypotension Secondary to Congestive Heart Failure in Response to Imbalance Between Myocardial Oxygen Supply and Demand*
- *SA/AV Node Ischemia*
- *IVC Defects*
- *Heart Block*

Intravenous access must be established immediately in individuals with alterations in cardiac output related to conduction disturbances, hypotension, or both. Dextrose and water at a keep-open rate (if hypotension is not related to fluid volume loss) is usually the solution of choice for the administration of emergency medications. Patients will often question the necessity of this invasive procedure. An explanation stating that the prophylaxis is in case of emergency is generally acceptable. Blood for routine laboratory analysis (i.e., CBC and electrolytes, and cardiac enzyme assays) should be drawn prior to or concurrent with starting the IV line. Continuous close monitoring of the patient with alterations in cardiac output is a priority nursing function, and the patient should be immediately placed on a cardiac monitor, and a 12-lead EKG should be done.

Cardiac dysrhythmias represent a common and often serious problem. The patient's hemodynamic status is the key to determining the urgency of treatment. Identification of dysrhythmias in the setting of an acute MI, although necessary, is but a small part of total patient care. Without correlation of symptomatology, physical findings, history, and chief complaint, rhythm identification is insignificant. (Specific drugs for treatment of dysrhythmias are discussed in Chap. 10; see the sections on dysrhythmia interpretation, and management.)

Ongoing assessment and monitoring of vital signs are critical nursing interventions for patients with alterations in cardiac output. Blood pressure is a key factor in evaluating the patient's clinical status. Hypotension may indicate decreased perfusion secondary to a dysrhythmia, a recurrence of ischemia and pump failure, or a response to medications. Since coronary artery perfusion is dependent upon adequate blood pressure, hypotension may well worsen the patient's condition. Of primary concern in the MI patient are left-sided heart failure and consequent pulmonary edema. Parameters reflective of left-sided heart failure include crackles, dyspbe felt cutaneously at the electrode sites. The pads are positioned anteriorly and posteriorly. The positive electrode is attached to the anterior pad, the negative electrode to the posterior pad.

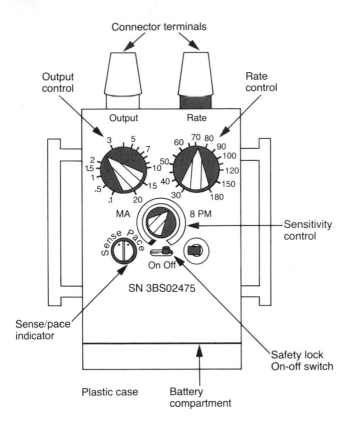

FIGURE 9-8. External pacemaker device.

The patient with an alteration in cardiac output related to SA or AV node ischemia, intraventricular conduction defects, or heart block may require a pacemaker. Transvenous or transthoracic pacemakers, both internal pacemakers, may be inserted as a temporary means of stimulating myocardial electrical activity. The route of entry for a transvenous pacemaker is generally the brachiocephalic or the external-internal jugular vein, although the femoral or subclavian vein may be used. The catheter is advanced by venous blood flow to the desired position in the right atrium or ventricle.

The transthoracic approach involves the passage of a spinal needle (20-gauge) with a stylet in place percutaneously through the left chest directly into the right or left ventricle. The stylet is removed and is replaced by a pacing catheter that is advanced until endocardial contact is made. The needle is removed, leaving the pacer wire in place. Coronary artery trauma, pericardial tamponade, and dysrhythmias are risks incurred by this approach.

Regardless of the means of pacing wire insertion, the external pulse generator is similar in each situation (Fig. 9-8).

The unit is battery operated and has two electrode connections, one positive and the other negative. The settings to be adjusted once the pacemaker is in place are rate, output, sensitivity, and mode. Rate refers to the number of beats per minute. Output signifies power to be generated by the pacemaker. Sensitivity reflects the ability of the pulse generator to sense the patient's intrinsic myocardial electrical activity. This

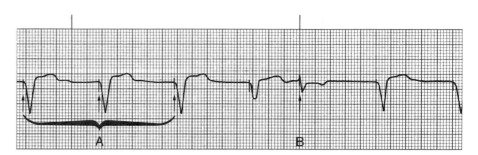

FIGURE 9–9. Pacemaker-driven rhythm: *(A)* Pacemaker spikes rate: 60, *(B)* intrinsic junctional escape beat.

setting is turned to "asynchronous" when demand mode is not being used. The mode relates to two manners of pacing: demand (synchronous) and fixed rate (asynchronous). In demand pacing, the pacer is utilized only when there is a demand for it. This type of pacing is useful when the patient has intermittent drops in heart rate. The pacer senses the patient's myocardial electrical activity. If the heart rate drops below a predetermined parameter, the pacer takes over and discharges at the preset rate. Fixed rate, or asynchronous, pacing represents a continuous form of electrical stimulation of the myocardium. Patients with bradycardia refractory to drug therapy or asystole are candidates for this type of pacing mode. Nursing care is focused toward monitoring pacer function by noting spikes on the EKG rhythm strip prior to the QRS complex and assessing vital signs to evaluate peripheral perfusion (Fig. 9–9).

External pacing devices are finding increasing use in emergency situations. Although this means of pacing does not substitute for transvenous or permanent pacing devices, it does provide a quick and easy method of pacing temporarily. Most external pacing devices are part of a standard monitor and defibrillator unit. The pacing portion of the unit is designed to function as either a fixed rate or demand system. Electrodes are attached to special skin pads. Current can be adjusted between 1 and 200 millivolts. Generally, 50 to 125 millivolts is sufficient to capture the myocardium. This current is enough to stimulate cardiac activity yet not enough to cause patient discomfort. Patients should be warned of the tingling sensation that will be felt cutaneously at the electrode sites. The pads are positioned anteriorly and posteriorly. The positive electrode is attached to the anterior pad, the negative electrode to the posterior pad.

Pain, Related to Lactic Acidosis, Secondary to

• *Imbalance Between Myocardial Oxygen Supply and Demand*

Nitroglycerin (NTG) and morphine sulfate (Mso$_4$) are the preferred agents for pain relief in persons experiencing alterations in comfort related to an imbalance between myocardial oxygen supply and demand. Both serve to increase perfusion of coronary vessels, although by different mechanisms.

Nitroglycerin works by relaxing vascular smooth muscle and, to a lesser extent, by dilating the coronary arteries. The effect on venous capacity serves to decrease

TABLE 9-4
Characteristics of Commonly Used Nitrate Preparations

Form	Onset of Action (min)	Peak (hours)	Duration (hours)
Isosorbide Dinitrate (Isordil)			
Sublingual	2–5	1	1–2
Chewable	3–4	1	3–4
Oral	20–40	1–2	4–6
Tembids	Sustained release	6	8–10
NTG Ointment (Nitro-Bid; Nitrol)	20–40	1–2	2–12
NTG Topical (Nitrodisc; Nitro-Dur; Transderm-Nitro)	30	Slow release	24

Source: From Conley SK, Small RE, eds. 1983. Dimensions of Critical Care, JB Lippincott, 20.

preload or the amount of blood returning to the heart, thereby benefiting those patients in particular who have signs of congestive heart failure. As venous return is reduced, the ventricular filling pressures likewise fall, resulting in lessened ventricular workload and a fall in myocardial oxygen demand.

NTG is supplied in many forms (Table 9–4), each of which has unique characteristics. Sublingual nitroglycerin is the most commonly used form. It is supplied in 0.3, 0.4, and 0.6 mg tablets and should act in 3 to 5 minutes for a period of 1 to 2 hours (Conley 1983). Because of potential hypotension related to venous dilation, vital signs should be monitored prior to and during the first few minutes after NTG administration. NTG is usually not given if the blood pressure is less than 90 mmHg systolic. The patient should also be warned of possibly feeling lightheaded, dizzy, or flushed or of having a headache. Patients may present to the ED with transdermal NTG patches in place. It is important to check for these patches and remove them before administering sublingual or IV NTG in order to avoid a precipitous fall in blood pressure.

Intravenous NTG has joined sublingual and cutaneous administration as a means of reducing the pain of myocardial ischemia. Although the goal of therapy is the same as with other nitrates, the IV route allows titration of the solution based on the myocardial response to the drug. Titration and maintenance of the infusion are dependent upon the S-T segment response, the patient's subjective interpretation of the pain, and hemodynamic response (Chyun 1983). An improvement in coronary artery perfusion is reflected by normal S-T segments and a diminished sense of pain. Should the patient's systolic blood pressure drop below 90 mmHg, the drip rate must be diminished.

Special IV tubing and glass IV bottles are necessary for use with NTG solutions because of the absorption occurring with polyvinyl chloride tubings and plastic bags. Commercially prepared NTG solutions are packaged with special tubing. Mixture of other drugs in or through the same line should be avoided, since little is known about compatibility of NTG with other drugs (Chyun 1983). An infusion pump is necessary to assure accurate infusion rates. Solutions are generally started at 5 μg/min and increased in 5 μg increments every 3 to 5 minutes. Continuous monitoring of blood pressure is necessary whether manually, by arterial line pressure monitoring, or by a noninvasive automatic blood pressure monitor.

When nitroglycerin has not been effective in relieving chest pain resultant from myocardial ischemia, MSO_4 is used. Intravenous analgesics are the most effective means of relieving severe pain and avoiding the confusion from elevated serum enzymes that may result from intramuscular injection (Eliot 1982). Additionally, medications may not be absorbed readily into the blood stream when a decreased cardiac output exists. Mso_4 has excellent analgesic as well as sedative effects. The latter serves to reduce the apprehension so often associated with myocardial pain. Mso_4 is also known to cause peripheral vasodilation, which contributes to venous pooling and a resultant reduction in preload. Reduced diastolic filling pressures translate into reduction in workload of the heart. With less blood to pump in each stroke volume, the oxygen requirements of the myocardium are reduced. The usual dosage for Mso_4 is 2 to 4 mg as an intravenous bolus over 1 to 2 minutes and repeated as necessary for pain relief (Rosen 1988, 1377).

Ongoing evaluation of the effectiveness of pain control is imperative. A ten-point scale is often utilized to allow patients to quantify, or rate, their perception of the pain; one equals pain-free, and ten represents maximum pain. This method allows a means of judging the effect of vasodilator or analgesic or both therapies. One can also assess pain by noting objective manifestations. Patients who consistently grimace or have a "beaten" look are obviously continuing to experience pain. Increased muscle tone may indicate intense pain in some, whereas listlessness may indicate intense pain in others. Ongoing and periodic assessments are crucial to appropriate management. The autonomic response to pain — evidenced by diaphoresis, slight elevations in blood pressure and heart rate, pupillary dilation, and increased respiratory rate — although frequently present initially should abate with appropriate therapy.

Injury, Actual or Potential, Related to Myocardial Ischemia Secondary to

• *Imbalance Between Myocardial Oxygen Supply and Demand*

When actual or potential myocardial injury occurs as the result of a decreased cardiac blood supply, coronary artery blockage from a clot, atherosclerotic lesion, or spasm has occurred. Streptokinase and urokinase have recently been investigated and deemed safe and efficient in achieving re-perfusion and alleviating ischemia in a majority of patients in the acute phase of myocardial infarction (Bullas 1983). However, the ability of such restoration of flow to preserve myocardial function has not yet been demonstrated (Missri 1984).

Streptokinase is a thrombolytic agent that is derived from the group C hemolytic streptococci. It converts plasminogen to the proteolytic enzyme plasmin, which is responsible for clot lysis (Anderson 1985). Urokinase, often used in patients with hypersensitivity to streptokinase, is an enzymatic protein and a direct plasminogen activator.

Although streptokinase and urokinase are effective in achieving coronary thrombolysis, the activation of plasminogen leads to generalized lysis of blood components and possibly to bleeding. Alternatively, tissue plasminogen activator (T-PA), a naturally occurring protease, converts plasminogen to plasmin primarily after binding to fibrin clots. The plasmin concentration increases mainly at the clot rather than in the systemic circulation (Sobel 1984).

The initiation of thrombolytic therapy should be as prompt as possible. Emergency nurses, aware of guidelines for patient selection, can promptly identify suitable candidates for this therapy and thus can expedite care. Generally, patients who (1) are seen within 4 hours of onset of chest pain, (2) have EKG evidence of acute MI (S-T segment elevation or depression of greater than 2 mm and new Q waves) and (3) have no contraindication to anticoagulant therapy are selected. Postthrombolytic patients are kept on anticoagulants to minimize the possibility of rethrombosis. Invasive procedures such as arterial blood gas sampling should be avoided, as they provide a potential source for hemorrhage.

Although thrombolytic agents are generally administered in intensive care settings, they may be initiated in the emergency department. Ventricular dysrhythmias are commonly encountered after thrombolysis and in fact are evidence that reperfusion has occurred. These dysrhythmias are treated with lidocaine.

Intracoronary streptokinase must be given in the cardiac catheterization laboratory under fluoroscopy. The emergency nurse's role is to prepare the patient by brief explanations of what is to be done, to obtain admission for laboratory tests and radiography, and to assure that an informed consent has been obtained by the physician.

Knowledge Deficit, Potential, Related to

• *Etiology, Pathophysiology, Treatments, Complications, and Prognosis of Illness*

It is the responsibility of the emergency nurse to educate cardiac patients regarding their disease. Although this may be impossible with respect to the acutely ill or unstable patient, many patients present without complications and in stable condition. Patients should be aware of the events that precipitated their chest pain or discomfort. They should also be informed of what is being done in the emergency department — rationales and the intended plan of care. Friends, family members, or both should be included in these explanations.

Evaluation

Close patient monitoring is critical to the nursing care of patients experiencing myocardial ischemia or infarction. The focus is on frequent assessment of vital signs, cardiac rhythm, fluid intake and output, and pain or comfort levels. The nurse is alert to changes based on his or her assessments and prioritizes actions and interventions in accordance with the often-changing clinical picture of the patient. In short, evaluation of nursing interventions is ongoing, based on the patient's total experience.

Desired outcomes, suggesting stabilization of the patient's condition, include the following: (1) an effective breathing pattern demonstrated by arterial blood gas values within normal limits, a statement by the patient of ease in breathing, and clear bilateral breath sounds on auscultation; (2) decreased patient anxiety; (3) effective cardiac output reflected by blood pressure within normal limits and clear mentation; (4) absence of pain or discomfort; and (5) a stable and effective cardiac rhythm on the monitor.

CONGESTIVE HEART FAILURE

Congestive heart failure (CHF) refers to a symptom complex representing a decrease in cardiac function. Congestive heart failure may be right- or left-sided; however, most commonly both right- and left-sided failure occur together. A diminished cardiac output as well as pulmonary or venous congestion or both are usually present.

Etiology

There are multiple causes of congestive heart failure, the most common in adults being valvular disease such as mitral and aortic stenosis or regurgitation. Hypertension, pericarditis, and myocardial infarction are other well-known causes in adults. Children most commonly develop heart failure secondary to a congenital cardiac anomaly.

Pathophysiology

Since congestive heart failure involves an alteration in blood flow dynamics, a brief review of blood flow through the heart is in order. Venous blood from the inferior and superior venae cavae flows to the right atrium at a mean pressure of 4 to 12 mmHg. Blood flow is from a region of greater pressure to a region of lesser pressure. Therefore, most of ventricular filling occurs passively in early diastole as blood flows from the right atrium (where the pressure is 4 to 12 mmHg) to the right ventricle (where the pressure is 0 to 5 mmHg). Near the end of diastole, the atria contract and eject approximately 30% more blood into the ventricles. When this "atrial kick" is absent, as in certain rhythm disturbances such as atrial fibrillation, the decreased diastolic filling of the ventricles may result in a significantly reduced stroke volume and cardiac output.

The right ventricle ejects blood through the pulmonic valve into the pulmonary artery. During systole the right intraventricular pressure increases to 25 mmHg. As seen in Figure 9–10, the pulmonary vasculature is a low-pressure system. Once again, blood flows down a pressure gradient from the right ventricle, where the pressure during systole is 25 mmHg, to the pulmonary vasculature, where the pressure is approximately 15 mmHg. Elevated pulmonary vascular pressures occur when either flow or resistance to blood flow is increased. Left-sided congestive heart failure and pulmonary edema, pulmonary embolus, or pulmonary fibrosis result in elevated pulmonary pressures.

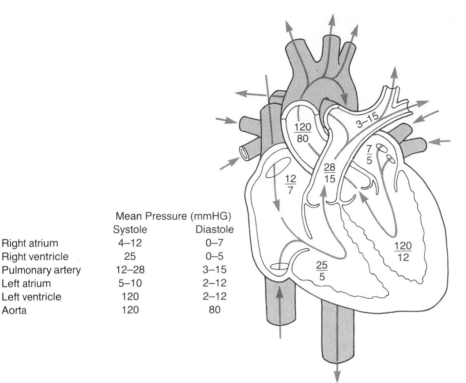

Mean Pressure (mmHG)		
	Systole	Diastole
Right atrium	4–12	0–7
Right ventricle	25	0–5
Pulmonary artery	12–28	3–15
Left atrium	5–10	2–12
Left ventricle	120	2–12
Aorta	120	80

FIGURE 9–10 Cardiac chambers and mean systolic and diastolic pressures within them. (Redrawn from Abeloff D. Medical Art: Graphics for Use, Vol. 4, p. 10. © by Williams & Wilkins, 1982.)

A pressure gradient is also responsible for blood flow from the pulmonary system into the left atrium. As Figure 9–10 demonstrates, the left side of the heart is a high-pressure system.

Preload and afterload are terms used to define elements of blood flow that affect myocardial filling and ejection. Preload refers to myocardial fiber stretch, which is in part affected by the volume of blood returning to the heart. Blood return to the heart is determined by total blood volume, vascular capacity, ventricular contractility, and ventilation.

Afterload is determined by the systemic vascular resistance or any obstruction to outflow of blood from the ventricles, as in hypertension and aortic stenosis.

In congestive heart failure, end-diastolic intraventricular chamber pressures become elevated. When this occurs, the ventricles cannot empty adequately during systole, and the left end-systolic intraventricular pressures become elevated. During diastole, the ventricle continues to receive additional blood from the atria, which further increases the intraventricular pressure. This increase in intraventricular pressure (i.e., preload) in addition to the increase in fluid retention (triggered by a reduction in glomerular filtration rate that stimulates the renin-angiotensin system in response to a reduced cardiac output) augments cardiac output via the Frank-Starling mechanism. The relation, stated simply, is that the force of myocardial contraction is dependent upon the amount of fiber stretch. It reflects the heart's ability to adjust to changing blood flow; the greater the heart is filled in diastole, the greater will be the quantity of blood ejected (stroke volume) during systole. However, there is a limit to this compensatory mechanism wherein additional stretch does not improve the stroke volume and in fact causes a deterioration in the amount of blood ejected from the ventricles with each contraction. Transmission of elevated pressures from the ventricles to the atria and subsequently to the pulmonary capillary bed on the left side and the vena cava on the right side is responsible for the characteristic signs and symptoms of CHF.

Pulmonary congestion is responsible for dyspnea. As the left atrial pressure increases beyond 18 mmHg, fluid leaves the pulmonary capillaries and enters the interstitial space. The accumulation of interstitial edema reduces pulmonary compliance and increases airway resistance, producing the sensation of dyspnea. As pulmonary compliance is lessened and airway resistance increases, the right ventricle has greater difficulty ejecting blood through the pulmonic valve into the pulmonary vasculature. Right-sided CHF may then result. Elevated right-sided pressures are reflected by jugular venous distention and peripheral edema as noted especially in the lower extremities. Liver engorgement in right-sided failure can be determined by eliciting the hepatojugular reflex. This reflex results in jugular venous distention when pressure is exerted on the liver by palpation. Right-sided heart failure refers to the symptom complex associated with elevated heart pressures and systemic venous congestion. Left-sided heart failure is the clinical state produced by elevated left-sided heart pressures and pulmonary congestion.

Clinical Manifestations

Left ventricular dysfunction results in elevated left ventricular end-diastolic pressure (LVEDP) with subsequent pulmonary congestion. Patients may subjectively describe the pulmonary congestion as shortness of breath (SOB), dyspnea on exertion (DOE), orthopnea, and paroxysmal nocturnal dyspnea (PND). When right-sided CHF is present, an increase in systemic circulatory volume and subsequent organ congestion are responsible for the patient's subjective complaints of weight gain, extremity swelling, and abdominal pain. Abdominal pain and shortness of breath are most likely related to ascites and subsequent diaphragmatic displacement. Palpitations, lightheadedness, dizziness, and loss of consciousness in addition to constitutional symptoms (i.e., lethargy, anorexia, nausea and vomiting, and anxiety) may also be described by the patient.

As with subjective symptomatology, objective findings may also be quite varied in patients with CHF and are dependent upon the severity as well as on whether left- or right-sided failure or both is present. Physical examination of a patient with moderate-to-severe CHF usually reveals an ill-appearing individual who is tachycardic, has a weak, thready pulse, and is hypotensive, with a narrowed pulse pressure. Pulse rate and blood pressure vary depending on the degree of cardiac dysfunction and compensatory mechanisms in play. He or she may exhibit pale, cool, and diaphoretic skin, and possibly even an altered mental status.

When left-sided heart failure is present, some form of respiratory distress is nearly always present. Most commonly, this respiratory distress is manifested as rapid, labored, and shallow breathing. Blood-tinged, frothy sputum may also be evident, especially in the face of pulmonary edema. Cheyne-Stokes respirations are an ominous sign. Pulmonary auscultation will reveal crackles bilaterally, audible

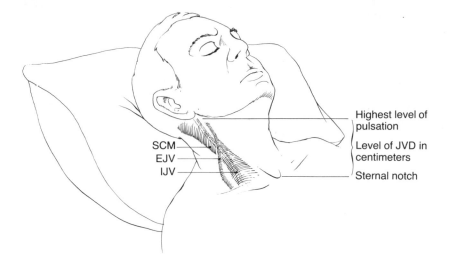

SCM
EJV
IJV

Highest level of
pulsation

Level of JVD in
centimeters

Sternal notch

FIGURE 9–11 Jugular venous distention. Note the vertical distance between the highest point at which pulsation of the jugular can be seen and the angle of Louis (sternal notch). In the figure, jugular venous distention can be seen as the highest level of pulsation at the angle of the mandible. The patient with a normal central venous pressure will have an approximately 2-cm difference between the sternal notch and the highest level of pulsation.

wheezing, or both. Arterial blood gases typically demonstrate hypoxemia with varying degrees of respiratory acidosis or alkalosis, depending on the patient's rate and depth of ventilations and degree of metabolic compensation. Chest radiographs usually show evidence of cardiomegaly and often of pulmonary edema, depending on the severity of left-sided failure. When right-sided failure is present, objective findings usually demonstrate abdominal organomegaly, jugular vein distention (Fig. 9–11), elevated central venous pressures (higher than 12 cm H_2O), and peripheral pitting edema.

Patients with symptoms suggesting CHF often have a multitude of medical problems. They may exhibit behavior that reflects frustration with the chronic nature and frequent exacerbations of their heart disease. Additionally, patients are often anxious as they are aware of the seriousness of their illness and the relationship that exists between a functional heart and quality of life.

Treatment and Nursing Care

The interventions for the patient in congestive heart failure relate mainly to strengthening ventricular function in an effort to increase cardiac output, reducing intravascular volume, aiding the patient's oxygenation status, and reducing cardiac workload. Although patients who present to the emergency department may be experiencing varying degrees of CHF, stage I nursing care needs to be instituted in most instances. Intravenous access should be immediately established, and supplemental oxygen, ventilatory assistance, or both should be provided when indicated. Arterial blood gas analysis and chest radiography should also be ordered as soon as possible. Continuous cardiac monitoring is initiated, and a 12-lead EKG is obtained. Emergency equipment (i.e., intubation tray, crash cart, and so forth) and drugs must be readily available should the patient experience pulmonary edema or cardiogenic shock.

Decreased Cardiac Output Related to Left Ventricular Dysfunction Secondary to

- *Myocardial Infarction*
- *Valvular Disease*
- *Pericarditis*
- *Hypertension*
- *Other (e.g., Hypotension, Shock, Dysrhythmias)*

Initial interventions for the patient who presents with an alteration in cardiac output related to left ventricular dysfunction are similar to those relating to any individual with a cardiac problem. Stage I nursing interventions, previously described, should be instituted. Nursing care, as with most cardiovascular emergencies, must be dynamic and alternate between stage I and stage II care. Medical therapeutics to optimize cardiac function and diminish symptomatology associated with cardiac dysfunction include the administration of diuretics, vasodilators, and positive inotropic agents.

The most commonly used diuretic is furosemide (Lasix), which decreases the circulating blood volume, thus decreasing preload and the work of the heart. Nitroglycerin and Mso_4 are commonly used vasodilators. By decreasing afterload, nitroglycerin decreases cardiac workload; morphine sulfate, in addition to having sedative properties, also acts to reduce cardiac workload by decreasing venous return (preload) via systemic vasodilation. Digoxin works to strengthen cardiac contractility by its positive inotropic properties.

Impaired Gas Exchange Related to Elevated Pulmonary Capillary Pressure Secondary to

- *Alteration in Cardiac Output (Decreased)*

Supplemental oxygen therapy should be anticipated for the patient with impaired gas exchange related to elevated pulmonary capillary pressures. As in the myocardial infarction patient, 5 to 6 liters through nasal cannula is adequate. Blood gas analysis and subjective clinical response to therapy will dictate changes in the amount and method of oxygen administered. Respiratory assessment is performed as often as necessary to determine changing patterns of ventilation and pulmonary congestion. Intubation equipment should be readily available. Elevating the head of the bed to 45 degrees will allow optimal lung expansion and ventilation and promote patient comfort.

Fluid Volume Excess Related to Decreased Cardiac Output Secondary to

- *Ventricular Dysfunction*

Monitoring of fluid volume status is extremely important for the patient with fluid volume excess related to decreased cardiac output. Measurements of intake and output, jugular venous distention, and respiratory findings reflect the total fluid volume balance. The administration of furosemide (Lasix) will decrease preload by its diuretic effect. Exertion necessary to use the bedpan for frequent urination may be taxing for the compromised individual. An indwelling urinary catheter may aid in patient comfort and safety and provide an ongoing means of assessing diuretic effect. Intravenous fluid administration should be limited to a keep-open rate. Serum electrolytes, especially potassium and sodium, must be monitored for depletion related to diuresis.

Tissue Perfusion, Potential Alteration in, Related to Cardiogenic Shock Secondary to

• *Alteration of Cardiac Output*

Therapies designed to increase the strength of ventricular contractions should be anticipated for the patient with potential alteration in tissue perfusion related to cardiogenic shock. The effect of dopamine (Intropin) on alpha, beta, and dopaminergic receptor sites causes an increase in heart rate and contractility. It also causes peripheral vasoconstriction and promotes blood return to the heart. Vasodilation of the renal and splanchnic vasculature promotes increased renal perfusion and improved diuresis. A potential complication of inotropic agents in the patient with myocardial dysfunction is the extension of myocardial injury. Since the desired effects of increasing cardiac output require additional myocardial work and consequent oxygen supply, the already taxed heart may be unable to provide the necessary ingredients to promote myocardial function.

The intraaortic balloon pump (IABP) is a counterpulsation device that may be used to assist the failing heart by decreasing afterload and increasing coronary artery perfusion. The balloon, placed within the aorta just distal to the aortic valve (where the coronary arteries fill), inflates during diastole to allow improved coronary artery filling. During systole, the balloon deflates, causing reduced resistance to blood flow through the aorta and therefore reduces afterload.

Evaluation

Once the patient is out of the acute stage of illness, stage II nursing care may dominate the remainder of the hospital stay. Frequent monitoring of vital signs, EKG rhythm, and intake and output must continue. Patients recovering from congestive heart failure should exhibit a decreased heart rate, normal blood pressure, increased urine output, reduced jugular venous distention, improved breath sounds, reduced dyspnea and hypoxemia, and a diminished anxiety level.

AORTIC ANEURYSM AND DISSECTION

A true aortic aneurysm is an abnormal widening that involves all three layers of the aortic wall. The basic defect is destruction of elastic fibers in the medial layer, which

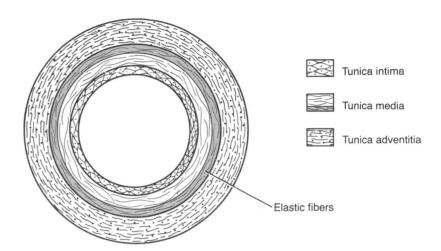

	Tunica intima
	Tunica media
	Tunica adventitia

Elastic fibers

FIGURE   9–12.   Anatomic
layers of the aorta.

permits the remaining fibrous tissue to stretch and leads to an increase in diameter
that in turn raises wall tension. As this process leads to further enlargement, rupture
becomes increasingly possible (Dalen 1983). Acute aortic dissection occurs secondary to a tear in the intima, or inner lining of the aorta, which allows blood to dissect
between this and the medial layer. As the dissection progresses, blood flow through
arterial branches of the aorta becomes blocked, and blood flow to the organs they
serve is compromised. The outer (adventitial) layer remains intact (Fig. 9–12).

Pathophysiology

Nearly all aneurysms in the abdominal aorta are caused by arteriosclerosis. The
majority of victims are men over age 60 and more than half are associated with
hypertension (Dalen 1983). The primary defect permitting dissection is necrosis of
the medial layer caused by increased hemodynamic stress within the vessel from
hypertension, pregnancy, bicuspid aortic valve, and coarctation (Marfan's syndrome
has also been associated) (Woods 1986).

   Aortic dissection can be classified into either three or two categories, based upon
anatomic location involved (Fig. 9–13).

Clinical Manifestations

Patients who have an aortic aneurysm or a dissecting aortic aneurysm may complain
of a sudden onset of severe anterior chest pain radiating to the interscapular area. Low
back and abdominal pain may occur if the area affected is the abdominal aorta. There
may be variation in right- and left-sided blood pressures. A murmur of aortic regurgitation can be heard if the dissection proceeds proximally. Hemopericardium and
pericardial tamponade can occur in type A (Cooley classification) dissections. A
widened mediastinum on chest radiographs suggests a diagnosis of aortic dissection.

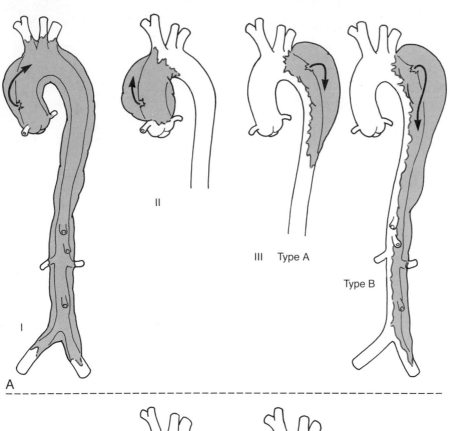

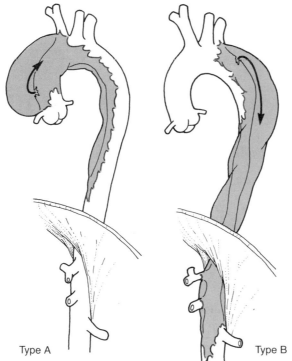

FIGURE 9-13. *A*, DeBakey classification of dissecting aneurysms of the thoracic aorta. *B*, Cooley classification of dissecting aneurysms, based upon site of origin. Indications for surgical intervention vary between the two types, especially in the acute cases. In type A aneurysms, the intimal tear occurs transversely above the level of the coronary orifices. Type A cases may have extension of the dissection into the descending and abdominal aortas or beyond. In this type, aortic valve regurgitation frequently results. Injury to coronary arteries may occur. In type B aneurysms, the site of origin is distal to the aortic arch, and the dissection proceeds distally. In some instances, the dissection may extend proximally into the ascending aorta. (Redrawn from Cooley DA. 1986. Surgical Treatment of Aortic Aneurysm. WB Saunders, 44–45.)

Treatment and Nursing Care

When an aortic dissection is suspected in the emergency setting, the patient must be monitored closely. The diagnostic evaluation should proceed quickly. A large-bore intravenous line should be initiated and the patient's blood should be typed and cross-matched for transfusion should surgery become necessary. The patient should be placed on the cardiac monitor. Blood pressure, if elevated, is reduced to normal by intravenous infusion of sodium nitroprusside (Nipride). A chest radiograph should be ordered immediately and the patient should be scheduled for angiography.

Anxiety, Potential, Related to

- *Sudden Change in Health Status*

Patients who have experienced a sudden change in health status will be anxious. Answering questions and responding to concerns regarding the diagnostic phase of care may help to allay anxiety. The patient needs support of friends and family and should be allowed to see them as requested.

SUMMARY

The patient presenting to the emergency department with cardiovascular disease presents a challenge to the emergency nurse. A thorough understanding of cardiovascular assessment and clinical manifestations associated with cardiovascular disease contributes to expeditious care and sets the framework for an optimal patient experience. By using a nursing diagnosis framework, interventions can be methodically addressed. Psychosocial support is extremely important in reducing the anxiety and discomfort that so often accompanies an acute cardiovascular event.

In order to contribute to the reduction in incidence, morbidity, and mortality of heart disease in the United States, information on community programs related to prevention of heart disease and health promotion is vital. Patients who are in the high-risk category for development of cardiovascular disease should be informed of such programs. Such teaching is probably best done when patients present with minor emergencies. One of our overall nursing goals for all patients treated in the emergency setting should be prevention of cardiovascular disease.

REFERENCES

Alpert JS. 1984. Physiopathology of the Cardiovascular System. Boston, Little, Brown & Company.

Alpert JS, Rippe JM. 1985. Manual of Cardiovascular Diagnosis and Therapy, 2nd ed. Boston, Little, Brown & Company, 36.

Anderson C. 1985. Patient with acute myocardial infarction receiving streptokinase therapy in the emergency department. J Emerg Nurs 2:14.

Andreoli KG, Zipes DP, Wallace AG, et al. 1987. Comprehensive Cardiac Care, 6th ed. St. Louis, CV Mosby.

Blowers MG, Sims RS. 1984. How to Read An

EKG. Oradell, N.J., Medical Economics Books, p. 6.

Bullas J, Pfister S. 1983. Are you listening? Crit Care Nurse 3:16.

Bullas J, Talmadge E. 1983. Thrombolytic therapy in acute evolving myocardial infarction. Crit Care Nurse 3:34–37.

Chung EK, Chung LS. 1983. Introduction to Clinical Cardiology, Continuing Education Series. New York, Karger, 140.

Chyun DA. 1983. IV nitroglycerin in ischemic heart disease. Dimen Crit Care 2:10.

Conley SK, Small RE. 1983. Administering IV nitroglycerin: nursing implications. Dimens Crit Care 2:20.

Crumpley LA, Rinkenburger RL. 1983. An overview of antiarrhythmic drugs. Crit Care Nurse 3:58.

Dalen J. 1983. Diseases of the aorta. In Harrison's Principles of Internal Medicine, 10th ed. Braunwald E, Isselbacher KJ & Petersdorf RG, et al, eds. New York, McGraw-Hill Book Co, 1448.

DeWood MA, Spores J, Notske R, et al. 1980. Prevalence of total coronary occlusion during the early hours of transmural myocardial infarction. N Engl J Med 303:897–901.

Eliot RS, 1982. Cardiac Emergencies. Mount Kisco, N.Y., Futura Publishing Co, 147.

Froelicher Victor F, Atwood Edwin J. 1986. Cardiac Disease. A Logical Approach Considering DRGs. Chicago, Year Book Medical Publishers, 90.

Guyton AC. 1981. Textbook of Medical Physiology, 6th ed. Philadelphia, WB Saunders, 13.

Hammond BB, Lee G. 1984. Quick Reference to Emergency Nursing. Philadelphia, JB Lippincott, 163.

Hudak CM, Gallo BM, Lohr T. 1986. Critical Care Nursing, 4th ed. Philadelphia, JB Lippincott, 112.

Jourard S. 1963. Personal Adjustment, 2nd ed. New York, Macmillan, 121–146.

Lie KL, Wellens JH, et al. 1974. Lidocaine in the prevention of primary ventricular fibrillation: a double-blind, randomized study of 212 consecutive patients. N Engl J Med 291:1324–1326.

Madias JE, Hood WB, Jr. 1976. Reduction of precordial ST segment elevation in patients with anterior myocardial infarction by oxygen breathing. Circulation 53:198–200.

Maroko PR, Radvany P, Braunwald E, et al. 1975. Reduction of infarct size by oxygen inhalation following acute coronary occlusion. Circulation 52:360–368.

Missri JC, Ide PA, Williams CB. 1984. A New Therapeutic Approach in Fibrinolytic Therapy: Intra-Coronary Streptokinase. Heart Lung 13:177.

Oliva PB, Breckenridge JC. 1977. Arteriographic evidence of coronary arterial spasm in acute myocardial infarction. Circulation 56:366.

Pantridge JF, Geddes JS. 1967. A mobile intensive care unit in the management of myocardial infarction. Lancet 2:271–273.

Rose RM, Lewis AH, Fewkes J, et al. 1974. Occurrence of arrhythmias during the first hour in acute myocardial infarction (abstract). Circulation 50 (suppl 3):111–121.

Rosen P, Baker F, Barkin R, et al. 1988. Emergency Medicine: Concepts and Clinical Practice. St. Louis, CV Mosby.

Smith CE. 1984. Assessment under pressure: when your patient says, "My chest hurts." Nursing 144:36–37.

Sobel BE, Gross RN, Robison AK. 1984. Thrombolysis, clot selectivity, and kinetics. Circulation 70:160–164.

Sweetwood HM. 1983. Clinical Electrocardiography for Nurses. Rockville, MD, Aspen, 62.

VanMeter M, Lavine P. 1977. Reading EKGs Correctly. Jenkintown, Intermed Communications, 148.

Williams ES. 1981. Supraventricular tachycardias. Heart Lung 10:634–643.

Woods JW. 1986. Hypertension in adults. In Edlich RF, Spyker DA, eds. Current Emergency Therapy, 3rd ed. Rockville, Md, Aspen, 339.

Wyman MG, Hammersmith L. 1974. Comprehensive treatment plan for the prevention of primary ventricular fibrillation in acute myocardial infarction. Am J Cardiol 33:661–667.

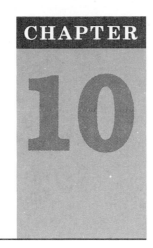

Stephanie Kitt, RN MSN

Dysrhythmia Interpretation and Management

Cardiac dysrhythmias represent a common and often serious problem in emergency department patients. The patient's hemodynamic status is the key to determining the urgency of treatment. Identification of dysrhythmias in the setting of an acute myocardial infarction (MI), although necessary, is but a small part of total patient care. Without correlation of behavior, physical findings, history, and chief complaint, therapeutic modalities cannot be determined. This chapter reviews the characteristics, significance, and treatment of dysrhythmias. Cardiac monitoring provides a means to evaluate physiologic processes. The effects of interventions are readily demonstrated. Once an intervention is instituted, it is critical that immediate evaluation begin and continue throughout the crisis period.

ASSESSMENT

There are several groups of patients who require cardiac monitoring. Patients with complaints that suggest cardiac dysfunction should be monitored for cardiac dysrhythmias (refer to Chap. 9). In addition, individuals with a change in mental status, drug overdose, seizure activity, respiratory distress, or who are in shock require close and continuous monitoring for rhythm disturbances. In short, anyone who is acutely ill, who has the potential to deteriorate in clinical status, or who is receiving therapy that may alter the cardiovascular status should be placed on the cardiac monitor.

Once the patient is attached to the monitor, the rhythm should be evaluated and a rhythm strip should be obtained and attached to the emergency department record. Cardiac rate, rhythm, PR interval, and QRS duration should be noted. Since patients who require cardiac monitoring may deteriorate in clinical condition, establishing intravenous access is crucial. Assessment should proceed as discussed in other chapters for individual conditions.

ETIOLOGY AND PATHOPHYSIOLOGY

There are numerous precipitating causes of dysrhythmias. Cardiac rhythm disturbance may occur as a result of a primary cardiac disorder, as a secondary response to a systemic problem, or as a complication of drug toxicity or electrolyte imbalance (Canobbio 1986).

The pathogenesis of cardiac dysrhythmias may be classified into abnormalities of impulse formation (sinus, atrial, ventricular) or impulse conduction or a combination of both (Hoffman and Cranefield 1964). Electrophysiologic mapping, a specialized procedure performed to identify origins of dysrhythmia formation and pathways of impulse conduction, has led to more precise medical and surgical management of patients with highly refractory tachydysrhythmias.

It is thought that automaticity and reentry are the two primary mechanisms for formation of premature beats—whether atrial, junctional, or ventricular in origin. Increased automaticity occurs when a myocardial cell develops a leaky membrane

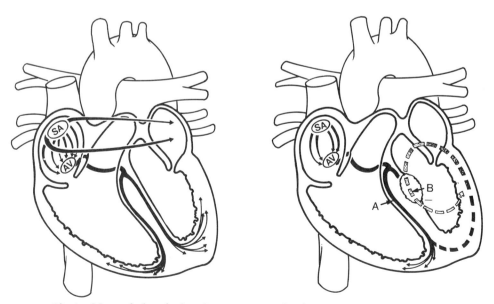

FIGURE 10–1. Normal electrical and reentrant conduction.

allowing passage of ions, particularly Na, into the cell (Guyton 1981). This cell reaches threshold and depolarizes prior to sinus node depolarization. A premature beat results. The second phenomenon related to the development of premature complexes is reentry whereby an ischemic area causes a unidirectional block in one of the fibers of a conduction pathway (Fig. 10–1). The electrical impulse cannot pass through the blocked area (*B* in the figure). The unaffected pathway *(A)* allows the impulse to spread through the normal pathway. The impulse then makes a circuit and travels in a retrograde fashion through the ischemic area to depolarize the tissue above the blocked site, which is in a relatively refractory state. This gives rise to an ectopic impulse.

TREATMENT AND NURSING CARE

All patients who exhibit cardiac dysrhythmias warrant the following nursing diagnosis.

Decreased Cardiac Output, Potential or Actual, Related to

- *Heart Rate (Bradycardia or Tachycardia)*
- *Cardiac Rhythm Abnormality*
- *Conduction Disturbance*

Any dysrhythmia may have a significant negative hemodynamic effect, making early recognition and treatment vital. Unrecognized or untreated dysrhythmias may lead to a fall in cardiac output, an increase in myocardial oxygen consumption, more lethal dysrhythmias and pump failure (Lewis 1987). Appropriate nursing interventions may include the following (adapted from Lewis 1987, 30):

1. Continuous cardiac monitoring noting heart rate, rhythm, frequency and progression of rhythm abnormalities.

2. Treatment of precipitating causes of dysrhythmias—pain, anxiety, fever, hypoxia, electrolyte and acid-base imbalances, drugs, congestive heart failure, hypotension.

3. Maintenance of a patent IV line for administration of antidysrhythmic medications.

4. Administration of antidysrhythmics as ordered.

5. Monitoring of effects of medications that may affect heart rate, rhythm, or conduction.

6. Monitoring of hemodynamic effects of dysrhythmias, including vital signs, sensorium, level of consciousness, manifestations of peripheral hypoperfusion, and urinary output.

The listed interventions relate to any patient with a dysrhythmia and may be thought of as the basis for a standardized approach to evaluation and management of the patient with a potential for alteration in cardiac output. In addition, individualized therapies may be indicated for treatment of specific dysrhythmias.

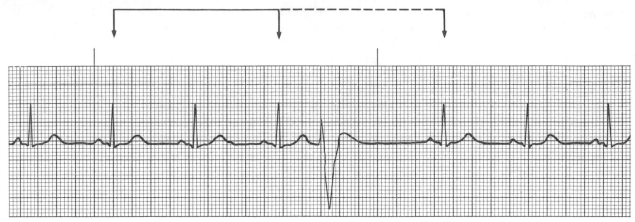

FIGURE 10-2. The dotted line represents compensatory pause; the solid line, the distance between three regular beats.

Premature Ventricular Contractions

A premature ventricular contraction (PVC) or premature ventricular beat (PVB) can be described as a complex occurring prematurely and exhibiting a wide (>0.12-second) and bizarre QRS complex. Depolarization may originate from either ventricle. Because of the unusual depolarization there is abnormal repolarization causing T wave inversion (Rosen et al 1988, 1272). A compensatory pause usually occurs and can be determined by measuring the distance between the R wave before the PVC and the R wave following the PVC. This distance should equal the distance between three normal sinus beats (Fig. 10-2).

Characteristics

PVCs may be uniformed or multiformed. That is, the premature beats may originate in one section of myocardium, travel the same pathway with each impulse, and reflect identical EKG configurations for each beat. These are called uniformed PVCs (Fig. 10-3). Multiformed PVCs originate in varying areas of the myocardium, travel a variable pathway through the conduction system with each beat, and create varying configurations on the EKG (Fig. 10-4).

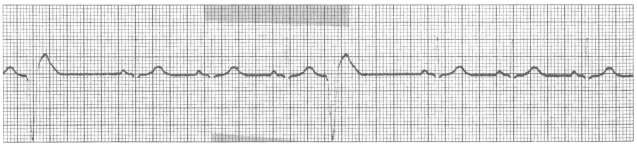

FIGURE 10-3. Uni-formed PVC.

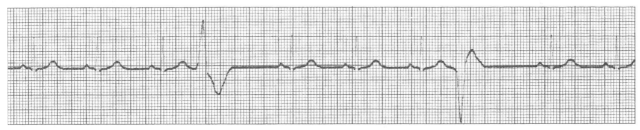

FIGURE 10-4. Multiformed PVCs.

PVCs are significant because they may compromise cardiac output. Generally, PVCs do not produce the stroke volume of a normal cardiac contraction. In addition, PVCs may precede dysrhythmias such as ventricular tachycardia and ventricular fibrillation. A life-threatening dysrhythmia is more likely to occur if the premature ventricular contractions are multiformed, occur in couplets, occur close to the preceding T wave, or occur at a rate of five or more per minute (Rosen et al 1988, 1274). The T wave signifies the relative refractory period and indicates that a small stimulus will cause impulse conduction, ventricular irritability, and ectopy.

Treatment

In the setting of chest pain highly suggestive of an evolving MI, antidysrhythmic therapy should be started at the earliest possible time following symptom onset (Lie et al 1974; Wyman 1974). There is controversy in the literature as to whether or not lidocaine should be given prophylactically in the setting of an acute myocardial infarction (MI). It is thought that a certain number of life-threatening dysrhythmias occur without warning and could be ameliorated if treated before evident. Based upon that hypothesis, some believe that lidocaine should be administered on the basis of history alone rather than in response to ectopic ventricular beats (Wyman and Gore 1983).

Lidocaine is a local anesthetic agent with physiologic actions that appear to be different depending on whether tissue is ischemic or nonischemic. Lidocaine decreases conduction velocity in ischemic Purkinje cells or myocardial tissue. In nonischemic tissue, lidocaine has little effect on conduction velocity but decreases duration of action potential (Andreoli et al 1987, 317).

Lidocaine should be initiated as a bolus of 1 mg/kg IVP at a rate of 50 mg/minute. The half-life of lidocaine is short— about 20 minutes; therefore readministration may be necessary until a therapeutic serum level is reached. Administration of half-normal adult dosages should be considered when giving lidocaine to the elderly, patients in congestive heart failure, and those with liver or renal disease. These patients do not metabolize drugs as efficiently as those with normal liver function. Careful monitoring is necessary to detect drug toxicity. Untoward effects of lidocaine therapy are mainly related to central nervous system disturbance. Patients may become confused or may develop slurred speech, paresthesias, and hypotension. Should any of these effects occur, lidocaine should be discontinued. Refer to Table 10-1 for information on other antiarrhythmic drugs.

TABLE **10–1**
Clinical Pharmacology of Antiarrhythmic Drugs

Agent	Administration and Dosage	Elimination Half-Life	Usual Plasma Concentrations	Comments
Lidocaine	IV: Load: 2 mg/kg Maintenance: 1–4 mg/min	100 min	1.5–6 μg/ml	Clearance depends on hepatic perfusion
Quinidine	IV: Load: 0.5 mg/kg/min Average loading dose: 9 mg/kg Oral: 1200–2400 mg/day	6–11 hr	3–5 μg/ml	Active metabolites Anticholinergic effects
Procainamide	IV: Load: 10–15 mg/kg at 20–50 mg/min Maintenance: 2–6 mg/min Oral: 2–8 gm/day	3–4 hr 6 hr for sustained release form	4–8 μg/ml	Active metabolite, NAPA, accumulates in renal insufficiency
Disopyramide	Oral: 400–1200 mg/day	4–8 hr 8–12 hr for sustained release form	3–8 μg/ml	Anticholinergic effects
Tocainide	Oral: 1200–1800 mg/day	12 hr	6–12 μg/ml	Electrophysiologic effects similar to lidocaine
Propranolol	IV: 0.1 mg/kg in 1 mg increments Oral: 40–1000 mg/day	4 hr	>40 μg/ml	Beta-adrenergic antagonist
Verapamil	IV: 5–10 mg bolus Oral: 240–480 mg/day	3–7 hr	15–100 mg/ml	Ca^{++} channel antagonist alpha-adrenergic antagonist
Bretylium	IV: Load: 5–10 mg/kg Maintenance: 1–2 mg/min	8–10 hr	0.8–2.4 μg/ml	Biphasic adrenergic effects: initial adrenergic agonist effect followed by depressant effects
Phenytoin	IV: Load: 12 mg/kg at 20 mg/min Oral: Load: 900–1200 mg/24 hr Maintenance: 300–400 mg/day	24 hr	10–20 μg/ml	Nonlinear kinetics
Amiodarone	IV: 2.3 mg/kg × 12 hr, then 0.7 mg/min × 36 hr Oral: Load: 800–1600 mg/day × 7–10 days Maintenance: 200–400 mg/day	45–60 days during chronic therapy	1.5–3.5 μg/ml	Antiadrenergic effects
Flecainide	Oral: 200–600 mg/day	16–20 hr	0.2–1.0 μg/ml	New antiarrhythmic agent with "local anesthetic" effects
Mexiletine	Oral: 600–1200 mg/day	12 hr	0.5–2 μg/ml	Effects similar to lidocaine
Encainide	Oral: 100–240 mg/day	3–4 hr	variable	Active metabolites account for much of antiarrhythmic effects
Propafenone	Oral: 450–900 mg/day	3–6 hr	0.2–3.0 μg/ml	Nonlinear kinetics; has weak beta-blocking effects

Ventricular Tachycardia

Ventricular tachycardia is described as three or more PVCs occurring consecutively. The ectopic impulse originates in the ventricular myocardium, occurs at a rate of 100 to 250 beats/minute, and is usually regular (Brooks 1987) (Fig. 10–5). It is sometimes difficult to differentiate ventricular tachycardia from aberrant supraventricular tachycardia. Both dysrhythmias have wide QRS complexes. The important point to consider is the patient's clinical presentation and hemodynamic stability. Ventricu-

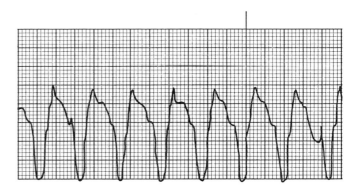

FIGURE 10-5. Ventricular tachycardia.

lar tachycardia can be seen in the patient with acute MI. It often precedes ventricular fibrillation and usually signifies an unstable cardiac rhythm.

Treatment

Therapy should be instituted as soon as possible. If available direct current (DC) cardioversion at 50 to 100 watt-seconds (joules) may be administered. This should be reserved for unconscious patients who are hypotensive. Lidocaine can be given as an intravenous bolus of 1 mg/kg, followed by a drip of 1 to 4 mg/minute in the patient who is awake (Fig. 10-6).

   Bretylium tosylate (Bretylol), which exerts a direct effect prolonging the duration of action potential and the effective refractory period of cardiac cells, may also be used for ventricular tachycardia. It can be administered intravenously with an initial dose of 5 to 10 mg/kg, followed by a maintenance drip of 1 to 2 mg/kg. Side effects of bretylium relate to the drug's interference with catecholamine release and uptake. The blood pressure frequently shows an immediate rise, followed by a hypotensive period. Other side effects include nausea and vomiting (Crumpley 1983).

Ventricular Fibrillation

Ventricular fibrillation originates in the ventricular myocardium and has no organized format on the electrocardiogram. Since the ventricles do not contract in an organized fashion, there is no cardiac output. A life-threatening situation ensues (Fig. 10-7).

   The treatment consists of mechanical defibrillation at 200 watt-seconds times two, followed by a lidocaine bolus and drip. Bretylium may be used if lidocaine is ineffective. Cardiopulmonary resuscitation (CPR) and advanced life-support regimens must be initiated (Fig. 10-8).

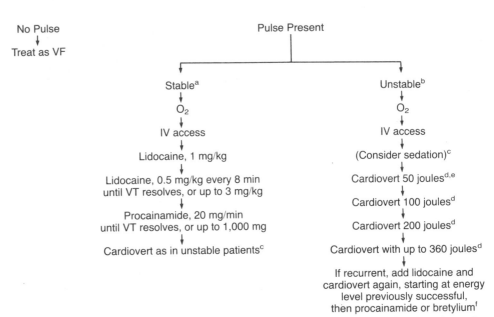

FIGURE 10–6. Sustained ventricular tachycardia (VT). This sequence was developed to assist in teaching how to treat a broad range of patients with sustained VT. Some patients may require care not specified herein. This algorithm should not be construed as prohibiting such flexibility. Flow of algorithm assumes that VT is continuing. VF indicates ventricular fibrillation. (Reproduced with permission. © Textbook of Advanced Cardiac Life Support, 1987, American Heart Association.)

a. If patient becomes unstable (see b for definition) at any time, move to "Unstable" arm of algorithm.

b. Unstable indicates symptoms (e.g., chest pain or dyspnea), hypotension (systolic blood pressure <90 mmHg), congestive heart failure, ischemia, or infarction.

c. Sedation should be considered for all patients, including those defined in b as unstable, except those who are hemodynamically unstable (e.g., hypotensive, in pulmonary edema, or unconscious).

d. If hypotension, pulmonary edema, or unconsciousness is present, unsynchronized cardioversion should be done to avoid delay associated with synchronization.

e. In the presence of hypotension, pulmonary edema, or unconsciousness, a precordial thump may be employed prior to cardioversion.

f. Once VT has resolved, begin intravenous (IV) infusion of antiarrhythmic agent that has aided resolution of VT. If hypotension, pulmonary edema, or unconsciousness is present, use lidocaine if cardioversion alone is unsuccessful, followed by bretylium. In all other patients, recommended order of therapy is lidocaine, procainamide, and then bretylium.

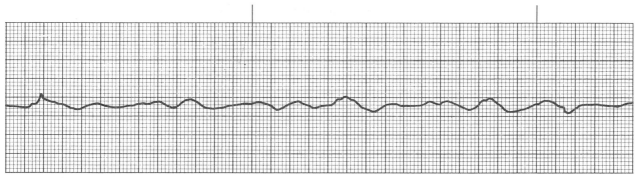

FIGURE 10–7. Ventricular fibrillation.

FIGURE 10–8. Ventricular fibrillation (and pulseless ventricular tachycardia).

This sequence was developed to assist in teaching how to treat a broad range of patients with ventricular fibrillation (VF) or pulseless ventricular tachycardia (VT). Some patients may require care not specified herein. This algorithm should not be construed as prohibiting such flexibility. Flow of algorithm assumes that VF is continuing. CPR indicates cardiopulmonary resuscitation. (Reproduced with permission. © Textbook of Advanced Cardiac Life Support, 1987, American Heart Association.)

a. Pulseless VT should be treated identically to VF.

b. Check pulse and rhythm after each shock. If VF recurs after transiently converting (rather than persists without ever converting), use whatever energy level has previously been successful for defibrillation.

c. Epinephrine should be repeated every 5 minutes.

d. Intubation is preferable. If it can be accompanied simultaneously with other techniques, then the earlier the better. However, defibrillation and epinephrine are more important initially if the patient can be ventilated without intubation.

e. Some may prefer repeated doses of lidocaine, which may be given in 0.5-mg/kg boluses every 8 minutes to a total dose of 3 mg/kg.

f. Value of sodium bicarbonate is questionable during cardiac arrest, and it is not recommended for routine cardiac arrest sequence. Consideration of its use in a dose of 1 mEq/kg is appropriate at this point. Half of original dose may be repeated every 10 minutes if it is used.

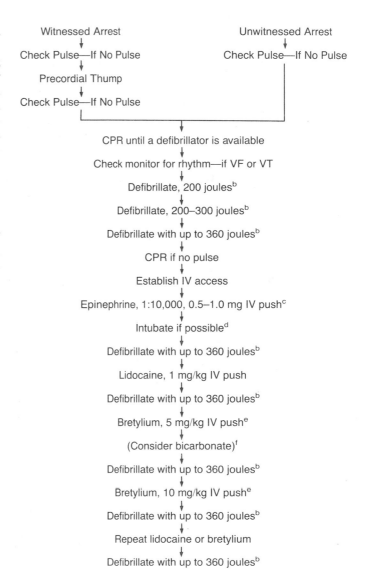

If rhythm is unclear and possibly ventricular fibrillation,
defibrillate as for VF. If asystole is present,[a]
↓
Continue CPR
↓
Establish IV access
↓
Epinephrine, 1:10,000, 0.5–1.0 mg IV push[b]
↓
Intubate when possible[c]
↓
Atropine, 1.0 mg IV push (repeated in 5 min)
↓
(Consider bicarbonate)[d]
↓
Consider pacing

FIGURE 10–9. Asystole (cardiac standstill). This sequence was developed to assist in teaching how to treat a broad range of patients with asystole. Some patients may require care not specified herein. This algorithm should not be construed to prohibit such flexibility. Flow of algorithm presumes asystole is continuing. VF indicates ventricular fibrillation; IV, intravenous. (Reproduced with permission. © Textbook of Advanced Cardiac Life Support, 1987, American Heart Association.)

    a. Asystole should be confirmed in two leads.

    b. Epinephrine should be repeated every five minutes.

    c. Intubation is preferable; if it can be accomplished simultaneously with other techniques, then the earlier the better. However, cardiopulmonary resuscitation (CPR) and use of epinephrine are more important initially if patient can be ventilated without intubation. (Endotracheal epinephrine may be used).

    d. Value of sodium bicarbonate is questionable during cardiac arrest, and it is not recommended for the routine cardiac arrest sequence. Consideration of its use in a dose of 1 mEq/kg is appropriate at this point. Half of original dose may be repeated every 10 minutes if it is used.

Asystole

Asystole represents a total lack of cardiac rhythm on the EKG, cessation of ventricular activity, and a lack of cardiac output. The patient is in need of CPR and advanced life support (Fig. 10–9; Table 10–2).

Sinus Dysrhythmia

A sinus dysrhythmia occurs when the P–P or R–R cycles vary by 0.16 second or more. This rhythm is frequently associated with sinus bradycardia, particularly in children and young adults. Generally, sinus dysrhythmias are related to the respiratory cycle. The sinus rate increases with inspiration and slows with expiration. This change is caused by a variation in vagal tone secondary to reflex mechanisms in the pulmonary and systemic vascular systems that respond to respiratory cycle variations. Vagal tone is accentuated by expiration, whereas it is lowered by inspiration (Fig. 10–10).

    A wandering pacemaker may frequently be associated with a sinus dysrhythmia. A characteristic feature of the wandering pacemaker rhythm is that the P wave changes configuration from beat to beat. This occurs because the pacemaker shifts from one part to another in the atrium or AV node (Kelly 1984).

TABLE **10-2**
Drugs Commonly Used in Cardiac Arrest: How Supplied, Usual Dose (average adult)*

Drug	Concentration and Volume of Prefilled Syringe	Dose	Infusion Rate	Remarks
Atropine sulfate	0.1 mg/ml in 10-ml syringe	0.5–1.0 mg = 5–10 ml		Repeat at 5-minute intervals to achieve desired rate. Generally, do *not* exceed 2 mg.
Bretylium tosylate	50 mg/ml in 10-ml ampule	5 mg/kg 350–500 mg as initial dose	500 mg in 5% dextrose in water (in 250 ml = 2 mg/ml; in 500 ml = 1 mg/ml) Infusion: 1–2 mg/min	Infusion started after loading dose to control recurrent ventricular tachycardia or ventricular fibrillation
Calcium chloride 10%	100 mg/ml in 10-ml syringe	500 mg = 5 ml		May repeat dose every 10 minutes as needed
Dopamine	200 mg in 5-ml ampule		200 mg in 250 ml dextrose in water = 800 μg/ml Infusion: 2–10 μg/kg/min	
Epinephrine 1 : 10,000	0.1 mg/ml in 10-ml syringe	0.5 mg–1.0 mg = 5–10 ml IV or intratracheal	1 mg in 5% dextrose in water (in 250 ml = 4 μg/ml; in 500 ml = 2 μg/ml) Infusion: 1 μg/min for maintenance of BP	Avoid intracardiac injection. Repeat dose every 5 minutes as needed in cardiac arrest
Isoproterenol	0.2 mg/ml in 5-ml ampule		1 mg in 5% dextrose in water (in 250 ml = 4 μg/ml; in 500 ml = 2 μg/ml) Infusion: 2–20 μg/min Titrate	Beware of PVCs
Lidocaine	For IV bolus: 1% (10 mg/ml) in 10 ml = 100 mg 2% (20 mg/ml) in 5 ml = 100 mg For infusion after bolus: 4% (40 mg/ml) in 25 ml = 1 g	1%: 75 mg = 7.50 ml 2%: 75 mg = 3.75 ml	2 g in 500 ml 5% dextrose in water (or 1 g in 250 ml) = 4 mg/ml Infusion: 1–4 mg/min	For breakthrough ventricular ectopy: additional 50 mg bolus every 5 minutes to suppress, or total of 225 mg. Increase drip to 4 mg/min
Procainamide	For IV bolus: 100 mg/ml in 10-ml ampule For infusion after bolus: 500 mg/ml in 2-ml ampules	20 mg/min until: a) Dysrhythmia suppressed b) Hypotension c) QRS widens by 50% d) Total 1 g administered	1 g in 250 ml 5% dextrose = 4 mg/ml Infusion: 1–4 mg/min	Monitor ECG and blood pressure. Administer cautiously in patients with acute myocardial infarction
Sodium bicarbonate	1 mEq/ml in 50 ml = 50 mEq	1 mEq/kg or 75 ml initial dose (average-size adult) or preferably according to pH		Repeat according to pH. If not available, use 1/2 initial dose every 10 minutes

Source: Data from Textbook of Advanced Cardiac Life Support. 1987. American Heart Association.
* For additional information refer to Standards and Guidelines for Cardiopulmonary Resuscitation and Emergency Cardiac Care. JAMA 255:2938–2942.

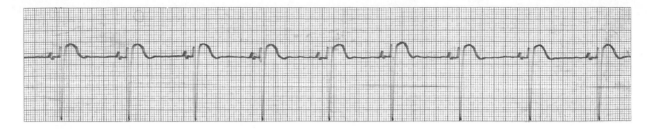

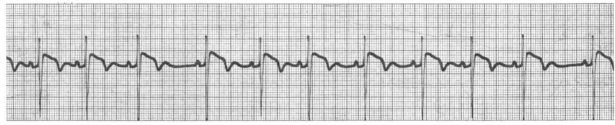

FIGURE 10-10. Sinus dysrhythmia. (Courtesy of Linda Hellstedt, R.N., M.S., Clinical Specialist, Medical Intensive Care, Northwestern Memorial Hospital, Chicago.)

Treatment

Treatment is not required for this dysrhythmia unless a bradycardia significant
enough to cause hypotension is present. In such cases atropine is the drug of choice
(Blowers 1984).

Sinus Bradycardia

Sinus bradycardia is defined as a rhythm originating in the sinus node and occurring
at a rate of less than 60 beats per minute. All other rhythm parameters are within
normal limits (see Fig. 10-6). Sinus bradycardia may be normal for the well-condi-
tioned athlete. In the emergency setting, it is often associated with acute MI, particularly inferior wall MIs. The right coronary artery supplies the inferior portion of
myocardium as well as the SA node in most people. Ischemia of the SA node can
result in sinus dysrhythmias (Fig. 10-11).

Treatment is unnecessary unless the patient with sinus bradycardia is symptomatic with one or more of these: syncope, light-headedness, hypotension, and chest
pain. Atropine, a parasympatholytic drug, is the drug of choice in symptomatic
patients. The dose is generally 0.5 to 1 mg IVP rapidly and may be repeated every 5
minutes to a total of 2.0 mg. If pushed slowly, a rebound bradycardia may occur.

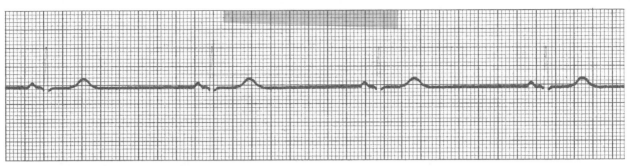

FIGURE 10–11. Sinus bradycardia.

Sinus Tachycardia

Sinus tachycardia, seen in Figure 10–12, is characterized by a heart rate of more than 100 and less than 160 beats/minute. The P wave originates in the sinus node. The P, QRS, and T waves are normal.

Sinus tachycardia may occur normally as in exercise, or abnormally as in certain illnesses and injuries. The rhythm may be a response to increased metabolism (e.g., from exercise, anxiety, caffeine intake, fever) or decreased cardiac output (as in hypovolemia or cardiogenic shock). The normal physiologic response to hypoxia, hypoxemia, or both is an increased heart rate. The cause may range from poor perfusion at the cellular level to inadequate oxygenation in the lungs. Regardless, the net result is the same: oxygen deprivation and a physiologic need to improve oxygen delivery to the tissues.

Treatment

Treatment is based on the cause of the tachycardia. In the hypovolemic patient, fluid replacement is necessary. The patient in cardiogenic shock will require vasopressors such as dopamine to increase blood pressure and venous return to the heart. The

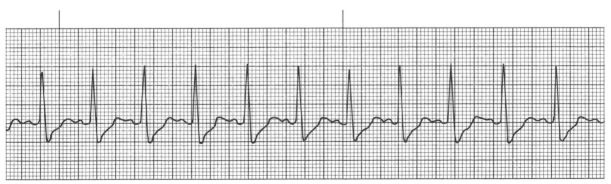

FIGURE 10–12. Sinus tachycardia.

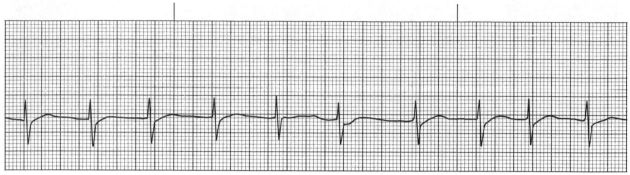

FIGURE 10–13. Atrial fibrillation.

patient in pulmonary edema will require diuretics and Mso_4 to decrease venous return to the heart and decrease fluid in the lungs. The febrile patient will require antipyretics.

Atrial Fibrillation

Atrial fibrillation is characterized by a rapid atrial rate depicted on the EKG as irregular, rapidly occurring waves instead of clearly definable P waves. The ventricular response to the erratic firing of the many foci in the atria is inconsistently irregular — that is, there is no pattern in the irregularity of the ventricular response to atrial activity in atrial fibrillation (Fig. 10–13).

Atrial fibrillation is a dysrhythmia commonly seen in patients with arteriosclerotic or rheumatic heart disease. These conditions lead to scarring of the atrium, which disrupts the normal course of the P wave (Blowers 1984). Emboli are possible complications that occur secondary to incomplete emptying of the atria and consequent stasis of atrial blood. Because of the irregular electrical pattern, the atria are unable to fully eject the blood within. The net result is stagnation of blood within the atria and the possibility of clot formation.

Treatment

If the patient is stable, digoxin 0.25 to 0.50 mg given slowly through an intravenous line is the treatment of choice. In unstable patients synchronized cardioversion should be attempted using 20 to 50 watt-seconds. One should be aware that ventricular fibrillation or asystole may result from cardioversion if the patient is sensitive to the toxic effects of digitalis.

Atrial Flutter

Atrial flutter refers to rapid regular firing of an irritable ectopic focus in the atrium. The accelerated atrial rate causes a sawtoothed baseline configuration in place of the

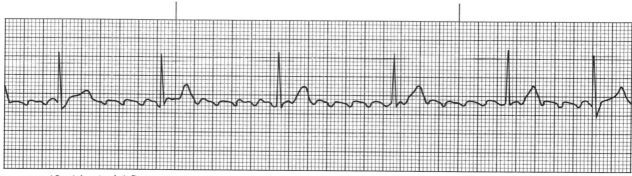

FIGURE 10–14. Atrial flutter.

normally occurring P waves of the EKG. The atrial rate is usually 250 to 350 beats/ minute. Since many impulses fail to conduct to the ventricles, the ventricular rate is slower than the atrial rate and may be regular or irregular in rhythm (Fig. 10–14). Atrial flutter may be associated with valvular heart disease, coronary artery disease, or thyrotoxicosis.

Treatment

If untreated, the ventricular rate is usually 100 to 150 beats/minute. Treatment is directed at either slowing the ventricular rate or totally converting the dysrhythmia to a normal sinus rhythm. Unstable patients are treated with synchronized cardioversion at 50 to 100 watt-seconds. Stable patients are treated with digitalis.

Premature Atrial Contractions

Premature atrial contractions are complexes initiated by an ectopic atrial focus causing a premature beat to occur in the normal sinus cycle. The P wave occurs prematurely and is commonly superimposed on the preceding T wave. The P-R interval is usually the same or longer than the sinus P-R interval. The QRS is usually similar to the normal sinus rhythm complex. There is no compensatory pause (Fig. 10–15). PACs indicate atrial irritability and may be warnings of more serious atrial

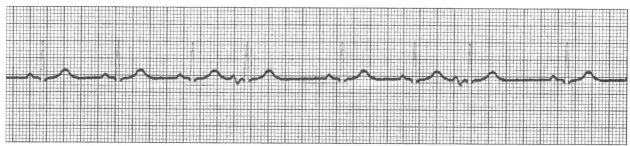

FIGURE 10–15. Premature atrial contractions.

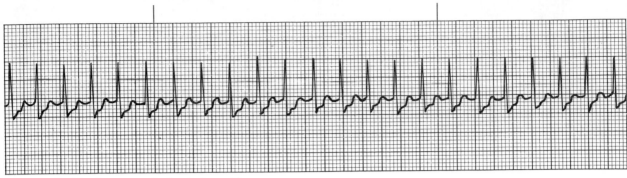

FIGURE 10-16. Supraventricular tachycardia.

dysrhythmias. They may stimulate reentrant tachydysrhythmias or signal the first indication of atrial dilation associated with congestive heart failure, COPD, or pulmonary embolus.

Treatment

Usually no treatment is required. Specific treatment for the underlying abnormality may abolish the dysrhythmia. Since stimulants may be the cause, patients are advised to avoid caffeine.

Supraventricular Tachycardia

Paroxysmal supraventricular tachycardia (PSVT) is a rapid rhythm that originates above the level of the bundle of His. The onset is usually abrupt, and the heart rate is 150 to 250 beats per minute. The P wave may be buried in the preceding T wave and may not be apparent on the EKG. P waves, when visible, may be abnormally shaped. The QRS appears normal (Hammond 1984) (Fig. 10-16).

PSVT may be seen in young adults with no evidence of organic heart disease, acute MI, myocarditis, rheumatic heart disease, digitalis toxicity, advanced COPD, pulmonary embolus, or thyrotoxicosis. The main hemodynamic consequence of a rapid ventricular rate is shortening of diastolic filling time. Reduced diastolic filling results in a 15% to 20% decrease in cardiac output (Hammond 1984). Because the coronary arteries fill during diastole, myocardial ischemia may result from this rhythm (Sweetwood 1983).

Treatment

Treatment usually consists of vagal stimulation in an effort to slow the ventricular response to the rapid atrial rate. This can be accomplished by having the patient

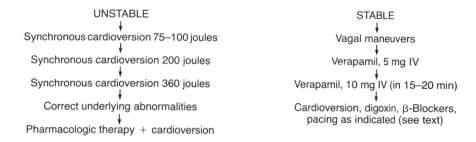

UNSTABLE	STABLE
↓	↓
Synchronous cardioversion 75–100 joules	Vagal maneuvers
↓	↓
Synchronous cardioversion 200 joules	Verapamil, 5 mg IV
↓	↓
Synchronous cardioversion 360 joules	Verapamil, 10 mg IV (in 15–20 min)
↓	↓
Correct underlying abnormalities	Cardioversion, digoxin, β-Blockers, pacing as indicated (see text)
↓	
Pharmacologic therapy + cardioversion	

If conversion occurs but PSVT recurs, repeated electrical cardioversion is *not* indicated. Sedation should be used as time permits.

FIGURE 10–17. Paroxysmal supraventricular tachycardia (PSVT). This sequence was developed to assist in teaching how to treat a broad range of patients with sustained PSVT. Some patients may require care not specified herein. This algorithm should not be construed as prohibiting such flexibility. Flow of algorithm presumes PSVT is continuing. (Reproduced with permission. © Textbook of Advanced Cardiac Life Support, 1987, American Heart Association.)

perform Valsalva's maneuver such as forced expiration against a closed glottis (bearing down). Carotid sinus massage is another method of direct vagal stimulation. Verapamil (Isoptin, Calan), 5 to 10 mg, can be administered intravenously over 2 minutes. It blocks slow channel calcium influx, resulting in slowed conduction through the AV node. Digitalis may also be used to decrease conduction through the AV node in hopes of slowing the ventricular response to atrial conduction. Synchronized cardioversion at low energy levels may be necessary if hemodynamic instability results from the dysrhythmia (Fig. 10–17).

Junctional Rhythms

Junctional rhythms originate within AV node tissue. The junction takes over as a pacemaker secondary to failure or slowing of the sinus node impulse. Although the intrinsic junctional firing rate is 40 to 60 beats/minute, junctional rhythms may accelerate to 70 to 90 beats/minute. This is referred to as an accelerated junctional rhythm. An increase to 150 beats per minute is termed junctional tachycardia.

AV junctional rhythms are usually regular. QRS complexes are generally the same contour as the normally conducted QRS. Junctional P waves may have one of the three characteristics. The P wave may have a negative deflection and precede the QRS complex (antegrade); it may have a negative deflection and occur after the QRS (retrograde); or it may not be seen at all (Andreoli et al 1987, 179). P wave characteristics are related to the spread of the impulse from the AV node to the ventricular and atrial conduction systems (Fig. 10–18).

Slow junctional rhythms may occur secondary to increased vagal tone. Junctional escape beats generally occur during pathologic slow sinus discharge or heart block. An ectopic foci within the junction fires to cause an escape beat or complex. Accelerated and tachycardic junctional rates generally are a result of conduction system ischemia or digitalis toxicity.

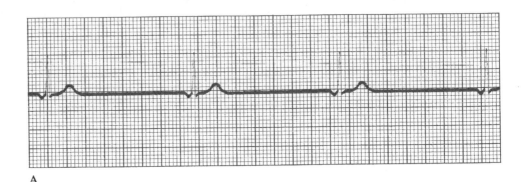

A

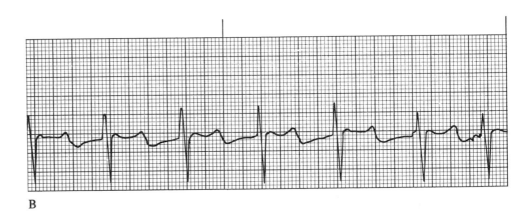

B

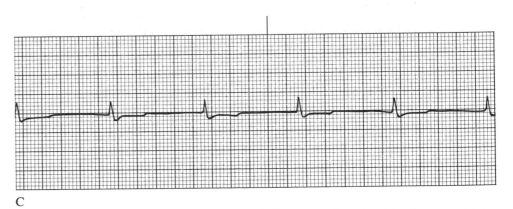

C

FIGURE 10–18. *A,* Junctional rhythm antegrade P waves; *B,* junctional rhythm — unable to identify P waves. *C,* Retrograde P waves, junctional rhythm.

Treatment

Chemotherapeutic treatment in hemodynamically compromised individuals includes atropine or isoproterenol. Atropine blocks parasympathetic (vagal) tone and increases the rate of impulse discharge from pacemakers above the AV junction. Isoproterenol (Isuprel), a pure beta agonist, increases heart rate (chronotropic effect), improves myocardial electrical conduction, and strengthens myocardial contractions (inotropic effect). Pacing is rarely indicated.

First-Degree Heart Block

First-degree heart block is characterized by prolongation of the PR interval in an otherwise normal-appearing cardiac rhythm. Although impulses originate within the sinus node, electrical conduction from the atria to the ventricles is abnormally prolonged. This is reflected on the EKG as a prolonged (>0.20 second) PR interval (Fig. 10–19).

In most instances first-degree heart block does not compromise cardiac function. If, however, the block is associated with a bradycardic rhythm, cardiac output may fall. Patients may exhibit signs and symptoms of hemodynamic compromise such as syncope, chest pain, or hypotension, and treatment is necessary. Although this dysrhythmia may occur in healthy individuals, there are pathologic causes as well. These include increased vagal tone, hypokalemia, myocardial ischemia, and degenerative disease of the conduction system.

Treatment

Atropine and isoproterenol are drugs of choice in treatment of first-degree heart block. They are used only when the patient's clinical status is compromised. Continuous cardiac surveillance is necessary to monitor drug effectiveness and untoward side effects that may occur, such as myocardial irritability and tachydysrhythmias.

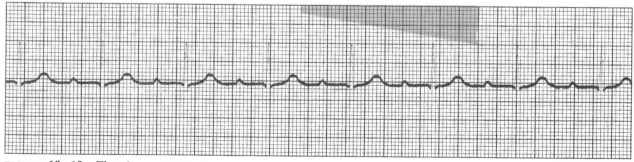

FIGURE 10–19. First-degree AV block.

Second-Degree Heart Block

Failure of some atrial impulses to conduct to the ventricles at a time when physiologic interference would not be expected constitutes second-degree AV block (Sweetwood 1983). The atrial rate is therefore greater than the ventricular rate. The pattern of dropped ventricular beats may be regular or irregular, creating either a fixed or a variable ratio of atrial to ventricular complexes. There are two types of second-degree AV block: Mobitz's type I, or Wenckebach, and Mobitz's type II.

Mobitz's Type I (Wenckebach)

Mobitz's type I heart block is characterized by a prolongation of the P-R interval. The P-R interval may initially be normal or prolonged but gradually increases until an impulse fails to conduct to the ventricles. This type of block is often associated with AV conduction abnormalities. The QRS complex is usually of normal width (Fig. 10–20).

Mobitz's type I rarely occurs among persons with normal hearts. It may occur with rapid supraventricular rates, digitalis toxicity, coronary artery disease, rheumatic fever, or degenerative disease of the conduction system (Andreoli et al 1987).

When the AV block results from diaphragmatic infarction, it usually occurs in the region of the AV node, owing to inflammation or edema that results from ischemia or infarction of neighboring myocardium. Blocks within the AV node are generally more likely to be transient than those in the ventricular conduction system (Andreoli et al 1987).

Treatment

Treatment may be necessary for patients who are symptomatic with very slow ventricular rates. Atropine, 0.5 mg IV, repeated every 5 minutes to a total of 2 mg, or isoproterenol (Isuprel), 1 to 2 mg, in 500 D₅W and titrated to obtain a heart rate of 60, may be indicated.

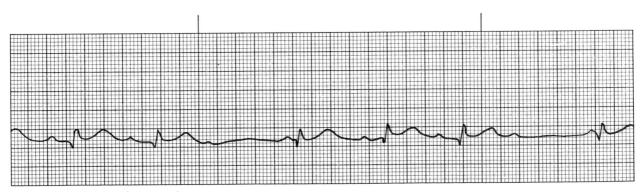

FIGURE 10–20. Mobitz's type I.

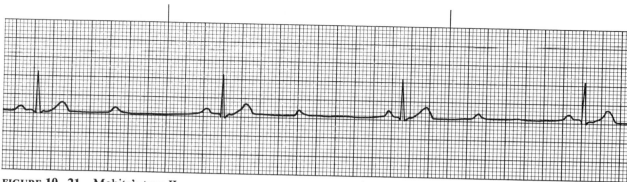

FIGURE 10–21. Mobitz's type II.

Mobitz's Type II

Mobitz's type II heart block is characterized on the electrocardiogram by a sudden and unexpected, nonconducted P wave. The atrial rate is regular and faster than the ventricular rate. The PR interval may be prolonged or normal but is always of constant duration when impulses are conducted to the ventricles. The ratio of atrial to ventricular conduction may vary, making the ventricular rhythm irregular. The QRS complexes may be normal but are usually wide as a result of ventricular conduction system defects (Fig. 10–21).

When an anterior wall infarction produces AV block, it is usually the result of extensive necrosis of the interventricular septum, which spares the AV node and bundle of His but inflicts severe damage to the bundle branches (VanMeter and Lavine 1977). Complete AV block may develop.

Treatment

Because Mobitz's type II is often associated with ominous dysrhythmias, it is imperative that a pacemaker be available for insertion. Asystole or a life-threatening bradycardia is possible. Otherwise, the treatment is similar to that of Mobitz's type I.

Third-Degree Heart Block

Third-degree heart block is characterized on the electrocardiogram by completely separate atrial and ventricular activity. Atrial impulses occur regularly and appear as P waves on the EKG. The atrial pacemaker may be of sinus or ectopic atrial origin and usually fires at a rate of 60 to 100 beats/minute. The ventricular pacemaker is generally in the bundle branch/Purkinje system and discharges at a rate of 30 to 40 times per minute. There is no observable relationship between atrial and ventricular activity (Fig. 10–22).

The slow ventricular rate during complete heart block may not be sufficient to support cardiac output, and hemodynamic compromise may occur. Angina, conges-

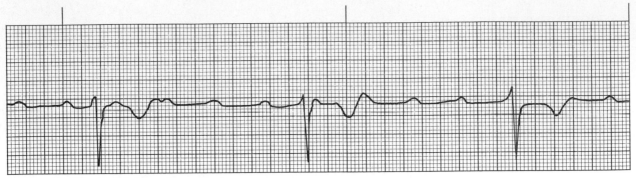

FIGURE 10–22. Third-degree heart block.

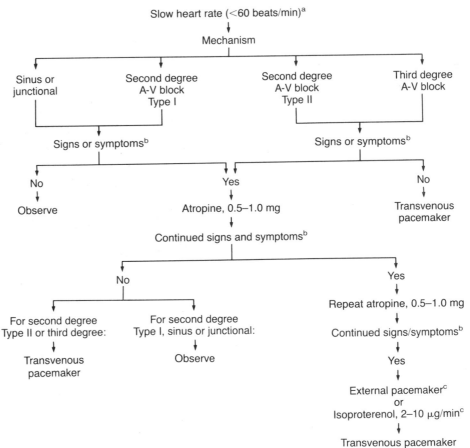

FIGURE 10–23. Bradycardia. This sequence was developed to assist in teaching how to treat a broad range of patients with bradycardia. Some patients may require care not specified herein. This algorithm should not be construed to prohibit such flexibility. AV indicates atrioventricular. (Reproduced with permission. © Textbook of Advanced Cardiac Life Support, 1987, American Heart Association.)

a. A solitary chest thump or cough may stimulate cardiac electrical activity and result in improved cardiac output and may be used at this point.

b. Hypotension (blood pressure < 90 mmHg), premature ventricular contractions, altered mental status or symptoms (e.g., chest pain or dyspnea), ischemia, or infarction.

c. Temporizing therapy.

216

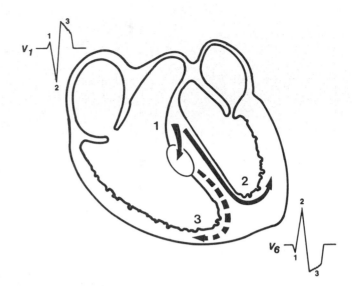

FIGURE 10-24. Right bundle branch block. The initial septal activation is from left to right and anteriorly, as normal (vector 1). Right ventricular activation (vector 3) occurs following completion of the left ventricular activation (vector 2). Delayed activation of the right ventricle is responsible for the production of the RR′ pattern in lead V1 and the round and deep S wave in lead V6. (Chung EK. Principles of Cardiac Arrhythmias, 3rd ed, 242. © Williams & Wilkins, 1983.)

tive heart failure, hypotension, or syncope may result. The slow ventricular rate may also allow escape tachydysrhythmias to occur.

Treatment

Drug treatment with atropine and isoproterenol is similar to that for second-degree heart blocks (Fig. 10-23). In the emergency setting, transvenous or transthoracic pacers are inserted as a temporary means of stimulating or supplementing intrinsic myocardial activity. See Chapter 9 for a thorough discussion on internal and external pacing devices.

Bundle Branch Block

Bundle branch block is a common form of intraventricular conduction disturbance. Although it has been reported in healthy individuals, there is a close relationship to ventricular hypertrophy and acute MI. In acute MI, conduction system damage is responsible for the bundle branch blocks. Right and left bundle branch blocks indicate a delayed activation of right and left ventricular conduction networks, respectively (Figs. 10-24 and 10-25).

The development of a bundle branch block warrants concern, because AV block may occur. Artificial pacing may be required as the patient's clinical condition deteriorates.

Idioventricular Rhythm

An idioventricular rhythm refers to cardiac electrical activity that originates within the ventricular conduction system. Idioventricular rhythms occur when the normal

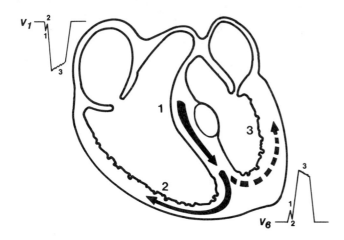

FIGURE 10-25. Left bundle branch block. The most important finding in left bundle branch block is the alteration of the initial septal force, which is directed from right to left, either anteriorly or posteriorly (vector 1). Left ventricular activation (vector 3) occurs after completion of right ventricular activation (vector 2). Delayed left ventricular activation is responsible for the production of the broad S wave in lead V1 and the broad R wave in lead V6. In left bundle branch block, physiologic (septal) Q waves in leads V4 to V6 are absent because of an abnormal septal activation. (Chung EK. Principles of Cardiac Arrhythmias, 3rd ed, 247. © Williams & Wilkins, 1983.)

cardiac pacemakers fail and ventricular pacemakers prevail. The ventricular rate is usually 30 to 40 beats/minute; however, acceleration to 110 beats/minute is not unusual. An idioventricular complex is generally wide (> 0.12 seconds) (Fig. 10-26). This rhythm occurs most often in myocardial infarction and digitalis toxicity. The slow rate is usually ineffective in maintaining cardiac output. Often cardiopulmonary support is necessary.

Treatment

Diagnosis and treatment of underlying problems is necessary in order to alleviate causal factors. Atropine, 0.5 mg intravenously, repeated as necessary, may be given in attempt to speed the sinus rate of discharge and capture electrical conduction within the ventricles.

AV Dissociation

AV dissociation is never a primary disturbance of rhythm. It is rather a consequence of a more basic disorder (Andreoli et al 1987, 215). The term means that the atria and

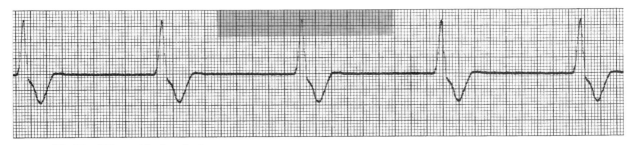

FIGURE 10-26. Idioventricular rhythm.

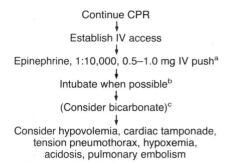

Continue CPR
↓
Establish IV access
↓
Epinephrine, 1:10,000, 0.5–1.0 mg IV push[a]
↓
Intubate when possible[b]
↓
(Consider bicarbonate)[c]
↓
Consider hypovolemia, cardiac tamponade,
tension pneumothorax, hypoxemia,
acidosis, pulmonary embolism

FIGURE 10-27. Electromechanical dissociation. This sequence was developed to assist in teaching how to treat a broad range of patients with electromechanical dissociation. Some patients may require care not specified herein. This algorithm should not be construed to prohibit such flexibility. Flow of algorithm assumes that electromechanical dissociation is continuing. CPR indicates cardiopulmonary resuscitation; IV, intravenous. (Reproduced with permission. © Textbook of Advanced Cardiac Life Support, 1987, American Heart Association.)

a. Epinephrine should be repeated every 5 minutes.

b. Intubation is preferable. If it can be accomplished simultaneously with other techniques, then the earlier the better. However, epinephrine is more important initially if the patient can be ventilated without intubation.

c. Value of sodium bicarbonate is questionable during cardiac arrest, and it is not recommended for routine cardiac arrest sequence. Consideration of its use in a dose of 1 mEq/kg is appropriate at this point. Half of original dose may be repeated every 10 minutes if it is used.

ventricles are controlled by separate escape foci that have overtaken primary pacemakers.

The physiologic causes of AV dissociation include any measure that increases vagal tone such as Valsalva's maneuver or carotid stimulation. It may also be caused by beta blockers and excessive digitalis. Chronic ischemic heart disease, myocarditis, and increased intracranial pressure can also lead to AV dissociation (Brooks 1987).

Three mechanisms may produce AV dissociation: (1) slowing of a primary pacemaker, allowing a lower pacemaker to usurp control; (2) acceleration of a lower pacemaker, which then usurps control over higher pacemakers; (3) failure of normal conduction, allowing two pacemakers to function independently (Brooks 1987). AV dissociation is not a form of heart block although AV block is one of the several mechanisms that can be responsible for AV dissociation. Treatment is based upon alleviating the cause.

Electromechanical Dissociation

Electromechanical dissociation (EMD) is a condition characterized by seemingly organized cardiac electrical activity on the EKG in conjunction with a lack of cardiac output. It is caused by severe ventricular dysfunction or disorders of calcium transport (Missri 1984). Common causes include cardiac tamponade, tension pneumothorax, and hypovolemic shock. Cardiopulmonary resuscitation and advanced life support are immediately indicated. Treatment is geared toward alleviating the cause of the compromised hemodynamic state (Fig. 10-27).

CONCLUSION

In summary, the patient presenting to the emergency department with cardiac dysrhythmias requires close monitoring and astute observation. A thorough understanding of dysrhythmia characteristics, etiologic factors, and treatment modalities for the individual with a potential alteration in cardiac output related to a rhythm disturbance is essential for emergency nursing personnel.

REFERENCES

Andreoli KG, Zipes DP, Wallace AG, et al. 1987. Comprehensive Cardiac Care, 6th ed. St. Louis, CV Mosby.

Blowers MG, Sims RS. 1984. How to Read an EKG. Oradell, N.J., Medical Economics Books, 6.

Brooks JL, Chapman PD, Troup PJ. 1987. Atrioventricular conduction abnormalities. In: Electrocardiography: 100 Diagnostic Criteria. Chicago, Year Book Medical Publishers, 151.

Canobbio NN. 1986. Cardiovascular system. In Thompson JM, McFarland GK, Hirsch JE, et al, eds. Clinical Nursing. St. Louis, CV Mosby, 25.

Crumpley LA, Rinkenburger RL. 1983. An overview of antiarrhythmic drugs. Crit Care Nurse 3:58.

Guyton AC. 1981. Textbook of Medical Physiology, 6th ed. Philadelphia, WB Saunders, 13.

Hammond L. 1984. Quick Reference to Emergency Nursing. Philadelphia, JB Lippincott, 163.

Heger JJ, Faust S. 1987. Cardiovascular drugs. In: Andreoli KG, Zipes DP, Wallace AG, et al, eds. Comprehensive Cardiac Care, 6th ed. St. Louis, CV Mosby.

Hoffman BF, Cranefield PF. 1964. The physiological basis of cardiac dysrhythmias. Am J Med 37:670.

Kelly SJ. 1984. ECG Interpretation: Identifying Arrhythmias. Philadelphia, JB Lippincott, 44.

Lewis VC. 1987. Monitoring the patient with acute myocardial infarction. Nurs Clin North Am 22:29.

Lie KL, Wellens JH, van Capelle SJ, et al. 1975. Lidocaine in the prevention of primary ventricular fibrillation: a double-blind, randomized study of 212 consecutive patients. N Engl J Med 291:1324–1326.

Missri JC, Ide PA, Williams CB. 1984. A new therapeutic approach in fibrinolytic therapy: intra-coronary streptokinase. Heart Lung 13:177.

Rosen P, Baker F, Barkin R, et al. 1988. Emergency Medicine: Concepts and Clinical Practice. St. Louis, CV Mosby.

Sweetwood HM. 1983. Clinical Electrocardiography for Nurses. London, Aspen Publishers, 62.

Van Meter M, Lavine P. 1977. Reading EKGs Correctly. Jenkintown, PA, Intermed Communications, 148.

Wyman MG, Gore S. 1983. Lidocaine prophylaxis in myocardial infarction: a concept whose time has come. Heart Lung 12:360.

Wyman MG, Hammersmith L. 1974. Comprehensive treatment plan for the prevention of primary ventricular fibrillation in acute myocardial infarction. Am J Cardiol 33:661–667.

Zipes DP, Maloy LB. 1987. Arrhythmias. In: Andreoli KG, Zipes DP, Wallace AG, et al. Comprehensive Cardiac Care, 6th ed. St. Louis, CV Mosby, 131–278.

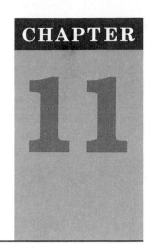

Janet Buckley, RN MSN
Timothy Buckley, RRT

Pulmonary Emergencies

Pulmonary emergencies are common occurrences in most emergency department (ED) settings. The inability to breathe is probably the most anxiety-provoking event that an individual can experience. The human organism can exist for only a few minutes without adequate oxygen and ventilation. Prompt recognition, accurate diagnosis, and effective management of pulmonary emergencies are skills valuable for ED nurses to possess.

This chapter begins with an overview of respiratory assessment. Anxiety is then discussed because it is so frequently present in persons experiencing respiratory emergencies. Discussions of the causes, pathophysiologies, clinical manifestations, and treatment modalities for a variety of pulmonary emergencies then follow.

RESPIRATORY ASSESSMENT

The ability to assess the function of the respiratory system adequately is a skill that can be gained only by constant practice and upgrading of techniques. None of the techniques are particularly difficult to master, and some are more useful than others. Probably the most valuable lesson to be learned from this section is to take a deliberately systematic approach to examination and assessment of the patient's lungs, thorax, and airway.

As with the assessment of other systems, a careful, detailed history is vital. In addition to taking the history, the practitioner must learn to conduct four basic steps

TABLE **11–1**
Information Obtained in the History

Age	Chest pain
Occupation	Wheezing
Hazardous exposures	Increased secretions
Frequency and duration of exposure	Past medical or surgical history
Family history	Asthma
Parents or siblings with lung disease,	Emphysema
asthma, emphysema, cystic fibrosis,	Cystic fibrosis
interstitial pulmonary fibrosis, pneumonia,	Pneumonia
tuberculosis, cancer, COPD	Tuberculosis
Cigarette-smoking history	Cancer
Pack-years (number of packs/day	COPD
× number of years)	Last chest radiograph
Alcohol or drug abuse	Last tuberculin skin test
Signs and symptoms	
Onset and duration	
Cough	
Sputum production (color, quantity)	
Dyspnea	
Hemoptysis	

in the examination of the respiratory system. They are (1) inspection, (2) palpation, (3) percussion, and (4) auscultation. These steps should be learned and practiced in this order so that no details are overlooked. Practitioners will learn to conduct these steps and modify them for use in their specific practices, but none of the steps should be deleted or skipped.

A careful history is elicited from the patient or other reliable person (Table 11-1). Details of the present illness should be sought, including onset, symptoms, and duration. The patient's past medical and medication history should be reviewed as well. Diseases of the pulmonary system as well as other systems should be recorded. Special attention should be paid to work history and potential exposure to toxic substances. Rarely are all the details of a history completely normal. At this point you will start to mesh the history with the physical findings.

The first step in the physical assessment of the respiratory system is inspection. Inspection of the patient starts when you first view the patient. What is his or her general state of health? How is he or she breathing? How much effort does it take for him or her to inhale and exhale? Is he or she sitting forward and using accessory muscles? All of these questions can be answered as you approach the patient. Other pertinent observations include the patient's color, symmetry of chest wall movement, obvious scars or surgical sites, the presence or absence of diaphoresis, cough, clubbed digits, and the patient's nutritional status. Standing at the foot of the patient's cart or bed is a good position from which to make such observations (Table 11–2).

Palpation is the next step. Palpation simply means to touch the patient. In touching the patient, we can begin to gather data about temperature, diaphoresis, anxiety level, and perfusion. Palpation of the chest is usually performed by placing one hand on each side of the chest, starting at the top. The palms should be in contact with the chest wall, with the thumbs toward the middle of the chest. As the patient breathes, each hand should move equally if aeration is the same on both sides.

Through palpation, the quality of the air entry may be judged. If air is moving

TABLE 11-2
Observations to be Noted During Inspection at Respiratory Assessment

Symmetry of chest wall	Distress
Size	General state of health
Shape	Surgical sites or scars
Movement	Posture of patient
Use of accessory muscles	COPD: slumped forward on elbows
Length of inspiratory and expiratory time	Level of consciousness
(normally 1:2)	Clubbing
Color	
Diaphoresis	

past secretions in the airways, fremitus can often be felt. The hands are moved down the chest until the diaphragm is reached. With practice and concentration, diaphragmatic movement can be assessed. Rib fractures and flail chest may be detected by palpation. Subcutaneous emphysema may also be noted on palpation; it is the result of air bubbles in the subcutaneous tissue and indicates that the pulmonary system is not intact.

Palpation may reveal tenderness or masses. Localized lack of air entry also may be obvious over areas of the lung that are consolidated, collapsed, or atelectatic. By placing a finger in the suprasternal notch, the position of the trachea can be palpated. The trachea will shift toward a collapsed or atelectatic area and away from a space-occupying lesion.

The relative density of underlying tissue can be assessed by performing percussion. Percussion is the act of sending a sound wave through the chest wall and evaluating the sound that is reflected back. Percussing over dense tissue such as the liver results in a very dull or hyporesonant sound. When percussion is performed over a hollow organ, such as an empty stomach, a very hollow echo, or hyperresonant sound, is heard. Normal lung has an air-tissue ratio that returns a characteristic sound. This sound should be somewhere in the middle of the sounds made by percussing the liver and the empty stomach.

Classically, percussion is performed by placing the distal portion of the middle finger flat over the area to be percussed. This area is struck with the tip of the middle finger of the other hand with a snapping motion of the wrist. It is a difficult technique to learn, but once mastered yields much information. Lung hyporesonance results from percussing over denser tissue, such as fluid, or a consolidated area, as in pneumonia. A very hollow, hyperresonant sound occurs when you percuss over a hyperinflated area of the lung, such as in chronic obstructive pulmonary disease (COPD), asthma, or pneumothorax.

The last step in the physical examination of the respiratory system is auscultation. The entire lung field should be auscultated, with special emphasis to areas that have aroused suspicion in the earlier spots of the examination. Again a systematic approach is recommended, starting at the top and comparing each side as you move down the chest wall. Normally, air entry should be heard as a quiet whoosh of air into and out of the lung. The sound and duration should be equal bilaterally.

Many terms have been used to describe breath sounds, and there has been much confusion regarding their meanings. In general, use terminology that describes what you are hearing. Crackles (formerly called rales) are sounds that are made as air passes through fluid or secretions in airways. The character of the crackle can be described as well. Fine crackles are heard in early congestive heart failure (CHF) or COPD. Coarse crackles are heard when air is rasping past thick secretions. Crackles can be simulated for the novice by rubbing hair between your fingers over your ear. The sound made is very close to what you will hear when listening to crackles through a stethoscope.

The other general category of sounds you will hear from a chest is wheezes. Wheezes occur when air is passing through constricted airways. The tighter the constriction, the higher pitched is the wheeze. Fine wheezes are characteristic of asthma. Coarse wheezes may be heard with an aspirated foreign body.

Not all of the auscultation is done with a stethoscope. Listen to the patient's breathing without one. Upper airway swelling is associated with inspiratory stridor, a high-pitched "crowing" sound. Often the wheezes in a severe asthma attack are audible even standing at a distance from the patient.

The key to a successful assessment is to be able to compile, sort, and make sense of what you have heard. Correlate your physical findings with the patient's history, and a picture should begin to emerge (Table 11–3). This will lead to choosing appropriate laboratory examination and to prompt and effective treatment of the patient's disorder.

Anxiety, Related to

• Dyspnea

As already stated, the most frightening event that an individual can experience is the feeling of being unable to breath. With all respiratory disorders, patients experience some degree of dyspnea (the subjective feeling of shortness of breath) and the fear associated with it. In many cases this fear may be exaggerated, although it is very realistic to the patient. As a result, anxiety and fear associated with pulmonary disorders or emergencies and their related nursing interventions must be addressed. Nurses are reminded to keep these interventions in mind as they care for persons with various types of respiratory emergencies.

In general, the nursing interventions center on reducing the patient's anxiety and fear. In this respect, the ED staff must reinforce to the patient that his or her fears and concerns are understandable, and that the staff is there to help and assist the patient. Patients with mild to moderate anxiety are very receptive to new information. They welcome information about procedures and equipment. Explanations should be conveyed in a calm manner; the nurse should use simple explanations and therapeutic touch as appropriate. Because these patients will encounter a variety of stimuli in the ED environment, the nurse must be keenly aware of the patient's perceptions and keep him or her informed about little things, such as how the cool moisture of humidified oxygen feels and how the bubbling of the oxygen humidifier might sound. Staff members should introduce themselves to patients and their families, particularly because they will encounter many people in the ED.

Patients with severe anxiety require additional interventions. A single nurse should communicate with the patient and family. Explanations should be given in a calm, low voice, as procedures are performed; terminology should be simple and concrete. Only essential information should be provided to decrease the amount of

TABLE 11-3
Physical Examination in Acute Respiratory Illness

Suspected Diagnosis	General Inspection	Lung Sounds	Associated Physical Findings
Asthma (severe)	Tachypnea Labored respirations Use of accessory respiratory muscles Cyanosis	Audible wheezing Diffuse high-pitched rhonchi throughout both lungs Decrease in breath sounds	Prolonged expiration Increase in pulsus paradoxus Tachycardia Hyperresonant thorax
Acute bronchitis	Normal (if mild); increase in respiratory rate (if severe)	Normal breath sounds Low and medium, occasional high-pitched rhonchi and rales	Fever Purulent sputum
Pneumonia	Increase in respiratory rate with shallow breathing Splinting of affected side Cyanosis (if severe)	Localized bronchial breath sounds, high-pitched inspiratory rales, occasional egophony ("E → A" changes) Whispered pectoriloquy Pleural friction rub	Fever Tachycardia
Pulmonary embolism (with infarction)	Increase in respiratory rate Splinting of affected side Central cyanosis	Bronchial breathing, localized rhonchi or rales, or both	Tachycardia Pleural friction rub Arrhythmias Phlebitis Dullness to percussion over affected area
Pleural effusion (large)	Increase in respiratory rate Decreased expansion of thorax on affected side	Decreased breath sounds over affected area Bronchovesicular or bronchial breathing (directly above effusion)	Dullness to percussion Tracheal shift to opposite side Decreased vocal and tactile fremitus Shifting dullness on percussion in decubitus position
Tension pneumothorax	Increase in respiratory rate Shallow labored respirations Cyanosis	Diminished or absent breath sounds over affected area	Shock, signs of associated trauma Bulging rib spaces Shift of trachea and apical cardiac impulse to opposite side Hyperresonant thorax Neck vein distention
Pulmonary edema (cardiogenic)	Increase in respiratory rate Diaphoresis Cyanosis Noisy breathing	Diffuse moist rales	Tachycardia Cardiomegaly Gallop rhythm Cardiac murmur Hepatojugular reflux or neck vein distention or both Peripheral edema
Complete lobar atelectasis	Increase in respiratory rate	Bronchial breathing, or diminished or absent breath sounds over affected area	Narrowing of rib spaces and decreased chest expansion on affected side Absent or increased vocal fremitus Dullness to percussion over area Tracheal shift

Source: Zagelbaum GL, Paré JA. 1982. Manual of Acute Respiratory Care. Little, Brown and Co.

information the patient must process. A high anxiety level may not allow the patient to hear initial instructions. Instructions may need to be repeated, and may be preceded by touch to offer reassurance (Kim et al 1987).

Patients with difficulty breathing may also experience fear of being left alone. The nurse should not only check on the patient very frequently but also make him or her aware of the nurse's presence in the room often and availability at any time by use of the call bell or simply by calling out. Frequently the family can provide emotional support for the patient if allowed to remain with their loved one. Too frequently the family is left in the waiting room, when their presence could help to alleviate much of the patient's fear and anxiety.

DISORDERS OF THE AIRWAY

Acute Airway Obstruction Resulting from External Compression

Etiology and Pathophysiology

Air flow through the airway may be partially or totally obstructed by external compression. This can be the result of enlarged lymph nodes or tumors compressing the airway. Airway obstruction can also result from foreign bodies externally compressing the airway. Examples might include missiles or penetrating objects from gunshot wounds, automobile accidents, or construction accidents. The obstruction can create atelectasis distal to the obstruction, retention of secretions, and the possibility of check-valve obstruction, which allows air to enter a particular area but not leave it. This results in air-trapping and overdistention, which can occur with any episode of airway obstruction resulting from external compression.

Clinical Manifestations

The presenting signs and symptoms in persons who come to EDs with acute airway obstruction secondary to external compression may vary depending on the severity of obstruction. In general, nonspecific complaints, such as cough, dyspnea, shortness of breath on exertion, and wheezing, will be present.

On physical examination the patient will exhibit some degree of respiratory distress, which will depend on the size of the area affected, as well as on pre-existing lung disease. Chest wall movement will be asymmetric, with less movement noted over the affected area. Palpation may reveal decreased air entry over the affected side if there is limited expansion and flow. If the area is consolidated or collapsed, palpation will reveal tactile fremitus and the region will be dull to percussion. On the other hand, check-valve obstruction will show hyperresonance to percussion. If the collapse or check-valve obstruction is significant, there will be deviation of the trachea toward the collapse or away from the check valve. Breath sounds will be decreased or absent, and wheezing will also be noted, particularly in the event of partial obstruction. Tachycardia will be present at rest if hypoxemia is significant. The patient may be febrile, especially if secretions are retained.

Arterial blood gases (ABGs) may show decreased Pao_2, whereas the $Paco_2$ and pH generally are normal. Chest radiographs (CXR) may show atelectasis or consolidation distal to the obstruction. Hyperinflation may be evident in a check-valve obstruction.

Treatment and Nursing Care

Airway Clearance, Ineffective, Related to

- *Acute partial or total airway obstruction secondary to external compression*

Treatment of acute airway obstruction secondary to external compression depends on the nature and severity of the obstruction. Total or near total obstruction will require stage I care. Endotracheal intubation, cricothyroidotomy, and tracheotomy equipment should be available but is of little use unless the obstruction is at or above the larynx. Because both tracheostomy and cricothyroidotomy increase morbidity and mortality rates significantly, very rarely are these necessary when an endotracheal tube is available. Obstruction resulting from tumors, enlarged lymph nodes, or a penetrating foreign body generally requires surgical intervention. Traumatic pneumothoraces require chest tubes. Oxygen therapy to combat a decreased Pao_2 may also be required.

Stage II interventions usually begin after the immediate cause of the airway obstruction is removed or the life-threatening situation treated. Humidity therapy and pulmonary hygiene to mobilize retained secretions may be required. Close observation for recognition of tracheal edema, swelling, or any additional pulmonary compromise is advised.

Anxiety, Related to

- *Ineffective airway clearance secondary to external compression*

As discussed previously (Anxiety, Related to Dyspnea), anxiety will be experienced in different degrees by patients with an acute airway obstruction. Stage I nursing care centers on reducing the anxiety and preventing a panic attack, in an attempt to prevent further respiratory decompensation. Interventions include staying with the patient and providing only essential information in a calm manner, using concrete terms.

Stage II intervention usually begins after the imminent threat has been removed. Patients may then be ready for more information about procedures and equipment.

Acute Airway Obstruction Resulting from Internal Factors

Etiology and Pathophysiology

Air flow through the airways may be partially or totally obstructed by internal factors. This sort of obstruction may result from a variety of factors, such as anatomic structures, secretions, or aspirated foreign bodies. The tongue is the most common anatomic structure that can cause upper airway obstruction. Swelling and inflammation of the epiglottis, vocal cords, and the laryngotracheal area can also cause airway obstruction. Upper or lower airway obstruction may be caused by an increase in the amount, viscosity, or volume of secretions (Parey and Youtsey 1981). Generally, obstruction by secretions is the result of an existing pulmonary or neuromuscular disease such as amyotrophic lateral sclerosis (ALS) or myasthenia gravis; that makes removal of the secretions difficult.

Aspiration of a foreign body may lead to respiratory failure if a major airway is occluded. Food is the most common foreign object aspirated for adults. Usually this is due to the common experience of talking or laughing while trying to chew food (referred to as a "cafe coronary"). In children, the offending object commonly is a peanut. Peanuts are among the more dangerous foreign bodies to be aspirated because they are small enough to go deep into the tracheobronchial tree. In children younger than 2 years old, aspiration of small plastic parts may occur because many toys for this age group are composed of small parts that are easily aspirated (Berté 1986).

Regardless of the cause, obstruction may result in the loss of lung volume distal to the obstruction, consolidation, and infection. A tumor or foreign body in the airway itself may also lead to a check-valve obstruction and hyperinflation distal to the obstruction.

Clinical Manifestations

Clinical signs and symptoms in patients who come to EDs with interal airway obstruction will vary depending on the severity and location of the obstruction. Partial obstruction may cause a patient to exhibit varying degrees of respiratory distress, indicated by snoring, expiratory stridor, gurgling, inspiratory squeaking, and audible breathing. Tachypnea and tachycardia may also be noted (Parey and Youtsey 1981). However, with partial obstruction the patient is still able to cough effectively and speak. With complete airway obstruction, patients experience severe respiratory distress, and they are unable to cough or speak. They may make extreme efforts to move air into the lungs, as evidenced by deep retractions of the sternum. These patients will appear anxious and diaphoretic. If the obstruction is not removed, loss of consciousness and respiratory arrest rapidly ensue.

Patients with chronic pulmonary diseases, such as cystic fibrosis, or neuromuscular diseases, such as amyotrophic lateral sclerosis (ALS), Guillain-Barré syndrome, or myasthenia gravis, are likely to have airway obstruction owing to the inability to manage secretions. These patients will complain of dyspnea, cough, shortness of breath on exertion, and wheezing. The onset of symptoms in aspiration is usually sudden, and the patient or a witness can often detail the event. A history of seizures, drug or alcohol abuse, or inability to coordinate oral and pharyngeal functions should cause the practitioner to have a high index of suspicion concerning aspiration. Children playing with small toys or food may also be likely candidates for aspiration.

Physical examination will reveal various symptoms of respiratory distress consistent with the amount of lung involved. Chest movement may be diminished over the affected area, and the trachea may be deviated away from a check-valve obstruction or toward an area of collapsed tissue. Likewise, there will be dullness to percussion over a collapsed or consolidated area. Hyperresonance will occur over a hyper-inflated area distal to a check-valve obstruction. Auscultation reveals coarse crackles or wheezes over the affected area. Diminished or absent breath sounds indicate a total obstruction or consolidation of the area.

Initial ABG values show a decreased Pao_2 while the $Paco_2$ and pH remain normal unless there is hyperventilation to compensate for the decreased Pao_2, in which case the decreased $Paco_2$ will accompany an increased pH (respiratory alkalosis). If the patient is unable to compensate, respiratory failure ensues, and ABG values will show an increased $Paco_2$ and decreased pH. This is an ominous sign, and prompt intervention is necessary. Chest radiograph may show obstruction or foreign body. It may also show nonspecific atelectasis or hyperinflation.

Treatment and Nursing Care

Airway Clearance, Ineffective, Related to

- *Acute partial or total obstruction secondary to internal factors*

Treatment of acute airway obstruction secondary to internal factors depends on the nature and severity of obstruction. Nearly total or total obstruction requires immediate stage I care. If foreign body aspiration results in a total obstruction, the Heimlich maneuver may be of use.

With the conscious victim who is standing, the Heimlich maneuver is performed by standing behind the person to support him or her, and placing your arms around the victim (Fig. 11–1). If the victim is sitting, the chair is used as a support. One fist is

FIGURE 11–1. Heimlich maneuver. (Redrawn with permission from Effron DM. © Cardiopulmonary Resuscitation [CPR], 3rd ed, 1986. CPR Publishers, 30).

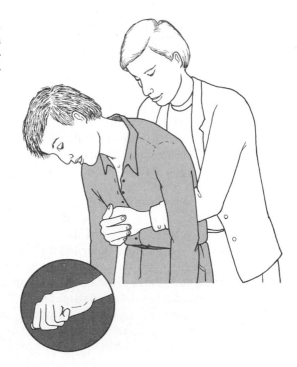

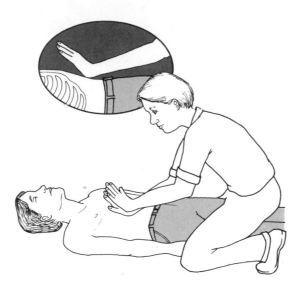

FIGURE 11–2. Heimlich maneuver. (Redrawn with permission from Effron DM. © Cardiopulmonary Resuscitation [CPR], 3rd ed. 1986. CPR Publishers, 28).

placed between the lower ribcage and the navel, and the palm of the other hand is placed on top of the fist. A quick inward and upward compression expels the remaining air in the victim's lung and, it is hoped, also expels the object. The thrusts are repeated in rapid sequence until the obstruction is cleared or the victim becomes unconscious. In the latter event, place the patient in the supine position. Straddling the victim's thighs, with one hand over the other, place the heel of your bottom hand midline, just above the patient's navel. Quickly thrust inward and upward toward the head (Fig. 11–2). Each thrust has the potential of relieving the obstruction. The thrusts are done more gently in smaller adults and children. This technique is useful in the prehospital setting. With children it is especially important to be aware of the probable cause of airway obstruction. Two conditions should exist before manual thrusts are used on a conscious child: (1) you should actually see him or her become obstructed after ingesting food or a foreign object or find the child in a situation in which that is apparent—for example, a toddler playing with a toy with small pieces; (2) you must also have evidence of poor air exchange, such as an ineffective cough and increasing difficulty in breathing. If obstruction results from swelling in the airway in an illness such as croup or from a severe allergic reaction, the Heimlich maneuver would be ineffective and could be harmful (Effron 1986, 30).

The maneuver for infants consists of back blows and chest thrusts. To administer back blows, the infant is placed face down on the nurse's forearm. Head and neck support are provided by resting the infant's chin in a curve between the thumb and index finger. The heel of your hand is used to deliver four forceful blows to the infant's back between the shoulder blades (Fig. 11–3).

To deliver chest thrusts, one hand is positioned behind the infant's head and neck. Two or three fingers of the other hand are placed on the midsternum to apply the chest thrusts at a rate of approximately one per second (Fig. 11–4).

This technique is useful in the prehospital setting but of limited value in the ED. Endotracheal intubation, cricothyroidotomy, or tracheotomy may be necessary, so equipment and skilled personnel should be available. Oxygen to correct hypoxemia

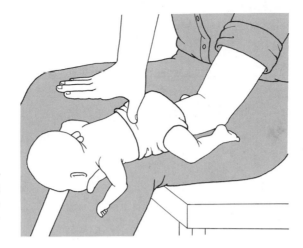

FIGURE 11–3. Back blows. (Redrawn with permission from Effron DM. © Cardiopulmonary Resuscitation [CPR], 3rd ed. 1986. CPR Publishers, 34).

should also be available. Chest physical therapy and postural drainage are *contraindicated* in foreign body aspiration. In addition, humidity therapy may cause movement of the foreign body within the lung. Usually the safest method for extraction of foreign bodies not expelled by the previously described methods is by bronchoscopy.

Obstruction resulting from secretions is generally managed by vigorous pulmonary hygiene, humidity therapy to mobilize secretions, and oxygen therapy to correct hypoxemia.

As was stated previously, the obstruction may be the result of an anatomic

FIGURE 11–4. Chest thrusts. (Redrawn with permission from Effron DM. © Cardiopulmonary Resuscitation [CPR], 3rd ed. 1986. CPR Publishers, 34).

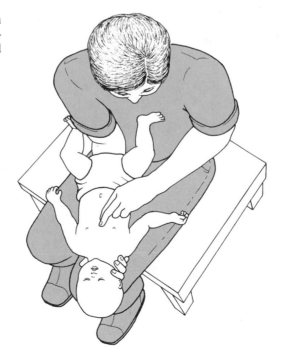

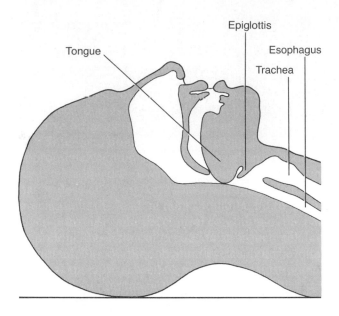

FIGURE 11–5. Upper airway obstruction caused by soft tissue (tongue). (Redrawn with permission from Shapiro B, Harrison R, Trout C: Clinical Application of Respiratory Care. © 1982 by Year Book Medical Publishers, Inc., Chicago, 236.)

structure. The most common airway emergency is caused by the lack of patency between the base of the tongue and the posterior wall of the pharynx (Fig. 11–5).

Treatment of soft tissue airway obstruction is obvious: Relieve the obstruction. This should be accomplished by the simplest maneuvers possible (Shapiro et al 1985, 214). The neck extension and chin manipulation maneuvers are done provided that cervical spine injury is ruled out (Fig. 11–6).

An oropharyngeal airway may be used to maintain the airway. The device lies between the posterior pharynx and the root of the tongue and thereby maintains a

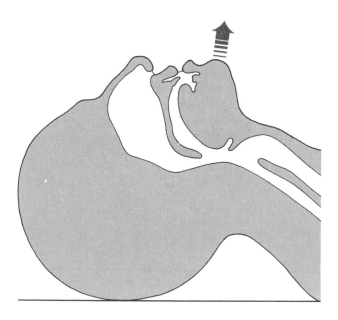

FIGURE 11–6. Clearing soft tissue upper airway obstruction by neck extension and chin elevation. (Redrawn with permission from Shapiro B, Harrison R, Trout C: Clinical Application of Respiratory Care. © 1982 by Year Book Medical Publishers, Inc., Chicago, 236.)

patent airway. This type of airway frequently causes stimulation of the oropharynx and will activate the gag reflect if it is intact. Thus, an oropharyngeal airway is well tolerated by an unconscious patient, but as consciousness returns, the stimulation of this airway may produce gagging, vomiting, and even laryngospasm (Shapiro et al 1985, 216).

It should be noted that an artificial airway should *not* be inserted while a patient is actively seizing. Teeth can become dislodged from forceful insertion of the airway. This in itself can cause an obstruction. The patient may also regain consciousness quickly.

Stage II care for airway obstruction involves continued close observation of vital signs and assessment of respiratory status, including laboratory findings. Initiation of treatment with broad-spectrum antibiotics and steroids is common after removal of the foreign body. Antibiotics are useful in the treatment of bacterial pneumonitis associated with aspiration, and steroids are valuable in dealing with the inflammation associated with aspiration (Berté 1986).

Chronic Obstructive Pulmonary Disease (COPD)

Chronic obstructive pulmonary disease (COPD) is a condition that affects millions of people. An insult such as infection or exposure to an allergen upsets the normal balance that exists in these patients. Because their cardiorespiratory system is already compromised, a relatively small insult can have drastic effects on the patient. If the insult persists or is severe, it can lead to acute respiratory failure.

Etiology and Pathophysiology

COPD actually refers to a group of diseases in which the movement of oxygen and carbon dioxide throughout the pulmonary system is altered. These diseases include chronic bronchitis, pulmonary emphysema, and a mixture of the two. Asthma was formerly grouped in the category of COPD; however, this is erroneous because asthma, although it is an obstructive disease, is better characterized by increased responsiveness of the airways that changes in severity, either spontaneously or as a result of treatment (West 1987). In general, these diseases result in narrowing or obstruction of the small airways leading to the terminal respiratory unit. This narrowing may be the result of bronchospasm, thick mucus, or lack of elasticity of the airways. The effect of this obstruction is reduced expiratory flow rates, leading to air trapping, CO_2 retention, and hypoxemia.

Clinical Manifestations

Patients experiencing respiratory distress resulting from COPD usually will present to the ED with a history of such distress. Dyspnea, dyspnea on exertion, increased sputum production, increased sputum viscosity, and changes in color of sputum are common complaints. The patient may report decreased exercise tolerance and changes in appetite or sleep habits. Marked changes in mental status or loss of consciousness may be signs of advanced carbon dioxide retention or hypoxemia. Cyanosis is generally a poor sign to rely on as an early indicator of symptom severity, because the COPD patient is usually profoundly hypoxemic before cyanosis would be evident.

On physical examination the patient appears in respiratory distress and is working hard to breathe. Usually the patient will be sitting, leaning forward, and exhaling through pursed lips to prolong the expiratory phase. The increased anteroposterior (AP) diameter of the chest and the low flattened diaphragm are characteristic of COPD. Some COPD patients exhibit digital clubbing, but this is of little value in diagnosing the acute episode. Use of accessory muscles, particularly those of the neck and upper chest, is common. The patient may be cyanotic. The quality of breath sounds is generally decreased. Crackles and wheezes may be heard throughout the lung fields, and hyperresonance is noted on percussion. The patient may be febrile, especially if infection is the cause of exacerbation.

Chest radiographs may show chronic changes: a flattened lowered diaphragm, increased AP diameter, and cor pulmonale. ABG values show increased $Paco_2$ with a partially compensated pH, and a decreased Pao_2. Complete blood count (CBC) may show increased numbers of white blood cells and eosinophils, if infection is present.

Treatment and Nursing Care

Airway Clearance, Ineffective, Related to

- *Obstruction of small airways secondary to COPD*

Stage I treatment consists of administration of low-flow oxygen, 1 to 2 L, to achieve a Pao_2 of 55 to 60 mmHg. Increasing the Pao_2 above 60 mmHg may decrease the patient's respiratory drive. Because the COPD patient has a chronically high $Paco_2$ level, the normal drive to breathe may be inactivated and the patient may breathe on a drive triggered by hypoxia. Overcorrection of hypoxemia will result in decreased minute ventilation and increased $Paco_2$.

Beta agonist drugs may be administered by aerosol to relieve bronchospasm. Aminophylline, IV, should be administered as a loading dose of 5 mg/kg over 30 minutes and followed by a continuous infusion of 0.5 to 0.9 mg/kg/hour. Sedatives should be avoided as they may result in respiratory depression, unless the patient is being mechanically ventilated.

If despite therapy the patient's clinical condition continues to deteriorate (increasing $Paco_2$, decreasing pH, and decreasing Pao_2), an endotracheal tube should be placed and mechanical ventilation should be instituted.

A device that is particularly useful in the management of the COPD patient during an acute crisis is the Venti-mask (Venturi mask). This device works to deliver a specific concentration of gas to the patient. Normally the Fio_2 delivered by a nasal cannula or oxygen mask will vary with the flow as well as the respiratory pattern of the patient. The Venti-mask will always deliver the precise concentration of oxygen that it is set to deliver. Fio_2 values of 24 to 28 percent are useful in the management of the COPD patient.

Once life-threatening respiratory failure is no longer imminent, stage II care may be initiated. This involves continual assessment of laboratory data (ABGs), vital signs, and general respiratory status. During this time, patients and their families need to be assessed for any possible knowledge deficits that they may have related to COPD.

Allergic Airway Disease: Asthma

• *Etiology and Pathophysiology*

Asthma is a common disease that affects millions of children and adults. It results in widespread bronchoconstriction, reduced airflow, and increased air trapping. Mucosal edema adds to the decreased airflow, as do thickened secretions. The asthmatic patient may always have some degree of bronchoconstriction, but acute episodes are triggered by a wide variety or combination of factors, including immunologic, environmental, and psychologic factors.

Clinical Manifestations

The patient may report a sudden or gradual onset of wheezing, chest tightness, dyspnea, and cough. This may be the result of exposure to known or unknown stimuli. Often attacks accompany a cold or upper respiratory infection. Patients with acute episodes may have a previous history of the disease. Care should be taken to assess medication that the patient has taken prior to admission. It is not uncommon to find that overuse of medication has caused the patient to become tachyphylactic to certain drugs, resulting in the patient's requiring higher doses of the drug to achieve the desired effect.

On physical examination the patient will appear to be experiencing some degree of respiratory distress. Usually the patient will be sitting, and he or she may be leaning forward. Cough will usually be irritating, dry, and nonproductive. Sputum that is produced is generally clear or white, thick, and mucoid. The patient will be dyspneic and tachypneic. Breathing is shallow, with a prolonged expiratory phase, and wheezing may be audible without a stethoscope. Auscultation reveals wheezes and crackles, a prolonged expiratory phase, and possibly poor air entry. Pulsus paradoxus (a decrease of 10 mm Hg or more in the systolic blood pressure during inspiration) is characteristic of acute episodes of asthma. Palpation reveals decreased chest wall movement, and percussion reveals hyperresonance.

ABGs will change with the severity of the attack. $Paco_2$ increases with air trapping, Pao_2 decreases, and the pH will decrease as a result of increasing $Paco_2$. Bedside pulmonary function tests (PFTs) will reveal decreased vital capacity (VC) and increased functional residual capacity (FRC) and residual volume (RV). Flow rates are diminished as evidenced by the decreased forced expiratory volume at one second (FEV_1). There is generally an increase in eosinophils in both the blood and the sputum. Electrocardiogram (EKG) may show a right axis deviation. Chest radiograph (CXR) generally is nonspecific, or it may show some air trapping or an increased AP diameter.

Treatment and Nursing Care

Airway Clearance, Ineffective, Related to

  • *Narrowing or obstruction of airways secondary to asthma*

Goals of stage I treatment for persons experiencing acute asthma attacks are generally to relieve bronchoconstriction and air trapping (Zagelbaum and Paré 1982). When the episode of bronchospasm is judged to be severe, some or all of the following therapeutic interventions may be employed to relieve bronchoconstriction: administration of aerosolized bronchodilators, parenteral bronchodilators, and sympathomimetics; oxygen; and intravenous fluids. Blood for CBC, theophylline levels, and ABGs are also commonly obtained.

Aerosolized bronchodilators are often the first line of treatment for persons experiencing severe asthma in the ED setting. Doses of the bronchodilators vary with the particular drug selected. Metaproterenol, 5% (Alupent), or salbutamol, 0.5% (Ventolin), are two commonly used beta-2 selective agonists. These drugs have fewer side effects than isoproterenol (Isuprel) and isoetharine (Bronkosol) while providing effective bronchial smooth muscle relaxation.

Parenteral bronchodilators are then indicated if the patient does not respond to appropriately administered aerosolized bronchodilators. Aminophylline, 5 to 7 mg/ kg as a loading dose over a 30-minute period, may be administered, with a maintenance dose of 15 mg/kg/24 hours. If the patient is currently taking a theophylline preparation, the loading dose should be up to 3 mg/kg, depending on the amount given previously and the clinical condition of the patient. Aminophylline functions to prolong the action of beta-agonist bronchodilators and also acts as a respiratory stimulant. Blood aminophylline levels should be followed in an attempt to determine optimal therapy, as well as safeguard against potentially toxic effects of the drug. Signs and symptoms of toxicity include cardiac dysrhythmias, nausea, vomiting, diarrhea, abdominal pain, confusion, and seizures.

Sympathomimetics, such as epinephrine or terbutaline (Brethine), have been used in the treatment of severe bronchoconstriction. Doses of 0.1 to 0.3 ml of a 1 : 1000 epinephrine solution may be given subcutaneously and repeated two to three times at 20-minute intervals. If *terbutaline* (0.25 to 0.5 mg subcutaneously every 6 to 8 hours) is administered, it has the advantage of more specific beta-2 activity and longer duration of action (Zagelbaum and Paré 1982).

Oxygen should be administered to relieve hypoxemia. Some asthmatic patients may show signs of chronic CO_2 retention (high $Paco_2$, with a partially compensated pH). Low-flow oxygen to these patients must be closely monitored to prevent respiratory depression.

Intravenous fluids should be maintained and replaced to correct dehydration, which may thicken bronchial secretions and promote mucous plugging. Usually during an acute episode oral intake is poor. The solution and rate of infusion are determined by the individualized needs of the patient. "Some asthmatic patients, particularly the elderly with some cardiac decompensation, are susceptible to developing superimposed congestive heart failure from excessive fluid administration. Patients who are volume depleted should be constantly monitored with serial objective measurements of pulse rate, blood pressure, urinary output, and central venous pressure" (Zagelbaum and Paré 1982, 75).

Various steroids may be administered when typical treatment fails. Therapeutic responses to corticosteroids, however, may not be evident for several hours after administration. Nonetheless, in some cases corticosteroids can give dramatic relief. It is thought that they may potentiate the action of beta-2 adrenergic drugs. In acute situations, when asthma cannot be controlled by intravenous aminophylline, 125 mg of hydrocortisone (IV) or an equivalent is administered every 4 to 6 hours (Mitchell and Petty 1982).

Intubation with mechanical ventilation should only be used as a last resort. Mechanical ventilation is associated with a high incidence of complications in the asthmatic patient. Sedation and muscle paralysis (with Pavulon) is sometimes indicated in the management of these patients. Positive end expiratory pressure (with PEEP) and expiratory retard are generally *contraindicated* in these patients.

An attempt is made to identify and treat the precipitating cause of the attack in stage II care. Vigorous pulmonary hygiene is indicated, after the acute phase has passed. Caution should be exercised, as many patients will react adversely to the administration of aerosolized saline or water solutions. Certain positions in postural drainage may be poorly tolerated.

DISORDERS OF PULMONARY CIRCULATION

Pulmonary Edema

Etiology and Pathophysiology

Pulmonary edema may be the result of one or more factors that result in fluid accumulating in the lungs. Fluid from the pulmonary circulation crosses into the alveolar space, which normally is occupied with air. This may be the result of an increase in pulmonary artery pressure, increased blood volume load, left ventricular failure, increased capillary permeability, or changes in capillary pressure. A distinct disorder that presents the same set of symptoms and problems is high-altitude pulmonary edema. Patients can become acutely ill at higher altitudes, but the situation usually reverses when the patient is returned to a lower altitude.

Clinical Manifestations

The patient will have a history of COPD, cor pulmonale, or congestive heart failure (CHF). Presenting symptoms include dyspnea, anxiety, diaphoresis, tachycardia, hypertension, and possibly cyanosis.

On physical examination patients in pulmonary edema usually are sitting in an upright position and are in general distress. The patient appears diaphoretic, dyspneic, and extremely anxious. Air entry is coarse, but likely equal in both lungs. Respirations are quick and shallow. Cough is productive of pink frothy secretions that are characteristic of pulmonary edema. Auscultation reveals diffuse fine and coarse crackles and wheezes throughout the lung fields. A gallop rhythm is common on auscultation of the heart.

ABG values show a marked decrease in the Pao_2. In an attempt to compensate for hypoxemia, the patient's respiratory rate may increase, causing the $Paco_2$ to be low with respiratory alkalosis (increased pH). The CXR shows increased pulmonary vascular markings, cardiomegaly, or possible right-sided hypertrophy. A pulmonary artery catheter (Swan-Ganz) will show a high pulmonary artery wedge pressure.

Treatment and Nursing Care

Impaired Gas Exchange, Related to

- ### Pulmonary edema

Stage I treatment is usually required for patients with pulmonary edema. Relief of hypoxemia and improvement of ventricular performance are primary goals. Oxygen will both relieve the hypoxemia and reduce pulmonary artery pressure. Ventricular performance is enhanced by decreasing the preload. Venous return is reduced by elevating the patient's head and administering diuretics. Morphine sulfate, 3 to 5 mg intravenously, should be administered carefully to decrease anxiety and decrease preload. Careful monitoring is necessary to prevent respiratory depression or hypotension, or both. Adverse side effects of morphine should be promptly treated with reversal (naloxone [Narcan], 0.4 mg intravenously) and respiratory support.

Vasodilators such as nitroglycerin (0.3 to 0.6 mg sublingually) will improve ventricular performance by decreasing ventricular preload and decreasing peripheral vascular resistance (afterload). Vasodilators are contraindicated in the hypotensive patient. Digitalis will improve myocardial contractility in an attempt to decease the preload.

Hypoxemia, acidosis, and hypokalemia should all be corrected before administering digitalis, and the dose should be conservative if acute myocardial infarction is suspected. Electrocardiogram (EKG) should be monitored for dysrhythmias.

A Swan-Ganz catheter is very useful in the stage II management of these patients. Generally the goal is a pulmonary artery wedge pressure (PAWP) of 12 to 14 mmHg. A PAWP of 18 mmHg and above indicates poor left ventricular function, whereas a PAWP of less than 12 mmHg indicates shock.

Pulmonary Embolus or Pulmonary Infarction

Etiology and Pathophysiology

In a strict sense, pulmonary embolism (PE) is a circulatory disorder with pulmonary manifestations. In severe cases, these pulmonary manifestations can be life threatening. Prompt recognition, and rapid, effective management are the keys to successful treatment.

Pulmonary embolism develops when a thrombus or clot arises in the venous system, passes through the right side of the chest and lodges in the pulmonary circulation. The pulmonary circulation is the point with smallest diameter before the blood reaches the left side of the heart. Thus, any clots or debris will lodge somewhere in the pulmonary circulation. The magnitude of the cardiopulmonary disruption is directly related to the size, number, and location of the clots as well as the patient's baseline cardiopulmonary status. The resultant blockage prevents blood flow from the right side of the heart (pulmonary arterial) from passing through the affected area of the pulmonary vasculature. This flow is shunted through other areas of the lung that are not blocked. If the blockage is small, there is very little effect on the overall picture.

However, when the blockage is large or there are small and numerous clots, a greater percentage of the blood flow is affected. This results in an increased percentage of the right heart output reaching the left side of the heart without participating in gas exchange. This is termed percentage shunt. As the percentage shunt increases, the patient's condition deteriorates, as he or she is no longer able to compensate for the deficiency in gas exchange.

Another expression of the underlying problem can be seen in terms of ventilation-perfusion mismatch. In the resting state, the total alveolar ventilation roughly matches the cardiac output, so that in the healthy adult the ratio of ventilation to perfusion is $1:1$. When circulation disturbance decreases the theoretical match between ventilation and perfusion, a condition exists in which ventilation exceeds perfusion. The resulting mismatch alters gas exchange and ultimately blood gas values. As the patient responds to this alteration by increasing his or her minute ventilation, the classic picture of decreased $Paco_2$, decreased Pao_2, and increased pH (respiratory alkalosis) with hypoxemia results.

The emergent condition is frequently preventable and potentially fatal. Small emboli are common and often go undiagnosed. Most pulmonary emboli arise as detached portions of venous thrombi from deep veins of the lower extremities. Other sites include the right side of the heart associated with atrial fibrillation. Nonthrombotic emboli, such as air, fat from a long bone fracture, or amniotic fluid from childbirth, can also occur but less frequently (West 1987).

Because nutrition to the lung tissue is partially derived from the pulmonary blood flow, continued blockage can result in infarction and loss of effective lung tissue. Pulmonary infarction can be over a small or large area depending on the site and magnitude of the blockage.

Clinical Manifestations

Most cases of significant pulmonary embolism arise in patients with very well defined predisposing factors (Table 11–4). The patient will report sudden shortness of breath, possibly chest pain, anxiety, and possibly hemoptysis.

TABLE 11–4
Factors Predisposing to Pulmonary Embolism

Immobilization	Trauma
Thrombophlebitis	Pregnancy state,
Recent surgery	postpartum
Myocardial infarction	Birth control pill
Atrial fibrillation	Obesity
Congestive heart failure	

Often the patient's presenting sign is profound respiratory distress with a general absence of other pulmonary symptoms. The patient may be diaphoretic, anxious, febrile, and cyanotic, and may report pleuritic pain. A cough may be present that is either nonproductive or productive of blood. The patient will be tachypneic and tachycardic. Breath sounds are usually clear and equal bilaterally.

Most laboratory results are nonspecific and tend only to support a suspected diagnosis of pulmonary embolism. ABG values may show hypoxemia (decreased Pao_2), a compensatory hyperventilation with a lowered $Paco_2$, and respiratory alkalosis (increased pH). The EKG shows nonspecific changes. Chest radiograph (CXR) usually is normal, but it may show an enlarged pulmonary artery, pleural effusion, or consolidation. Lung scans may show diminished perfusion with normal ventilation patterns, depending on the size and distribution of the embolus(i). Pulmonary angiography is the most definitive diagnostic tool.

Treatment and Nursing Care

Impaired Gas Exchange, Related to

- *Perfusion imbalance secondary to pulmonary embolus(i)*

Stage I therapy includes relief of hypoxemia, maintenance of cardiopulmonary function, and relief of pain and respiratory distress. Oxygen therapy should relieve the hypoxemia associated with embolization. The oxygen should be delivered to maintain the Pao_2 between 60 and 90 mmHg. Correction of the hypoxemia may not relieve the subjective feeling of shortness of breath. Vasoactive drugs may be used if cardiac failure with depression of cardiac output occurs. Fibrinolytic therapy such as streptokinase or urokinase may be used to dissolve fibrin clots and for rapid resolution of large emboli in pulmonary arteries. Because of potential adverse side effects, careful monitoring of the patient is essential.

Stage II care is aimed at reducing the risk of further venous thrombosis and embolization. Specific treatment will be based on the patient's presenting condition. Parenteral anticoagulation with heparin is initiated in many cases of suspected pulmonary embolism without a firmly established diagnosis. An initial bolus of 5000 to 15,000 units is given intravenously. Therapy is maintained by a continuous intravenous infusion at 20 units/kg/hour or approximately 1000 units/hour. Heparin therapy is best monitored by obtaining an initial and then serial partial thromboplastin times (PTT).

DISORDERS OF CONTROL OF BREATHING (HYPOVENTILATION): HEAD TRAUMA, SPINAL CORD INJURY, CEREBROVASCULAR ACCIDENT (CVA)

Etiology and Pathophysiology

The act of breathing is controlled by cells in the brain stem and influenced by various peripheral chemoreceptors. Injury to the brain stem, peripheral receptors, or the

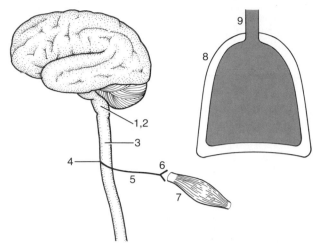

FIGURE 11-7. Causes of hypoventilation. They include (1) depression of the respiratory center by drugs (especially barbiturate and morphine derivatives) or anesthesia, (2) diseases of the medulla including encephalitis, trauma, hemorrhage, or neoplasm (rare), (3) abnormalities of the spinal conducting pathways, as following high cervical dislocation, (4) anterior horn cell diseases such as poliomyelitis, (5) diseases of the nerves to the respiratory muscles including the Guillain-Barré syndrome and diphtheria, (6) diseases of the myoneural junction such as myasthenia gravis and anticholinesterase poisoning, (7) diseases of the respiratory muscles, for example, progressive muscular dystrophy, (8) thoracic cage abnormalities such as crushed chest, (9) upper airway obstruction such as tracheal compression by a thymoma or aortic aneurysm. (Redrawn from West J. Pulmonary Pathophysiology—The Essentials, 3rd. ed. pp. 23-24. © by Williams & Wilkins, 1987.)

nervous pathway to the respiratory muscles can have a profound effect on the patient's cardiorespiratory status. When the volume of fresh gas going to the alveoli per minute (alveolar ventilation) is reduced, hypoventilation results. *Hypoventilation* is the accepted term for these disorders that affect gas exchange. "Hypoventilation is commonly caused by diseases outside the lung; indeed, very often the lungs are normal" (West 1987, 23) (Fig. 11-7). A spinal cord injury is usually the result of trauma. Impulses generated in the brain stem cannot be transmitted to the respiratory muscles via the damaged spinal cord. Indirect injury to the brain stem can be caused when intracranial pressure is increased either by injury, such as closed head trauma, or by diseases, such as hydrocephalus. Because there may be no way for this pressure to be relieved in the closed cranium, the increased pressure can actually push the brain stem down through the hole at the bottom of the skull. The damage caused by herniation of the brain stem is usually fatal and always debilitating. A cerebrovascular accident (CVA) may infarct the area responsible for controlling respiratory function, resulting in apnea or abnormal breathing patterns.

Clinical Manifestations

Because respiratory insufficiency and failure ensue as the result of hypoventilation, regardless of the cause, physiologic pulmonary manifestations for each of these disorders are similar (Emanuelsen and Densmore 1981; Hopp and Williams, 1987; West 1987). The patient's level of consciousness may range from alert to comatose. The patient may complain of dyspnea and will exhibit anxiety if alert. A traumatic event will usually be involved or suspected. A history of drug use or attempted suicide might also be considered.

Ventilation may be labored and muscles of the neck and upper chest may be in use. The patient is dyspneic and may be tachycardic. There is poor chest excursion and air entry, and few specific pulmonary signs are present. Secretions may accumulate and the patient may have a weak ineffective cough. The patient may exhibit muscle weakness or sensory loss depending on the nature of the injury.

ABG values will indicate a decreased Pa_{O_2}, and if ventilatory failure is present there will be an increased Pa_{CO_2} and decreased pH. Depending on the nature and the duration of the disorder, the CXR may show scattered atelectasis. In spinal cord injury, the diaphragm may be high on one or both sides.

Treatment and Nursing Care

Breathing Pattern, Ineffective, Related to

- **Disorders of Control of Breathing (Hypoventilation)**

The word *management* is more appropriate for this section rather than *treatment,* because hypoventilation is not a specific disease but rather results from multiple disorders. The pulmonary manifestations must be handled as part of each of these disorders.

Respiratory supportive measures are the focus of the stage I care when respiratory insufficiency or failure occurs. The goal of all treatments is to ameliorate or modify disabling symptoms of the ineffective breathing pattern and to ensure adequate gas exchange (Hopp and Williams 1987, 205). Stage I care required for respiratory or ventilatory failure secondary to a spinal cord injury, CVA, drug overdose, or neuromuscular disorder will be immediate intubation and mechanical ventilation. The tidal volume and Fi_{O_2} will be individualized for each patient's needs. For example, the patient with a neuromuscular disorder may require only a low Fi_{O_2} but a full tidal volume, whereas the postoperative patient with a CVA may require a higher Fi_{O_2}, if he or she has superimposed pulmonary complications.

If narcotic overdose is suspected, the patient should be given naloxone (Narcan) intravenously in doses of 0.2 to 0.4 mg and 50 ml of a 50% dextrose solution. If this initial dose provides no improvement, it is repeated after 5 minutes using 0.4 to 1.6 mg. More invasive measures, such as gastric lavage and purging, may be instituted (Brenner 1985).

Stage II care would center on obtaining drug toxicology screening for the drug overdose patient. Supportive therapy for this if aspiration is suspected would include sending sputum cultures, performing chest physical therapy, and administering antibiotics. The neuromuscular patient may also require these measures, as aspiration is common.

As was stated previously, the pulmonary manifestations are just part of the problems these patients have. Specific stage I and stage II treatment of the injury or disorder is discussed elsewhere in this book.

DISORDERS OF GAS EXCHANGE

Carbon Monoxide Poisoning

Carbon monoxide (CO) is an odorless, colorless gas that is generally formed as the result of combustion. Inhalation of the gas results in a severe hypoxia that can be rapidly fatal. The relative level of CO in the blood determines the severity of the disorder. Hemoglobin, the chemical compound in the red blood cell (RBC) that binds and carries the oxygen, has 240 times more affinity for CO than oxygen. Thus, CO rapidly replaces the oxygen that is carried by the RBCs, resulting in severe tissue hypoxia. Because the affinity of hemoglobin for carbon monoxide is so high, it is difficult to displace the CO from the hemoglobin molecule once it is bound.

Clinical Manifestations

The patient generally is found in a closed environment in the presence of combusted gases, such as smoke, automobile exhaust, or fumes from a faulty furnace. The patient's level of consciousness will range from alert to comatose, depending on the blood level of CO. Patients who smoke or are exposed to automobile exhaust may run baseline CO levels of 12 to 18%. The normal is considered to be under 12%. Ideally 0% would be best, but all of us are affected by environmental factors that influence the CO level. Manifestations of CO levels of 20 to 25% include headache, dizziness, nausea, and dyspnea. A level of 40% to 50% can lead to coma. The patient may exhibit the characteristic "cherry-red" color of the skin and mucous membranes. Depending on the source of the CO, the patient may also have airway burns and a cough that is dry and productive of dark debris-filled sputum. Tachycardia and dehydration may also be seen. Carboxyhemoglobin levels are key to the management of these patients.

Treatment and Nursing Care

Impaired Gas Exchange, Related to

- *Carbon monoxide poisoning*

Depending on the degree of carbon monoxide poisoning, stage I care may be required. Treatment consists primarily of exposure to high concentrations of oxygen for prolonged periods of time. Moderate cases can be treated with exposure to humidified oxygen with an Fio_2 of 1.0 (100%) for 4 to 6 hours. Higher CO levels can be treated with hyperbaric oxygenation. However, treatment should not be delayed to move a patient to a hyperbaric chamber. In a hyperbaric chamber the atmospheric pressure is increased to two to three times normal. With an Fio_2 of 1.0, it is possible to achieve very high Pao_2 levels in the patient and thus reverse the tissue hypoxia more quickly and effectively.

Stage II treatment involves continued observation of the patient's vital signs and neurologic signs and observation of the CO level. Additionally, some events leading to CO exposure may require stage II assessment to prevent future injuries.

Cyanide Poisoning

Etiology and Pathophysiology

Cyanide is a poison that prevents removal of oxygen from the RBCs at the tissue level. The patient will not appear cyanotic, despite the fact that his or her organs and tissues will be severely hypoxic. Cyanide poisoning can occur from purposeful or accidental ingestion or inhalation of cyanide compounds, such as potassium cyanide, hydrocyanic acid, or vinyl cyanide, to name a few.

Clinical Manifestations

The diagnosis of cyanide poisoning is not definitive but is rather based on a high level of suspicion. The patient may have attempted suicide or have been exposed in an industrial setting. He or she may have unexplained changes in mental status or may be comatose. Severe tissue hypoxia may cause cardiac excitability and rhythm disturbances. Air entry and tidal volume appear to be adequate. Cardiac irritability and dysrhythmias are common. A characteristic "almond" odor is present. Toxicology screen is vital to diagnosis. ABG values and CXR will seem normal.

Treatment and Nursing Care

Impaired Gas Exchange, Related to

- *Cyanide poisoning*

    Stage I treatment involves the administration of the antidote for cyanide, which is amyl nitrite. It is inhaled for 30 to 60 seconds every 5 minutes until symptoms disappear. Sodium nitrite and sodium thiosulfate may then be given intravenously as necessary. Stage II care involves close observation of the patient and toxicology profiles.

Pulmonary Infection

The respiratory system usually functions in harmony with the pathogens to which it is exposed. The respiratory system has a very effective set of defenses that maintain nearly sterile conditions within the lower respiratory tract. A breakdown in these defenses can result in an infection in the respiratory tract, with response by the body to this infection. Even in the modern era of antibiotics, pneumonia is the leading cause of death from infectious disease in the United States (Donowitz and Mandell 1983; McKellar 1985).

Clinical Manifestations

Patients with a preexisting or chronic alteration in their immune systems are most commonly affected. Usually the patient's presenting complaints will be a gradual onset of general and then specific symptoms. The patient may complain of a recent or current "cold" or "flu." Pleuritic chest pain and aching ribs may also be reported. Usually, cough and sputum production are presenting symptoms. Pathogens can be viral, bacterial, mycobacterial, or fungal.

The patient will have varying degrees of respiratory distress that may be mild or severe, or perhaps occur only on exertion. Usually, respiratory infections are associated with another primary illness that has made the patient susceptible to the infectious agent. Also to be considered is aspiration or acute injury, such as pulmonary contusion. Typically, the patient is febrile. Character and severity of the fever should be noted, as should the duration and nature of the cough and the amount, consistency, and nature of sputum produced. Auscultation may reveal crackles, wheezes, or a combination of both over an affected area or areas of the lung(s). Breath sounds may be normal or absent in some cases. Dullness to percussion over consolidated areas is characteristic.

ABG values may be normal. In patients with pre-existing pulmonary disease there may be significant alteration of ABGs. Normally a decrease in the Pao_2 would be expected if there were any changes at all. CXR may show the abnormality, especially if it is well established. "Radiologic abnormalities may be diffuse or localized and should be compared with physical examination of the chest. Infections can produce cavitations or loss of lung volume, pleural fluid or building interlobar fissures" (Zagelbaum and Paré 1982, 112). Chest radiograph changes may lag 24 hours behind the disease process. In general, fluid, consolidations, or changes in air volume should be noted. Also, it should be noted whether the abnormality is widespread or localized. Sputum should be obtained for Gram stain and staining for acid-fast bacilli (AFB). Blood cultures and white count should also be obtained. Leukocyte counts of 15,000 to 25,000 mm³ and presence of neutrophils are associated with bacterial pneumonia. A low or normal count is characteristic of viral or mycobacterial (tuberculosis, leprosy) pneumonia.

Treatment and Nursing Care

Impaired Gas Exchange, Related to

• *Pneumonia*

Stage I treatment for most pulmonary infections usually is not required. Treatment is directed toward identifying and treating the specific infectious agent. The next step is dealing with the symptoms and response to the infection. This includes oxygen therapy to treat hypoxemia and aerosolized bronchodilators to treat bronchospasm. Aggressive pulmonary hygiene is used to treat excessive secretions and consolidation. Adequate systemic hydration and humidity therapy will help to thin and mobilize secretions. Fever and pain should be controlled with appropriate drugs.

CONCLUSION

The inability to breathe is probably the most anxiety-provoking event a person can experience. Caring for patients with this problem is one of the biggest challenges a nurse will face. To meet this challenge, it is essential that nurses have a good understanding of the pathophysiology and symptoms associated with pulmonary disorders. Nurses must also possess excellent assessment skills to be able to identify problems and anticipate the care required for this type of patient.

REFERENCES

Berté JB. 1986. Critical Care of the Lung, 2nd ed. Norwalk, CT, Appelton-Century-Crofts.

Brenner BE. 1985. Comprehensive Management of Respiratory emergencies. Rockville, MD, Aspen Publications.

Donowitz GR, Mandell GL. 1983. Empirical therapy for pneumonia. Rev Infect Dis 5:S40–S51.

Effron DM. 1986. Cardiopulmonary Resuscitation (CPR), 3rd ed. Tulsa, OK, CPR Publishers.

Emanuelsen KL, Densmore MJ. 1981. Acute Respiratory Care. Bethany, CT, Fleschner Publishing Co.

Hopp LJ, Williams M. 1987. Ineffective breathing pattern related to decreased lung expansion. Nurs Clin North Am 22:193–205.

Kim MJ, McFarland GK, McLane AM. 1987. Pocket Guide to Nursing Diagnoses. St. Louis, CV Mosby Co.

McKellar P. 1985. Treatment of community acquired pneumonias. Am J Med 79 (Suppl 2A):25–31.

Mitchell RS, Petty TL. 1982. Synopsis of Clinical Pulmonary Diseases. St. Louis, CV Mosby Co.

Parey KP, Youtsey JW. 1981. Respiratory Patient Care. Englewood Cliffs, NJ, Prentice-Hall.

Shapiro BA, Harrison RA, Kacmarek RMT, et al. 1985. Clinical Application of Respiratory Care, 3rd ed. Chicago, Year Book Medical Publishers.

West J. 1987. Pulmonary Pathophysiology: The Essentials, 3rd ed. Baltimore, Harper.

Zagelbaum G, Paré JA. 1982. Manual of Acute Respiratory Care. Boston, Little, Brown and Co.

Respiratory Care Devices and Procedures

OXYGEN THERAPY

---

cannula: An oxygen delivery device that administers oxygen through nasal prongs that are positioned in the patient's nares. Generally this device is used to deliver oxygen at flows of 1 to 6 L/minute.

Venti-mask: An oxygen delivery device that consists of a mask that fits over the patient's nose and mouth and incorporates a Venturi device. The Venturi device takes a flow of oxygen and entrains a precise amount of room air, resulting in the delivery of a specific oxygen concentration. These devices are useful when an exact concentration of oxygen must be delivered, and they can provide concentrations of 24% to 40%.

non-rebreather mask: An oxygen delivery device that consists of a mask that fits over the patient's nose and mouth, with a reservoir bag. It is used to deliver high concentrations of oxygen. The reservoir bag fills with oxygen when the patient exhales, and this reservoir supplements the flow of oxygen during inspiration to deliver a higher concentration of oxygen to the patient. Flow rates of 8 to 15 L/minute should be used with this device and can provide a concentration of oxygen of 21% to 90% or more. The flow should be adequate to prevent the complete collapse of the bag during inspiration.

high-flow system: An oxygen delivery system that provides a precise concentration of oxygen at a flow rate that meets or exceeds the patient's inspiratory demand. This ensures that the patient will receive the set Fio_2. High-flow systems can provide concentrations of 24% to 100% oxygen. These systems are commonly used by patients with tracheostomies and endotracheal tubes.

hyperbaric therapy: A chamber in which the atmospheric pressure can be changed. Patients can be placed under pressures of several times the normal atmospheric pressure. This chamber is used in the treatment of carbon monoxide poisoning, air embolism, diving accidents, and anaerobic infections. Often these chambers are large enough to accommodate a surgical team along with the patient being treated.

AEROSOL OR HUMIDITY THERAPY

drug administration: A liquid medication can be made into a mist (aerosolized) that is inhaled by a patient. This allows deposition of the drug directly in the patient's airways. Drugs delivered by aerosol are generally those that are used as bronchodilators or to thin secretions, although it is possible to deliver other drugs for absorption to the blood stream by this route. In general, solutions of 3 to 5 ml of the drug is placed in a nebulizer. The nebulizer is powered by a compressed gas such as air or oxygen, and it aerosolizes the medication for inspiration by the patient.

pneumatic aerosol: This refers to large-volume aerosol generators that make a mist of sterile water or saline solution to be inhaled by a patient. The purpose is generally to humidify the respiratory tract and thin secretions.

ultrasonic aerosol: This device generates an aerosol mist by use of high-frequency sound waves. The mist that is produced contains droplets of a very small particle size. This allows for deposition in the smaller airways, but caution must be exercised because these units are capable of delivering large volumes of water to the respiratory tract in a relatively short period of time. Overliquefication of secretions in a debilitated patient can lead to "drowning" in one's own secretions.

heated humidity: A device that adds both heat and humidity to a flow of gas. Usually gas is passed through a reservoir that contains water and a heat source. The most common device of this type is the cascade type humidifier. These are generally used with patients on ventilators with artificial airways, although they can be used with face masks.

PULMONARY HYGIENE

suction: A catheter is passed into the patient's airway, and a vacuum is applied to the catheter. This will draw fluid and secretions, as well as air, through the catheter and into a reservoir. This procedure is used to remove secretions from a patient's airway or to obtain samples of sputum (Lukens tube). Suctioning is a stressful procedure for the patient and is associated with cardiac irritability. Patients should be well oxygenated and ventilated prior to suctioning.

chest physical therapy: A procedure in which rhythmic clapping and vibration over specific segments of the lung is used to help loosen and mobilize secretions. It is commonly used in the long-term management of patients with chronic lung diseases.

postural drainage: A procedure often associated with chest physical therapy, in which gravity is utilized to drain specific segments of the lung. By positioning the patient so that the bronchi that drain a segment of the lung are pointed down, movement of secretions to the main stem bronchi is enhanced.

MECHANICAL VENTILATION

manual ventilation: A procedure in which air is forced into the patient's airways and lungs through a tight-fitting mask or via an artificial airway. This is done to replace or supplement a patient's own spontaneous ventilation. It is used in conjunction with CPR, to hyperventilate the patient, or in place of mechanical ventilation. Usually a resuscitator bag is used. A reservoir attached to the end of the bag will allow higher concentrations of oxygen to be delivered. Manual ventilators are usually self-inflating and allow use of either room air or supplemental oxygen. Pressure and volume are delivered by manually squeezing the bag. The bigger the squeeze, the higher the volume or pressure delivered.

positive pressure ventilation: A procedure in which all or a portion of the patient's work of breathing is assumed by a mechanical device. Many different devices are available that vary in complexity. In general, they can be set to deliver pressure, a set tidal volume, a preset respiratory rate, a specific Fio_2, and a variety of other variables.

negative pressure ventilation: A procedure in which negative pressure is exerted over the patient's thorax or upper abdomen, pulling up and down on the thorax and down on the diaphragm. The resulting change in pressure creates a passive inspiration by the patient. Iron lungs, "turtle" shells, and chest cuirasses are the devices commonly used. For a time these devices fell into disuse, but recently they have found a new life in the management of the patient with chronic lung and neuromuscular diseases.

ARTIFICIAL AIRWAYS

endotracheal tube: A device that can be inserted orally or nasally through the larynx and into the patient's trachea. In adults, a cuff seals the outer edge of the tube. The distal tip of the tube should be positioned above the patient's carina so that both lungs will be ventilated. Suction catheters can be passed through the tube to remove secretions from the lungs. Positive pressure ventilation can be delivered through the tube as well.

tracheotomy: A surgical procedure in which an opening is created in the patient's trachea. This is usually done to pass a tracheostomy tube into the airway, but it can be done as an emergency procedure to relieve airway obstruction.

tracheostomy tube: A device made of metal or plastic that is placed into the patient's trachea by a surgical procedure. The tube allows suction catheters to be passed into the airway to remove secretions. It also allows positive pressure ventilation to be delivered to the patient's airways and lungs. This artificial airway is preferred to the endotracheal tube for long-term use (more than a few days).

transtracheal catheter: A device that is placed through the wall of the trachea in a surgical procedure. It is used to deliver low flows of oxygen to the patient suffering from a chronic disease that requires continous oxygen therapy. The tube will not interfere with normal breathing or emergency procedures, such as CPR, or with endotracheal intubation.

BEDSIDE SPIROMETRY

Tests are done with hand-held and portable devices to assess the function of the patient's pulmonary system. Commonly performed tests include the following:

tidal volume: The volume of air inhaled or exhaled during a normal breath. Normally it is 500 to 750 ml in a normal adult.

vital capacity: The amount of air that is exhaled after a maximal inspiration and exhalation by the patient. Normally it is 4 to 5 L in the adult.

peak flow: The flow rate in L/minute at the peak of a forced expiratory maneuver. Generally used to assess the effectiveness of bronchodilators in the asthmatic patient.

FEV_1: Forced expiratory volume after 1 second. The patient performs a forced expiratory maneuver after a maximal inspiration. The volume that is exhaled in the first second is measured and compared against the predicted value, and reported as percentage predicted. Normal is greater than 80% predicted. Used to assess air trapping in COPD and asthma.

incentive spirometry: A procedure that utilizes a device that measures the patient's inhaled or exhaled volume. The patient is encouraged to achieve this volume repeatedly. This procedure is used in postoperative patients to encourage deep breathing.

LABORATORY

arterial blood gases: A sample of arterial blood is obtained from a peripheral artery. It is analyzed for its Pao_2, $Paco_2$, and pH, which allows for the calculation of metabolic values. This allows assessment of the ability of the cardiorespiratory system to deliver oxygen to the tissues and remove waste products (CO_2) and maintain a balanced pH (acid-base ratio).

carboxyhemoglobin: A sample of blood, usually arterial, is analyzed for carbon monoxide content. CO content is expressed as a percentage of the hemoglobin that is saturated with CO. Normal CO content varies because smoking and air pollution affect the value. Sometimes values as high as 17% to 18% are considered normal.

Linda Clemmings, RN MA MS
Jane Duda, RN MSN
Joan Duda, RN MS

Gastrointestinal Emergencies

Gastrointestinal (GI) emergencies encompass a multitude of problems, including appendicitis, cholecystitis, pancreatitis, and upper and lower GI bleeding. These emergencies range from life-threatening overt GI bleeding to a more subtle presentation of abdominal pain. Astute assessment by the emergency clinician is necessary to facilitate the diagnostic phase of care and expedite emergency interventions. This chapter discusses the causes, pathophysiology, clinical manifestations, and treatment of selected nontraumatic GI emergencies. An overview of GI assessment is presented first, however.

GASTROINTESTINAL ASSESSMENT

The patient who arrives in the emergency department (ED) with an abdominal complaint may be physiologically unstable. Therefore, the first priority in assessing this patient, or any patient, is to determine whether airway, breathing, or circulation (ABCs) is compromised. If there is evidence or suspicion of compromise in these areas, the patient must be brought directly to the treatment area for immediate intervention.

If the patient's airway, breathing, and circulation are adequate, a thorough history, including the patient's chief complaint, history of present illness, and his or her past medical and surgical history should be sought out. A medication and allergy history should also be obtained.

The most common chief complaint of a patient experiencing a GI emergency is abdominal pain. A complete description of the pain characteristics must be obtained, as often this can greatly assist in determining its cause. Pain characteristics that should be assessed include the location, quality, severity, and chronology of the pain. Additionally, aggravating and alleviating factors, along with associated or concurrent manifestations of the pain, also should be sought out.

In assessing the location of pain, the patient should be asked to point to the site of the pain with one finger. Note if he or she is able to localize the pain or if it is diffuse and scattered. Visceral pain characteristically is poorly localized, whereas parietal pain is specific to the area of the abdomen involved (Way 1978, 398). Ask the patient if the pain radiates in any direction. The presence of referred pain should also be established. Referred pain is defined as pain perceived in an area outside the pathologic process, resulting from stimulation of the same neurosegment that supplies the diseased organ. Referred pain in GI disease is usually well localized and may be reported in the scapula (Kehr's sign), the flank, or the groin.

Quality of pain should be assessed by asking the patient to describe the pain. Common descriptions include adjectives such as crampy, sharp, dull, burning, and aching. Also question whether or not the quality of pain has changed and whether it is continuous or intermittent. Intestinal pain from an obstruction is often described as crampy and intermittent, whereas pain from acute appendicitis is described as steady and continuous (Way 1978, 401). Pain associated with ulcers often is characterized by burning. The nurse should be aware that severe pain that is described as "unbearable" can indicate an acute problem, such as a vascular emergency, pancreatitis, or a kidney stone.

Asking the patient to rate the pain on a scale from 1 to 10 (being sure the patient understands 1 is mild and 10 is severe) is helpful in assessing pain severity or intensity. The patient should be asked again at subsequent intervals so that changes in pain severity or intensity can be quantified.

The chronology of the patient's pain is determined by asking when the pain began, how long it has lasted, how it has progressed or changed, and what the patient was doing when it first began.

Assessment of factors that aggravate or alleviate a patient's abdominal pain often are crucial in the differential diagnosis of abdominal pain. Differentiating abdominal pain of truly GI origin from abdominal pain of obstetric, gynecologic, genitourinary, and even cardiac origin is imperative. Therefore, patients must be asked which factors make their pain better, which make it worse, and which have no effect on the pain. Factors to consider include changes of pain in response to activity, changes in position, inspiration, food, and medications (e.g., antacids, nitroglycerin).

The nurse should also inquire about the presence or absence of associated or concurrent symptoms. Ask the patient whether or not he or she has experienced nausea, vomiting, diarrhea, constipation, excessive gas, dysuria, anorexia, or weight loss. Ask when the patient's last bowel movement was, and inquire whether or not any blood was present in the emesis or stools. An obstetric and gynecologic history should be obtained in women to rule out related causes of abdominal pain. Other questions should determine when the patient's last normal menses was, what birth control measures she currently uses, and whether or not she has any abnormal vaginal discharge.

Once the details of the patient's chief complaint and the history of the present illness have been obtained, questions relating to the patient's past significant medical and surgical history should be asked. These questions should establish whether or not the patient has had any abdominal surgeries, and whether or not he or she has ever had ulcers, diverticulitis, inflammatory bowel diseases (e.g., Crohn's disease, ulcerative colitis), hepatitis, cirrhosis, kidney stones, GI bleeding, or hemorrhoids. Women should be asked about any history of pelvic inflammatory disease, ovarian cysts, and ectopic pregnancies. The frequency of alcohol ingestion and amount of consumption also should be asked of all patients.

Medications that may cause or contribute to abdominal complaints or disorders include aspirin, steroids, anticoagulants, and iron pills. Therefore, ask the patient if these have been used and how often.

The physical examination for a patient experiencing GI complaints (or any patient requiring an abdominal examination) should proceed in the following order: inspection, auscultation, percussion, and palpation.

Inspection should include the patient's general appearance in addition to inspection of the abdomen. Note if the patient is in obvious distress. Is he or she clenching at the abdomen or moaning? What position is he or she assuming? Is the patient lying quietly, afraid to move because movement causes pain if peritoneal irritation is present, or is he or she pacing with pain and unable to lie down, often seen in patients with renal calculi? Patients who are lying with their hips flexed and knees pulled up to the abdomen may have appendicitis. Note the patient's overall skin and scleral color. Is he or she pale or cyanotic, suggesting significant blood loss and inadequate oxygenation, or is he or she jaundiced, suggesting hepatic disease? Does the patient have a reddened nose or spider angiomas, suggestive of alcoholism? Dry mucous membranes noted in the mouth or tongue can indicate poor oral intake or vomiting.

Vital signs are important indicators of the severity of the disease process. An elevated temperature indicates an inflammatory process is likely present. One should suspect that the kidneys, pelvic organs, or thorax may be involved when temperatures are elevated between 103 and 105°F.

The patient's blood pressure, pulse, and respiratory rates help identify the need for emergency intervention. Changes noted in the patient's blood pressure and pulse relating to posture, hypotension, tachycardia, and dizziness associated with abdominal pain signal significant fluid loss. Bleeding and sequestration of fluid into the third space are two serious sequelae of GI emergencies. An alteration in respiratory rate can indicate cardiopulmonary involvement or severe GI disease that causes abdominal pain (Trott 1988, 1394). When assessing the abdomen, findings should be reported and described as to their respective quadrants or sections (Fig. 12–1).

Inspection of the abdomen includes the rating and describing of skin markings (e.g., scars, bruises, petechiae, striae, spider angiomas), masses, pulsations, visible peristalsis, and contour. Protuberant abdomens may indicate simple obesity, pregnancy, gas, tumors, and/or ascites.

Abdominal auscultation should always be performed prior to percussion and palpation as these latter two maneuvers may stimulate or exaggerate baseline bowel sounds. All four quadrants and the epigastrium should be auscultated for the presence of bowel sounds, noting their frequency and pitch. Bowel sounds should never be considered absent unless they cannot be auscultated for at least 2 consecutive minutes (normally, 10 to 20 peristaltic sounds/minute should be auscultated).

Upper right quadrant   Upper left quadrant

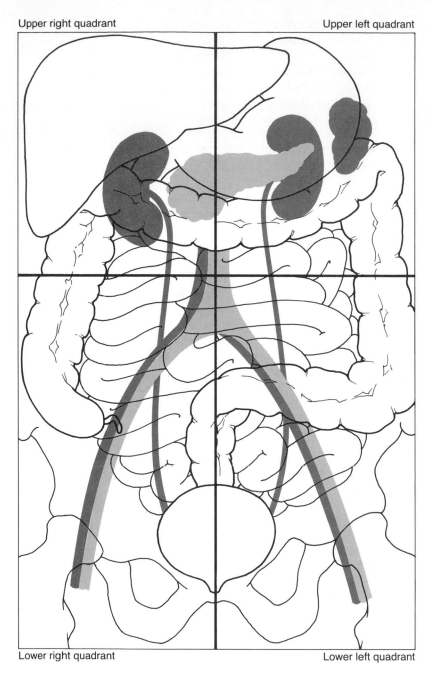

FIGURE 12-1. Location of organs within the abdomen.

Lower right quadrant   Lower left quadrant

Bowel sounds are often normal early in the course of an abdominal emergency. With peritonitis, they may only become decreased 6 to 8 hours after the onset of pain or injury. On the other hand, bowel sounds are generally high-pitched and hyperactive early in small bowel obstruction as the bowel works to overcome the obstruction; later, as the bowel tires, bowel sounds diminish. (High-pitched bowel sounds are

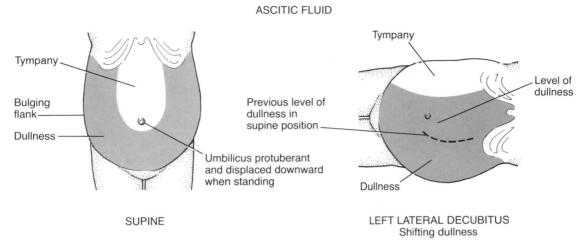

ASCITIC FLUID

Tympany

Bulging flank

Dullness

Previous level of dullness in supine position

Umbilicus protuberant and displaced downward when standing

Tympany

Level of dullness

Dullness

SUPINE

LEFT LATERAL DECUBITUS
Shifting dullness

FIGURE 12-2. Shifting dullness associated with ascites. (Redrawn from Bates B. 1979. A Guide to Physical Examination, 2nd ed. JB Lippincott, 214.)

indications of intestinal fluid and air under tension in a dilated bowel.) Bowel sounds are generally hyperactive and steady in patients with gastroenteritis (Rosato 1983, 28).

Vascular bruits should be listened for in the areas of the renal and iliac arteries and aorta. They suggest turbulent or obstructed flow, which may be indicative of an aneurysm.

Percussion should be performed in all four quadrants of the abdomen to identify the nature of the matter underlying the area(s) percussed. Solid matter (e.g., organs such as liver and spleen), air, and fluid create different sounds on percussion. Normally, tympany, which suggests the presence of gas or air, is the predominant sound heard with percussion of the abdomen. Dullness is normally present over the liver and spleen. Abdominal ascites yields dullness to percussion and may be detected by noting shifting dullness (Fig. 12-2).

The final portion of the abdominal examination is palpation. Both light and deep palpation should be performed. Light palpation identifies areas of tenderness, muscle guarding, and rigidity. Deep palpation identifies less superficial areas of pathology. Both light and deep palpation should begin at the farthest point away from the area of maximal pain. During palpation of the abdomen, it is recommended that the patient's thighs be flexed to provide optimal relaxation of the abdomen (Cope 1963, 25).

The presence or absence of tenderness also needs to be identified during the abdominal examination. Rebound tenderness indicates peritoneal irritation. It is detected by pressing slowly and deeply over the painful area and suddenly releasing the hand. If the patient complains of pain after releasing the hand, rebound tenderness is said to be present (Way 1978, 402). Visceral or organ pain that is elicited on palpation usually is not associated with rebound tenderness or muscular rigidity. Common causes of abdominal tenderness from visceral pain include acute salpingitis, pleurisy, and hepatomegaly. Rebound tenderness is commonly (but not always) present in acute appendicitis, diverticulitis, pancreatitis, and cholecystitis.

Dysfunction of other organ systems may be manifested by abdominal complaints. Upper abdominal tenderness or pain may result from pulmonary disorders, such as pneumonia or pulmonary embolism, or cardiovascular problems, such as acute myocardial infarction and pericarditis. Genital, rectal, and pelvic examinations should be performed to rule out genitourinary causes of abdominal pain.

A complete abdominal assessment, including progression of pain and changes in vital signs and physical findings, needs to be repeated frequently while the patient is in the emergency department. Symptoms often change, providing clues to the diagnosis in specific gastrointestinal emergencies.

GASTROINTESTINAL BLEEDING

Gastrointestinal bleeding, a common condition observed in the ED is associated with significant mortality. Blood loss may be overt and rapid or slow and occult. The source of the bleeding may be the upper or the lower portion of the GI tract. Upper GI bleeding is generally defined as that which originates within and proximal to the duodenum. Lower GI bleeding is defined as that which originates distal to the duodenum.

Upper GI Bleeding

Etiology and Pathophysiology

Common causes of upper GI bleeding include ulcerative conditions such as peptic ulcer disease; inflammatory conditions such as gastritis; esophageal and gastric varices; carcinomas; and Mallory-Weiss tears. Each of these conditions is discussed briefly so that the way in which they cause or contribute to upper GI bleeding is understood.

The term *peptic ulcer* is used to refer to a group of ulcerative disorders of the upper gastrointestinal tract. The major forms are chronic duodenal and gastric ulcer (McGuigan 1987, 1239). Peptic ulcers are produced when the aggressive effects of acid-pepsin dominate the protective effects of mucosal resistance (McGuigan 1987, 1239). Substances such as aspirin, alcohol, caffeine, and steroids may corrode the mucosal barrier, allowing acid backwash and mucosal destruction. If pyloric dysfunction exists, bile is allowed to reflux into the stomach and further irritate the mucosal lining. This may produce bleeding ulcerations.

Stress ulcers are frequently multiple and are most common in the antrum and duodenum. Acute stress erosions are usually superficial, with erosion limited to the mucosa (McGuigan 1987, 1252). The most common clinical finding is painless gastrointestinal bleeding. Blood loss is usually minimal.

Esophageal varices are dilated blood vessels in the esophagus caused by portal hypertension. Portal hypertension exists when there is a resistance to the flow of blood through the liver. Causes include parenchymal liver disease, cirrhosis, congenital obstruction of the portal vein, occlusion of the hepatic vein, and thrombosis of the splenic vein from acute pancreatitis (Broadwell 1986, 1166). When blood vessels around the esophagus become tortuous, variceal bleeding and rupture can occur. Bleeding is most common in varices in the region of the gastroesophageal junction. The degree of portal hypertension and size of the varices affect the tendency toward bleeding (Podolsky and Isselbacher 1987, 1347).

Gastritis is a term that describes generalized inflammation of the gastric mucosa. It may be acute or chronic. There are several drugs, stimuli, and circumstances associated with acute gastritis, including aspirin, anti-inflammatory agents, alcohol, corticosteroids, major physiologic stress, and intense emotional reactions (Broadwell 1986, 1168).

The term *gastrointestinal carcinoma* refers to the malignant neoplasms and tumors in the gastrointestinal tract. If the mucosa covering the carcinoma is irritated and becomes ulcerated, the patient may have signs of gastric or intestinal bleeding.

The Mallory-Weiss syndrome involves a tear at the cardioesophageal junction that occurs after repeated episodes of retching or vomiting. A history of alcohol ingestion and hiatal hernia has been associated with this lesion. The tear is the result of a sharp increase in intra-abdominal pressure, which causes the tissue to stretch and open. The first emesis may show no blood but after repeated episodes of retching or vomiting, bleeding can occur.

Hiatal hernias are clinically significant when accompanied by a reflux of acid. Upper gastrointestinal bleeding may occur secondary to reflux esophagitis and mucosal destruction. Anemia from chronic ulcerations is also possible.

Certain hematologic disorders may affect blood clotting and thus produce gastrointestinal bleeding. Patients with leukemia may have a decreased platelet count and thus are susceptible to increased clotting time and the potential for bleeding. Individuals with disseminated intravascular coagulation (DIC) exhibit clotting factor deficiencies secondary to the inordinate consumption of clotting factors associated with the intravascular coagulopathy. Massive bleeding throughout the gastrointestinal system occurs.

Lower GI Bleeding

Etiology and Pathophysiology

Common causes of lower GI bleeding include diverticulosis; inflammatory diseases such as enterocolitis, Crohn's disease, and ulcerative colitis; and polyps. Diverticulosis is an outpouching of the mucosa of the large colon through the muscle layers. If perforation of a diverticulum occurs, lower GI bleeding may be evident.

Inflammatory bowel disease is a term for a group of chronic inflammatory disorders (such as enterocolitis, Crohn's disease, and ulcerative colitis) of the GI tract of unknown cause that may induce lower GI bleeding. Enterocolitis is an inflammation and necrosis of the bowel that affects primarily the mucosa and occasionally the submucosa. It may be caused by antibiotic therapy that alters the normal bowel flora. Crohn's disease is a chronic inflammatory disorder that may occur in any part of the

GI tract, but the most common sites are the ileum and colon. The major clinical features of Crohn's disease are fever, abdominal pain, diarrhea (often without blood), and generalized fatigability (Glickman 1987, 1281). Ulcerative colitis is a chronic mucosal inflammatory disease limited to the colon and rectum. The major symptoms are bloody diarrhea and abdominal pain, often with fever and weight loss in more severe cases. Although the cause of ulcerative colitis and Crohn's disease remains unknown, certain features of these diseases have suggested several possible etiologic factors. These include familial or genetic, infectious, immunologic, and psychologic factors (Glickman 1987, 1277).

A polyp is a tumor with a pedicle or a tissue mass elevated above the mucosal surface. Although polyps may occur throughout the gastrointestinal tract, the predominant site is in the distal 25 cm of the colon (Broadwell 1986, 1217). Polyps may be neoplastic or non-neoplastic. Occult or overt rectal bleeding may be evident.

Bleeding throughout the gastrointestinal tract may occur slowly over an extended period of time or suddenly within minutes. When slow bleeding occurs, the body compensates by increasing production of red blood cells. Hypochromic red blood cells of microcytic origin suggest chronic blood loss. The patient may be asymptomatic for some time. In a rapidly developing ulceration, massive bleeding may develop as the vessel wall erodes. Signs and symptoms of hypovolemic shock will be evident within minutes.

Clinical Manifestations

The patient who experiences an episode of GI bleeding will have a chief complaint of vomiting blood or passing a bloody stool. He or she may describe the vomitus as bright red or consisting of coffee-ground material. Patient estimates of the amount of blood loss are generally inaccurate, but it may be helpful to ascertain the number of times the patient vomited.

Bloody stools may result from either upper or lower GI bleeding. The patient's description of the stool may vary from bright red with clots to dark red to black and tarry. Stool color depends on bleeding site, rapidity of bleeding, and intestinal motility. As blood passes through the GI tract, it becomes darker. Frank blood with or without clots indicates a recent or ongoing bleed. Reports of a single incident of rectal bleeding or numerous episodes of melena give some clue as to the quantity of blood loss.

Patients with GI bleeding may or may not complain of abdominal pain. If pain is an associated symptom, a complete description of its characteristics (see section on Assessment) should be elicited. Acute gastric mucosal lesions are often painless because of the buffering effect of blood in the stomach. The patient may describe a history of recurring episodes of ulcer-like pain. Localized tenderness in the right upper quadrant or epigastrium may also be present with peptic ulcer disease. On the other hand, a more constant discomfort may be associated with a malignancy. Pain that persists during a bleeding episode may indicate perforation (Clearfield 1976, 77). The presence of other associated symptoms, such as heartburn or vomiting, should be sought.

A history of significant alcohol ingestion alerts the clinician to the possibility of cirrhosis and esophageal varices as the cause of GI hemorrhage. These patients can also suffer from gastritis or duodenal ulcer disease, which may eventually lead to GI bleeding. Medications such as aspirin, steroids, anti-inflammatory agents, and particularly anticoagulants may also contribute to or be the cause of the bleeding episode.

The major concern in cases of GI bleeding is the possibility of hypovolemic shock due to blood loss. Therefore, once airway patency and breathing are established, assessment of the patient's hemodynamic status takes priority over other aspects of the initial history and physical examination. The patient may be pale and have cool, clammy skin. Capillary refill time may be prolonged to greater than 2 seconds. These signs are the result of the body's sympathetic response to hypovolemia and indicate decreased tissue perfusion. In addition, the patient may complain of weakness, dizziness, and thirst and may appear dehydrated.

Heart rate and blood pressure (BP) values are also important indicators of the patient's hemodynamic status. A systolic BP of less than 100 mmHg and a supine heart rate of greater than 100 beats/minute in a healthy adult may be the result of 25 to 50% blood volume loss. Determine if there are any orthostatic blood pressure changes. In addition, respiratory rate may increase owing to hypotension with acute blood loss (Barsan 1983, 1059).

An elevation of body temperature to 100 to 102°F is not uncommon in patients with an upper GI bleed. A temperature greater than 102°F is generally due to other causes, such as sepsis. Conversely, hypothermia may indicate sepsis or profound shock (Barsan 1983, 1059).

Anemia can be detected by hyperextending the fingers and examining the palmar creases. Loss of redness in the palmar creases indicates a hemoglobin level half the normal value (Barsan 1983, 1059).

Further inspection of the patient may reveal jaundice or spider angiomas, indicative of hepatic disease and a coagulopathy. Petechial and purpuric lesions may be associated with blood dyscrasias, which may also be the cause of bleeding (Barsan 1983, 1059). The patient may have dried blood around the lips or a malodorous smell from vomited blood or the passing of a bloody stool.

With an acute GI bleed, hyperactive bowel sounds are usually noted on auscultation owing to the cathartic effect of the bleed. Decreased or absent bowel sounds are indicative of perforation and the resulting ileus (Barsan 1983, 1060).

Baseline laboratory values, including a complete blood count, electrolytes, blood urea nitrogen (BUN), creatinine, and clotting studies, need to be determined. The BUN level may increase owing to the breakdown of blood in the GI tract and decreased liver metabolism secondary to decreased liver perfusion. A markedly elevated BUN level in association with a normal creatinine level indicates massive bleeding has occurred (Holloway 1984, 421).

Serial hemoglobin and hematocrit values are followed to monitor blood loss. In acute hemorrhage, plasma and red cells are lost proportionately and the hematocrit and hemoglobin values appear normal initially. In an attempt to compensate for volume loss, extracellular fluid enters the intravascular space and hemodilution occurs, causing the hematocrit level to drop eventually. Because of the likely need for volume replacement, the patient's blood should be typed and cross-matched.

As with any patient experiencing hypovolemia, arterial blood gas (ABG) values may reveal respiratory alkalosis as a result of compensation for diminished blood flow through the lungs. Metabolic acidosis, due to the accumulation of metabolic waste products, may signify inadequate liver function in addition to poor peripheral tissue perfusion.

With upper GI hemorrhage, an endoscopic examination will help visualize the site of bleeding and determine the degree of tissue injury. Angiography may be performed to examine the gastrointestinal vasculature if endoscopy is inconclusive or cannot be done. Barium swallow radiographic studies may be necessary to rule out other GI problems.

Plain abdominal radiographs can identify an unsuspected hollow organ perforation, abnormal mucosal configurations, which may suggest inflammatory bowel disease, or the distended bowel of toxic megacolon. A chest radiograph and an electrocardiogram are important diagnostic tests, especially in the elderly, to monitor pre-existing myocardial and respiratory problems.

With lower GI bleeding, a rectal examination may be necessary to detect occult bleeding. Sigmoidoscopy helps identify anal lesions, proctitis, or rectal mass lesion (Tedesco 1983, 93). If bleeding has stopped or slowed significantly without intervention, a barium enema may be performed unless contraindicated by other colonic problems, such as acute ulcerative colitis or perforation (Thomas 1983, 43).

Treatment and Nursing Care

Stage I care may need to be instituted for those patients with an acute GI bleed who have signs of severe hypovolemia due to blood loss, heart or renal failure, hollow organ perforation, or sepsis. Airway, breathing, and circulation must be supported and monitored. Restoration of intravascular volume and control of blood loss are priority management goals. Resuscitative equipment must be available for immediate use. The specific treatment plan will be dictated by the patient's clinical presentation.

Fluid Volume Deficit, Related to

• **Gastrointestinal Bleeding**

Patients with GI bleeding may be hypotensive or tachycardic or have other clinical signs of shock. Two large-bore (14-gauge) intravenous lines must be established immediately with either normal saline or lactated Ringer's solution. These crystalloid solutions are infused in 500- to 1000-ml boluses, and the patient's clinical response to fluid administration is closely monitored. If the patient fails to respond to rapid fluid infusion, the pneumatic antishock garment may be applied (Barsan 1983, 1050).

Because the patient is experiencing blood loss, the most appropriate fluid for volume replacement is blood. Fully cross-matched blood is preferred but type O RH negative, or type-specific blood can be administered. Packed red cells are used to avoid left ventricular volume overload in elderly patients and in patients with a history of congestive heart failure or heart disease. Because banked blood is deficient in clotting factors, fresh frozen plasma may be given in addition to whole blood or packed red cells.

The patient's clinical response to fluid volume replacement must be carefully monitored. Adequate tissue perfusion is indicated by warm, dry skin with a capillary refill time of less than 2 seconds. Other positive indicators of adequate fluid resuscitation are a heart rate of 80 to 100 beats/ minute, slowly rising central venous pressure (CVP), urine output of at least 30 ml/hour, and improving mentation.

In addition to volume replacement, stage I care focuses on control of blood loss. Gastric lavage using cool saline solution promotes local vasoconstriction and clot formation. Additional effects include the dilution and evacuation of gastric acids and a decrease in autodigestive activity. Iced saline is contraindicated, as the extreme temperature may stimulate hydrochloric acid production (Strange 1987, 109). To prevent fluid overload, the nurse must maintain accurate measurements of gastric fluid intake and output.

Drug therapy may be initiated in an effort to reduce or halt the bleeding process. Vasopressin (Pitressin) and vitamin K are the most commonly used chemotherapeutic agents in the emergency setting for massive gastrointestinal bleeding. Pitressin, a pituitary hormone, may be used to reduce portal and mesenteric blood flow. It causes contraction of smooth muscle of the GI tract and of all parts of the vascular bed. It is given intravenously or by intra-arterial infusion. Side effects of Pitressin include abdominal cramping, diarrhea, hyponatremia (secondary to the antidiuretic effect), peripheral vasoconstriction, hypertension, a fall in cardiac output, angina, and dysrhythmias. Precaution should be taken when administering Pitressin to patients with a history of cardiac disease.

Vitamin K (AquaMEPHYTON) may be administered via the intravenous, intramuscular, or subcutaneous route to aid in liver production of prothrombin (factor II), proconvertin (factor VII), plasma thromboplastin component (factor IX), and Stuart factor (factor X).

Balloon tamponade of the bleeding varices may be accomplished with a triple-lumen, Sengstaken-Blakemore (SB) tube (Fig. 12–3). The tube contains a gastric and an esophageal balloon which, when inflated, compresses bleeding vessels. One balloon is positioned against the gastric fundus and the other in the esophagus. The gastric balloon is inflated first with 200 to 250 ml of radiopaque dye and clamped. Gentle traction is next applied to the tube to wedge the balloon into the cardio-esophageal junction. The esophageal tube can then be inflated. Hemorrhage caused by esophageal or gastric varices can be controlled temporarily by this method. It is also utilized on patients who have massive, life-threatening hemorrhage and a history of varices, cirrhosis, or signs of alcoholic liver disease (Levinson 1982, 21).

Untoward side effects that can occur with utilization of the SB tube include aspiration, asphyxia, esophageal rupture, and erosion of the esophageal wall (De-Laurentis 1974, 67). Gastric suction must be readily available for evacuation of blood in the oropharynx and upper esophagus proximal to the esophageal balloon. Patients with an altered level of consciousness or inability to control the airway will require airway protection with an endotracheal tube. Constant assessment of respiratory status is necessary to prevent aspiration and associated complications. Respiratory distress related to occlusion of the airway by a balloon is possible. Scissors need to be kept at the bedside at all times. The tube needs to be cut immediately and removed if signs of respiratory distress or obstruction occur (Moorhouse et al 1987, 203).

Complaints of sudden back or upper abdominal discomfort may indicate an esophageal rupture secondary to the SB tube. Hypotension and tachycardia will accompany the complaints associated with esophageal rupture. Fluid resuscitation, blood replacement, and surgical interventions (portacaval shunt) can be anticipated.

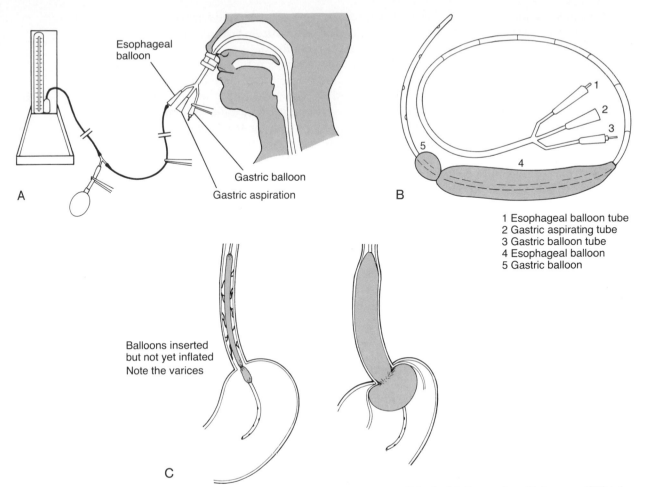

Esophageal balloon

Gastric balloon

Gastric aspiration

A

B

1 Esophageal balloon tube
2 Gastric aspirating tube
3 Gastric balloon tube
4 Esophageal balloon
5 Gastric balloon

Balloons inserted
but not yet inflated
Note the varices

C

FIGURE 12–3. Esophageal tamponade accomplished with Sengstaken-Blakemore (SB) tube. *A,* Schematic illustration of a method used to determine amount of intraballoon pressures. *B,* Diagram of balloons composing the SB tube. *C,* Inflated esophageal and gastric balloons. Note the asymmetric inflation of the gastric balloon. The upper, tapered portion of the self-retaining esophageal balloon is reinforced to prevent upward expansion and provide adequate hemostasis at the bleeding site. Separate airways for inflating the balloons are incorporated into the tube. (Redrawn courtesy of Davol Rubber Company, Providence, R.I.)

Fear, Related to

• Uncertainty Surrounding Prognosis

The patient who is vomiting blood or passing bloody stools is usually very frightened and fearful of what will happen next. Emotional and psychologic support can be provided in a variety of ways. Anticipating the events that will take place in the diagnostic phase of care and relaying information to the patient and family are important in fostering knowledge of and some sense of control over the situation. Explanations of procedures as they are being performed may help allay some anxieties. Frequent assurances and a calm and caring manner promote confidence in the health care givers. The person fearing death may request to see family or significant others. Although the patient may be seriously ill, untidy in appearance, or perhaps covered with blood, it is imperative that the patient's request be honored as soon as possible. Allowing for a short visit may alleviate much anxiety and provide some psychologic comfort.

A chaplain or a crisis, mental health, or social worker should be called to assist with supporting family members. Periodic updates on the patient's condition should be shared with waiting family members. If the patient requires surgery, the family should be allowed to visit the patient at least for a brief period prior to transfer to the operating room.

Self-Esteem, Disturbance in, Related to

- **Bloody Vomitus or Frequent Diarrhea Secondary to GI Bleeding**

The patient experiencing an acute episode of GI bleeding often becomes soiled from bloody vomitus or stool. The patient may be embarrassed because he or she cannot control the vomiting or diarrhea. The nurse can assist the patient by promptly changing bed linens if necessary and providing oral hygiene in an empathetic manner. Patient privacy must be ensured during episodes of bleeding as well as for all aspects of care.

Evaluation

Resuscitative measures are initiated immediately in patients with hypovolemic shock due to GI bleeding. Once the patient's condition is stabilized, continued evaluation of fluid replacement is essential. Results of peripheral tissue perfusion, urinary output, level of consciousness, and vital signs indicate the adequacy of intravascular volume. Control of blood loss must be accomplished to maintain hemodynamic stability.

ACUTE APPENDICITIS

Acute appendicitis accounts for more than 50% of surgical abdominal emergencies. Approximately 7% of the population experiences appendicitis during their lifetimes. The greatest frequency is between the second and third decades of life, but appendicitis can occur at any age (Shrock 1978, 1825).

Undiagnosed acute appendicitis is a life-threatening situation and should be considered in every patient with acute abdominal pain. Two thirds of patients with acute appendicitis come to the emergency department within 24 hours of symptom onset; however, approximately 28% of these individuals already have a perforated appendix. The frequency of perforation is highest in the first decade of life and after the age of 40 years. Three of four children with appendicitis under the age of 5 years will have had a perforation by the time they undergo surgery. These facts emphasize the importance of careful assessment and observation to rule out the possibility of appendicitis, especially in the young (Jones et al 1985, 282).

Etiology

The appendix is situated at the posterior medial wall of the cecum. In more than 50% of people, the appendix is not fixed in one position and is presumed free to move in response to cecal distention and postural changes (Shrock 1978, 1825–1826). The precipitating factor in the development of appendicitis is obstruction of the appendix owing to kinking, infection, or a hard mass of feces.

Pathophysiology

The exact function of the human appendix is not clearly understood. Its lumen is long and narrow and can easily become obstructed. When obstruction occurs, the mucosa continues to secrete fluid and the intraluminal pressure rises. Eventually the intraluminal pressure exceeds venous pressure, resulting in vascular compromise. The appendix becomes hypoxic and mucosal ulceration and necrosis follow. Bacteria of the normal GI flora invade the appendix wall. The infection produces more swelling and ischemia. Gangrene and perforation may result within 24 to 36 hours (Shrock 1978, 1826).

Clinical Manifestations

The chief complaint of the patient with acute appendicitis is usually abdominal pain. Many patients report a dull ache around the umbilicus or in the upper abdomen. Often the pain localizes between the umbilicus and the right iliac crest (McBurney's point).

The pain is often described as steady; coughing and movement may intensify the pain. Rebound tenderness, especially at McBurney's point, may be noted. If perforation and peritonitis have occurred, the abdominal wall is generally rigid. This finding is a serious sign that must be identified to expedite treatment (Jones et al 1985, 283).

Adhesions may form around the inflamed appendix and adjacent loops of bowel. When the appendix perforates, pus and exudate cannot spread, and a localized abscess results. A tender mass can then be felt in the right lower quadrant (Jones et al 1985, 283).

Progressively severe symptoms are characteristic of appendicitis. Other complaints associated with appendicitis include nausea and vomiting, which generally begin several hours after the onset of pain. Diarrhea may be present and, in conjunction with vomiting, may produce a clinical picture suggesting gastroenteritis (Jones et al 1985, 282–283).

The patient with appendicitis is generally hemodynamically stable. Vital signs are usually normal; the pulse rate is barely elevated in early appendicitis. Tachycardia is an important sign of local peritonitis (Jones et al 1985, 283). Markedly increased temperature and heart rate indicate septic complications (Boniface and Spadafora 1988, 1477).

An elevated leukocyte count greater than 10,000 cells/mm^3 is seen in 80% to 90% of patients with acute appendicitis. A left shift is often noted, with more than 75% neutrophils. Approximately 96% of patients have an elevated leukocyte count, abnormal differential cell counts, or both. However, a completely normal white cell count does not rule out the possibility of appendicitis (Shrock 1978, 1828).

Urinalysis is performed to rule out the presence of a urinary tract infection. A pregnancy test should be done on women of childbearing age to eliminate other possible causes for the abdominal pain, such as ectopic pregnancy (Boniface and Spadafora 1988, 1477).

Treatment and Nursing Care

Stage I care is not usually indicated in the patient with acute appendicitis unless there is hemodynamic instability. Most interventions relate to stage II care and include arranging for necessary laboratory studies and monitoring the course of the patient's pain. The treatment of appendicitis is immediate surgical removal if the inflammation is localized. If the appendix has ruptured and there is evidence of peritonitis or an abscess, antibiotic therapy and parenteral fluid administration may be implemented to prevent sepsis and dehydration. Therapy may be implemented for a 6- to 8-hour period prior to performing an appendectomy.

Fluid Volume Deficit, Actual or Potential, Related to

- ### *Vomiting or Inability to Tolerate Oral Intake Secondary to Abdominal Pain*

Patients with potential or actual fluid volume deficit require intravenous therapy of 0.9% normal saline or lactate Ringer's solution. The rate is adjusted according to hydration status as determined by urine output. Maintenance of a urinary output of at least 30 ml/hour is necessary.

Nothing should be taken by mouth to allow the stomach to empty in anticipation of anesthesia and surgery. Oral hygiene with sponge sticks should be offered. Ice chips provide relief from dry mouth and sensations of thirst.

Antiemetics may be helpful in relieving associated nausea and vomiting. Intramuscular prochlorperazine (Compazine) and intramuscular hydroxyzine (Vistaril) are the most commonly used antiemetics. A nasogastric tube may be ordered prior to surgery or for relief of vomiting associated with paralytic ileus. Monitoring of intake and output is necessary to determine fluid volume status.

Comfort, Altered, Related to

- ### *Abdominal Pain*

The course of the patient's pain must be monitored and changes in severity or location reported. With perforation and the development of peritonitis, the pain becomes constant and is increased by movement, breathing, coughing, and palpation. It is often described as a burning sensation, and it can be referred to the shoulder, back, and chest. In addition, there may be abdominal guarding, distention, and rigidity (Strange 1987, 244).

The patient usually feels more comfortable positioned with the hips slightly flexed because the inflamed appendix may irritate the iliopsoas muscle (Boniface and Spadafora 1988, 1466). Patient movement should be slow and deliberate, splinting the painful area. This helps reduce the muscle tension and guarding and minimizes the pain of movement. Lastly, the nurse should provide alternative comfort measures such as massage, breathing and relaxation exercises, and back rubs to help provide relaxation and pain relief (Moorhouse et al 1987, 195).

Knowledge Deficit

The patient will need psychologic preparation for surgery because the underlying cause (the inflamed appendix) must be eliminated. Questions regarding what has happened and what is expected after surgery must be anticipated and answered. Involving the patient's family as well will provide more insight and support to the patient.

Evaluation

Close monitoring of the patient's vital signs and pain status will help identify changes in the clinical picture. The goals of patient care include providing hydration, maintaining normal vital signs, and identifying or preventing peritonitis. Surgical evaluation is necessary to treat the underlying problem. Therefore, the patient and significant others must be prepared adequately.

ACUTE INTESTINAL OBSTRUCTION

Intestinal obstructions may be of a mechanical or neurogenic nature. With simple mechanical obstruction, intestinal contents cannot pass through the intestinal tract because of occlusion of the gut lumen. A strangulated mechanical obstruction occurs when the blood supply of the involved intestinal segment is interrupted; gangrene of the tissue can result. In a neurogenic intestinal obstruction, the intestinal contents do not traverse the bowel because of intestinal paralysis (Ellis 1982, 1–2).

Etiology

Intestinal obstructions can occur in all age groups but generally are rare in children and young adults. The incidence increases in middle age and reaches a peak in the fifth decade. Common causes of intestinal obstruction vary with age (Table 12–1).

TABLE 12–1
Causes of Intestinal Obstruction by Age Group

Age Group	Causes	Brief Description
Neonate	Congenital intestinal atresia	Pathologic closure of the normal opening of the intestines
	Volvulus	Twisting of the bowel on itself
	Meconium ileus	
	Hirschsprung's disease	Congenital anomaly; autonomic ganglia in smooth muscle of colon are absent
	Imperforate anus	Congenital anomaly; involving patency of anorectal area
Infant	Intussusception	Sliding of one part of the intestine into another part just distal to it
	Strangulated hernia	Congenital or acquired protrusion of bowel through an abnormal opening in the muscle wall, causing stricture of the intestine, loss of blood supply, and potential gangrene
	Meckel's diverticulum	Congenital sac or pouch found in the lower portion of the ileum
Young and Middle-Aged Adults	Postoperative adhesions	Fibrous bands that hold parts of the intestine together; adhesions develop as a result of inflammation or injury
	Crohn's disease	Regional inflammation of the intestine
	Strangulated hernia	Regional inflammation of the intestine
Older Adults	Large bowel cancer	
	Diverticular disease	Inflammation of a diverticulum
	Fecal impaction	

Source: Adapted from Ellis H. Intestinal Obstruction. 1982. Appleton-Century-Crofts, 2.

Pathophysiology

Bowel obstruction results in fluid accumulation within the intestine secondary to mechanical blockage and physiologic interference with fluid and electrolyte transport. Abdominal distention occurs as fluid and gas accumulate above and within the obstructed segment of bowel. Normally, 7 to 8 L of electrolyte-rich fluid — mostly saliva, gastric and intestinal juices, and biliary and pancreatic secretions — enter the small bowel each day. Most of this fluid is reabsorbed before reaching the colon, but abdominal distention impairs this process (McConnell 1987, 36). Distention of bowel also promotes secretions, further compounding the distention. Swallowed air and other intestinal gases similarly contribute to distention and bloating.

Interference with normal fluid and electrolyte transport, particularly sodium and water, from the intestinal lumen to the blood is evident during the first 12 to 24 hours after an obstruction develops (McConnell 1987, 36). As sodium, water, and gases accumulate within the intestinal lumen, intraluminal pressures rise. Increased pressure impedes arterial and venous blood flow and contributes to edema formation. The increased intraluminal pressure also causes plasma to transude into the peritoneal cavity. Obstructed capillary circulation leads to red blood cell sludging, hemolysis, and mucosal necrosis (McConnell 1987, 37) (Fig. 12–4).

Although stagnant, bacteria-laden, noxious fluid collects in the obstructed intestinal segment, it does not pose a risk because absorption from the distended bowel is absent. However, if the blood supply is compromised and gangrene develops, infected contents will pass from the strangulated bowel into the peritoneal cavity even without gross perforation. As a result of this bacterial invasion, peritonitis develops (McConnell 1987, 37).

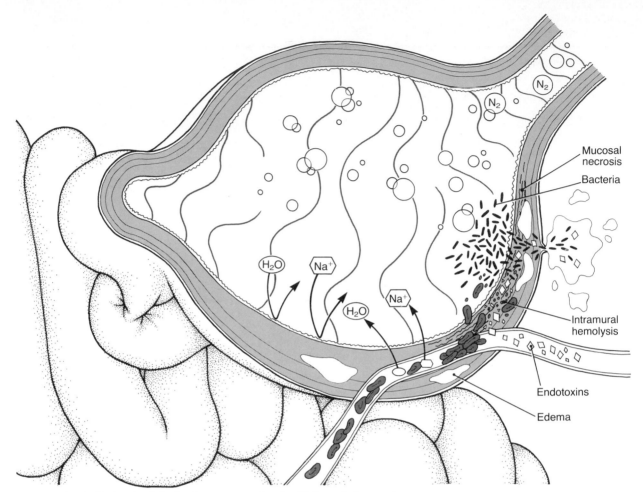

FIGURE 12–4. Pathophysiologic changes associated with bowel obstruction.

Severe hypovolemia may occur secondary to intestinal obstruction. Extracellular volume depletion is related to the loss of the bowel's absorptive capacity, increased bowel secretion, and transudation of plasma and fluid into the peritoneal cavity. In addition, blood loss may occur in strangulated segments of bowel where there is interruption of mesenteric blood flow. This contributes to volume depletion.

Clinical Manifestations

Patients with intestinal obstruction commonly complain of abdominal pain and vomiting. The pain is described as crampy or colicky and generally diffuse. Vomiting may be forceful with complete mechanical obstruction but is more effortless when associated with paralytic ileus (Currie 1979, 176).

The patient often reports constipation. However, bowel movements may occur after obstruction as the distal bowel empties its contents. Afterwards, neither feces nor gas is passed rectally. With incomplete bowel obstruction, some of the accumulated fluid passes through the obstructed area. Crampy abdominal pain and distention are associated with diarrhea (Currie 1979, 176).

Patients with intestinal obstruction may exhibit signs of dehydration. The skin, tongue, and mucous membranes of the mouth appear dry. The eyeballs are soft and sunken; skin turgor is decreased. The patient may complain of thirst and weakness (Currie 1979, 177–178).

Vital signs may be normal initially. However, with large fluid deficits, the blood pressure can drop and the pulse rate increase.

Abdominal inspection may reveal previous laparotomy scars, increasing the possibility of an adhesive obstruction (Williamson 1987, 135). If the patient's abdominal wall is thin, peristaltic waves may be visible. Generally, there is some degree of abdominal distention.

Auscultation may reveal hyperactive bowel sounds, which are the result of gas and fluid mixing. Percussion demonstrates tympany over gas-filled bowel. The abdomen is gently palpated to detect tenderness or masses.

Distended loops of gut and multiple fluid levels seen on plain abdominal radiographs are characteristic findings of bowel obstruction (Williamson 1987, 135). Routine laboratory studies such as BUN, creatinine, electrolytes, complete blood count, and differential count also provide important information.

Treatment and Nursing Care

Intravenous fluid replacement with an isotonic solution is necessary to replenish fluid losses. Incomplete bowel obstruction may be reversed with nasogastric suctioning. However, this more conservative treatment is indicated only for selected partial obstructions. Management of complete mechanical obstruction is surgical; a delay in surgery increases the risk of strangulation (Williamson 1987, 135–136).

Fluid Volume Deficit, Related to

- ### *Dehydration Secondary to Vomiting, Diarrhea, and Decreased Intestinal Absorption of Fluids*

Stage I care is implemented when hypovolemic shock secondary to fluid loss occurs. Intravenous administration of crystalloid and electrolyte solutions is necessary to replace the fluid and electrolytes lost with obstruction. Airway, breathing, and circulation may require support; resuscitative equipment must be readily available.

The amount of fluid replaced depends on fluid losses from vomiting, diarrhea, and nasogastric and urinary outputs. As discussed earlier in this chapter, fluid resuscitation is guided by the patient's clinical response. In older patients or patients with heart disease, rehydration should proceed slowly. Close clinical observation and monitoring of central venous pressure is necessary to prevent fluid overload.

Bowel Elimination, Altered: Diarrhea or Constipation, Related to

- *Obstruction*

A nasogastric tube is inserted to prevent further bowel distention. Gastric output is measured and replaced with intravenous fluids and electrolytes. Nasogastric intubation and intravenous fluids are maintained until the amount of nasogastric output diminishes and bowel sounds and flatus return.

Anxiety or Fear, Related to

- *Possible Surgery*

If the obstruction is complete, the patient must be prepared for surgical intervention. The nurse should explain the purpose of preoperative preparation, state where family members can wait during surgery, and describe postoperative procedures such as coughing and deep breathing. Providing specific information can help alleviate the patient's fears and concerns. Time should be spent answering the patient's and family's questions regarding surgery and hospitalization.

Infection, Potential for Septicemia, Related to

- *Complete Bowel Obstruction, Gangrene, and Possible Perforation*

Because of possible peritonitis and peritoneal contamination during the surgical procedure, a single dose or short course of prophylactic antibiotics is given. Strangulation and the potential for septicemia increase the need for appropriate antibiotic coverage.

Evaluation

Evaluation of patients with acute intestinal obstruction requires careful assessment to identify and prevent complications such as perforation and sepsis. Correction of fluid deficits is a priority, and the patient's hemodynamic status must be closely monitored.

ACUTE PANCREATITIS

Acute pancreatitis is defined as a sterile inflammation of the pancreas; its course can be mild or lethal. As the disease progresses, pancreatic and other digestive enzymes lose their normal inhibitory mechanisms. The result is activation of the enzymes within the pancreas, leading to permanent organ damage (Roberts 1985, 311).

Acute pancreatitis can be categorized as edematous (interstitial) or hemorrhagic. With edematous pancreatitis, the enzymes escape into the nearby tissues and peritoneal cavity. If complications occur, the acute edematous phase may advance to the severe form of pancreatitis, known as hemorrhagic pancreatitis (Roberts 1985, 311).

Etiology

In the United States, acute pancreatitis is estimated to occur at a rate of 1.5 per 100,000 people (Clark 1983, 1083). The factors that precipitate acute pancreatitis are varied. Approximately 30 per cent of patients have no identified cause for their pancreatitis; these cases are termed idiopathic. In the United States, the most common diseases associated with pancreatitis are biliary tract disease and alcoholism. However, trauma, hyperlipidemia, heredity, hyperparathyroidism, hypercalcemia, certain drugs (corticosteroids, thiazide diuretics, oral contraceptives), vasculitis, cancer, pregnancy, renal transplantation, duodenal disease, and some infectious diseases are also recognized as etiologic factors for acute pancreatitis (DiMagno and Bell 1982, 217).

Pathophysiology

Acute pancreatitis is an inflammatory process precipitated by activation of pancreatic enzymes. Neither the factors that mediate this activation nor the variables that determine the severity of inflammation are clear. With mild pancreatitis, the inflammation characteristically is confined within the pancreas. In severe pancreatitis,the response is more serious and leads to pancreatic necrosis and hemorrhage. Activated pancreatic enzymes, toxins, and vasoactive material pour into the retroperitoneal space and possibly the peritoneal cavity. Pancreatic ascites develops when the accumulation of active pancreatic enzymes and leukocytes irritates the peritoneal surfaces and fluid accumulates in the peritoneal cavity (Broadwell 1986, 1261). The exudate causes a chemical burn, which results in movement of protein-rich fluid into the third space. The same process leads to pleural effusion when lymphatics around the diaphragm are affected.

Proteolytic enzymes (phospholipase A and elastase) are responsible for pancreatic autodigestion. Elastase is implicated in the hemorrhage associated with necrotizing pancreatitis (Broadwell 1986, 1261). It dissolves the fibers of blood vessels, and hemorrhage occurs.

If the activated enzymes and toxins are reabsorbed into the vascular system, they produce many harmful effects; among these effects are an increased capillary permeability and systemic vasodilatation; and damage to end organs directly, which causes respiratory failure, renal failure, congestive heart failure, and coma (Banks 1986, 437).

Hypocalcemia develops as calcium binding to serum protein is reduced secondary to a drop in albumin levels. In addition, damage to islet cells decreases insulin release and causes hyperglycemia.

Clinical Manifestations

The majority of patients who have acute pancreatitis present with a chief complaint of abdominal pain. In fact, acute pancreatitis should be suspected in all patients with upper abdominal pain (Jones et al 1985, 105). Pain is noted in the epigastrium of left upper quadrant, often radiating through the back. The pain is described as constant and severe. The patient tends to lie still with the legs brought up so as to open the retroperitoneal space and help relieve the pain (Pops 1982, 299).

The patient may also complain of nausea and vomiting owing to a localized or generalized ileus. Diarrhea, melena, or hematemesis is rarely present but can confuse the clinical presentation of acute pancreatitis (DiMagno and Bell 1982, 224).

The patient's history may identify one of the etiologic factors associated with pancreatitis, such as alcoholism, biliary tract disease, or one of the other factors discussed previously under Etiology.

The patient's overall appearance may be one of agitation, restlessness, and apprehension. The skin is often pale, cool, mottled, or moist owing to peripheral vasoconstriction. Jaundice, secondary to associated liver or gallbladder disease, can be mild or obvious. Ascites and generalized edema may be present. The patient can experience coarse tremors of the extremities as a result of hypocalcemia.

Vital signs are variable with acute pancreatitis. Hypertension secondary to the pain may be present, or the patient may experience tachycardia and hypotension owing to hypovolemic shock. There may be a low-grade fever or a persistently elevated temperature, which can suggest complications such as pancreatic abscess or peritonitis (Moorhouse et al 1987, 180–181). Dyspnea and tachypnea may be due to acute respiratory distress syndrome, a serious complication of pancreatitis with high morbidity and mortality (DiMagno and Bell 1982, 224–225).

Physical examination may reveal breath sounds with basilar crackles owing to a pleural effusion (Moorhouse et al 1987, 181). Discoloration of the flanks (Turner's sign) or bruising discoloration around the umbilicus (Cullen's sign) may be noted on abdominal inspection in patients with hemorrhagic pancreatitis (Moorhouse et al 1987, 180).

Abdominal distention is frequently noted. Bowel sounds are diminished or absent owing to decreased peristalsis or ileus. Epigastric bruits may result from vascular compression and distortion by the swollen pancreas (DiMagno and Bell 1982, 226). Guarding, rigidity, and rebound tenderness are common findings on abdominal palpation. An epigastric mass may be noted, indicating the presence of a phlegmon (suppurative inflammation), pseudocyst, or abscess (DiMagno and Bell 1982, 226).

Laboratory values help confirm the diagnosis of acute pancreatitis. A serum amylase level above 1200 units/L strongly supports the diagnosis. However, other disease entities, such as perforated peptic ulcer or infarcted bowel, can also produce elevated serum amylase levels. A urinary amylase level greater than 3000 units/L (normal, 300 to 1500) is a helpful confirmation (Jones et al 1985, 105).

The complete blood count and differential count demonstrate an elevated hematocrit owing to dehydration or the effusion of fluid into the pancreas or retroperitoneal area. The white blood cell count also is elevated in the majority of cases. The serum calcium level is low, indicating fat necrosis. The potassium level can likewise be low because of gastric losses, or it may be elevated secondary to tissue destruction,

TABLE 12–2
Prognostic Signs in Acute Pancreatitis

At Admission or Diagnosis

Age over 55 years
White blood cell count over 16,000/mm³
Blood glucose over 200 mg/dl
Serum lactate dehydrogenase over 350 IU/dl
Serum glutamic oxaloacetic transaminase over 250 IU/dl

During Initial 48 Hours

Hematocrit fall greater than 10 percentage points
Blood urea nitrogen rise more than 5 mg/dl
Serum calcium level below 8 mg/dl
Arterial Po_2 below 60 mmHg
Base deficit greater than 4 mEq/L
Estimated fluid sequestration more than 6L

Source: Banks PA. Acute pancreatitis: medical considerations. In Bayless TM, ed. Current Therapy in Gastroenterology and Liver Disease, vol. 2. Toronto, BC Decker, 1986: 437–442.

acidosis, or renal insufficiency. BUN and creatinine levels similarly may be elevated. The serum glucose level can be elevated during the acute attack. However, sustained glucose levels higher than 200 mg/dl indicate beta-cell damage and pancreatic necrosis and are an ominous sign. Serum albumin and protein levels may be low owing to a loss in colloids secondary to increased capillary permeability with subsequent fluid shifts into the extracellular space. The prothrombin time is often delayed owing to liver involvement and fat necrosis. The ABG values may reveal hypoxemia and hypercapnia, indicating respiratory insufficiency (Moorhouse et al 1987, 181).

Increases in serum bilirubin, alkaline phosphate, and transaminases can also occur secondary to obstruction of the common bile duct by the edematous pancreas. Serial hematocrit determinations must be done to note a falling level, as is seen with hemorrhagic pancreatitis (Pops 1982, 302).

Prognostic signs (Table 12–2) can be useful as objective criteria for determining the severity of pancreatitis. If fewer than three of these 11 signs are present, the pancreatitis is considered to be mild and rarely fatal. On the other hand, the presence of three or more variables indicates severe pancreatitis, which is fatal in approximately 15 to 20% of patients (Banks 1986, 437).

The value of radiologic examinations in acute pancreatitis is to eliminate other diagnoses, such as perforation of a viscus. Ultrasound can identify an enlarged pancreas or pseudocyst and serve as a baseline study. Endoscopic retrograde cholangiopancreatography (ERCP) should not be performed during the acute phase (Pops 1982, 302).

Treatment and Nursing Care

The goals and priorities of nursing care for patients with acute pancreatitis are to restore and stabilize the respiratory and circulatory losses and provide pain relief and emotional support.

In mild pancreatitis, the mortality rate is less than 5%; in severe pancreatitis, it is approximately 30%. Approximately one half of all deaths occur early in the course of the disease as a result of cardiovascular instability or respiratory or renal failure (Banks 1986, 437). Patients who come to the ED in shock, with impending shock, or with respiratory compromise require immediate stage I interventions.

Impaired Gas Exchange, Actual or Potential, Related to

- *Pulmonary Complications of Acute Pancreatitis*

Stage I interventions include respiratory support activities, such as assisting with intubation, manual ventilation, and tracheal suctioning. Stage II activities focus on assessing and monitoring the patient's respiratory status. Deep breathing, coughing, and position changes enhance ventilation of all lung segments, promote drainage of secretions, and decrease pulmonary atelectasis and congestion. Placing the patient in a semi-Fowler's to high Fowler's position promotes lung expansion and improves diaphragmatic excursion. Supplemental oxygen, to improve tissue perfusion, is provided on the basis of ABG values. Lastly, the nurse may prepare the patient for and assist with a thoracentesis or pericentesis if pleural effusion or ascites compromises the patient's respiratory status (Moorhouse et al 1987, 182–188).

Fluid Volume Deficit, Related to

- *Fluid Losses from Vomiting and Gastric Suctioning*
- *Third-Space Losses*
- *GI or Pancreatic Bleeding*

The goal of stage I care is to stabilize the condition of the patient in hypovolemic shock. Two large-bore intravenous lines are started and crystalloid fluids are infused rapidly. Fluid for intravascular volume replacement may also include blood products and albumin.

Stage II care involves monitoring the patient for changes in hemodynamic status as well as continued correction of fluid volume and electrolyte deficits. Frequently, monitoring of blood pressure, pulse, respiratory rate, and cardiac rhythm is necessary. Dysrhythmias may result from hypovolemia or electrolyte imbalances, such as hypokalemia. Hypocalcemia should be suspected if twitching and a positive Chvostek's sign (local spasm following a tap on the cheek) or Trousseau's sign (muscular spasm from pressure applied to upper arm nerves and vessels) is observed. Calcium losses are replaced with intravenous calcium gluconate if necessary (Moorhouse et al 1987, 183).

Intake and output are calculated because severe fluid losses can occur. A urinary catheter is inserted, and urine output is measured to determine the adequacy of renal perfusion and fluid resuscitation. A nasogastric tube is inserted to relieve pain and reduce pancreatic activity. Fluid losses of gastric secretions can be large and need to be replaced with intravenous electrolyte solutions (Moorhouse et al 1987, 183).

Changes in sensorium, such as confusion or a slowed response, may be seen with hypovolemia, hypoxia, electrolyte imbalances, or impending delirium tremens secondary to chronic alcohol abuse. Toxic psychosis can also result from pancreatic disease (Moorhouse et al 1987, 183).

Pain Related to

• *Pancreatitis*

In mild pancreatitis, a nasogastric tube usually is not necessary. One should be inserted, however, if a gastric or intestinal ileus is present or if nausea and vomiting are intractable. In severe pancreatitis, a nasogastric tube reduces the risk of aspiration and improves nausea and vomiting by draining gastric contents (Banks 1986, 438–439).

Pain relief is provided by administering meperidine hydrochloride (Demerol), 50 to 100 mg intramuscularly, as needed. Morphine sulfate should not be administered because it causes spasm of the sphincter of Oddi and aggravates acute pancreatitis (Kannan 1986, 418).

Positioning the patient on one side with the knees flexed may promote comfort by reducing abdominal pressure and tension. Providing a quiet environment can help decrease the patient's metabolic rate and GI stimulation and reduce pancreatic activity (Moorhouse et al 1987, 184).

Antispasmotics such as dicyclomine (Bentyl) or propantheline bromide (Pro-Banthine) are indicated for patients with bowel function. These drugs decrease vagal stimulation, intestinal motility, and pancreatic outflow. Enzymatic secretion is therefore interrupted and associated pain abated. Carbonic anhydrase inhibitors such as acetazolamide (Diamox) also reduce bicarbonate concentration of pancreatic secretion. Antacids may be given to neutralize gastric secretions, and cimetidine (Tagamet) specifically decreases hydrochloric acid by inhibiting histamine.

Evaluation

The goal of treatment is to resuscitate and stabilize the patient's respiratory and cardiovascular status. Positive outcomes would be indicated by systolic blood pressure greater than 99 mmHg, heart rate less than 100 beats/minute, improved mentation, and urinary output greater than 30 ml/hour. Relief of pain is also a goal in care of the patient with acute pancreatitis. Emotional support should be provided to the patient and family by explaining the necessary procedures and discussing the patient's treatment plan with him or her.

GALLBLADDER DISEASE

Cholelithiasis (stones in the gallbladder) is the most common disorder of the biliary system. Cholecystitis (inflammation of the gallbladder) is usually associated with cholelithiasis. Gallbladder disease affects approximately 4% of adult Americans; approximately 800 new cases are diagnosed each year (Clark 1983, 1076).

Etiology

Certain factors increase the risk of gallstone formation. Women are affected eight times more frequently than men (Clark 1983, 1076), and multiparous women are more often affected than nulliparous women (Kaplowitz 1982, 281). Obesity, a sedentary lifestyle, a familial tendency, and the use of oral contraceptives are other factors associated with gallbladder disease (Kaplowitz 1982, 281). Whites are more commonly affected than Asians and blacks, and there is an especially high incidence in Navajo and Pima Native Americans (Elrod 1987, 1122).

Pathophysiology

The function of the gallbladder is to concentrate and store bile. Secretion of bile is increased by parasympathetic (vagal) stimulation and the action of secretin, cholecystokinin-pancreozymin, vasoactive intestinal peptide (VIP), gastrin, and glucagon. The entrance of fatty foods into the duodenum stimulates secretion of these substances. When stimulated, the gallbladder contracts, forcing bile through the cystic duct into the common bile duct and the duodenum (Fig. 12–5). The sphincter of Oddi, located at the opening of the common bile duct and the pancreatic duct, serves to regulate the one-way flow of bile and pancreatic secretions into the duodenum.

Bile, formed by the liver, is composed of bile acid, phospholipids, cholesterol,

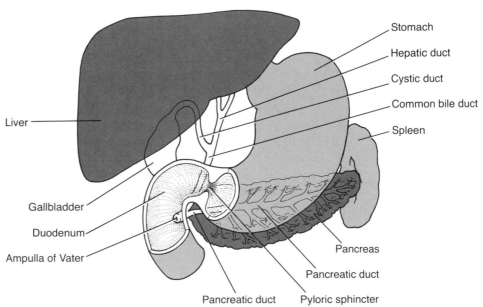

FIGURE 12–5. Anatomic relationships among liver, gallbladder, and pancreas.

and bile pigments. Bile is an emulsifying agent that facilitates fat metabolism. It also increases intestinal peristalsis.

Cholecystitis

Although cholecystitis commonly occurs in conjunction with stone formation, it may evolve alone as a result of bacteria reaching the gallbladder via the vascular or lymphatic route or from chemical irritants in the bile. *Escherichia coli* is the most common bacterium involved.

Inflammation of the mucous lining or the entire wall of the gallbladder may occur. The gallbladder becomes edematous and hyperemic and may be distended with bile or pus. Scar formation associated with healing may reduce gallbladder function.

Cholelithiasis

Gallstone formation occurs when cholesterol, bile salts, and calcium precipitate within the biliary tract. Patients with cholelithiasis are known to have increased cholesterol concentrations in the bile. Stasis of bile leads to progression of the super-saturation and changes in the chemical composition of the bile (Elrod 1987, 1122). Factors that decrease bile flow include immobility, pregnancy, and inflammatory or obstructive lesions of the biliary system. Hormonal factors during pregnancy may cause delayed emptying of the gallbladder.

Gallstones may be found in the cystic duct or in the common bile duct. Pain is manifested as the stones move through the ducts and an obstruction may occur if they become lodged within the ducts. If blockage occurs in the cystic duct, bile will continue to flow into the duodenum directly from the liver. However, if bile flow from the liver is obstructed, obstructive jaundice and an increased BUN will occur. Faulty absorption of fat-soluble vitamins (A, D, E, and K) also takes place because bile is not present in the small intestine to emulsify fat. Bleeding tendencies occur as a result of lack of absorption of vitamin K with decreased production of prothrombin.

Clinical Manifestations

The diagnosis of acute cholecystitis is usually based on clinical presentation. The classic chief complaint of the patient with gallstones is recurrent right upper quadrant or epigastric abdominal pain. This pain typically begins suddenly, and the patient usually remembers the initial onset. It progresses quickly to its peak intensity and lasts one to several hours; it then subsides more slowly than it began (Kaplowitz 1982, 281).

The pain may vary from mild, nonradiating to constant and colicky depending on the degree of inflammation or cystic duct obstruction. Severe pain is usually referred along the costal margins and toward the right scapular area. Twenty percent of patients experience pain to the left of the midline or into the chest (Trotman 1983, 400).

Nausea and vomiting usually accompany the pain; the patient usually feels better after vomiting. Episodes of pain, nausea, and vomiting often occur after meals or at night. As the gallbladder disease progresses, the attacks occur more frequently, often daily (Trotman 1983, 400).

Murphy's sign is often present in acute cholecystitis. This sign is elicited by palpating the abdomen while the patient takes a deep breath. If the patient is unable to breathe deeply because of pain, the sign is said to be positive. With inhalation, the liver moves downward, bringing the gallbladder closer to the examiner's hand. With an inflamed gallbladder, this maneuver causes pain (Patrizzi and Tackett 1984, 219).

The patient with cholecystitis may gradually develop fever, leukocytosis, and signs of local peritonitis. Severe cholecystitis can result in septic shock (Ihse and Isaksson 1987, 82).

After a history and physical examination are completed, appropriate laboratory tests, including urinalysis, liver and clotting profile, serum electrolytes, BUN, and creatinine, are performed. Complete blood count with differential count demonstrates leukocytosis. An elevated serum amylase level may be present even if the patient does not also have pancreatitis (Kaplowitz 1982, 282). Radiographs of the abdomen and chest are important because they may determine the presence of perforated viscus, intrathoracic problems, or calcified gallstones (Trotman 1983, 401). When gallstone disease is considered, the most useful tests are oral cholecystography and ultrasonography (Kaplowitz 1982, 282).

Treatment and Nursing Care

Persons who come to the ED with suspected gallbladder disease will usually be admitted to the hospital for further evaluation and treatment. Definitive management may involve surgical removal of the gallbladder, gallstone lithotripsy, or chemotherapeutic interventions. Chenodeoxycholic acid may be given to dissolve cholesterol stones. The patient with biliary colic who is not dehydrated, febrile, or experiencing excessive pain can be referred for follow-up care and treated in the outpatient setting. However, the patient who appears acutely ill and who has the potential for fluid volume deficit, pain, or infection will require the following emergency interventions.

Fluid Volume Deficit, Related to

• *Vomiting Secondary to Biliary Disease*

Restoration of fluid and electrolyte balance is attained by giving an isotonic solution intravenously. Stage I interventions may be required if fluid deficits are excessive and the patient is in hypovolemic shock. Stage II interventions involve patient monitoring and replacement of fluid losses noted in nasogastric drainage or emesis.

Pain, Related to

• *Inflammation of the Gallbladder*

Pain relief is a goal in the acute management of cholecystitis or cholelithiasis. Meperidine hydrochloride (Demerol) is the preferred analgesic because it has less spasmogenic effect on the biliary tract and small intestine than opiates such as morphine sulfate. Anticholinergics such as atropine or other antispasmotics may be used to relax smooth muscle of the biliary ducts. A nasogastric tube is inserted and placed to suction to relieve nausea and vomiting and associated discomfort.

Knowledge Deficit, Related to

• *Etiology, Pathophysiology, and Treatment of Gallbladder Disease*

Patients discharged to home may require dietary instructions. The major dietary modification for a person with gallstone disease is a low-fat diet. Foods to be avoided include dairy products such as whole milk, cream, butter, whole milk cheese, and ice cream; fried foods; rich pastries; gravies; and nuts. If obesity is a problem, a reduced calorie diet is indicated and referral to a weight loss program may be appropriate.

Evaluation

The expected outcome for the emergency patient with gallstone disease is correction of fluid deficits from vomiting and fever. Relief of pain, by administering analgesics and antispasmotics and instituting nasogastric suctioning, is also an important goal.

CONCLUSION

The nurse clinician plays a key role in assessing the patient with a GI emergency. Goals for nursing management of this patient are to identify and treat life-threatening situations, prevent potential complications, and meet the patient's psychosocial needs. Lastly, the nurse continually monitors and evaluates interventions and modifies the plan of care on the basis of the evaluation.

REFERENCES

Balint J, Sarfeh I, Fried M. 1977. Gastrointestinal Bleeding: Diagnosis and Management. New York, John Wiley.

Banks P. 1986. Acute pancreatitis: Medical considerations. In Bayless T, ed. Current Ther-apy in Gastroenterology and Liver Disease — 2. Toronto, BC Decker, 437–442.

Barsan W. 1983. Upper gastrointestinal tract disorders. In Rosen P, Baker F, Braen G, et al, eds. Emergency Medicine: Concepts and

Clinical Practice, vol 2. St. Louis, CV Mosby, 1036–1060.

Bitterman R. 1983. General disorders of the large intestine. In Rosen P, Baker F, Braen G, et al, eds. Emergency Medicine: Concepts and Clinical Practice, vol 2. St. Louis, CV Mosby, 1108–1122.

Boniface K, Spadafora M. 1988. Disorders of the small intestine. In Rosen P, Baker F, Barkin R, et al, eds. Emergency Medicine: Concepts and Clinical Practice, vol 2. St. Louis, CV Mosby, 1459–1478.

Broadwell DC. 1986. Gastrointestinal system. In Thompson JM, McFarland GK, Hirsch JE, et al, eds. Clinical Nursing. St. Louis, CV Mosby, 1105–1282.

Clark J. 1983. Disorders of the liver, biliary tract, and pancreas. In Rosen P, Baker F, Braen G, et al, eds. Emergency Medicine: Concepts and Clinical Practice, vol. 2. St. Louis, CV Mosby, 1067–1088.

Clearfield H. 1976. Diagnosis and management of upper gastrointestinal hemorrhage. In Clearfield H, Dinoso V Jr, eds. Gastrointestinal Emergencies. New York, Grune & Stratton, p. 75–81.

Cooperman A, Geiss A. 1982. Acute abdomen and intestinal emergencies. In Gitnick G, ed. Handbook of Gastrointestinal Emergencies. Garden City, NY, Medical Examination Publishing Co, 102–153.

Cope Z. 1963. The Early Diagnosis of the Acute Abdomen. London, Oxford University Press.

Currie D. 1979. Abdominal Pain. New York: McGraw-Hill.

DeLaurentis D. 1974. Management of Bleeding Esophageal Varices. In Clearfield II, Dinoso V Jr, eds. Gastrointestinal Emergencies. New York, Grune & Stratton, 65–73.

DiMagno E, Bell J. 1982. Acute pancreatitis and pancreatic injuries. In Gitnick G, ed. Handbook of Gastrointestinal Emergencies. Garden City, NY, Medical Examination Publishing Co, 215–259.

Ellis H. 1982. Intestinal Obstruction. New York, Appleton-Century-Crofts.

Elrod R. 1987. Problems of the liver, biliary tract, and pancreas. In Lewis SM, Collier IC, eds. Medical Surgical Nursing Assessment and Management of Clinical Problems, 2nd ed. New York, McGraw-Hill, 1089–1128.

Given B, Simmons S. 1984. Gastroenterology in Clinical Nursing, 4th ed. St. Louis, CV Mosby.

Glickman RM. 1987. Inflammatory bowel disease. In Braunwald E, Isselbacher KJ, Peterdorf RG, et al, eds. Harrison's Principles of Internal Medicine, 11th ed, vol 2. New York, McGraw-Hill, 1277–1290.

Holloway N. 1988. Nursing the Critically Ill Patient. 3rd ed. Menlo Park, CA, Addison-Wesley.

Ihse I, Isaksson G. 1987. Biliary emergencies. In Imrie CW, Moossa A, eds. Gastrointestinal Emergencies. Edinburgh, Churchill Livingstone, 76–92.

Imrie C. 1987. The management of severe acute pancreatitis. In Imrie CW, Moossa A, eds. Gastrointestinal Emergencies. Edinburgh, Churchill Livingstone, 93–107.

Jones P, Brunt P, Mowat N. 1985. Gastroenterology. London, William Heinemann Medical Books.

Kannan C. 1986. Gastroenterology: A Problem Oriented Approach. Garden City, NY, Medical Examination Publishing Co.

Kaplowitz N. 1982. Cholelithiasis. In Koretz RL, ed. Practical Gastroenterology. New York, John Wiley, 280–290.

Kennedy T. 1980. Clinical evaluation of the bleeding adult. In Fiddian-Green R, Turcotte R, eds. Gastrointestinal Hemorrhage. New York, Grune & Stratton.

Kim S. 1980. Pain: theory, research and nursing practice. Adv Nurs Sci 2:43–59.

Lamphier T, Lamphier R. 1981. Upper GI hemorrhage: Emergency evaluation and treatment. Am J Nurs 81:1814–1816.

Law D, Watts H. 1978. Gastrointestinal bleeding. In Sleisenger N, Fordtran J, eds. Gastrointestinal Disease: Pathophysiology, Diagnosis, and Management, 2nd ed. Philadelphia, WB Saunders, 217–240.

Levine G. 1983. Upper gastrointestinal hemorrhage, In Cohen S, ed. Clinical Gastroenterology: A Problem Oriented Approach. New York, John Wiley, 55–79.

Levinson S. 1982. Insertion of the Sengstaken-Blakemore tube. In Drossman D, ed. Manual of Gastroenterologic Procedures. New York, Raven Press, 21–27.

McConnell EA. 1987. Meeting the challenge of intestinal obstruction. Nursing 87 17(7):34–42.

McGuigan JE. 1987. Peptic ulcer. In Braunwald E, Isselbacher KJ, Peterdorf RG, et al, eds. Harrison's Principles of Internal Medicine, 11th ed, vol 2. New York, McGraw-Hill, 1239–1253.

Moorhouse M, Geissler A, Doenges M. 1987. Critical-Care Plans: Guidelines for Patient Care. Philadelphia, JB Lippincott.

Patrizzi J, Tackett M. 1984. Emergency Nursing: A Case Study Approach. Bowie, MD, Brady.

Podolsky DK, Isselbacher KJ. 1987. Cirrhosis. In Braunwald E, Isselbacher KJ, Peterdorf RG, et al, eds. Harrison's Principles of Internal Medicine, 11th ed, vol 2. New York, McGraw-Hill, 1341–1351.

Pops M. 1982. Pancreatitis. In Koretz RL, ed. Practical Gastroenterology. New York, John Wiley & Sons, 298–321.

Rice V. 1981. Shock: A clinical syndrome. IV. Nursing interventions. Crit Care Nurse 1(6):34–43.

Roberts S. 1985. Physiological Concepts and the Critically Ill Patient. Englewood Cliffs, NJ: Prentice-Hall.

Rosato E. 1983. Clinical approach to the patient with acute abdominal pain. In Cohen S, ed. Clinical Gastroenterology: A Problem Oriented Approach. New York, John Wiley, 21–37.

Shrock T. 1978. Acute appendicitis. In Sleisenger M, Fordtran J, eds. Gastrointestinal Disease: Pathophysiology, Diagnosis and Management, 2nd ed. Philadelphia, WB Saunders, 1825–1833.

Strange J. 1987. Shock Trauma Care Plan. Springhouse, PA, Springhouse Corporation.

Tedesco F. 1983. Lower gastrointestinal hemorrhage. In Cohen S, ed. Clinical Gastroenterology: A Problem Oriented Approach. New York, John Wiley & Sons, 81–100.

Thomas F. 1983. Differential Diagnosis of Abdominal Problems. New York, Arco Publishing Co.

Trotman B. 1983. Clinical approach to the patient with suspected gallstones or biliary tract disease. In Cohen S, ed. Clinical Gastroenterology: A Problem-Oriented Approach. New York, John Wiley & Sons, 399–412.

Trott AT. 1988. Acute abdominal pain. In Rosen P, Baker F, Barkin R, et al, eds. Emergency Medicine: Concepts and clinical practice, vol. 2, 2nd ed. St. Louis, CV Mosby 1389–1402.

Utley R, Carter D. 1987. Gastric duodenal emergencies. In Imrie CW, Moossa AR, eds. Gastrointestinal Emergencies. Edinburgh, Churchill Livingstone, 46–61.

Way L. 1978. Abdominal pain and the acute abdomen. In Sleisenger M, Fordtran K, eds. Gastrointestinal Disease: Pathophysiology, Diagnosis, Management, 2nd ed. Philadelphia, WB Saunders, 394–410.

Williamson R. 1987. Small bowel emergencies. In Imrie CW, Moossa AR, eds. Gastrointestinal Emergencies. Edinburgh, Churchill Livingstone, 132–149.

Stephanie Kitt, RN MSN

Abdominal Trauma

Abdominal injuries account for a large number of trauma-related injuries and deaths. Intraabdominal trauma seldom occurs as a single system injury. As would be expected, morbidity and mortality increase in direct proportion to the number of systems injured. The mortality associated with abdominal trauma has decreased significantly over the past decade, largely owing to the lessons learned from treatment of trauma during military conflicts.

Abdominal trauma may be blunt or penetrating in origin. Both types of injury may be associated with damage to abdominal viscera resulting in massive blood loss. Blunt intraabdominal injuries many times are not obvious externally, are concealed physiologically by intense compensatory mechanisms, and are masked anatomically by overlying skin, muscle, and fat. Blunt injuries are, therefore, more difficult to identify than other forms of trauma. Penetrating injuries to the abdomen can be classified as low velocity, as in stabbings, or high velocity, as in gunshot wounds. Open trauma to the abdomen may result in a variety of injuries ranging from innocuous to life threatening.

This chapter covers the assessment and management of blunt and penetrating abdominal trauma.

REVIEW OF ABDOMINAL ANATOMY

The abdomen extends from the diaphragm superiorly, the pelvis inferiorly, the vertebral column posteriorly, and the abdominal and iliac muscles anteriorly. The peritoneum is a serous membrane reflected over the viscera and lining the abdominal cavity. The visceral peritoneum envelops the abdominal organs. The parietal peritoneum lines the abdominal and pelvic walls and the undersurface of the diaphragm. A small amount of serous fluid is contained between the parietal and visceral layers of the abdomen. The fluid provides lubrication for the organs and the abdominal wall (Thompson et al 1986).

The organs contained within the peritoneal cavity include the stomach, small intestine, liver, gallbladder, spleen, transverse colon, sigmoid colon, upper third of the rectum, and, in women, the uterus. Retroperitoneal structures include part of the duodenum, ascending colon, descending colon, kidneys, pancreas, and major vessels (Fig. 13–1).

The omentum is a double fold of peritoneum attached to the stomach and connecting it with certain abdominal organs.

The mesentery is a peritoneal fold connecting the intestine with the posterior abdominal wall. The blood vessels and nerves of the small intestine flow through the mesentery.

The abdomen can be divided into four quadrants for physical assessment purposes (Fig. 13–2).

MECHANISMS OF INJURY

The most crucial factor in determining abdominal injuries is suspecting them. An accurate and detailed history of the accident will assist in identifying potential intra-abdominal injuries. Whenever he or she is conscious and capable, the patient is the best source of information. Emergency medical teams, relatives, or bystanders can aid in establishing facts related to the accident.

Mechanisms of injury must be identified as part of the history. The most common mechanisms of injury to the abdomen are blunt and penetrating forces. Blunt trauma occurs when the abdomen is struck by or against an object, creating internal bruising of organs, lacerations of solid organs from shear forces on acceleration and deceleration, rupture of hollow organs, and avulsion of organs and blood vessels from their supporting connective tissue. Motor vehicle accidents, assaults, falls, and sporting accidents account for a large portion of cases of blunt trauma to the abdomen. The nurse should determine the object causing the injury, the speed of force against the object, and the specific area of the abdomen where pressure was applied. For example, if the patient was a motorist involved in a motor vehicle accident (MVA), was he or she wearing a seat belt? This type information can help predict specific injuries such as chest, patellar, and hip injury in the nonrestrained driver and bowel and bladder rupture in the driver wearing a lap belt (Arajarvi et al 1987). The victim of assault who is struck in the abdomen just below the left ribs should be presumed to have a splenic or stomach injury until proved otherwise. A person who falls onto an object and sustains right lower rib fractures is suspected to have a liver injury. With few exceptions, the greater the distance of the fall, the greater the potential for injury.

Penetrating injuries result in direct disruption of internal organs and bone. Gunshot wounds and stabbings are the most frequent cause of penetrating abdomi-

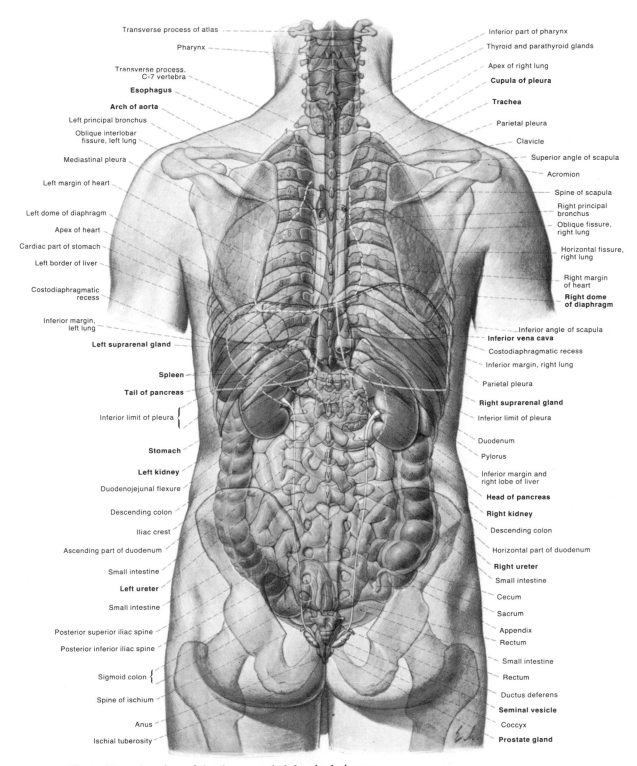

Transverse process of atlas
Pharynx
Transverse process, C-7 vertebra
Esophagus
Arch of aorta
Left principal bronchus
Oblique interlobar fissure, left lung
Mediastinal pleura
Left margin of heart
Left dome of diaphragm
Apex of heart
Cardiac part of stomach
Left border of liver
Costodiaphragmatic recess
Inferior margin, left lung
Left suprarenal gland
Spleen
Tail of pancreas
Inferior limit of pleura
Stomach
Left kidney
Duodenojejunal flexure
Descending colon
Iliac crest
Ascending part of duodenum
Small intestine
Left ureter
Small intestine
Posterior superior iliac spine
Posterior inferior iliac spine
Sigmoid colon
Spine of ischium
Anus
Ischial tuberosity

Inferior part of pharynx
Thyroid and parathyroid glands
Apex of right lung
Cupula of pleura
Trachea
Parietal pleura
Clavicle
Superior angle of scapula
Acromion
Spine of scapula
Right principal bronchus
Oblique fissure, right lung
Horizontal fissure, right lung
Right margin of heart
Right dome of diaphragm
Inferior angle of scapula
Inferior vena cava
Costodiaphragmatic recess
Inferior margin, right lung
Parietal pleura
Right suprarenal gland
Inferior limit of pleura
Duodenum
Pylorus
Inferior margin and right lobe of liver
Head of pancreas
Right kidney
Descending colon
Horizontal part of duodenum
Right ureter
Small intestine
Cecum
Sacrum
Appendix
Rectum
Small intestine
Rectum
Ductus deferens
Seminal vesicle
Coccyx
Prostate gland

FIGURE 13–1. Posterior view of the thorax and abdominal viscera.

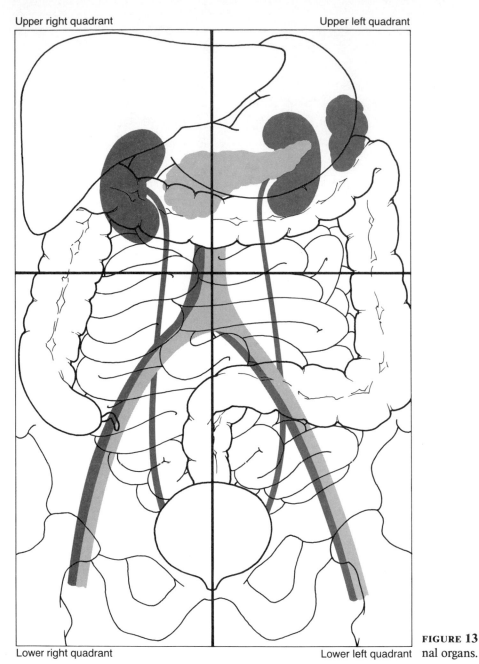

Lower right quadrant

Lower left quadrant

FIGURE 13–2. Anterior view of abdominal organs.

nal trauma. Damage to internal organs depends largely on the implement causing the injury; type, caliber, and distance of the gun from the victim when it was fired; size and length of stabbing implement; and direction of force.

Penetrating insults to the abdomen from stabbing implements generally are less severe than those involving ballistic weapons. Stab wounds are relatively benign

TABLE 13–1
Examples of Muzzle Velocity

Weapon	Velocity (ft/sec)
.22 Long rifle	1,335
.22 Magnum	2,000
.220 Swift	2,800
.270 Winchester	3,580
.357 Magnum	1,550
.38 Colt	730
.44 Magnum	1,850
.45 Army Colt	850

Source: From Trunkey DD. Trauma principles and penetrating neck trauma. In: Trunkey DD, Lewis FR, editors. Current Therapy of Trauma: 1984–1985. Toronto: BC Decker, 1984:80.

injuries unless a major blood vessel has been lacerated or unless a particularly vital structure has been injured (Trunkey 1984). Stab wounds produce straight-line injury with tissue disruption along the path of the implement only. The direction of force and length of the implement are key determinants of potential injuries.

Gunshot wounds may cause devastating injury, particularly if they are from high-velocity weapons or close-range shotguns. The extent of injury is directly related to the amount of kinetic energy that is imparted to the tissue (Ordog et al 1988). The amount of energy imparted to the tissue is equivalent to the kinetic energy on impact minus the kinetic energy on exit. V1 in the equation below relates to impact velocity and V2 to exit velocity.

$$\text{Kinetic energy released to tissues} = \frac{\text{mass} \times (V1^2 - V2^2)}{2 \times \text{gravitational force}}$$

Because kinetic energy equals mass times velocity squared, it follows that small increases in velocity produce massive increases in damage. Weapons capable of generating a missile velocity in excess of 3000 ft/sec are considered high-velocity weapons (Swan 1980) (Table 13–1). High-velocity weapons cause cavitation around the bullet, defined as a temporary cavity produced around a missile as tissues are stretched and compressed. Yaw and tumbling are associated with high-velocity missiles and contribute to massive injury. Yaw is the deviation of the nose of the bullet from a straight path. The bullet angles through the tissue, imparting great kinetic energy as it travels. Tumbling is the circular rotation of a bullet through tissue. Both yaw and tumbling create massive tissue injury (Weigelt and McCormack 1988, 105) (Fig. 13–3).

Close-range shotgun blasts cause the most devastating injuries of any weapon to which civilians are normally exposed (Trunkey 1984). Shotgun shells often contain pellets that disseminate on impact, cause large cavernous wounds, and draw contaminated particles into the wound as a suction effect is created by the velocity along the path of the bullet. This creates an increased risk of infection for the patient. Prophylactic antibiotic therapy generally consists of a cephalosporin given intravenously.

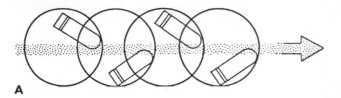

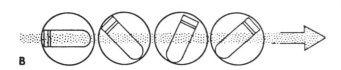

FIGURE 13–3. Effect of yaw and tumbling on wounding potential. *A,* Yawing is the deviation of the bullet in its longitudinal axis from the straight line of flight. *B,* Tumbling is the action of forward rotation around the center of mass. (From Weigelt JA, McCormack A. 1988. In Cardona VD et al, eds. Trauma Nursing: From Resuscitation through Rehabilitation. WB Saunders, 119.)

Evisceration can occur as a result of penetrating abdominal trauma. Protrusion of viscera from the wound is evidence of evisceration. Eviscerated omentum and other abdominal contents should be covered with sterile saline-soaked dressings. Care should be taken to avoid manipulation of any eviscerated material.

ASSESSMENT OF THE ABDOMINALLY INJURED PATIENT

The chief complaint will vary depending upon the organ injured. If the patient with abdominal injuries is able to communicate, he or she will usually complain of pain in the abdomen. The pain is generally dull and diffuse, with increased tenderness on palpation of involved organs. Specific assessment findings are discussed under clinical manifestations for selected organ injuries.

A thorough examination of the abdomen can be initiated once the airway, breathing, and circulation (ABCs) are stabilized. The abdomen should be examined in the following order; inspection, auscultation, percussion, and palpation. The abdomen is inspected, noting obvious contusions, abrasions, open wounds, or scars from previous injuries or surgery. Any abnormality should be noted with respect to region, size, and pattern. Ecchymosis about the flanks and abdomen (Grey Turner's sign) indicates infiltration of blood into the extraperitoneal tissues, usually implying injury to the spleen. The color, which appears 6 to 24 hours post injury, may be variable shades of blue-red, purple, or greenish-brown, depending upon the age of the hemorrhage (Cahill 1986). A slight bluish discoloration about the umbilicus (Cullen's sign) is a sign of hemoperitoneum. This generally indicates injury to the duodenum, gallbladder, or pancreas. It also may result from rupture of an ectopic pregnancy or abdominal aneurysm (Cahill 1986).

The contour of the abdomen should be noted. The abdomen may be distended and tense owing to trapped gas from the bowel or rupture of a hollow viscus. It is thought by some authorities that abdominal distention is difficult to discern. Because the abdomen is a cylinder and a 1-cm change in radius of a typical 70-kg person's abdomen would account for approximately 2.9 L of fluid, it is unlikely that any clinician can detect a 1-cm change in the radius of an abdomen (Trunkey 1984). In light of this concept, abdominal girths are not thought to be helpful in detecting changes in abdominal radius.

Auscultation of the abdomen is performed prior to palpation and percussion to avoid alterations in bowel sounds caused by manual compression. Trauma typically causes a paralytic ileus, characterized by abdominal distention and decreasing or absent peristaltic sounds.

Percussion yields information regarding the nature of matter within the abdomen. Air, fluid, and solid matter create varying sounds on percussion. Tympany, a hollow sound, suggests the presence of air or gas within the intestines or abdomen. Free air is usually associated with hollow organ perforation. Dullness on percussion may indicate a fluid-filled cavity, such as occurs in intra-abdominal hemorrhage or with a full bladder.

Palpation of the abdomen should be performed in two manners; light and deep. Light palpation defines areas of tenderness and involuntary abdominal muscular rigidity or guarding. Both are signs of peritoneal tenderness. The examination should be done systemically, saving the immediate area of pain for last. With the heel of the dominant hand placed over the umbilicus, the examiner can begin palpation with the finger pads at a point farthest from the pain, moving clockwise and using light, gentle touch. Masses in the upper abdominal area may indicate splenic or liver hematomas. Suspected masses or areas of tenderness may be circumscribed with a povidone-iodine swab for future reference.

Deep palpation is useful in identifying less superficial masses, organs, or areas of tenderness. With one hand placed over the other, the examiner can proceed in the same clockwise manner as in light palpation. However, a greater amount of pressure is applied, with the examiner's top hand allowing the hand in direct contact with the patient's abdomen to sense underlying structures.

Methodic and periodic examinations of the abdomen are essential in evaluation of the patient with potential disruption of intraabdominal integrity. Examinations should be performed at least every one-half hour initially when internal injury is suspected.

SPECIFIC INJURIES

Diaphragmatic Injury

The diaphragm, situated at the upper abdominal border formed by the intercostal angle, is a musculotendinous structure attached posteriorly to the first, second, and third lumbar vertebrae, anteriorly to the sternum, and laterally to the costal margins. It is susceptible to either penetrating or blunt trauma. Blunt trauma may occur with high-speed deceleration forces that cause an increase in intraabdominal pressure and diaphragmatic rupture. Herniation of bowel through the opening in the diaphragm may occur, and entrapment of bowel may produce strangulation. Penetrating injuries between the nipple and below the costal margins should be assumed to have penetrated the diaphragm (Trunkey 1984, 95). Hemothorax and pneumothorax frequently accompany this injury. Very often diaphragmatic injury is found on surgical exploration of the abdomen for other injury or may be diagnosed months post injury, after a diagnostic work-up for much more subtle symptoms relating to gastrointestinal distress.

Clinical Manifestations

Patients with diaphragmatic injury often have multiple associated injuries. They may be asymptomatic initially, or symptoms may be overlooked because of the critical nature of associated injuries. As bowel herniates through the diaphragmatic opening, dyspnea, gastrointestinal irritation, pain radiating to the left shoulder, and nausea and vomiting may be evident. Bowel sounds may be heard over the left lung field. Decreased breath sounds and heart sounds shifted to the side opposite the rupture may be apparent. Chest radiograph may show the presence of abdominal viscera or a nasogastric tube within the chest. An elevated right hemidiaphragm may indicate liver protrusion through the tear.

Treatment and Nursing Care

Impaired Gas Exchange, Related to

• **Compression of Lung Secondary to Bowel Herniation Through the Diaphragm**

Gas exchange may be impaired in the patient with massive diaphragmatic injury. The patient should be positioned in a semi-Fowler's position to facilitate breathing, if possible. Supplemental oxygen should be initiated, blood gases monitored, and the patient prepared for chest tube insertion and definitive surgical repair of the diaphragmatic opening.

The following section covers gastrointestinal, liver, spleen, and aortic injuries. Principles of treatment and nursing care for the injuries are discussed after consideration of the specific injuries.

Gastrointestinal Injuries

This discussion of gastrointestinal injuries includes the stomach, small bowel, and colon. The stomach is located within the peritoneal cavity in the left upper quadrant of the abdomen and joins the esophagus just below the diaphragm. It is most often affected by penetrating rather than blunt trauma. As with most hollow organs, the notable exception is the full or distended stomach that ruptures as a result of blunt insult. The stomach wall contains glands that secrete digestive enzymes, mucus, hydrochloric acid, intrinsic factor, pepsinogen types I and II, and serotonin. If perforating injury occurs, these gastric contents are released into the peritoneal cavity and cause peritonitis.

The duodenum or first section of the small bowel is attached to the stomach and posterior abdominal wall. It is positioned over the vertebral column and may be compressed between the vertebral column and the offending object. When the py-loric sphincter of the stomach is closed, increased intraluminal pressure causes bowel perforation. The jejunum lies in the umbilical region, making it vulnerable to seat belt injury. Sudden deceleration produces shearing forces in which the bowel and mesentery are torn from their attachments or crushed between the vertebrae and offending objects. The small bowel contents are generally sterile and, with the exception of the duodenum, have a neutral pH, making rupture less likely to cause a bacterial or chemical peritonitis.

The colon is divided into ascending, transverse, descending, and sigmoid segments. Septic complications make the colon one of the most lethal sites of abdominal injury. Colon injury can be suspected in patients with blunt abdominal trauma or a penetrating wound near the colon or rectal structures.

Clinical Manifestations

Injury to the stomach, small bowel, or colon will be manifested by guarding on physical examination and by generalized and or rebound tenderness. The patient will also be reluctant to change position, and any jarring of the cart may induce severe abdominal discomfort. Rigidity of the abdomen also may occur as bowel contents spill into the peritoneal cavity. Hypotension and tachycardia are associated with hypovolemic shock when intraabdominal hemorrhage occurs. Air outside the gastro-intestinal tract, commonly known as free air, will be evident on abdominal films.

Liver Injury

The liver is the organ injured most commonly by penetrating abdominal trauma and is second only to the spleen in being injured by blunt abdominal trauma (Anderson and Ballinger 1985). Death frequently is related to uncontrollable hemorrhage.

The liver, located in the right upper quadrant of the abdomen, is the largest intraabdominal organ. The right and superior surfaces of the liver follow the under-surface of the diaphragm (Stern 1988). The liver detoxifies metabolic byproducts, synthesizes many proteins, serves as an immunologic organ, and metabolizes fat, carbohydrate, and protein. The liver is a highly vascular organ that bleeds profusely when injured.

Liver injury should be suspected in patients who have a fracture of the right lower six ribs. The patient with an enlarged liver from cirrhosis, congestive heart failure, recent hepatitis, or other hepatic problem is particularly vulnerable. Even a minor fall may cause an enlarged liver to rupture. Falls from heights, especially in those who land on their feet, may avulse the hepatic veins from the vena cava.

Clinical Manifestations

Pain is typically located in the right upper quadrant and may be referred to the shoulder. Guarding, abdominal tenderness and rigidity, and signs of hypovolemic shock provide clues to liver injury.

Peritoneal tap and lavage are still used in some institutions to determine the presence of intraperitoneal blood. The tap can be performed using a closed (no incision) or open (incision) technique. In either case, a lavage catheter is placed into the peritoneum. Indications for peritoneal lavage include a history of abdominal trauma, equivocal findings on examination, neurologic impairment making abdominal examination impossible, and drug or alcohol intoxication. Blood withdrawn immediately from the tap site is considered a positive tap and reflects the need for surgery. When blood is not returned immediately, lavage with either normal saline (pH 5.3) or lactated Ringer's solution (pH 6.3) is initiated. Returns are sent to the laboratory and considered positive if there are greater than 100,000 red blood cells (RBCs) in blunt trauma, more than 10,000 RBCs in penetrating trauma, intraabdominal contents, bacteria, or bile (Dunham and Cowley 1986).

Computed tomographic (CT) scanning has been found very useful as a less invasive means of detecting intraabdominal injury. It allows assessment of the retroperitoneum, including the pancreas and duodenum (Trunkey 1984). In addition, it is more accurate, is more comfortable for the patient than peritoneal lavage, and affords less risk of invasive procedural complications.

Splenic Injury

The spleen, located in the left upper quadrant of the abdomen, lies deep to the ninth, tenth, and eleventh ribs posterior to the left midaxillary line (Stern 1988, 271). It is the most commonly injured organ in blunt trauma. The spleen functions to filter bacteria, aged erythrocytes, and particulate matter from the circulation. It also clears platelets from the circulation, manufactures immunoglobulin M (IgM) antibodies against circulating bacterial antigens, and provides storage for blood cells. The highly vascular nature of the spleen is evidenced by the volume of blood that circulates through it: approximately 350 L daily (Ramzy 1987).

Blunt and penetrating trauma to the left upper quadrant region of the abdomen or fractures seen on radiographs of ribs 9, 10, and 11 posteriorly may indicate splenic injury. To assess for rib fractures, the patient should be asked to inspire deeply. If pain is elicited, rib fracture and splenic injury are possible. The enlarged spleen is most susceptible in pregnancy when the capsule is very thin and the organ profusely engorged. It is also more susceptible to injury in patients with mononucleosis or a recent history of such.

Clinical Manifestations

The patient with splenic injury will complain of left upper quadrant pain that may radiate to the left shoulder (Kehr's sign). Manifestations of acute blood loss and hypovolemia are common as significant hemorrhage occurs. However, if subcapsular hemorrhage occurs, the bleeding source may be temporarily tamponaded by the capsule. The patient may be hemodynamically stable until splenic rupture and circulatory collapse occurs. It is extremely important to closely monitor patients with a history suggesting spleen injury. Occasionally individuals will return to emergency several days after being evaluated for trauma only to find a splenic injury is present.

An enlarging area of left flank dullness on percussion (Ballance's sign) or neck pain related to phrenic nerve irritation (Seagesser's sign), or both, suggests splenic injury. Bruising or abrasions over the left upper quadrant should also arouse suspicion of spleen injury.

Traumatic Aortic Dissection

The aorta, although not considered purely an abdominal organ, does enter the abdomen through the diaphragm. Motor vehicle accidents are a leading cause of traumatic aortic dissection. Extreme deceleration forces are capable of rupturing, shearing, or transecting the artery. Patients with traumatic aortic dissections often exsanguinate rapidly and if brought to the hospital are dead on arrival. Patients with partial disruptions or traumatic aneurysms may survive the initial insult.

Although the most common site of traumatic aortic dissection is in the vicinity of the descending aorta immediately distal to the left subclavian artery at the ligamentum arteriosum (Fig. 13–4), disruption can occur at any portion of the vessel. Tears found in the arch or lower descending aorta near the diaphragm occur less frequently (Cowley and Turney 1987). A tear in the abdominal aorta due to blunt trauma is seldom seen (Moncure and Brewster 1988, 195). Penetrating insults to the chest or abdomen can also injure the aorta directly.

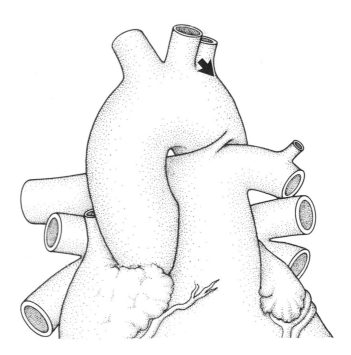

FIGURE 13–4. Aorta (arrow) is the most common site of traumatic rupture.

Clinical Manifestations

The patient who has suffered traumatic aortic disruption will be in profound hypovolemic shock. Hypotension that is unresponsive to massive fluid resuscitation, tachycardia, cold and clammy skin, diaphoresis, an altered mental status, and no other obvious source of hemorrhage are highly suggestive of aortic injury.

Blood pressure, when audible or palpable, may vary between upper and lower extremities. When the dissection disrupts blood flow to the lower extremities, femoral pulses may be diminished or absent. If the dissection is along the ascending aorta, perfusion to either upper extremity may be compromised, causing variation in left and right extremity pulses. A pseudocoarctation syndrome may occur, causing elevation in upper extremity blood pressure and diminished or absent femoral pulses. This syndrome is uncommon and is seen with partial aortic transection. It occurs secondary to partial aortic occlusion by a torn flap of intima or a periaortic hematoma compressing the aortic lumen (Symbas 1978). Sympathetic afferent nerve fibers located in the aorta are capable of causing reflex hypertension as a response to this stretching stimulus.

TREATMENT AND NURSING CARE

Because the abdominally injured patient frequently has multisystem injuries, stage I care—which consists of stabilizing the airway, breathing, and circulation—is the first priority. Supplemental oxygen should be administered to all patients with potential abdominal injuries. Because blood loss and hemorrhagic shock are of concern, two large-bore, 14 gauge or greater, intravenous lines (IVs) should be initiated immediately if not done in the prehospital setting. Crystalloid solutions should be infused rapidly and blood ordered for transfusion. Laboratory studies for the abdominally injured patient include hemoglobin, hematocrit, white blood count, serum electrolytes, amylase, blood urea nitrogen, and creatinine. Initial hemoglobin and hematocrit levels in the trauma patient are normal and only provide a basis for later comparisons. In addition, coagulation studies and typing and cross-matching of blood should be ordered in preparation for operative intervention. If a urethral injury is not suspected, a urinary catheter should be inserted and urine tested for blood before sending the specimen to the laboratory for further analysis. A nasogastric tube is necessary to evacuate the stomach and to determine the presence of blood in the upper gastrointestinal tract. To avoid bladder or stomach perforation, the urinary catheter and nasogastric tube must be inserted prior to peritoneal lavage.

Emergency diagnostic evaluation may include peritoneal lavage, computed tomography, abdominal flat-plate radiographs, or an abdominal series. The particular diagnostic test is determined by the physician on the basis of patient acuity, associated injuries, and physician preference.

Ongoing monitoring of the patient's vital signs is necessary. Blood pressure, pulse, and respiratory rate should be monitored at least every 5 minutes in the critically ill person. Early signs of shock include a decreased level of consciousness, decreased urine output, and delayed capillary refill. A rectal temperature should be obtained as soon as possible and care taken to avoid hypothermia. Blankets should cover the patient whenever examinations or procedures are not being performed.

Fluid Volume Deficit, Related to

• *Intra-abdominal Hemorrhage*

The abdominal trauma patient will demonstrate actual or potential fluid volume deficit and will require fluid resuscitation. The type of fluid (crystalloid or colloid) used for resuscitation depends on individual hospital protocols. Fluid should be infused to maintain the patient's blood pressure at or above 90 mmHg systolic pressure. Although patients may respond to initial fluid resuscitation favorably, a subsequent fall in blood pressure is significant. It is thought that a patient who becomes hypotensive and is unable to remain stable after fluid resuscitation requires immediate surgical repair of the internal pathology.

The pneumatic antishock garment (PASG) may be applied initially to elevate peripheral perfusion pressure. The suit should not be deflated until there is evidence of stabilization with fluid therapy, the surgeon is on hand to deal with the particular pathology that may be unmasked when the suit is removed, and the operating room is ready to accommodate the patient should he or she require operative intervention. The PASG is often left in place until the patient is in the operating room.

If possible, it may be helpful to place the patient in a modified Trendelenburg position (Fig. 13–5). This promotes venous return and may increase circulating blood volume within the vital organs yet avoids diaphragmatic compression that occurs with the traditional Trendelenburg position.

A central venous pressure (CVP) line may be inserted to guide fluid resuscitation. CVP measurements of 5 to 12 cm water pressure are considered normal. Monitoring the variation in measurements, rather than the actual values, is most useful in guiding volume repletion.

Several intravenous set-ups are available for massive volume infusion. Most devices include a fluid warming device, which is essential when large volumes of fluids at room temperature or refrigerated blood are given to the patient. Use of these devices will prevent iatrogenic hypothermia.

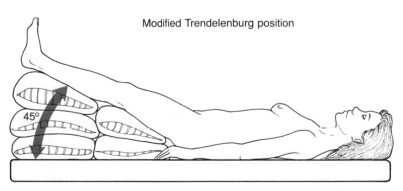

Modified Trendelenburg position

45°

Lower extremities elevated

Patient flat

FIGURE 13–5. Modified Trendelenburg position to increase venous return without compromising diaphragmatic excursion.

Tissue Perfusion, Altered (Peripheral), Related to

- *Hypovolemia*

Patients with intraabdominal hemorrhage will exhibit an alteration in tissue perfusion related to hypovolemia. Adequate cellular oxygenation depends, in part, on the ability of the RBCs (hemoglobin) to carry oxygen to the tissues. The patient in hypovolemic shock is in need of RBC replacement. Blood transfusions with packed RBCs or whole blood is in order. Type O negative blood can be given to the patient prior to determination of blood type, Rh, and antigen cross-match. Once type-specific blood is available, it should be used for transfusion.

Supplemental oxygen will enhance the diffusion of oxygen across the cell membrane to the blood. A non-rebreather oxygen mask connected to 12 to 15 L of oxygen flow is desirable and will ensure approximately 90 per cent FIO_2.

Pain, Related to

- *Disruption of Abdominal Integrity*

When they are conscious, persons with abdominal trauma generally experience pain. Because of the multiplicity and severity of associated injuries, generally it is impossible to position the patient in a way to alleviate pain associated with abdominal trauma. In addition, to avoid masking symptoms that might lead to defining the injury, analgesics are prohibited prior to definitive diagnosis. Therefore, much of the nurse's responsibilities with respect to pain management focuses on serial assessments and psychologic support. It is important to encourage verbalization of the pain and offer explanations for withholding medications. Anticipatory guidance can be offered in terms of the planned diagnostic tests, time frames for each, and expected feelings during procedures. This often helps the patient cope with the pain and anxiety associated with internal injuries. Additionally, family members and relatives should be allowed to converse with the patient whenever possible.

EVALUATION

Improved fluid volume status and hemodynamic stabilization are indicated by improved cardiac rate and rhythm, improved level of consciousness, stable CVP between 5 and 12 cm H_2O, urinary output greater than 30 ml/hour, warm and dry skin, and capillary refill less than 2 seconds.

Although often it is not possible to abate pain and anxiety totally, evaluation of the patient's response to the pain may indicate improved tolerance and decreased anxiety. Reduction in anxiety may be indicated by patient's statement of reduced anxiety and understanding of diagnostic evaluation phase, as well as decreased signs of agitation.

CONCLUSION

Persons who have sustained abdominal trauma may appear either stable or unstable initially. It is important to assess, resuscitate, and monitor each patient as though there is the potential for severe intraabdominal injury until proved otherwise. Although the medical management revolves around determining and defining injuries, the nursing focus is toward assessment and monitoring the patient's response to resuscitation and diagnostic procedures. Serial assessments and continuous monitoring assist in identifying injuries. Preparing the patient for surgery is a key point in nursing care because operative intervention often is required for a definitive diagnosis. Frequently persons with abdominal trauma are awake, alert, and very anxious. Informative explanations and anticipatory guidance with respect to the emergency evaluation and resuscitation are helpful in allaying anxiety and ensuring the best possible outcome physiologically and psychologically.

REFERENCES

Anderson CB, Ballinger WF. 1985. Abdominal injuries. In Zuidema GB, Rutherford RB, Ballinger WF, eds. The Management of Surgery, ed. 4. Philadelphia, WB Saunders Co, 449–504.

Arajarvi F, Santavirta S, Tolonen J. 1987. Abdominal injuries sustained in severe traffic accidents by seatbelt wearers. J Trauma 27:393–397.

Blaisdell FW, Trunkey DD. 1982. Abdominal Trauma, vol 1. New York, Thieme-Stratton.

Cahill M. 1986. Nurse's Reference Library, Signs and Symptoms. Springhouse, PA, Springhouse Corporation.

Cooley A. 1986. Surgical Treatment of Aortic Aneurysms. Philadelphia, WB Saunders Co, 44–45.

Cowley RA, Turney SZ. 1987. Blunt thoracic injuries: The ruptured aorta. In Cowley RA, Conn A, Dunham CM, eds. Trauma Care Surgical Management, vol 1. Philadelphia, JB Lippincott Co, 172–181.

Cummings PH, Cummings SP. 1987. Abdominal emergencies. In Rea RE, Bourg PW, Parker JG, Rushing D, eds. Emergency Nursing Core Curriculum, 3rd ed. Philadelphia, WB Saunders Co, 60–70.

Donohue JH, Federle MP, Griffiths BG, Trunkey DD. 1987. Computed tomography in the diagnosis of blunt intestinal and mesenteric injuries. J Trauma, 27:11–17.

Dunham CM, Cowley RA. 1986. Shock Trauma/Critical Care Handbook. Rockville, MD, Aspen Publishers.

De La Roche AG, Creel RJ, Mulligan GW, Burns CM. 1982. Diaphragmatic rupture due to blunt abdominal trauma. Surg Gynecol Obstet 154:175–180.

Frame SB, Timberlake GA, McSwain NE Jr. 1988. Trauma rounds, problem: abdominal stab wound. Emerg Med March 15, 59.

Mariadason JG, Parsa MH, Ayuyao A, Freeman HP. 1988. Management of stab wounds to the thoracoabdominal region: A clinical approach. Ann Surg 207:235–240.

Mattox KL. 1987. Decelerating aortic injury. In Bergan JJ, Yao JST, eds. Vascular Surgical Emergencies. Orlando, Grune & Stratton, 341–358.

Meredith JW, Trunkey DD. 1988. CT scanning in acute abdominal injuries. Surg Clin North Am 68:255.

Moncure AC, Brewster DC. 1988. Vascular trauma. In Burke JF, Boyd RD, McCabe CJ (eds). Trauma Management: Early Management of Visceral, Nervous System, and Musculoskeletal Injuries, 176–207.

Ordog GJ. 1988. Wound ballistics. In Ordog GJ (ed). Management of Gunshot Wounds. New York, Elsevier Science Publishing Co., 34.

Ramzy AI. 1987. Spleen: Save or sacrifice? In Cowley RA, Conn A, Dunham CM, eds. Trauma Care: Surgical Management, vol 1. Philadelphia, JB Lippincott Co, 152.

Richardson JD, Polk HC Jr, Flint L. 1987. Trauma Clinical Care Pathophysiology. Chicago, Year Book Medical Publishers.

Rosen P, Baker FJ, Barkin R, et al. 1988. Emergency Medicine: Concepts and Clinical Practice, 2nd ed, vol 1. St. Louis, CV Mosby Co.

Stern JT Jr. 1988. Essentials of Gross Anatomy. Philadelphia, FA Davis Co.

Swan KG, Swan RC. 1980. Gunshot wounds–Pathophysiology and management. Littleton, MA, PSG Publishing Co., 9.

Symbas PN. 1978. Traumatic Injuries of the Heart and Great Vessels. New York, Grune and Stratton.

Thompson JM, McFarland GK, Hirsch JE, Tucker SM, Bowers AC. 1986. Gastrointestinal system. In Clinical Nursing. St. Louis, CV Mosby Co. 1105–1182.

Trunkey DD. 1984. Abdominal trauma. In Trun-key DD, Lewis FR, eds. Current Therapy of Trauma. Toronto, B.C. Decker Co, 93–100.

Weigelt JA, McCormack A. 1988. Mechanism of injury. In Cardona VD, Hurn PD, Mason PB, et al (eds). Trauma Nursing: From Resuscitation Through Rehabilitation. Philadelphia, WB Saunders, 105–126.

Thomas Keeler, MD
Michael Carter, MD

Genitourinary Emergencies

Genitourinary tract diseases frequently lead people to emergency departments to seek medical care. Approximately 10 per cent of patients arriving at a busy emergency department (ED) will have some form of genitourinary pathology (Neih and Dretler 1984). A great many others are managed as outpatients. An increasing number of these patients are discharged with urethral catheters or may have returned because of some type of catheter malfunction. This chapter attempts to provide a basic fund of knowledge about a variety of diseases, both traumatic and nontraumatic. It will also provide guidelines for the proper management of genitourinary pathology by emergency nursing personnel.

GENITOURINARY TRACT ASSESSMENT IN TRAUMA

The patient who seeks emergency services following trauma requires evaluation for genitourinary trauma. Because isolated renal and genitourinary injuries are uncommon, patients coming to EDs with a history of multiple trauma must be evaluated initially to determine and manage life-threatening conditions. Refer to Chapter 6 for details on stage I care for the multiple trauma patient.

299

Etiology

Information on mechanism of injury is crucial in determining potential problem areas. Renal injuries must be suspected when the mechanism of trauma is consistent with rapid deceleration or a direct blow to the flank. The most common cause of bladder injury, accounting for 80 per cent of cases, is a direct blow to the abdomen. Urethral injuries are frequently associated (90 per cent) with pelvic fracture (Weems 1979). External genitalia are most commonly injured as a result of direct blunt or penetrating trauma.

Pathophysiology

The kidneys, situated in the upper retroperitoneum, are well protected by the vertebral column, overlying muscles, and ribs posteriorly and the intra-abdominal organs anteriorly (Fig. 14–1). The kidneys are surrounded with a generous layer of perinephric fat and a firm fascial envelope called Gerota's fascia, which also provides protection. However, the kidneys are mobile, secured only by the renal pedicle, which contains the renal artery, vein, lymphatics and neural tissue. This allows bruising and vascular injuries to occur as the kidney is thrust within its niche or torn away from the vascular attachments. Blunt trauma to the kidneys can cause superficial lacerations, hematomas, contusions, or severe injury, such as a deep cortical laceration.

The bladder, an extraperitoneal organ, is protected by the pubic symphysis. The dome of the bladder, however, is in contact with the peritoneum, and this is the most common site for intraperitoneal rupture. Rupture usually occurs with great blunt force and most commonly when the bladder is full.

The urethra, or outflow tract from the bladder, which emerges from the inferior aspect of the bladder, is approximately 4 cm long in women and passes through the pelvic muscular diaphragm anterior to the vagina. In men, the much longer urethra passes through the prostate gland and then exits the pelvis through the pelvic diaphragm and ventral aspect of the penis. The prostate gland lies inferior to the bladder and surrounds the proximal urethra (Fig. 14–2). The prostate is firmly attached by fascial connections to the pelvic side walls and to the symphysis pubis. Blunt forces to the pelvis can cause a tearing of the urethra at this site. A hematoma around the prostate, which gives the prostate a boggy feeling on physical examination, indicates urethral trauma.

Assessment of Genitourinary Tract

The chief complaint described by the patient gives an idea of the injured area. Pain should be described in type and location. Associated signs and symptoms relating to urinary elimination are key in evaluating genitourinary tract trauma. Does the patient have hematuria? Is there a change in voiding ability such as urgency or inability to void? Is there pre-existing renal disease or injuries?

Physical assessment focusing on the potential genitourinary tract injury begins with observation of the area of concern. Painful and contused areas should be noted. Bruises, abrasions, and surface lacerations about the flank and abdomen may signal

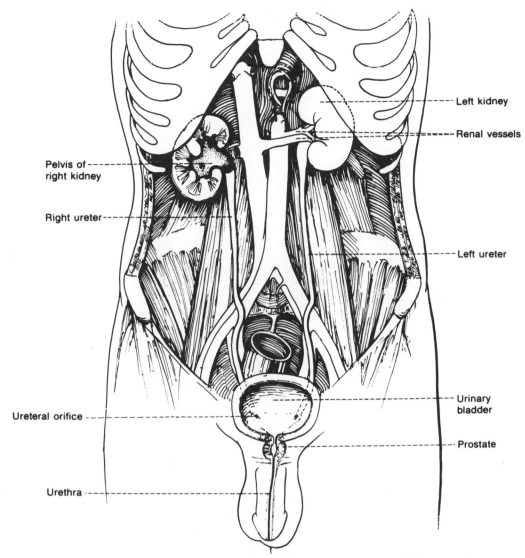

FIGURE 14–1. Anatomy of the urinary tract. (Copyright 1981. Urban and Schwarzenberg, Baltimore-Munich. Reproduced with permission from Basic Anatomy for the Health Sciences, edited by RL Montgomery. All rights reserved.)

underlying injury of the kidney and bladder, respectively. Blood noted at the external meatus is specific for urethral injuries. If blood is noted at the external meatus, a rectal examination should be performed to determine whether or not a boggy prostate is present, which would indicate a urethral hematoma and laceration. Palpation of tender areas and pressure exerted on the ischial tuberosities of the pelvis can indicate the presence of pelvic fracture.

A urinalysis is one of the primary diagnostic tests required in the emergency phase of evaluation. Conscious patients may be able to void. If there is no indication of urethral injury, multiply traumatized individuals or those unable to void will require catheterization. Initially a dipstick test for blood is sufficient until the re-

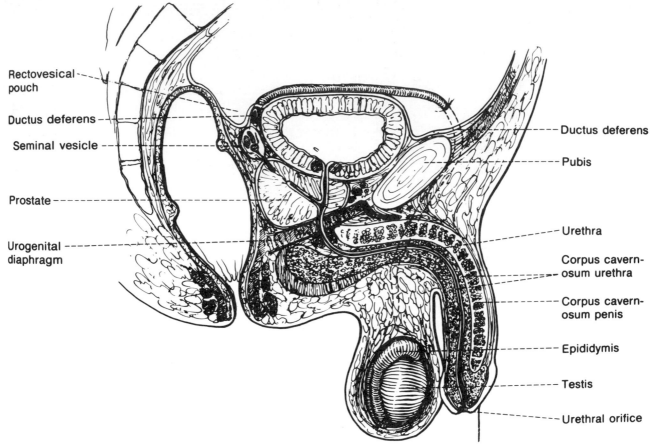

Rectovesical pouch

Ductus deferens

Seminal vesicle

Prostate

Urogenital diaphragm

Ductus deferens

Pubis

Urethra

Corpus cavern-osum urethra

Corpus cavern-osum penis

Epididymis

Testis

Urethral orifice

FIGURE 14–2. The male genital tract. (Copyright 1981. Urban and Schwarzenberg, Balti-more-Munich. Reproduced with permission from Basic Anatomy for the Health Sciences, edited by RL Montgomery. All rights reserved.)

mainder of the specimen can be sent to the laboratory for analysis. The presence of hematuria in any amount mandates further evaluation.

Other laboratory studies should be undertaken depending on the patient's condition and associated injuries. Blood for complete blood count (CBC), blood urea nitrogen (BUN), creatinine, and typing and cross-matching should be obtained in all multiple trauma victims.

Because significant bleeding in the pelvis may occur after pelvic trauma, hypovolemic shock is always a consideration. Frequent monitoring of vital signs is in order. Urinary output measurements at least every one half hour will provide information on kidney perfusion and fluid volume status.

Clinical Manifestations

As stated earlier, most genitourinary tract injuries occur in conjunction with other organ injuries. It is not uncommon for patients to have several associated injuries and be in hypovolemic shock. There are, however, cases involving an isolated genitourinary tract injury, and often these patients are in stable condition with a specific complaint on presentation.

Specific organ injuries have characteristic chief complaints and symptoms. Injury resulting from a direct blow to the flank or rapid deceleration is responsible for 80 per cent of renal injuries (Carlton et al 1968). These patients may complain of flank pain or grossly bloody urine, or they may have no specific complaints. Signs of renal injury include changes in vital signs suggesting blood loss, a flank mass, or flank ecchymosis. Hematuria is found in 90 per cent of renal injuries.

Bladder injuries are most likely to occur when the bladder is distended. A direct blow to the abdomen when the bladder is distended can result in rupture. Symptoms of bladder rupture include inability to void, urgency, and suprapubic pain. Hematuria, abdominal distention, and nausea and vomiting secondary to a paralytic ileus may also be present. Low or absent urinary output may be noted in the patient who has a bladder injury.

The patient with a urethral injury will usually complain of difficulty or inability to void. Blood at the meatus is common. Rectal examination may reveal a large hematoma obscuring palpation of the prostate in males.

Testicular injuries most often are a result of blunt trauma and are generally contusions. These patients may have severe scrotal pain and nausea. Scrotal discoloration, rapid swelling, or a palpably abnormal testicular contour is indicative of testicular rupture and constitutes a surgical emergency.

Rupture of the corpora cavernosa of the penis is rare but usually occurs during intercourse or self-stimulation. Patients report a snapping noise followed by intense pain and rapid detumescence. The penis will be edematous and ecchymotic. There is nearly 30 per cent incidence of associated urethral injury (Hudson 1975).

Treatment and Nursing Care

The focus for patients coming to EDs with complaints and signs or symptoms of potential genitourinary tract injury is on cardiovascular stabilization during stage I care. Stage II care involves the diagnostic work-up phase in an effort to determine the injuries present. Because the clinical presentations are varied, so too may be the portion of nursing time spent on stage I and stage II care. Emphasis throughout is on psychosocial support through explanations of the diagnostic tests being performed.

Fluid Volume Deficit, Related to

- *Hemorrhage Secondary to*
- *Renal Injury*
- *Pelvic Fracture*
- *Other Organ Injury*

Patients who come to EDs with actual or potential fluid volume deficit will require one or more large-bore intravenous lines for infusion of lactated Ringer's or normal saline solution as used routinely for resuscitation of patients in hypovolemic shock. Ongoing assessment and frequent monitoring of vital signs are critical nursing interventions for patients with alterations in fluid volume status. Hypotension, tachycardia, and delayed capillary refill indicate insufficient resuscitation efforts.

Potential for Injury, Related to

- *Blunt Forces to the Abdomen or Flank*
- *Deceleration Forces*
- *Trauma to Genitalia*

The patient with a history of blunt abdominal or flank trauma will require evaluation for genitourinary tract injuries. To evaluate the kidneys and ureters, an intravenous pyelogram (IVP) is the study of choice. The IVP may be done in the radiology department or possibly in the emergency services area when rapid evaluation is required. Iodinated contrast medium is given by intravenous push in a 150-ml bolus. The patient should be asked about allergy to contrast material before administration. The patient should be informed that the study may take as long as one hour to perform, and numerous radiographs will be taken. The patient may feel warm, flushed, or nauseated when the contrast agent is given. In unconscious patients or in those without an obtainable history, it is best to proceed with epinephrine and diphenhydramine (Benadryl) on hand in the unlikely event of an anaphylactic reaction. Ultrasound or nuclear renal scans can be done if the patient has an allergy to contrast agents.

Renal injuries can be placed into two categories (Fig. 14–3).Patients with minor injuries can be put on bedrest until their hematuria clears, are given analgesics, and have vital signs checked frequently. The patients with major injuries may require immediate exploration and repair of the injured kidney. Preparation for surgery is necessary.

The diagnostic test for determining a bladder injury is a gravity cystogram (Fig. 14–4). Contrast material (300 to 400 ml) is dripped into the bladder through a catheter. Precontrast, full bladder, and postcontrast (empty bladder) views of the pelvis are taken. The postcontrast view is crucial. Extravasation that otherwise may be hidden during the full bladder view may be evident. Small extraperitoneal injuries are frequently managed by catheter drainage and bed rest (Mulkey 1974). Larger tears may require open surgical drainage and primary repair of the bladder.

If pelvic fracture and voiding difficulties, blood at the urethral meatus, or any other physical finding raises the suspicion of urethral injury, the nurse must not attempt to pass a urethral catheter. A partial urethral disruption may be converted to a complete disruption by indiscriminate attempted catheterization. The study to evaluate for urethral injury is a retrograde urethrogram. Radiopaque contrast medium (30 ml) is injected into the urethra through a catheter-tipped syringe and a radiograph of the pelvis is taken (Fig. 14–5). Complete disruption of the posterior urethra is an indication for either a suprapubic catheter and delayed definitive repair or immediate surgical repair (DeWeerd 1977; Morehouse and MacKinnon 1985). For the patient with a partial disruption, a urologist may attempt to pass a catheter to splint the lesion.

Patients with testicular contusions will be managed with analgesics, elevation of the scrotum, iced compresses, and limited physical activity. All of these patients can be reassured that in almost all instances there will be no compromise of fertility.

Men with a ruptured penis are generally treated with sedation, elevation of the penis, and ice packs. Surgery may be advised to decrease penile deformity. Patients should know that impotence can occur but is not common after healing.

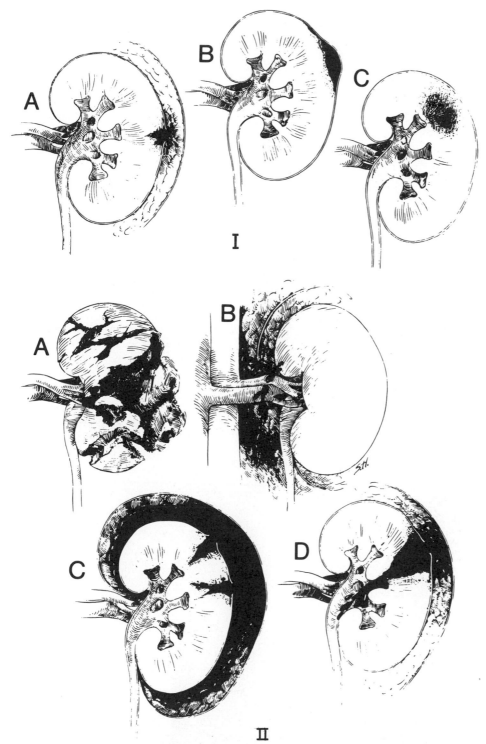

FIGURE 14–3. Classification of renal injuries. *I*, Minor renal injuries: *A*, superficial laceration; *B*, subcapsular hematoma; *C*, contusion. *II*, Major renal injuries: *A*, shattered kidney; *B*, renal pedicle injury; *C*, deep cortical lacerations with a perinephric hematoma; *D*, deep cortical laceration extending into the renal pelvis. (From Peters PC, Bright TC III. Blunt renal injuries. Urol Clin North Am 4:19, 1977.)

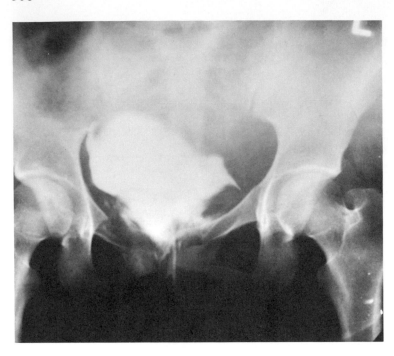

FIGURE 14–4. Cystogram demonstrating a ruptured bladder with extraperitoneal contrast extravasation.

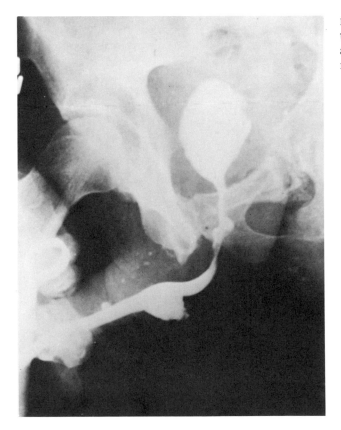

FIGURE 14–5. A partial urethral disruption resulting from a straddle injury revealed by retrograde urethrogram.

For entrapment of the foreskin in a zipper, sedation, analgesia, and much reassurance are needed to attempt the release of the foreskin. Usually, this can be accomplished by slowly and methodically unzipping the zipper. When this is not effective, it has been recommended that the median bar of the zipper be cut to release the locking mechanism (Flowerdew et al 1977). Local anesthesia may be used but also may result in increased edema. Once the foreskin has been freed, a simple dressing and an ice pack are usually all that are needed to manage the wound. Large lacerations will require suturing. Tetanus prophylaxis is in order.

Pain, Related to

- *Injury*

Generally, during the ED stay, the patient who has sustained trauma and has potential genitourinary tract injuries will not be medicated for pain. During the diagnostic phase of care it is important not to mask pain, which reflects specific pathology. An explanation that conveys the rationale for withholding medications is appropriate. Patients will often require repeated explanations and reassurance that as soon as their injuries are identified, they will be given medication to alleviate the pain.

Urinary Elimination, Altered Patterns of, Related to

- *Loss of Bladder or Renal Integrity Secondary to Trauma*
- *Fluid Volume Deficit Secondary to Trauma*

The patient who has evidence of an alteration in urinary elimination will require ongoing monitoring. Urinary output of 30 ml/hour is evidence of adequate renal perfusion. Fluid resuscitation is adjusted in part according to the urinary output.

A dipstick urinalysis provides necessary information related to urine characteristics. Hematuria in any amount requires further evaluation. A specific gravity of greater than 1.025 suggests concentrated urine and possible hypovolemia. When an indwelling catheter has been inserted, a sudden lack of output in the patient with gross hematuria may signal a blood clot blocking the urinary catheter. Irrigation may be prescribed by the physician.

Anxiety, Related to

- *Potential Sexual Dysfunction*

For the patient who has sustained an injury to the penis or scrotum, reassurance is necessary to allay anxieties related to threats of infertility and loss of sexual function.

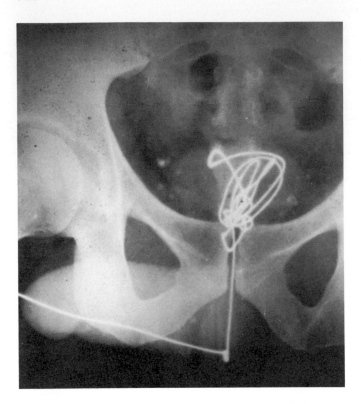

FIGURE 14-6. An adolescent youth came to medical attention with a small segment of electrical wire protruding from his urethra. This radiograph demonstrates the remaining wire coiled within the bladder. Suprapubic exploration and a vesicostomy were required to remove the foreign body.

FOREIGN BODIES

Over 566 different kinds of foreign bodies have been reported in the urethra and bladder in the literature (Aycinema 1986). They result from acts of masturbation or eroticism, assault while inebriated, psychiatric illness, and other causes. Some patients will deny knowledge of their presence whereas others are truly unaware of the cause of their symptoms.

Clinical Manifestations

Presenting complaints include gross hematuria, irritative symptoms, lower abdominal pain, and possibly urinary retention. Physical examination may reveal the foreign body palpable in or protruding from the urethra. There may be a urethral discharge, mass, or genital edema. Urine and urethral discharge cultures should be obtained.

Treatment

Intravesical foreign bodies can mostly be handled by transurethral removal on an outpatient basis. Larger objects may require general anesthesia and possibly a cystostomy to remove them (Fig. 14-6). This is especially true for objects in place for long periods of time that have been encrusted with stone debris. Many intraurethral objects can be removed in the ED. Sedation and local anesthesia are usually necessary. A broad-spectrum antibiotic may be given parenterally or orally. Psychiatric referral is appropriate in some cases.

NONTRAUMATIC EMERGENCIES

The most common nontraumatic genitourinary tract emergencies result from primary pathology of the genitourinary system. This section covers urolithiasis, inflammatory states, urinary retention, renal failure, hematuria, and priapism. The cause, pathophysiology, assessment, and management will be discussed for each.

Generally, patients with nontraumatic genitourinary problems are hemodynamically stable. An exception is the patient in septic shock. Refer to Chapter 5 for details of stage I care for the patient in septic shock. In most cases, treatment and nursing interventions are focused on stage II care.

Urolithiasis

The prevalence of renal stone disease in the general population has been estimated to be between 5 and 14 per cent. Frequency varies according to geographic region. The southeastern states, southern California, and an area just south of the Great Lakes are known for their increased frequency of renal calculi. Men tend to outnumber women by two to one. Blacks have a much lower incidence than whites, and industrialized nations have higher rates than third world nations. Diet has been evaluated extensively, and foods that contain high amounts of oxalate, purines, and calcium will increase urinary levels of these substances and may predispose to stone formation. Another major influence is the state of hydration. Dehydration promotes stone formation, and this may partially explain the differences seen when comparing geographic and occupational influences. Finally, family history plays a role, with some predisposition to development of renal stones being hereditary (Drach 1985).

Etiology

Approximately 75 per cent of calculi are composed of calcium combined with oxalate or phosphate, or both (Herring 1962). Hypercalciuria is an important predisposing factor. It is generally accepted that 300 mg/day in men and 250 mg/day in women are the upper limits of normal calcium excretion. A number of causes of hypercalciuria have been identified. Elevation in serum calcium level (hypercalcemia) can cause hypercalciuria. Table 14–1 lists the most common causes of hypercalcemia. Another cause of hypercalciuria is hyperabsorption of calcium by the intestinal mucosa. This increases the amount of calcium excreted by the kidney without elevating serum calcium levels. A third cause is an error in renal function whereby the tubules fail to reabsorb calcium. Finally, renal tubular acidosis results in hypercalciuria because calcium ions are lost in the urine along with bicarbonate ions.

Some patients may have no discernible error in calcium metabolism; they have normal blood and urine calcium levels but still form calcium stones. This occurs in 20 per cent of patients who develop calcium stones (Goldwasser et al 1986).

TABLE 14–1
Causes of Hypercalcemia

Primary hyperparathyroidism
Sarcoidosis
Neoplasms (primary or metastatic)
Milk-alkali syndrome
Paget's disease or other bone disorders
Immobilization
Vitamin D toxicity
Myxedema
Addison's disease
Hyperthyroidism

Renal stones may also consist of oxalate, which is a byproduct of metabolism. Elevated urinary oxalate levels can occur as an inborn error of metabolism, secondary to increased bowel absorption of oxalate as in Crohn's disease, and after small bowel bypass. There are idiopathic causes of hyperoxaluria that may be affected by diet. Table 14–2 provides a list of foods with high oxalate content.

Magnesium ammonium phosphate stones, occurring in 10 per cent of cases, are a result of chronic urinary tract infections that are capable of splitting urea to ammonia. This creates an alkaline environment suitable for magnesium stone formation (Fig. 14–7). The most common causative organisms are *Proteus* and occasionally *Klebsiella.*

Uric acid stones account for 7 per cent of calculi. They form when hyperurico-

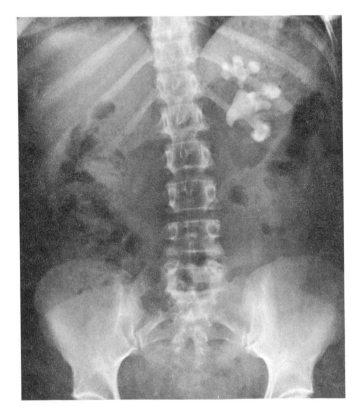

FIGURE 14–7. Kidney-ureter-bladder (KUB) film of a woman with recurrent *Proteus* urinary tract infections. A large staghorn calculus is identified on the left.

TABLE 14–2
Foods with High Oxalate Content

Tea
Cocoa
Grapefruit juice
Cranberries
Asparagus
Spinach
Rhubarb
Almonds
Greens

suria is present, urine volume is low, and the urine pH is less than 5.5. Elevated urinary uric acid occurs in gout, during chemotherapy for malignancies, with certain medications (salicylates, sulfinpyrazone, probenecid), and in idiopathic states (Fig. 14–8).

Clinical Manifestations

Most patients with urinary calculi are asymptomatic. When symptoms do occur, they may vary widely. The classic clinical manifestation of nephrolithiasis or ureter-

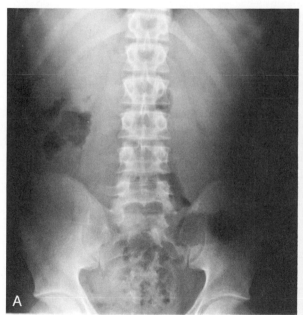
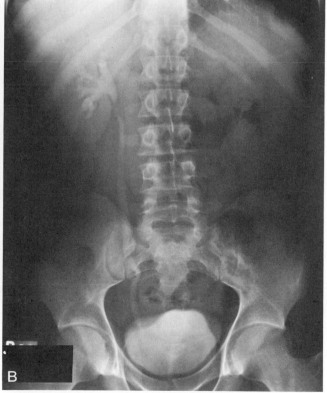

FIGURE 14–8. A 46-year-old man with a history of gout had right flank pain and microhematuria. A kidney-ureter-bladder (KUB) film *(A)* revealed no calculus, but an intravenous pyelogram (IVP) *(B)* demonstrated obstruction at the right ureterovesical junction. A small uric acid calculus subsequently was passed.

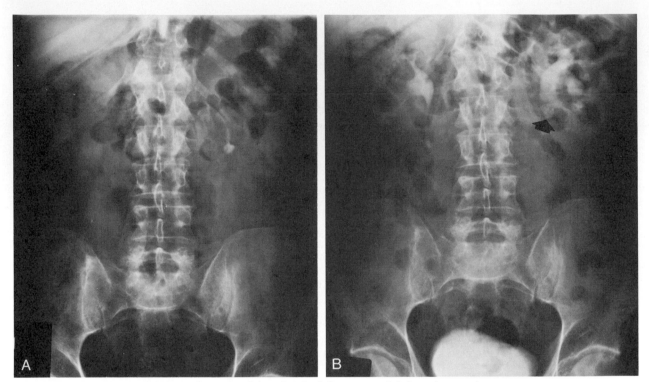

FIGURE 14–9. A large calcium oxalate stone located at the left ureteropelvic junction causing flank pain, obstruction, and hydronephrosis. *A,* Kidney-ureter-bladder (KUB) film. *B,* Pyelogram. Arrow points to the stone.

olithiasis is the sudden onset of excruciating pain. The pain may differ in location, depending on the site of the stone. A stone at the ureteropelvic junction (Fig. 14–9) tends to produce flank pain radiating anteriorly around the loin. As the stone progresses down the ureter, the pain can radiate to the ipsilateral testicle, labia, or inner thigh. Low ureteral stones may cause only lower quadrant abdominal pain and low back pain. Distal ureteral calculi at the level of the bladder wall or a stone in the bladder may induce irritative voiding symptoms as well as pain radiating to the urethral meatus. Nausea and vomiting usually result from distention of the collecting system and renal swelling or gastrointestinal ileus. The patient is frequently diaphoretic, restless, and unable to find a position of comfort, as opposed to diseases causing intraabdominal peritoneal inflammation, in which the patient tends to keep still. Fever is not common unless there is associated urinary tract infection.

Physical examination may reveal tenderness in the costovertebral angle. Diminished bowel sounds and abdominal tenderness may also be present. Orthostatic changes in the patient's vital signs may indicate dehydration.

Laboratory evaluation should include CBC, serum calcium, uric acid, creatinine, and BUN.

Treatment and Nursing Care

The experienced triage nurse will frequently suspect a renal stone on the basis of the symptom complex. These patients should be taken immediately to the treatment area. Pain relief is of primary importance.

Pain, Related to

- **Nephrolithiasis or Ureterolithiasis Secondary to Calcium Oxalate, Magnesium, or Uric Acid**

Patients with pain related to renal calculi will appear extremely uncomfortable and require analgesics. Some patients will require multiple and high doses of narcotics, generally meperidine (Demerol), to alleviate the pain. An important aspect of nursing care is evaluation of the effectiveness of analgesics. Patients may become quite lethargic once the medication takes effect. Frequent determinations of vital signs are in order.

The pain of renal colic is so excruciating that patients may become apprehensive, agitated, and restless. Lying down may be impossible. It is important to provide explanations of care and encourage positions that maximize comfort.

Urinary Elimination, Altered Patterns of, Related to

- **Urinary Obstruction Secondary to Kidney Stone**
- **Fluid Volume Deficit Secondary to Dehydration**

The patient with an alteration in urinary elimination patterns related to urinary obstruction will require diagnostic evaluation for evidence of stone formation. A clean-catch urine should be obtained for analysis and the presence of RBCs determined. A portion of urine should be saved in case a culture is deemed necessary. Menstruating women require catheterization to minimize contamination. All urine should be strained and stone debris saved for analysis. In rare cases, anuria may be present as a result of bilateral obstructing stones. These patients will require admission to the hospital and prompt relief of the obstruction.

An IVP will be necessary to confirm the diagnosis of urolithiasis. It is not unusual for a stone to pass at the time of an IVP. The patient may relate a sudden relief of pain shortly after injection of contrast agent if this has occurred. Refer to the section on trauma for nursing care associated with the patient undergoing an IVP.

All patients with signs and symptoms of urolithiasis require intravenous (IV) hydration. The IV line provides access for administration of analgesics. Isotonic fluid supplements improve hydration and may even hasten passage of the stone.

Knowledge Deficit, Related to

- **Lack of Information on Renal Calculi**

Many patients, especially those with a past history of urolithiasis, will be discharged from the ED. They should be supplied with a strainer and instructed to strain all urine until the stone has passed. Fluid intake of 4 L/day (six 8-oz glasses) is recommended. One half the total intake should be water and one half other liquids. Stone analysis for content determines the specific fluid to be avoided. It must be emphasized to patients that they follow up with their doctor or with the referral services recommended to them. This is important even if symptoms resolve. Resolution of symptoms does not guarantee the stone has been passed. Some patients may require a metabolic evaluation to determine the cause of the stone formation. All stones passed should be saved and given to the patient's physician for analysis.

Inflammatory Processes

The genitourinary tract is susceptible to infection. It has been estimated that 10 to 20 per cent of women will be afflicted with a urinary tract infection (UTI) during their lifetime. Men are infected much less frequently and usually have prostatitis or an associated urinary tract abnormality. The frequency of infection varies with age, with those over 50 years having the highest incidence. Most infections result from retrograde migration of bacteria up the urethra. Bacterial colonization of the vaginal introitus and the short length of the female urethra have been implicated in the higher rates of urinary tract infection in women. Factors that predispose to infection include sexual intercourse, diabetes mellitus, pregnancy, instrumentation, and urologic abnormalities (Stamey 1980).

Pyelonephritis is bacterial infection of the upper urinary tract, including the renal paranchyma. These infections are usually a result of ascending organisms from the lower tract, most often gram-negative in nature.

The most common urinary tract infection in men is prostatitis. The prevalence increases with advancing age and is uncommon under the age of 30 years. The offending organisms are the same as those seen in other urinary tract infections. Nonbacterial infections with *Trichomonas, Chlamydia,* and *Mycoplasma* have also been documented in the younger age group and are sexually transmitted. Urologic instrumentation is a common source of bacterial prostatitis.

Urethritis or inflammation of the urethra is usually the result of a sexually transmitted disease. Gonococcal and chlamydial infections are two main offenders.

Clinical Manifestations

Patients with cystitis, an inflammation of the bladder, complain of urgency, frequency, and dysuria. Gross hematuria (hemorrhagic cystitis) is seen primarily in women. Urge incontinence may result from the irritation. Low abdominal pain or pelvic pain and a low-grade fever may be seen. Passage of air (pneumaturia) may result from gas-forming bacteria.

Pyelonephritis is characterized by urinary frequency, dysuria, flank or back pain, fever, and malaise. Chills, nausea, and vomiting may also be present. Costovertebral angle tenderness or a palpable flank mass may be noted. Nausea and vomiting are common.

Symptoms of prostatitis include urinary frequency, dysuria, perineal aching, low back pain, fever, and malaise. Swelling of the prostate may obstruct the urethra and result in a weak stream or urinary retention. Physical findings are unremarkable except for prostatic tenderness.

Persons with urethritis will complain of urethral discharge and pain or burning on urination.

Treatment and Nursing Care

Urinary Elimination, Altered Patterns of, Related to

- **Infectious Process**

A clean-catch urinary specimen for analysis and possibly culture should be obtained from all patients with alterations in urinary elimination patterns related to infection. Fever or chills is an indication for obtaining a complete blood count with differential count. Blood cultures, obtained prior to antibiotic therapy, are in order for patients with shaking chills, a history of high fever, or risk of septicemia and for those who are debilitated, who have an indwelling urinary catheter, or who have suprapubic drainage device. Symptoms of septicemia and significant leukocytosis are indications for parenteral antibiotics.

For patients with urethral discharge, a culture and Gram stain of the discharge are obtained, best done prior to voiding. Voiding may cleanse the urethra enough to result in a false-negative culture. The presence of intracellular gram-negative diplococci indicates gonococcal infection. Treatment consists of 4.8 million units of procaine penicillin intramuscularly and 1 g of probenicid orally. The probenecid acts to delay the renal excretion of penicillin. The absence of gonococci implies nonspecific urethritis, and therapy consists of oral tetracycline, 500 mg four times per day for 10 days. Ceftriaxone sodium (Rocefin) is an antibiotic currently recommended because of its usefulness against penicillin-resistant strains of gonococcus. A single dose of 250 mg intramuscularly is recommended. The reconstituted form of Rocefin is not oil based, as is penicillin, and is therefore less painful for the patient on injection. Whether or not gonococci are present, patients should be instructed to avoid sexual contact until cleared by a repeat evaluation and until their sexual partners have also been evaluated.

Pain, Related to

- **Infection**

Generally, the patient with pain related to a urinary tract infection will experience relief once the infection is under control with antibiotics. An increased fluid intake will help flush the system and rid the tract of infection. Patients should be informed that the symptoms of infection generally last at least 24 hours after antibiotic therapy has begun. Severe symptoms may be relieved by phenazopyridine (Pyridium), which has a local anesthetic effect on the lining membranes of the bladder and urethra. This drug will change the urine color to orange and will stain clothing. Sitz baths may provide symptomatic relief for individuals with cystitis and prostatitis.

Evaluation

The effectiveness of therapy is shown by absence of chills, fever, urgency, dysuria, frequency, urethral discharge, and flank or abdominal pain. A statement by the patient that he or she understands the importance of following instructions on follow-up and taking all prescribed medications is important.

Urinary Retention

Urinary retention can be defined as the inability to adequately empty the bladder. The amount of retained urine can vary from small amounts of 30 ml to the entire bladder capacity of 350 to 450 ml.

Etiology and Pathophysiology

The cause of urinary retention can be one of many disease states. Most commonly, benign prostatic enlargement found in older men is the cause. Other causes in men include prostatic carcinoma, prostatitis, and urethral stricture. Both men and women may have retention because of neoplasms, calculi, and neurogenic dysfunction resulting from trauma, diabetes, or other nervous system afflictions.

Certain medications may result in urinary retention because of their anticholinergic or sympathomimetic properties. Anticholinergic effects weaken the bladder muscular contractions. Sympathomimetic effects result in an increased muscle tone at the bladder neck region and consequently increased resistance to emptying. Some medications with anticholinergic properties include antihistamines, tricyclic antidepressants, and phenothiazines. Many "over-the-counter" cold medications and diet aids may have anticholinergic effects. Ephedrine, pseudoephedrine, and propanolamine are specific compounds that have sympathomimetic properties.

Urinary retention may also have psychogenic origins, occurring more commonly in women and during periods of severe stress.

Clinical Manifestations

Patients unable to urinate may have mild to severe suprapubic discomfort. Other complaints may include an alteration in voiding pattern, such as frequency, urgency, hesitancy, inability to void, or incontinence. Frequency and urgency are commonly associated with the inability to completely empty the bladder during urination, with a consequent sensation of a full bladder and unrelenting urgency to urinate. Patients may dribble small volumes of urine with great frequency, and this can be associated with overflow incontinence. Overflow incontinence occurs when the patient can empty only small volumes from the bladder, and the addition of small amounts of urine from the kidneys stimulates another urge to void. Patients may also have a nearly normal voiding pattern, a distended abdomen, and a large residual urine volume in the bladder.

Abdominal evaluation to determine bladder size is necessary. A distended bladder is considered when dullness to percussion is noted above the symphysis pubis.

Men with complaints suggestive of urinary retention require a rectal examination for evidence of prostatic hypertrophy as a cause.

Treatment and Nursing Care

Urinary Elimination, Altered Patterns of, Related to

- **Inability to Empty Bladder**
- **Frequency**
- **Urgency**
- **Discomfort**

Secondary to

- *Prostatic hypertrophy*
- *Neuromuscular dysfunction*
- *Bladder calculi*
- *Bladder carcinoma*
- *Psychogenic origin*

Patients with alteration in urinary elimination related to the foregoing causes will require urinalysis. If the patient can void, a voided specimen is helpful to identify infection. If the patient cannot void, urethral catheterization should be performed using a Foley catheter. Usually, abundant lubricant is all that is needed to facilitate catheterization. Xylocaine jelly and, rarely, sedation may be useful to help alleviate anxiety. If the catheter does not pass easily, the site of obstruction is noted and attempts should not be made to pass the catheter. Further manipulation may traumatize the urethra and create a false passage. Urologic consultation should be obtained. When the distal portion of the urethra is the site of blockage, a smaller catheter may pass because a stricture is the likely cause of the obstruction. If the prostatic urethra cannot be negotiated, a coudé-tipped catheter may enter the bladder more easily. Suprapubic puncture is the last resort and should be done with great care to avoid bowel or rectal injury. In patients who have had previous lower abdominal surgery, bowel may overlie the bladder.

Once urine begins to flow from the catheter, the output should be noted. Because hemorrhagic cystitis, evidenced by gross hematuria, may occur when the bladder is emptied quickly, clamping of the catheter after every 500 to 800 ml has been obtained is recommended.

Urinary Elimination, Altered Patterns of, Related to

- **Gross Hematuria**
- **Diuresis**

Secondary to

- *Bladder decompression*

When the bladder is decompressed it is not uncommon to note gross hematuria. The bleeding is usually limited in nature but may become a problem and require irrigation to remove any accumulating clots. Irrigation with normal saline solution in 50-ml amounts is recommended and should proceed until the return is clear.

Postobstructive diuresis may also occur after relief of the obstruction. This phenomenon consists of an increased urinary output that can be as high as several hundred milliliters per hour. It is thought to be caused by at least two mechanisms. The first is an osmotic diuresis owing to the elevation of BUN and other solutes. The other mechanism is a temporary renal tubular defect that results in solute loss and diuresis. Patients with chronic retention, elevated BUN and creatinine levels, peripheral edema, or congestive heart failure are more likely to develop a diuresis. The urine output may be so great that the patient may become hemodynamically unstable. Occasionally intravenous fluids may be required to maintain the intravascular volume.

Knowledge Deficit, Related to

- **Rationale for and Management of Indwelling Urinary Catheter**

Patients sent home with an indwelling urinary catheter should be instructed in routine catheter care. Increasing numbers of patients are being managed as outpatients with some form of catheter drainage. Patients with neurogenic bladders and various kinds of bladder outlet obstruction may have temporary or chronic urethral or suprapubic catheters (Fig. 14–10). More frequently people are being sent home

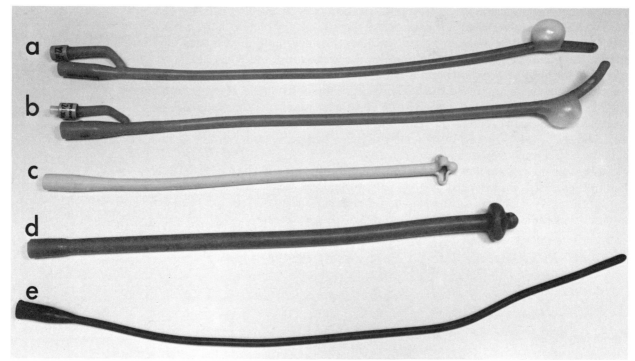

FIGURE 14–10. Types of catheters commonly used for transurethral or suprapubic bladder drainage: *a,* Foley balloon catheter; *b,* Foley balloon catheter with curved coudé tip; *c,* Malecot retention catheter; *d,* de Pezzer retention catheter; *e,* straight Robinson catheter.

between surgical procedures with urethral or percutaneous nephrostomy tubes. These tubes can become occluded or dislodged, putting some patients at risk for infectious complications because all catheters become colonized with bacteria in a short period of time.

The catheter will be attached to a leg bag or bedside drainage bag. Leg bags are used during the day and are changed to the larger bedside drainage bag for nighttime use. The catheter should be secured with tape or a commercially available device to prevent traction on the catheter, which can result in discomfort or dislodgement. The patient should clean around the urethral meatus twice daily with a mild soap and water solution to prevent mucus build-up and irritation. He or she should be instructed to inspect the tubing periodically to make sure no kinking occurs. Instructions to empty collection bags periodically to avoid overdistention and impedance to catheter drainage are important. The bag should be kept below bladder level to allow appropriate drainage. Leg bags should be washed with peroxide or soap and water and allowed to dry. This will prevent mucus and bacteria build-up.

If the catheter will not function properly even though there is no apparent mechanical problem, such as tubing kink, the catheter has either become occluded or become dislodged. Mucus, tissue, clots, or stone fragments may be causative. The patient should be instructed to contact his or her physician or seek immediate emergency attention should this occur.

A urethral or suprapubic catheter may be irrigated with 25 to 50 ml of saline. If the catheter is totally occluded or no saline will return, a new catheter generally is needed.

NEPHROSTOMY TUBES

A nephrostomy tube should be irrigated with only 5 to 10 ml because the renal pelvis has a smaller capacity. It must be stressed to a patient that these catheters are not meant to be permanent and require routine maintenance or must be changed every 4 to 6 weeks to prevent encrustation and occlusion.

An occluded or dislodged nephrostomy tube is an urgent problem. The affected kidney is usually obstructed and at risk for further damage. The tube tract will close quickly. In this situation immediate consultation with the patient's urologist is advised. An IV line should be inserted and broad-spectrum antibiotics begun because extensive instrumentation may be required to replace one of these tubes.

Infection, Potential, Related to

• *Indwelling Catheter*

Sepsis is more common in patients with indwelling catheters. The catheters and tubing become colonized with bacteria after a few days. The bacteria may enter the blood stream or cause pyelonephritis if the catheter does not drain well or becomes occluded. Patients must be made aware of this increased risk of infection and told to watch for fever and flank pain.

RENAL FAILURE

Renal failure occurs when renal function deteriorates sufficiently to cause an accumulation of nitrogenous wastes in the body (azotemia). The acute form occurs when renal function deteriorates over a period of days and may be reversible. Chronic renal failure is a condition that develops over months or years as a result of progressive and irreversible destruction of nephrons (Braunwald 1987).

Etiology and Pathophysiology

There are numerous causes of renal failure. A classification based on etiology is useful in defining the causes: prerenal, renal, and postrenal. Prerenal causes of renal failure result from a reduction in renal blood flow from processes that reduce intravascular volume or perfusion pressure: dehydration, hemorrhage, shock, heart failure, and so forth. Renal causes resulting from primary damage to the kidneys occur in acute tubular necrosis, pyelonephritis, glomerulonephritis, renal vein occlusion, nephrotoxic substances, and blood transfusion reactions. Postrenal causes relate to problems occurring in the urinary tract distal to the kidneys, such as ureteral obstruction from calculi or chronic urinary retention from BPH.

Damage to the nephrons results from ischemia, inflammation, necrosis, and scarring. The net result is an inability of the kidney to appropriately filter substrates and concentrate urine. Theories of pathogenesis of acute renal failure can be divided into two categories: those suggesting a tubular basis and those suggesting a vascular basis. It seems that both components interact to cause acute renal failure (Anderson and Schrier 1987).

Chronic renal failure implies a severe reduction in functional nephron mass, with eventual impact on every organ system. Uremia is the term applied to the clinical syndrome observed in patients suffering from a profound loss of renal function. Chronic renal failure is accompanied by malnutrition, impaired metabolism of carbohydrates, fats, and proteins, and defective utilization of energy (Brenner and Lazarus 1987).

Fluid, electrolyte, and red blood cell alterations generally are evident. Salt and water overloads are present and result in hyponatremia and edema. Hyperkalemia, hyperphosphatemia, and hypermagnesemia result from decreased renal elimination. Hypocalcemia occurs and is related to the hyperphosphatemia. Because endogenous metabolic acids cannot be eliminated by the inefficient kidney, metabolic acidosis occurs. Normocytic normochromic anemia follows the onset of azotemia. The factors that contribute to anemia include decreased erythropoiesis, shortened RBC survival, hemodilution, and gastrointestinal blood loss. Patients in renal failure also have a decreased ability to metabolize glucose.

Clinical Manifestations

Patients may arrive in the ED in acute or chronic renal failure. History may include short-term weight gain, edema, dyspnea, nausea and vomiting, hematemesis and melena, alteration in mental status, and general malaise. There may or may not be a change in amount of urinary output.

On physical assessment hypertension and distended neck veins may be present if the patient is hypervolemic. Fluid overload is the major cause of hypertension in patients with renal failure. Hypotension and flat neck veins indicate hypovolemia. Tachycardia, tachypnea, crackles, and wheezes on auscultation of lung fields, fever, and dry sallow skin may also be evident.

Treatment and Nursing Care

Treatment is based on identifying and possibly alleviating the cause of the immediate problem. Patients with complaints of dyspnea require a thorough evaluation to determine whether the cause is fluid overload or an acute cardiac or pulmonary event. Likewise, patients with neurologic abnormalities require evaluation to rule out extrarenal causes. Often dialysis is necessary to control fluid volume, electrolyte balance, acid-base balance, and nitrogenous waste elimination.

Fluid Volume Excess, Related to

• *Renal Failure*

The person with fluid volume excess related to renal failure will require careful monitoring of intake and output. If intravenous infusion of isotonic solution is required, it should be administered through a microtubing administration set to avoid further overload. If the patient is severely hyperkalemic, and particularly if there are EKG changes related to the elevated K^+ ions (hyperacute T waves), calcium chloride, sodium bicarbonate, insulin, and dextrose are administered intravenously (see Chap. 20 for a more detailed discussion). In less of an emergency situation patients may be treated with sodium polystyrene sulfonate (Kayexalate) orally or by enema. The usual dose is 15 g orally or 30 to 50 g via rectal tube.

Tissue Perfusion, Altered, Cerebral or Cardiopulmonary

Persons with altered tissue perfusion will require supplemental oxygen and cardiac monitoring. Dysrhythmias may be a result of electrolyte abnormalities, especially potassium. An EKG change typical of hyperkalemia includes peaked T waves. Cardiac arrest is a possibility.

Blood transfusions may be necessary if the patient is severely anemic. Ongoing assessment of vital signs, capillary refill, and mental status reflects the status of tissue perfusion.

Potential for Injury, Related to

• *Shunt or Fistula Disruption*

Patients with chronic renal failure may have a shunt or fistula in place for hemodialysis. Precautions to prevent damage to the shunt or fistula include medical record documentation of the site and warning against blood pressure measurement from the involved extremity. Although patients are generally aware of this precaution, a warning note on or around the patient's cart may be helpful.

Knowledge Deficit

Explanations should include what is happening, anticipated diagnostic tests and treatment, and expected outcomes for the emergency stay. Although anger and frustration may be evident, particularly in the patient with chronic renal disease, a caring attitude that allows venting of anger and time for questions is therapeutic. Referrals to social service or other support agencies may be necessary.

HEMATURIA

Gross hematuria can be a frightening experience. A minute quantity of blood can cause the urine to change color. It must be remembered that hematuria is only a sign of a disease process.

Etiology and Pathophysiology

The causes of hematuria include dozens of disease states. These causes vary with age and sex (Table 14–3). A dietary history also should be obtained because certain foods and dyes can cause red urine (Table 14–4). Blood dyscrasias may be familial or may result from cirrhosis or from anticoagulants. If bleeding has been chronic or quite heavy, anemia may be present. Large clots may cause an obstruction to urine flow.

Treatment and Nursing Care

Evaluation includes a urinalysis and culture. Black patients should be checked for sickle cell trait. A coagulation profile should be obtained in any case in which blood dyscrasia is suspected. A CBC will help determine anemia.

If large clots are noted and cause difficulty voiding, catheterization is in order. A large-bore catheter (greater than 24 French) should be used. All clots should be

TABLE 14–3
Most Common Causes of Hematuria by Age Group

	Males		
	1	**2**	**3**
Pediatric	Infection	Glomerulonephritis	
Adolescent	Glomerulonephritis	Infection	Calculus
Young Adult	Infection	Calculus	Neoplasm
Middle Age	Neoplasm	Calculus	Infection
Elderly	Benign prostatic hypertrophy	Neoplasm	Calculus

	Females		
	1	**2**	**3**
Pediatric	Infection	Glomerulonephritis	
Adolescent	Glomerulonephritis	Infection	Calculus
Young Adult	Infection	Calculus	Neoplasm
Middle Age	Infection	Calculus	Neoplasm
Elderly	Neoplasm	Infection	Calculus

Source: Modified from Grayhack JT. 1977. In Sabiston DC Jr, ed. Textbook of Surgery: The Biological Basis of Modern Surgical Practice. WB Saunders Co, 1720.

irrigated manually from the bladder using normal saline. This will allow the open vessels to retract and occlude.

Knowledge Deficit, Related to

• *Prevention or Relief of Hematuria, or Both*

Those patients being discharged should be instructed to increase their fluid intake to dilute the urine. Two or 3 L of water per day should be sufficient. Patients should avoid platelet-inactivating drugs such as aspirin and ibuprofen. Finally, they must be strongly encouraged to return to their physicians for follow-up and further evaluation, which generally will include an IVP and cystoscopy.

TABLE 14–4
Sources of Red or Dark Urine Without Hematuria

Aniline dyes
Beets
Blackberries
Crayons
Cascara
Phenolphthalein (laxatives)
Phenytoin
Rhubarb
Serratia marcescens (red diaper syndrome)
Other chemicals
Severe dehydration

PRIAPISM

Priapism is a prolonged erection, which can last for many hours. It is painful at times. Patients will lack sexual desire. Orgasm will not result in detumescence. Urination may be difficult to the point of requiring catheterization. Men of all age groups can be affected. The erection is also abnormal anatomically: the glans penis and corpus spongiosum are flaccid, whereas only the corpora cavernosa is turgid.

Etiology and Pathophysiology

The cause of priapism is not always clear. At times no source is identified. Some medications have been linked to this condition, including the psychotropic drug thioridazine and the phenothiazines. Anticoagulants, guanethidine, and marijuana also can induce the disorder. Sickle cell anemia, leukemia, and carcinomas invading the penis can be causes. Reports of trauma, infection, and neurologic disorders causing priapism are also found.

Aside from discomfort, the reason priapism is an emergency is the high incidence of impotence that follows untreated cases (Wendel and Grayhack 1981). The cause of impotence is fibrosis of the corpora cavernosa following resolution and healing. Sickle cell crisis may produce hemagglutination and subsequent priapism. Therefore, patients with potential for sickle cell disease (blacks, men with olive complexions) should be questioned on past medical history.

Treatment and Nursing Care

For patients with sickle cell disease, blood transfusions and oxygen may result in resolution of the erection. Most patients with other causes will require an operative shunting procedure. This allows drainage of stagnant blood. In these cases, preoperative laboratory studies should be obtained.

Pain, Related to

- *Prolonged Erection*

Narcotics and sedatives intramuscularly or intravenously may be administered to alleviate the pain and discomfort associated with priapism.

INTRASCROTAL EMERGENCIES

Torsion

This is a condition in which the vascular pedicle of the testis twists, resulting in ischemia of the testis. A congenital abnormality in the development of the testicular tunics allows the testis to turn within the scrotum (Klauber and Sant 1985). This lesion is frequently bilateral. Generally, it occurs in the adolescent and young adult population, but it can also occur in older men.

Clinical Manifestations

Pain is the predominant symptom. It usually is sudden in onset and may develop while at rest or with simple activity, such as crossing one's legs. Nausea, vomiting, and lower abdominal pain also may be present. There may be a history of similar episodes that have resolved spontaneously. Perhaps because of fear or some social stigma, young children and adolescents frequently withhold complaints and delay seeking treatment for several hours. Delayed presentation may allow for testicular enlargement, scrotal erythema, and edema.

Treatment and Nursing Care

A urinalysis and CBC should be performed as soon as possible to exclude infectious processes. Other diagnostic modalities include Doppler scanning of the testicular artery and nuclear scanning. Management of torsion consists of surgical exploration, detorsion, and fixation of the testis in a stable position. Sometimes detorsion of the testicle can be accomplished manually without surgery by elevation and rotation of the testis. Local anesthesia infiltrated into the spermatic cord by a urologist may facilitate this maneuver. Studies have shown nearly 100 per cent testicular salvage with detorsion less than 6 hours after torsion. A delay of more than 12 hours greatly increases the risk of necrosis (Parker and Robinson 1971).

Epididymitis

Epididymitis is an inflammatory process, usually infectious, of the epididymal tubule. It is a disease of adults and is rarely seen in children.

Etiology and Pathophysiology

Nearly all cases of epididymitis are caused by retrograde migration of organisms through the vas deferens. It may occur spontaneously, but is frequently seen in patients with prostatitis, cystitis, or other urinary tract abnormalities. It also occurs after instrumentation. The offending organisms are usually gram-negative bacteria. *Gonococcus, Mycobacterium tuberculosis,* and many other species can cause infection. *Chlamydia* has been implicated in sexually active young men. Heavy lifting and mild trauma are noninfectious causes.

Clinical Manifestations

Men with epididymitis will complain of testicular pain and a heavy sensation. Fever and malaise are also generally present. Scrotal erythema, edema, and possibly a hydrocele will appear. Abscess formation can occur. Elevation of the testis may relieve the discomfort temporarily (Prehn's sign).

Treatment and Nursing Care

Pain, Related to

- **Scrotal Infection and Edema**

Bed rest, ice packs, and scrotal elevation provide symptomatic relief. Antibiotics directed against gram-negative organisms are prescribed. In young men and in cases in which previous cultures have been sterile, tetracycline is the drug of choice to eradicate chlamydial infection. Antibiotics will not shorten the duration of symptoms but will sterilize the urine and prevent progression of the infectious process.

CONCLUSION

In conclusion, patients may come to the ED with one of a broad spectrum of genitourinary maladies. These problems range from life-threatening trauma and infection to asymptomatic hematuria. During initial triage, the nurse should be alert for symptoms suggesting a surgical emergency and be able to rapidly begin assessment and management of the problem. The indications and contraindications for urethral catheterization must be clearly understood. Finally, the nurse should have a thorough knowledge of the consequences of improper follow-up care or poor catheter management so that patients can be properly instructed at the time of discharge.

REFERENCES

Anderson RJ, Schrier RW. 1987. Acute renal failure. In Harrison P, ed. Principles of Internal Medicine, 11th ed, vol 2. New York, McGraw Hill Book Co, 1239–1252.

Aycinema JF. 1986. Foreign bodies in the urinary bladder and urethra. In Kaufman JJ, ed. Current Urologic Therapy. Philadelphia, WB Saunders, 252–253.

Baily RR. 1978. Treatment of urinary tract infection with a single dose of trimethoprim-sulfamethoxazole. Can Med Assoc J 118:551.

Braunwald E, Isselbacher KJ, Petersdorf RG, et al. 1987. Disorders of the kidney and urinary tract. In Harrison P, ed. Principles of Internal Medicine, 11th ed, vol 2. New York, McGraw Hill Book Co, 1139–1140.

Brenner BM, Lazarus JM. 1987. Chronic renal failure: Pathophysiological and clinical considerations. In Harrison P, ed. Principles of Internal Medicine 11th ed, vol 2. New York, McGraw-Hill Book Co, 1155–1161.

Bright TC, White K, Peters PC. 1978. Significance of hematuria after trauma. J Urol 120:445.

Brosman SA, Paul JG. 1976. Trauma of the bladder. Surg Gynecol Obstet 143:605.

Carlton CE Jr, Scott R Jr, Goldman M. 1968. The management of penetrating injuries of the kidney. J Trauma 8:1071.

DeWeerd JF. 1977. Immediate realignment of posterior urethral injury. Urol Clin North Am 4:75.

Drach GW. 1985. Urinary lithiasis. In Walsh PC, Gittes RF, Perlmutter AD, et al, eds. Campbell's Urology. Philadelphia, WB Saunders Co, 870.

Flowerdew R, Fishman IJ, Churchhill BM. 1977. Management of penile zipper injury. J Urol 117:671.

Goldwasser B, Weinerth JL, Carson CC III. 1986. Calcium stone disease: Overview. J Urol 135:1.

Grayhack JR. 1977. The urinary tract. In Sabiston

DC, ed. Davis-Christopher Textbook of Surgery. Philadelphia, WB Saunders Co, 870.

Guerriero WG. 1984. Urologic Injuries. Norwalk, CT, Appleton-Century-Crofts.

Hai MA, Pontes JE, Pierce JM Jr. 1977. Surgical management of major renal trauma: A review of 102 cases treated by conservative surgery. J Urol 118:7.

Herring LC. 1962. Observations in 10,000 urinary calculi. J Urol 88:545.

Heyns CF, DeKlerk DP, DeKock MSS. 1985. Nonoperative management of renal stab wounds. J Urol 134:239.

Hudson MJK. 1975. Rupture of the corpus cavernosum of the penis. Br J Clin Pract 29:191.

Klauber GT, Sant GR. 1985. Disorders of the male external genitalia. In Kelalis P, King L, Belman B, eds. Pediatric Urology. Philadelphia, WB Saunders Co, 848.

Meares EM. 1971. Traumatic injuries of the corpus cavernosum. J Urol 105:407.

Morehouse DD, MacKinnon KJ. 1985. In Blaisdell FW, Trunkey DD, McAninch JE, eds. Trauma Management, vol 2. Urogenital Trauma. New York, Thieme-Stratton, 1–121.

Mulkey AP Jr, Witherinton R. 1974. Conservative management of vesical rupture. Urology 4:426.

Neih PT, Dretler SP. 1984. Acute genitourinary disorders. In May HC, ed. Emergency Medicine. New York, John Wiley & Sons, 711.

Parker RM, Robinson JR. 1971. Anatomy and diagnosis of torsion of the testicle. J Urol 106:243.

Peters PC, Bright TC. 1977. Blunt renal injuries. Urol Clin North Am 4:17.

Pontes JE, Pierce JM. 1978. Anterior urethral injuries: Four years experience at the Detroit General Hospital. J Urol 120:563.

Stamey TA. 1980. Pathogenesis and Treatment of Urinary Tract Infections. Baltimore, Williams & Wilkins, 123, 59.

Tynberg P, Hoch WH, Persky L, et al. 1973. The management of renal injuries coincident with penetrating wounds of abdominal trauma. J Trauma 13:502.

Walker JA. 1969. Injuries of the ureter due to external violence. J Urol 102:410.

Weems WL. 1979. Management of genitourinary injuries in patients with pelvic fractures. Ann Surg 189:177.

Wendel EF, Grayhack JR. 1981. Corpora cavernosa–glans penis shunt for priapism. Surg Gynecol Obstet 153:586.

Nancy Jo Reedy, CNM MPH
Mary C. Brucker, CNM DNSc

Obstetric and Gynecologic Emergencies

More women seek health care for both preventive and emergency reasons than do men. A woman seeking care for either gynecologic or nongynecologic reasons has an inherent sense of being female. A woman's female identity permeates her interpretation of the care she has received. Common complaints for which women seek emergency services include pelvic or abdominal pain and vaginal bleeding, any of which may indicate a gynecologic (e.g., pelvic inflammatory disease, ovarian cysts, mittelschmerz, dysmenorrhea) or obstetric (e.g., abortion, ectopic pregnancy, abruptio placentae) problem. Other common conditions that cause women to seek emergency care are trauma of a gynecologic (i.e., rape) or an obstetric (i.e., trauma in pregnancy) nature. In all gynecologic and obstetric emergencies, the health care provider must use not only technical skills to affect a good outcome but also sensitivity to manage the psychologic implications of the insult.

This chapter will discuss the etiology, pathophysiology, clinical manifestations, and treatment modalities for a variety of gynecologic and obstetric emergencies for which women often seek emergency services. Those emergencies of a traumatic nature in each category are discussed first. The chapter closes with a discussion of emergency deliveries.

GYNECOLOGIC EMERGENCIES

Rape*

Rape is a violent crime against an individual. One of the myths about rape is that no one can be raped unless they wish to be. In reality, persons of all ages (including children) have been raped without provocation (Riesenberg 1987). Another misconception has been that the rapist is a faceless, anonymous individual who possesses great sexual prowess. In many cases, such as date rape, the rapist is not faceless but is actually known to the victim. Rather than sexual prowess, rapists have often been reported to have sexual dysfunctions such as impotence or premature ejaculation.

Etiology

In general, rape is a means to humiliate and injure a victim. Race, ethnic background, and age of rapists all vary. Their few identified characteristics in common include immaturity and the need to obtain sexual satisfaction within the context of violence (Riesenberg 1987).

Clinical Manifestations

State and legal definitions of rape vary. The common component of all definitions is sexual relations imposed against the victim's will. Vaginal intercourse, although common, is not the only form of rape. Oral-genital sex and sodomy also can occur. Physical trauma, such as bruising, lacerations, and fractures, is often associated with rape and may even be life-threatening. However, the lack of such physical trauma does not imply that the victim consented and thus negated the definition of rape (Cartwright 1987).

Psychoemotional responses to rape are varied and labile. Victims may demonstrate composure and calmness one minute and intense fear and crying the next. Any and all such responses should be accepted and support should be provided as necessary.

Treatment and Nursing Care

Health treatment of a rape victim has both medical and legal components. Medically, the victim's emotional and physical needs must be identified and attended. Legally, rape must be reported to the police, although the victim may choose whether or not she wants to give law enforcement officials information or press charges or both. Each

---

* Although the discussion of rape in this text is centered around women as victims, it should be recognized that men may also be victims of rape. Additionally, although rape is being discussed under the category of gynecologic emergencies, it should be evident throughout this content that victims of rape should be evaluated and treated holistically with regard to both their physical and emotional needs.

legal jurisdiction will require health care providers to gather specific evidence for later use in possible court proceedings. Although evidence collection along with thorough nonjudgmental documentation must be carefully and continuously done throughout the patient's stay in the emergency department (ED), the patient should never be made to feel that these matters supersede her emotional and physical well being.

Injury, Related to

- *Physical Trauma Resulting from Rape*
- *Psychologic Trauma Resulting from Rape*

Stage I nursing care is often required for victims of rape, if not because of physical trauma then because of psychologic trauma. Treatment of physical trauma depends on the nature and severity of the injury. Immediate interventions for psychologic trauma should include bringing the victim of rape to a quiet room, assuring her privacy and safety while details of the assault are elicited (in a nonjudgmental manner), and assisting her to regain a sense of control by providing opportunities to make decisions (e.g., regarding her health care, who should be notified, and so forth).

Victims of rape should not be left alone while awaiting care or during examination. Prior to an examination, counseling by a nurse or a rape victim advocate can assist in decreasing the anxiety engendered by the examination, in gathering required evidence, and in helping the victim begin to deal with the situation (Kille 1986). Whenever possible, the victim should be offered the option of a female health care provider.

Physical Examination and Evidence Collection

A careful physical examination and concurrent evidence collection should be done. Any and all signs of trauma should be identified and documented. Photographs taken with the patient's consent may be included in the chart and are important in the event of legal action against the rapist. All evidence collected must be properly labeled and sealed in containers, and a chain of evidence must be maintained. External evidence should be collected prior to obtaining internal cultures and evidence.

Clothing worn by the patient should be placed in clean paper bags for the police. Fingernail scrapings may be useful evidence and should be obtained and placed in two separate envelopes, marked according to the hand from which they were obtained. Combed head hair and miscellaneous debris (e.g., soil, fibers, and the like) should also be collected and placed in envelopes or bags.

An oral examination should be done, and gonorrhea culture, wet-mount for sperm and acid phosphatase, and two air-dried slides of fluid (collected from the oral cavity) should be obtained. Acid phosphatase will be present in semen even if the rapist has had a vasectomy, and blood typing can be done from saliva.

The pelvic and rectal examinations should identify pelvic or anal trauma or both. All perineal, vaginal, or anal lacerations may need rapid repair to limit hemorrhage. Samples of combed and plucked pubic hair should be obtained and placed separately in envelopes so that pubic combings can be used for comparison against the patient's own plucked hair. Dried semen in the perineal area should be removed with a saline-moistened swab. A Woods light can be used to identify semen. Samples of secretions should be taken for sperm and acid phosphatase. Two air-dried slides of fluids from the vagina and rectum should also be obtained and saved as routine police evidence (Heinrich 1987; Adkinson, Frost, and Peterson 1986).

Cultures for sexually transmitted diseases (STDs), including gonorrhea and chlamydia, should be performed. These cultures and the serum tests for syphilis, human immunodeficiency virus (HIV), and pregnancy, which are taken shortly after a rape, establish the baseline condition of the woman. Blood for type and Rh analysis are drawn to use in evaluation of the other samples taken. It is suggested that gonorrhea and chlamydia cultures be repeated in 3 to 6 weeks; syphilis and HIV tests, 12 weeks after the potential exposure. HIV serum testing may be repeated every three months for a year since guidelines are not yet well established.

Prophylactic treatment for STDs may include ceftriaxone sodium (Rocephin), 250 mg intramuscularly (IM) for gonorrhea and doxycycline (Vibramycin), 100 mg, orally twice a day for 10 days for chlamydia. Pregnancy prevention in the form of diethylstilbestrol (DES) may be administered after an informed consent is obtained. Nausea and vomiting are common side effects if such a treatment is given. However, the treatment is not universally successful in the prevention of a pregnancy and a woman should be so informed.

Psycho-Emotional Aspects of Care

Psycho-emotional needs of rape victims must be recognized and supports made available to them and, in some cases, their families. The rape-trauma syndrome described by Burgess and Holmstrom (1974), is divided into two phases. Common manifestations of the first, acute phase, include disorganized sleep patterns, eating disorders, fears, mood swings, feelings of degradation, guilt, and humiliation.

In the second, or reorganization phase, there is usually a disruption of lifestyle in which regression and isolation is usual. Some women have a silent reaction in which they refuse to share the experience with anyone.

Nursing intervention with rape victims is intended to diminish the effects of rape-trauma syndrome. Nursing actions include the following:

1. Verbal explanations in preparation for the physical examination, evidence collection, and necessary legal procedures.

2. Giving permission for ventilation of feelings about the rape, violence in general, and aspects of self concept.

3. Offering assistance in recognition of feelings regarding prophylactic treatment for STDs, prevention of pregnancy, and abortion.

4. Identifying the patient's personal support systems and referral for long-term counseling and support.

5. Explaining the importance of follow-up testing.

Pelvic Inflammatory Disease

Pelvic inflammatory disease (PID) is a generic term used to describe an acute or chronic infection of the fallopian tubes, ovaries, pelvic peritoneum, or pelvic connective tissue. PID may denote infection of one of these areas or any combination. The term *salpingitis* is often used synonymously with PID, since the most common single site of PID is the fallopian tube (Prepas 1984).

PID is a major gynecologic problem. It has been estimated that it is directly or indirectly related to almost 20% of all cases of infertility and has clearly been associated with the recent dramatic, nationwide rise of ectopic pregnancies (Eschenbach 1984).

Risk factors associated with the development of PID are related to age, race, socioeconomic status, and number of sexual partners. Although PID may occur in any woman, the most common profile for the PID patient is a black adolescent of a lower socioeconomic level who experiences sexual activity with multiple partners (Quan, Rodney, and Johnson 1983).

Etiology

Traditionally, the etiologic agent associated with PID has been *Neisseria gonorrhea* (GC). In fact, almost 20% of women with GC develop PID as a complication (Martin 1978). However, *Chlamydia trachomatis* is another potent etiologic agent. From 20% to 70% of the time, chlamydia has been found concomitantly with gonorrhea (Lumicao and Heggi 1979). Moreover, chlamydia itself has been estimated to be the causative organism for PID in approximately 20% to 50% of cases (Eschenbach 1984).

Pathophysiology

Pelvic infections are almost exclusively caused by organisms transmitted during sexual activity. Spread of the infection initially occurs by way of the mucosal surfaces. Therefore, a transient endometritis usually precedes the salpingitis. The ascending spread of lower genital tract organisms into the upper genital area varies in degree of severity as well as timing. In severe episodes, abscesses of the fallopian tubes or even peritoneal cavity are possible.

Clinical Manifestations

The most common symptom of PID is pain. Ninety-five per cent of women report some degree of abdominal or pelvic pain, usually immediately preceding or following menses. Other symptoms or signs characteristically include fever, a purulent vaginal discharge, dysuria, and dyspareunia. Severe nausea and vomiting are suggestive of peritonitis or abscess formation; guarding of the abdomen and hyperactive bowel sounds may be present. Pain upon cervical motion is characteristic. Laboratory data obtained from women with PID includes elevated white counts with a right-to-left shift and elevated sedimentation rates. Cervical cultures that are positive for gonorrhea or chlamydia or both are also commonly seen. Other conditions should be considered in a differential diagnosis. Noninfectious processes such as ectopic pregnancies, corpus luteum cysts, and torsion of ovarian cysts may mimic the pain of PID, but the characteristic laboratory findings of infection are absent. Appendicitis and urinary tract infections should also be ruled out. Pelvic ultrasound can add to the diagnostic ability of the practitioner by detecting changes such as fluid accumulation and mild hydrosalpinx.

Treatment and Nursing Care

All women should be aware of sexually transmitted diseases (STDs). Preventing STDs, especially gonorrhea and chlamydia, would decrease not only the incidence of PID but also the associated ectopic pregnancies and infertility. The degree of infection may be ameliorated by a general increase in host well-being with optimal nutrition and overall health promotion.

Infection, Related to

- *Neisseria gonorrhea*
- *Chlamydia trachomatis*

There are three grades of PID (Gomez-Carrian 1987). In all cases pelvic peritonitis may be either present or absent. Grade I is uncomplicated; the condition has not spread beyond one or both tubes or ovaries. For grade I outpatient treatment is possible, and hospitalization may not be necessary. Grade II is a complicated condition, commonly necessitating inpatient care. In this category the infection includes a mass or abscess of one or both tubes or ovaries. In grade III, the least common and most severe form of PID, the infection has spread to structures beyond the pelvis, as illustrated with a ruptured tubo-ovarian abscess. Grade III almost always requires hospitalization and surgical treatment.

The pharmacologic intervention for PID is determined by the etiologic agents as well as degree of severity. Cervical cultures need to be collected carefully to enhance accurate diagnosis. For example, the culture medium for gonorrhea should be room temperature when the culture is taken and should be quickly placed in an anaerobic environment, preferably at body temperature, to encourage growth of the organism.

Currently, nonhospitalized patients are usually treated for gonorrhea with 250 mg ceftriaxone sodium (Rocephin) IM and for chlamydia with an oral tetracycline. Any patient who receives intramuscular antibiotics should be observed for at least 30 minutes following the injection to be certain that an anaphylactic reaction does not occur. Hospitalized patients commonly have several parenteral medications administered simultaneously. Typical antimicrobial agents include clindamycin, gentamicin, and doxycycline (Mead 1987). Comprehensive pharmacologic treatment of PID includes (1) accurate diagnosis of the etiologic agent, (2) adequate treatment as demonstrated by negative follow-up cultures 48 to 72 hours after completion of treatment, and (3) patient education to decrease future episodes.

Knowledge Deficit (Possible), Related to

- *Etiology, Pathophysiology, and Treatment of PID*

The sexual transmission of gonorrhea and chlamydia should be stressed so that the woman's partner or partners can be promptly treated and precautions taken to decrease reinfection and future episodes. Patient education should include signs and symptoms of PID so that a reoccurrence can be diagnosed early. The importance of compliance with the full course of treatment and follow-up must also be stressed. Lastly, psychologic support needs to be an integral component of care, especially in view of the sexual nature of the disease and the potential problems of infertility or pregnancy loss through ectopic pregnancy.

Ovarian Cysts

Ovarian cysts are common, usually benign, conditions, most common among women of reproductive age, although they can occur anytime—even neonatally (Nussbaum, Saunders, Benator, et al 1987; Giacoia and Wood 1987). Typically, a woman experiencing an ovarian cyst is unaware of the condition since most cysts are functional and resolve spontaneously. Occasionally, ovarian cysts do not resolve but instead increase in size, and torsion may occur. Some women appear to have a predilection toward production of ovarian cysts. Alternatively, women who use oral contraceptives are unlikely to develop cysts.

Etiology and Pathophysiology

An ovarian cyst in the adult generally results from a mild dysfunction of the menstrual cycle in which excessive fluid is collected around the Graafian follicle or corpus luteum. Occasionally, ovarian cysts and possibly even otherwise normal ovaries and tubes can become ischemic as a result of torsion.

Clinical Manifestations

Most ovarian cysts less than 5 cm in size are asymptomatic (Fogel and Woods 1981). Large cysts (greater than 5 cm) or cysts with torsion are more likely to be symptomatic. The most common symptom is abdominal pain without any symptoms or laboratory signs of an infectious process. Menstrual irregularity, especially delayed or prolonged menstruation, is another common symptom. Vomiting has been characterized as an early symptom of torsion (Queenan 1983). Ectopic pregnancy must be ruled out. Definitive diagnosis is accomplished by pelvic ultrasonography on the affected side (Lavery, Koontz, Layman, et al 1986; Baltarowich, Kurtz, Pasto, et al 1987; Thornton and Wells 1987).

Treatment and Nursing Care

Ovarian cysts that remain symptomatic generally require operative intervention. Some cysts are managed by aspiration of the contents under ultrasonography before rupture occurs (Diernaes, Rasmussen, Sorensen et al 1987). Spontaneous rupture of a large ovarian cyst can result in peritonitis, dense adhesions from chronic leakage, or even severe hemorrhage (Queenan 1983). Ischemia from torsion can result in long-term damage to the ovary or tube. To prevent such complications, a laparoscopy allows surgical exposure of the site and the opportunity to manipulate the affected organs. Torsion can be resolved and cysts can be aspirated. In rare cases, a minilaparotomy may be needed so that necessary oophorectomy or salpingectomy can be performed.

Pain, Related to

- **Ovarian Cyst**

A major nursing challenge is adequate pain treatment for the woman with an ovarian cyst. Analgesia of adequate dosage may provide comfort once the diagnosis of an ovarian cyst is made. It is possible that the cyst may resolve spontaneously and medication will not be necessary.

Patient education needs to include the fact that ovarian cysts commonly reoccur. When such cysts have necessitated surgery in the past, the woman should have early signs and symptoms reviewed so that she can recognize and report a reoccurrence appropriately.

Mittelschmerz

Occasionally, a woman will notice a sharp pelvic or abdominal pain about the time of ovulation. This benign pain has been termed mittelschmerz. Some women experience mittelschmerz monthly, others occasionally, and some never.

Etiology and Pathophysiology

The etiologic agent for mittelschmerz remains unknown. It has been suggested that spasms in fallopian tubes may cause the pain. An alternative explanation has been escape of a small amount of ovarian fluid that culminates in irritation.

Clinical Manifestations

Mittelschmerz is usually one-sided pain lasting only a few hours or as much as 24 to 48 hours. It is diagnosed on the basis of the time of occurrence in the menstrual cycle and lack of any other explanation for the acute pain. Alternative gynecologic explanations for pain should be explored before the diagnosis of mittelschmerz is made. These explanations include infections (PID, appendicitis), uterine myomas, and ovarian cysts. Diagnosis is confirmed by ruling out both the infections (on the basis of laboratory data) and the gynecologic abnormalities (discoverable by ultrasound or clinical examination).

Treatment and Nursing Care

Pain, Related to

- **Mittelschmerz**

Mittelschmerz resolves spontaneously. Treatment is conservative and is centered on appropriate analgesia for the discomfort. Patient education should include the benign nature of the condition.

Dysmenorrhea

Until recently dysmenorrhea was commonly dismissed as a female psychologic rather than organic disease (Harlow 1986). Today dysmenorrhea is a recognized condition, although many of the nuances of the physiology remain to be understood. Most cases of dysmenorrhea are self-diagnosed and in large part self-treated. However, occasionally the symptoms of dysmenorrhea are so severe that a woman seeks emergency care.

Etiology

Dysmenorrhea is generally divided into two types: primary and secondary. Primary dysmenorrhea is due to uterine spasms most commonly experienced by the young, nulligravida woman (Kustin and Rebar 1987). Secondary dysmenorrhea usually occurs in women over thirty who have gynecologic problems such as uterine myomas, endometriosis, or premenstrual syndrome (Bayer and Seibel 1986).

Pathophysiology

The two major types of nerves involved in pelvic pain include cutaneous and muscle innervations with the A nerve fibers, which are responsible for acute pain, and visceral innervations involving C fibers, which are responsible for the chronic type of pain that is typically referred. Uterine spasms in primary dysmenorrhea can involve both types of nerves (Helms 1987). In fact, the types of nerve fibers, issue of referred pain, and personal implications of reproductive pain make accurate diagnosis of gynecologic pain difficult. Endocrine studies of the pituitary-ovarian axis are ongoing in an effort to identify the primary etiologic agent. Studies of prostaglandin and progesterone appear to engender the most interest.

Clinical Manifestations

Almost 80% of all women have reported a degree of dysmenorrhea at some point in their lives (Fogel and Woods 1981). Dysmenorrhea is characterized by pelvic pain. Primary dysmenorrhea most commonly occurs one to two years after menarche. At this time ovulatory function is established. Prior to onset of ovulation but after menarche, anovulatory cycles occur and are generally painless. Dysmenorrhea of primary or secondary type occurs either with onset of menses or 24 to 48 hours immediately before. Referred sensations include pain in the legs or suprapubic area. Accompanying signs or symptoms may include breast tenderness, headaches, nausea, vomiting, and abdominal distention.

Dysmenorrhea is diagnosed by the clinical picture and lack of any other diagnostic entity. For example, the alternative explanations for acute pelvic pain may include ectopic pregnancy, appendicitis, ovulatory cysts, or PID. These conditions need to be investigated prior to diagnosing dysmenorrhea.

Treatment and Nursing Care

Pain, Related to

- **Dysmenorrhea**

Once the diagnosis of dysmenorrhea is made, one of the most effective modalities is the new category of analgesics. Nonsteroidal antiprostaglandins actually inhibit intrauterine prostaglandin synthesis and decrease pain (Owen 1984; McCaffrey 1985; Amadio and Cummings 1986; United States Pharmacopia Dispensing Information 1987). Education of the patient that dysmenorrhea is an organic problem is also of benefit. For women with secondary dysmenorrhea, education should include the diagnosis and prognosis for the associated gynecologic condition.

OBSTETRIC EMERGENCIES

Management of the gravid woman and her fetus during emergencies is based upon an understanding of key anatomic and physiologic changes of pregnancy. The goal of management is the maintenance and restoration of both mother and fetus. Unless key principles are recognized, serious morbidity or mortality to mother and baby will result. Modified, Cruikshank's factors for management of pregnant trauma victims provide an excellent guidepost for management of all emergencies during pregnancy (1979). The following are the authors' modifications of Cruikshank's complicating factors:

1. The fact that the patient is pregnant may alter the pattern of severity of the injury or emergency condition.

2. The pregnancy may alter the signs and symptoms of the injury or condition and the results of laboratory tests used in diagnosis.

3. Management of the trauma victim who is pregnant needs to be modified to accommodate and preserve the physiologic changes induced by pregnancy.

4. The injury or condition may have initiated or have been complicated by pathologic conditions peculiar to pregnancy (e.g., abruptio placentae, amniotic fluid embolism, ruptured uterus), or a pregnancy-related disease may occur coincidental

to trauma and thus complicate the diagnosis and therapy (e.g., eclampsia complicating possible head trauma) (Cruikshank 1979).

Anatomic Changes in Pregnancy

During pregnancy, the heart is deviated upward and develops an outward rotation. As the uterus grows, the bowel is compressed upward into the upper abdomen increasing both the numbers of loops of bowel and overall bowel compression. Peritoneal signs diminish as the abdominal wall stretches and distends with the growing abdominal contents. In addition, the usual pain referral patterns may be altered as the abdominal organs are rearranged during pregnancy. The bladder moves anteriorly and superiorly out of the pelvis into the abdomen during pregnancy. Ureters and renal pelves are markedly dilated and dilation is more pronounced on the right.

Physiologic Changes in Pregnancy

Cardiovascular Changes

Maternal pulse increases as much as 15 beats per minute (BPM) in pregnancy. Because tachycardia is an important indicator of hypovolemia, it should be recognized that normal maternal pulse during the third trimester borders on tachycardia. Maternal blood pressure remains at prepregnant baseline level with only a small (5- to 15-mmHg) drop in the second trimester. Third trimester blood pressure should be at the baseline established in the first trimester. The most dramatic physiologic change occurs in maternal blood volume. From 10 to 34 weeks gestation, maternal blood volume increases from 40% to 45% above the prepregnant level. At term the gravid woman has a total blood volume in excess of 4000 ml. This increased volume is not matched by a corresponding increase in erythrocytes and as such a dilutional or "physiologic" anemia of pregnancy results. The normal gravida has a hemoglobin between 11 and 13 mg/dl. Approximately 500 to 700 ml of blood circulates through the uterus every minute, the total maternal blood volume circulating through the uterus every 8 to 11 minutes. As such, uterine trauma can result in massive blood loss. Because of the increased volume, clinical signs of shock (i.e., hypotension and tachycardia) may not appear until the woman has lost 35% of her total blood volume (1400 ml). Cardiac output rises in the first 10 weeks of pregnancy from 6.0 to 7.0 L/minute and remains at that level until delivery. Peripheral venous pressure rises in the lower extremities as a result of the weight of the pregnant uterus but remains unchanged in the upper extremities. Central venous pressure is 1 to 5 mmHg until 30 to 42 weeks when it rises to 10 mmHg.

Pulmonary Changes

Tidal volume in pregnancy increases 40% by increased excursion without any change in respiratory rate. The increased tidal volume lowers the partial pressure of carbon dioxide (Pco_2) to 30 mmHg in the second and third trimesters.

Gastrointestinal System Changes

Pregnancy causes a delay in gastric emptying time and intestinal transit time because of decreased motility. This decreased motility often results in heartburn, constipation, or both.

Nervous System Changes

It is not known what changes, if any, occur in the nervous system as a result of pregnancy. Neurologic signs during pregnancy must be carefully and completely evaluated because the literature is replete with examples of eclamptic women treated for seizure disorders or head injury. Misdiagnosis has resulted in mortality as well as serious maternal and fetal morbidity. Seizures in the third trimester of pregnancy must *always* be considered eclampsia until eclampsia has been ruled out.

Trauma in Pregnancy

The incidence of motor vehicle accidents, work-related injuries, domestic acts of violence, and active sports injuries is increasing. One half of the persons involved are women, and a significant number of these women will be pregnant. The number of deaths from trauma in pregnancy is equal to or greater than the deaths from hypertensive diseases in pregnancy (Crosby and Costiloe 1971). The incidence of serious wife or partner abuse is increasing, and women are particularly vulnerable during pregnancy. Forty-two per cent of residents of a shelter for battered women reported battering that occurred during a pregnancy (Stacey and Shupe 1983). The incidence of battering during pregnancy is so high that all injuries to pregnant women are suggestive of battering and must be investigated (Stark, Flitcraft, Zuckerman, et al 1981).

Etiology

As pregnancy progresses, women become increasingly awkward, with a resulting increase in minor trauma. They fall more easily, leading to bruises and perhaps fractures of small bones. Major trauma, such as motor vehicle accidents and acts of violence, remains constant throughout pregnancy. Maternal injury may be more severe and is complicated by the pregnancy. The fetus is dependent on maternal physiology for survival. The baby may be injured or die as a result of direct injury (gunshot to pregnant uterus) or indirect injury (maternal shock). Indeed, the leading cause of fetal death is maternal death. The second leading cause of fetal death is unrecognized or poorly managed maternal shock (Crosby and Costiloe 1971).

Clinical Manifestations

Trauma during pregnancy has two victims — mother and fetus. Each victim must be assessed independently. Maternal injury must be considered with the precepts of pregnancy in mind. For example, hypovolemia must be identified early without waiting for classic changes in vital signs. Changes in vital signs in pregnancy signal significant and potentially irreversible shock. Signs and symptoms of trauma may be altered because of the anatomy and physiology of pregnancy. Damage to the integrity of the uteroplacental unit will lead to life-threatening hemorrhage without visible bleeding. In the event of intrauterine hemorrhage, fetal distress may be the first indicator of trouble.

The status of the mother is not a clear indicator of the status of the fetus. Fetal ability to withstand and recover from insult is dependent upon gestational age and previous prenatal condition. The preterm (less than 37 weeks gestation) fetus is vulnerable to stress, and the fetus of a diabetic or hypertensive mother is already stressed and may be less able to tolerate a traumatic insult. On the other hand, the term fetus of a healthy pregnancy has metabolic reserve that will enable him or her to tolerate temporary or minor insult. Fetal tachycardia (above 160 BPM) or fetal bradycardia (below 110 BPM) indicates serious fetal stress and must be investigated immediately. Fetal heart range will change before the maternal vital signs, as the fetus is more sensitive to maternal hypovolemia and maternal hypoxia.

Treatment and Nursing Care

Treatment of the pregnant trauma victim and her fetus is dependent upon the nature and severity of injury or injuries sustained. Often, stage I care is required. In all cases of trauma during pregnancy, care must be rendered to both mother-to-be and the fetus. Cardiopulmonary resuscitation should be instituted as indicated for all victims of trauma and should be maintained in a terminal woman if delivery of her fetus is anticipated.

Fluid Volume Deficit, Related to

• Hemorrhage or Hypovolemia Secondary to Trauma

Uterine penetration (resulting from blunt or penetrating injuries), uterine rupture, bladder trauma, and pelvic fractures are common causes of hemorrhage in pregnant trauma victims. In such instances, increased maternal blood volume must be maintained. Immediately upon arrival in the ED, large-bore intravenous central or peripheral catheters or both should be placed for vigorous fluid replacement. Blood for typing, cross-matching, and for baseline coagulation and other studies should be drawn. If disruption of the uteroplacental unit is suspected, typing and cross-matching for at least six units of whole blood or packed cells is prudent. Blood loss should be replaced with blood, crystalloid solution, or both equal to three times the estimated amount lost. Blood will return fetal arterial oxygenation to normal levels without fetal tachycardia (Grais 1986). Other fluids may support the mother but will not support fetal oxygenation. For deep shock, the leg portion of a shock suit may be used but not the upper body section. Vasopressors should be avoided (they cause vasoconstriction within the uterus) unless required for maternal indications.

Cardiac Output, Decreased Related to

- **Hemorrhage or Hypovolemia Secondary to Trauma**
- **Supine Hypotension Syndrome**

Supine hypotension syndrome must be considered during the assessment of hypotension in the pregnant trauma victim. A pregnant woman should be positioned on her left side with a wedge placed under her right hip or the uterus should be manually deflected off the vena cava to prevent supine hypotension. A 15- to 20-degree elevation of the patient's right side should not interfere with endotracheal intubation, stabilization of the neck, or placement of intravenous lines (Morkovin 1986). Uterine displacement must be maintained at all times to assure adequate maternal and fetal circulation.

Impaired Gas Exchange, Potential, Related to

- **Trauma During Pregnancy**

Injured gravidas should be given oxygen at 8 L/minute by nasal canula or 15 L/minute via a non-rebreather mask to assure adequate oxygenation of mother and fetus.

Injury, Potential, Related to

- **Trauma**

A complete history (including details of the traumatic event and sustained trauma) and physical should be performed on all pregnant victims of trauma. The attending obstetrician or certified nurse-midwife should be contacted for current pregnancy information. A nasogastric (NG) tube, urinary catheter, or both may need to be placed if internal injury such as either gastric or bladder trauma is suspected. NG and urinary catheters may also be needed if close fluid monitoring or management is required. Diagnostic studies should be performed as indicated to assess maternal injury. If a test or procedure is essential to maternal diagnosis and treatment, it must be done regardless of potential fetal risk. Peritoneal lavage should be performed only by physicians experienced in performing the procedure in a pregnant patient.

Potential Fetal Compromise (Bobak and Jensen 1987),* Related to

- **Trauma During Pregnancy**

Fetal risk correlates with maternal shock, since homeostatic mechanisms of the gravid woman to maintain circulation may curtail uterine blood flow (VanderVeer 1984). The fetus must be assessed with an electronic fetal monitor. Both fetal heart rate and uterine activity should be evaluated initially for at least 24 hours and again for 24 hours after any episode of maternal instability. In addition, abruptio placentae

---

* Non–NANDA-approved nursing diagnosis.

is a danger for several days following a traumatic injury. Ultrasound will determine gestational age and placental indicators of fetal well-being.

Infection, Potential, Related to

- *Trauma*

Any alteration in skin integrity carries with it the risk of infection (which can lead to premature labor). Depending on the nature and severity of alteration in skin integrity, antibiotics and tetanus prophylaxis may be required. Wound care should be initiated in the ED. Education relating to wound care (i.e., care of wound, signs and symptoms of infection, and so forth) should be given to the patient prior to discharge.

Spontaneous Abortion

Abortion refers to termination of a pregnancy before viability of the fetus. The incidence of spontaneous abortion in the United States has been commonly estimated to be 10%, although such a number is most likely an underestimate because of the nature of such an early gestational event and even the debate as to when pregnancy begins (Ellish, Chen, Jason, et al 1986; Lind and McFayden 1986).

Etiology

The most common pathologic finding in an early spontaneous abortion is an abnormality of the embryo or fetus or of the placenta. Chromosomal abnormalities are found in the great majority of spontaneous abortions (Byrne and Blanc 1985). In addition to genetic influences on abortion, several other factors have also been implicated. Maternal infections, endocrine defects, malnutrition, substance abuse, immunologic incompatibility, surgery in pregnancy, and structural anomalies of the reproductive organs also have been found to be associated with abortion.

Clinical Manifestations

Six categories are used to describe types of spontaneous abortions (Bobak and Jensen 1987). Table 15–1 summarizes the clinical signs and symptoms of each of the categories. Diagnosis is based on history, clinical examination, serum pregnancy tests, and pelvic ultrasound.

Treatment and Nursing Care

Fluid Volume Deficit, Potential, Related to

- *Spontaneous abortion*

When a woman presents with active bleeding in early pregnancy, she should receive volume replacement, observation, and support. Additionally, blood tests should

TABLE 15-1
Categories of Abortion and Their Characteristic Symptomatologies

Type of Abortion	Amount of Bleeding	Uterine Cramping	Passage of Tissue	Tissue in Vagina	Internal Cervical Os	Size of Uterus
Threatened	Slight	Mild	No	No	Closed	Agrees with length of pregnancy
Inevitable	Moderate	Moderate	No	No	Open	Agrees with length of pregnancy
Incomplete	Heavy	Severe	Yes	Possible	Open with tissue in cervix	Smaller than expected for length of pregnancy
Complete	Slight	Mild	Yes	Possible	Closed	Smaller than expected for length of pregnancy
Septic	Varies; usually malodorous; fever present	Varies; fever present	Varies; fever present	Varies; fever present	Usually open; fever present	Any of the above with tenderness
Missed	Slight	No	No	No	Closed	Smaller than expected for length of pregnancy

Source: Reproduced by permission from Warner CG. Emergency Care: Assessment and Intervention (p. 553). St. Louis, 1983, The C.V. Mosby Co.

include blood group, RH status, coagulation profile, and a complete blood count. If the abortion is incomplete, surgical dilation and curettage is indicated. If it is a missed abortion, coagulation indicators should be carefully monitored until the uterus is empty. Disseminated intravascular coagulopathy is a life-threatening complication associated with retention of a dead fetus, especially for more than five weeks (refer to Chap. 21). Women with threatened abortions may be sent home with instructions to remain on bedrest and avoid coitus. They should be given follow-up and told to call their primary care providers or return to the ED if bleeding, abdominal cramping, or both increase, tissue is passed, or a fever develops.

In any case, when pregnancy loss occurs for the Rh-negative woman, anti-D serum should be administered within 72 hours. Administration of Rh immune globulin minimizes the possibility of isoimmunization.

Infection, Potential, Related to

• *Septic Abortion*

In women with a septic abortion, an immediate termination of the pregnancy is required for the health of the mother. Simultaneously, obtaining cervical secretions for cultures and for sensitivity testing allow identification of the etiologic agent and the appropriate antibiotic.

Grieving, Related to

• *Spontaneous Abortion*

Women who have experienced an abortion have experienced the death of a baby (Sandelowski and Pollock 1986). Professionals should be aware that laypersons associate the term *abortion* with voluntary termination of a pregnancy. *Miscarriage* is the lay term that implies unintentional loss of the pregnancy. In speaking to the grieving couple, *miscarriage* therefore is the preferred term. Regardless of length of gestation, a woman or couple will need support for the grief associated with the death of a child. Anticipatory guidance needs to include teaching a woman or couple to expect another period of depression to occur around the estimated date of confinement (EDC). Feelings of guilt, anger, and even denial are not uncommon and need to be recognized. This phenomenon is common and the woman and her family should be offered supportive care, including chaplaincy, community support groups for miscarriage, and individual support as necessary.

Ectopic Pregnancy

An ectopic pregnancy is a gestation in which the embryo or fetus is implanted outside the uterine cavity. It is estimated that approximately 1 of every 200 pregnancies is ectopic and that the rate has risen dramatically within the last two decades (Hemminki and Heinonen 1987). Of the ectopic pregnancies, more than 90% occur in the fallopian tubes, frequently on the maternal right side.

Etiology

In some ectopic pregnancies, there is no obvious etiologic agent. However, women with impaired tubal transport systems clearly have an increased incidence of ectopic pregnancies. High-risk factors include one or more previous ectopic pregnancies, infertility, prior salpingitis, intrauterine device (IUD) in situ, or pregnancy after tubal sterilization (Bisits and Woodhouse 1987).

Pathophysiology

In pregnancy, the zygote does not remain on the surface of an area, instead it burrows through the epithelium. Normally, this occurs within the uterine cavity. With an ectopic pregnancy, the implantation is usually into the muscular wall of the fallopian tube. As the products of conception expand, the oviduct may rupture and hemorrhage may ensue. As a result of the hormonal changes of the corpus luteum, regardless of ectopic placement, uterine growth and softening occur.

Clinical Manifestations

The most common signs and symptoms of an ectopic pregnancy are vaginal bleeding or spotting and abdominal pain. However, no single classic picture of ectopic pregnancy has yet emerged. For example, some of the more common signs or symptoms can include abdominal pain on the same side, different side, or even referred pain in the shoulder. The bleeding associated with an ectopic pregnancy can be simple spotting or can be similar to menses or even mild vaginal hemorrhage. A pelvic examination generally but not always reveals unilateral tenderness on the affected side, especially with cervical movement. These variations contribute to the difficulty in diagnosing ectopic pregnancy and relate to its description as the "mimicker" (Andolesek 1987).

Diagnosis is usually based on pelvic ultrasonography, the clinical picture, and a serum pregnancy test (Filly 1987). Differential diagnoses for ectopic pregnancy should include spontaneous abortion, ovarian cyst, appendicitis, and PID (Table 15-2).

TABLE 15-2
Differential Diagnosis of Ectopic Pregnancy

	Ectopic Pregnancy	Appendicitis	Salpingitis	Ruptured Corpus Luteum Cyst	Uterine Abortion
Pain	Unilateral cramps and tenderness before rupture	Epigastric, peri-umbilical, then right lower quadrant pain; tenderness localizing at McBurney's point; rebound tenderness	Usually in both lower quadrants with or without rebound; dysuria sometimes present	Unilateral, general with progressive bleeding	Midline cramps
Nausea & vomiting	Occasionally before, frequently after rupture	Usual; precedes shift of pain to right lower quadrant	Infrequent	Rare; no symptoms or signs of pregnancy	Almost never
Menstruation	Some aberration; missed period, spotting	Unrelated to menses	Hypermenorrhea or metrorrhagia or both	Period delayed; bleeding, often with pain	Longer amenorrhea, then spotting, then brisk bleeding
Temperature and pulse	37.2°–37.8°C (99–100°F); pulse variable: normal before, rapid after rupture	37.2°–37.8°C (99–100°F); pulse rapid	37.2°–40°C (99°–104°F); pulse elevated in proportion to fever	Not over 37.2°C (99°F); pulse normal unless blood loss marked, then rapid	To 37.2°C (99°F) if spontaneous; to 40°C (104°F) if induced (infected).
Pelvic examination	Unilateral tenderness, especially on movement of cervix; crepitant mass on one side or in cul-de-sac	No masses; rectal tenderness high on right side	Bilateral tenderness on movement of cervix; masses only when pyosalpinx or hydrosalpinx present	Tenderness over affected ovary; no masses; uterus firm and not enlarged	Cervix slightly patulous; uterus slightly enlarged irregularly softened; tender with infection
Laboratory findings	WBC to 15,000/ml; RBC strikingly low if blood loss large; sedimentation rate slightly elevated	Negative B-hCG. WBC: 10,000–18,000/μl (rarely normal) sedimentation rate slightly elevated	Negative B-hCG. WBC: 15,000–30,000/μl; RBC normal; sedimentation rate markedly elevated	Negative B-hCG. WBC normal to 10,000/μl; RBC normal; sedimentation rate normal	WBC: 15,000/μl if spontaneous; to 30,000/μl if induced (infection); RBC normal; sedimentation rate slightly to moderately elevated

Source: Reproduced, with permission, from Pernoll ML, Benson RC: Current Obstetric and Gynecologic Diagnosis and Treatment (p. 267). Copyright Appleton & Lange, 1987.

Treatment and Nursing Care

Fluid Volume Deficit, Potential, Related to

• *Rupture and hemorrhage at site of implantation*

Early diagnosis and treatment of an ectopic pregnancy is the most effective strategy in prevention of tubal rupture and subsequent hemorrhage. Once the diagnosis is made, intervention should be prompt. The typical treatment is laparoscopy — or a laparotomy, if more extensive surgery is indicated. With early diagnosis a salpingostomy may resolve the condition, and the tube may be saved (Hallat 1986). Research has suggested that upon early diagnosis of ectopic pregnancy by serial ultrasonography, patients may be treated medically with methotrexate (Ory, Villaneuva, Sand et al 1986). Methotrexate is an anticarcinogenic drug with a predisposition to destruction of gestational tissue. This treatment is limited to very early gestation and is still under investigation. Another similarly suggested medical treatment has been prostaglandin F_2-alpha-($PGF_{2\alpha}$) (Lindbloom, Hahlin, Kallfelt, et al 1987). In the event of tubal rupture or hemorrhage, large-bore intravenous lines should be placed and volume replacement should be initiated. Blood for typing and cross-matching, CBC, and coagulation studies should be obtained. When possible, orthostatic blood pressure should also be obtained. RH-negative women who have experienced an ectopic pregnancy should have anti-D serum administered within 72 hours as protection from isoimmunization.

Grieving, Related to

- *Loss of Pregnancy*

Ectopic pregnancies typically present both a surgical experience for the patient and the loss of a pregnancy. Not only does this situation involve the deep feelings described for spontaneous abortion, it also may connote serious impairment for future childbearing. For an infertile patient, for example, loss of a tube or ovary decreases her future childbearing potential. Thus a woman may grieve not only for the loss of the child but also the consequences for future childbearing.

Placenta Previa

When a placenta is abnormally implanted in the lower uterine segment, the term *placenta previa* is used. The type of placenta previa—partial, marginal, or central (total, complete)—describes the degree to which the placenta occludes the cervical os. Although it is estimated that during the second trimester, approximately 45% of women have a placenta previa, the incidence at term is less than 1%.

Etiology

The etiology of placenta previa remains unknown. Certain factors appear to be related to the development of the condition. Among factors related to development of placenta previa are advanced maternal age; previous uterine scarring, including that associated with a cesarean section birth; previous surgery for retained products of conception; and short spacing between pregnancies (Rose and Chapman 1986; Spellacy, Miller, and Winegar 1986; Page 1987).

Pathophysiology

Placental placement at term is related to insertion site, size of the placenta, and normal physiology of the uterus. In the second trimester, uterine growth is accomplished by an increase in uterine fiber size and number. Thus by term, the normal physiology of the uterus caused by these fiber changes results in the placental site being displaced upward. Typically, a previously low-lying placenta or placenta previa no longer exists (Townsend, Laing, Nyberg, et al 1986). For those situations in which the placenta continues to remain as a previa, the placenta commonly is larger than usual. The disproportionate size occurs because the circulation across the cervical os or in the lower uterine segment is less than optimal and the placenta increases in size to compensate. If a persistent placenta previa is not appropriately diagnosed, profound hemorrhage may occur when the cervix normally effaces (thins) and dilates in preparation for labor during the third trimester. As the cervix effaces and dilates, the placenta is traumatically separated from the uterine wall. Complications of the resulting hemorrhage can include fetal or maternal death from the hemorrhage or other complications, such as disseminated intravascular coagulopathy (DIC) (see Chap. 21). On rare occasions, the placenta previa not only is located in an abnormal place, but in addition this placement leads to abnormal adherence to the uterine wall. Therefore the adherent placenta (placenta accreta, increta, percreta) can result in uncontrollable hemorrhage with subsequent hysterectomy as the sole life-saving treatment modality.

Clinical Manifestations

In the second trimester of pregnancy, the silent placenta previa may be diagnosed when it appears as an incidental finding on ultrasonography. However, a placenta previa may also be diagnosed when a patient comes to the ED in an emergent state. The classic symptoms are painless hemorrhaging of bright red blood. Often the patient between 28 and 32 weeks of gestation awakens in a pool of blood. The first occurrence rarely is life-threatening unless it is a total placenta previa. However, if the first sign of bleeding has been ignored or incorrectly attributed to "spotting" or "bloody show," the woman may present in the third trimester with life-threatening bleeding. The hemorrhage may be of such a sudden nature that traditional laboratory data does not demonstrate the severity of the loss for several hours. Diagnosis is best accomplished by consideration of the clinical picture combined with pelvic ultrasonography.

Treatment and Nursing Care

Fluid Volume Deficit, Related to

• *Hemorrhage secondary to placenta previa*

Since critical bleeding rarely occurs with a one-time episode, conservative treatment for a preterm pregnancy may include hospitalization and close observation until fetal maturity is demonstrated. When the bleeding is severe or previa is diagnosed with a term infant, the treatment is delivery by cesarean section. Intravenous fluids are used for temporary fluid replacement, and two to four units of whole blood or packed cells should be obtained for replacement as needed. Although it was uncommon in the past, because of the risks of hepatitis and HIV through blood transfusions, it is no longer unusual for a pregnant woman to have blood ready for an autologous transfusion. Therefore, blood for autologous transfusion should be thawed and used as the primary vehicle for replacement. It has been recommended that the platelet counts are better indicators of the severity of the loss and the risk of DIC in pregnancy than other hematologic factors. Thus a minimum level of 100,000/cu mm is suggested. Pelvic examinations in placenta previa are contraindicated as they can further dislodge the previa and result in potentially life-threatening loss of blood.

Occasionally, a marginal previa will be discovered when a woman is in active labor. In those situations, rupture of the membranes can enhance the tamponade effect of the presenting part against the previa as labor progresses. A vaginal birth can occur when the previa is not severe and the labor is progressing quickly.

Patients who have experienced placenta previa should be carefully monitored postpartum (McShane, Heyl, and Epstein 1985). Blood loss may predispose the patient to infections in general and to endometritis in particular. Moreover, they can leave the new mother exhausted and unable to adequately care for herself and her infant. While the woman recuperates from a placenta previa, assistance in identifying her support at home can be invaluable.

Placental Abruptio

An abruptio placentae occurs when the placenta prematurely separates from the uterine wall. Although it occurs in less than 3% of the pregnancies, abruptio placentae is related to more than 15% of all perinatal deaths. Among the predisposing factors are pregnancy-induced hypertension (PIH) of any etiology, advanced maternal age, multiple gestation, substance abuse, and previous history of placenta previa (Martel, Wacholder, Lippman, et al 1987). A history of reproductive loss and the development of diabetes mellitus have also been implicated as high-risk factors for abruptio placentae (Krohn, Voigt, McKnight, et al 1987).

Etiology

An abruptio may occur for several reasons. Trauma in pregnancy is one etiologic agent involved in the condition (Higgins and Garito 1984). Ischemia or poor uteroplacental circulation associated with diabetes and hypertension can result in inadequate perfusion and even tissue death, culminating in separation.

Pathophysiology

After the twentieth week of pregnancy, separation usually occurs in the area of the decidua basalis. When separation occurs, the bleeding may dissect the decidua basalis from the membranes, and vaginal bleeding will be apparent, or it may spread between myometrial fibers and be concealed. In some cases, both scenarios occur (Hill, Breckle, and Gehrking 1985).

Clinical Manifestations

The signs and symptoms of an abruptio placentae vary. Based on the pattern of separation, bleeding may be absent. When bleeding occurs, it is usually painful in nature. The uterus generally has a rigid muscle tone, and a rise in fundal height is noticeable, especially should there be bleeding into the myometrium. Fetal distress is one of the earliest signs of an abruptio and may precede any other clue that the condition is occurring. Complications of an abruptio placentae include hypovolemic shock, fetal death, DIC, and even renal failure (Sibai, Taslimi, el-Nazer, et al 1986). Diagnosis is based on pelvic ultrasonography, but the clinical picture and predisposing causes often provide a clear assessment even without its use (Cardwell 1987; Nyberg, Cyr, Mack, et al 1987).

Treatment and Nursing Care

Fluid Volume Deficit, Related to

- *Hemorrhage secondary to abruptio placentae*

When an abruptio is diagnosed, the treatment of choice is delivery. In the case of a marginal abruptio, the method of delivery may be vaginal, whereas when a severe abruptio has occurred, especially with fetal distress, the treatment will be an emergency cesarean section (Shall 1987).

Fluid volume should be maintained as discussed with placenta previa. Since coagulopathy is a risk, platelet counts should be carefully monitored. Postpartum, every effort should be made to decrease the possibility of infection and promote health through nutrition and identification of support at home.

Pregnancy-Induced Hypertension

Hypertension in pregnancy has profound effects on the maternal-fetal dyad. The term pregnancy-induced hypertension (PIH) encompasses the conditions of pre-eclampsia, eclampsia, chronic hypertension, and chronic hypertension with superimposed preeclampsia. It is estimated that 6% to 8% of all women will demonstrate some evidence of PIH when they are pregnant. More important, PIH is the leading obstetric cause of maternal death in the United States (Hoffmaster 1983).

The American College of Obstetricians and Gynecologists have developed definitions for each category of PIH. The definitions are descriptive and essentially treat each category as a unique syndrome. For example, preeclampsia is a disease occurring after the 20th week of pregnancy and characterized by the development of hypertension, with proteinuria, alone or with facial, digital, or generalized edema. Preeclampsia may appear before the twentieth week of pregnancy in trophoblastic disease (molar pregnancy). Eclampsia is the development of seizures in association with progressive pre-eclampsia, provided that the convulsions are not attributable to another cause. Chronic hypertension is elevated blood pressure in the absence of trophoblastic disease that is independent of the pregnancy, precedes the twentieth week of pregnancy, and continues beyond six weeks postpartum. Superimposed preeclampsia or eclampsia is the development of either condition by a woman who already has chronic hypertension.

The cardinal signs of PIH are hypertension, proteinuria, and edema. Hypertension is defined as a sustained rise of 30 mmHg or more above the usual systolic level, or 15 mmHg above the usual diastolic level. The term *sustained* indicates that elevation is present on at least two occasions, six hours apart (Wheeler and Jones 1981). A sustained blood pressure of 140/90 or greater also indicates hypertension, regardless of baseline level. In all of these cases, the blood pressures are taken in a resting state without pressure on the vena cava (supine hypotension syndrome).

Similarly, proteinuria is the sustained urinary excretion of more than 1 g/L of protein in a clean random urine sample or the excretion of 0.3 g/L over 24 hours. Edema may appear in the face, fingers, or total body. Dependent edema of the legs or feet is usually of mechanical origin and generally has no importance in PIH. An indirect measure of edema has been suggested to be a weight gain of 2.25 kg within a week (Chesley 1985, 8).

Women at risk for PIH include nulliparous women and those with a familial history of PIH. Preexisting conditions such as diabetes, multiple pregnancy, and chronic hypertension that potentially compromise the uteroplacental circulation also predispose a woman to preeclampsia and eclampsia. Other factors, such as extremes of age (under 16 or over 35), hydatidiform mole, and fetal hydrops also increase a woman's chance of developing PIH. Contrary to popular belief, PIH does not appear to be linked to socioeconomic level (Wheeler and Jones 1981).

Etiology

The etiology of preeclampsia and eclampsia remains a mystery. Previous studies have centered on the immune system and a possible antigenic reaction to the fetus, the existence of an endogenous or exogenous substance causing a toxic-like reaction (hence the term *toxemia of pregnancy*), or a mysterious psychologic reaction to the pregnancy (Wheeler and Jones 1981). Today the most prevalent theory is that the susceptibility to preeclampsia and eclampsia is inherited, probably through a recessive single gene (Chesley 1985).

Pathophysiology

PIH is often a subtle disease with pathologic changes often occurring weeks before the clinical signs are manifested. Preeclampsia-eclampsia is a multisystem disease essentially summarized by the term *vasospasm*. All organ systems are affected. For example, the rise in blood pressure is a symptom of the vasospasm (Alonso 1985). In contrast to the normal increase in glomerular filtration rate (GFR) and renal blood flow found in pregnancy, in PIH GFR and renal blood flow decrease. As the disease progresses, major renal destruction can occur.

It has been suggested that vasospasm traumatizes the blood vessels and predisposes them to coagulopathy. A result of the coagulopathy is thrombocytopenia. The accompanying decrease in fibrinogen values and platelet counts can result in hemorrhage, especially at time of delivery. Prenatally, microhemorrhages can occur in the liver capsule. Hepatic hemorrhage is clinically evident by epigastric pain.

The central nervous system also is influenced by vasospasms. Irritability, clinically manifested through visual disturbances, hyperreflexia, headaches, and, in the case of eclampsia, seizures result. The generalized vasospasms directly influence uteroplacental circulation by decreasing perfusion. Thus infarction of the placenta and reduction of nutrients and oxygen to the infant can result. Even an abruptio placentae can result from severely damaged uteroplacental circulation.

Clinical Manifestations

Based on the described pathophysiology and definitions, the common symptom is hypertension. For preeclampsia, the other symptoms of edema and proteinuria may be accompanied by oliguria, intrauterine growth retardation, headaches, epigastric pain, hyperreflexia, and visual disturbances. Abruptio placentae is a complication of PIH. Eclampsia may occur in women with few if any of the classic signs of pre-eclampsia. For example, hypertension has been found to be an unreliable indicator for impending seizures (Alonso 1985).

Hemolysis, elevated liver enzymes, and low platelet count (HEELP) has been described as a common component of severe PIH, although this syndrome may also appear as a separate entity. When these signs are discovered, treatment is needed quickly to prevent serious maternal disease such as DIC (Sibai, Taslimi, el-Nazer, et al 1986).

Treatment and Nursing Care

Maternal and/or Fetal Compromise (Potential) (Bobak and Jensen 1987),* Related to

  • *Diminished uteroplacental perfusion secondary to PIH*

According to Chesley (1985), the two keys to management of PIH are early detection and vigilance. For the patient with chronic hypertension, close monitoring of mother and fetus is advised for the entire pregnancy. Fetal activity counts offer a noninvasive method of fetal assessment for the last half of the pregnancy. Diuretics should be avoided because of significant effect on the fetus. Antihypertensive drugs are used cautiously for similar reasons.

The woman with preeclampsia or preeclampsia superimposed on hypertension is treated according to the severity of the disease. Mild preeclampsia is generally treated with decreased activity to facilitate uteroplacental perfusion, increased protein in diet to counter the protein lost through the glomerulus, and close observation of the woman's condition through monitoring of blood pressure, urine protein, weight, and fetal well-being. The latter may be accomplished with nonstress testing (NST) and biophysical profiles (assessment of amniotic fluid volume, fetal activity, and fetal breathing patterns).

The woman with severe preeclampsia must be treated quickly and adequately. The usual treatment is administration of magnesium sulfate ($MgSO_4$), which is not an antihypertensive agent. It directly affects transmission of acetylcholine at the myoneural junction, decreasing the incidence of seizures (Foster 1981). Other effects of the drug include some relaxation of vessels and subsequent decrease in the hypertension, and reduction in cerebral edema. Levels of magnesium sulfate must be

---

* Non–NANDA-approved nursing diagnosis.

drawn from the maternal serum every 4 to 6 hours to guard against toxicity. Clinically, toxicity is first evidenced by a loss of deep tendon reflexes, followed by coma and eventual respiratory arrest. The effects of $MgSO_4$ can be reversed by calcium gluconate. Even in nontoxic levels, magnesium passes freely to the fetus. Fetal bradycardia and decreased umbilical cord levels of calcium occur; mild neonatal depression can be seen.

Fluid Volume Excess, Related to

- *Fluid overload secondary to diminished renal function resulting from PIH*

One of the complications of PIH is fluid overload. For a woman with PIH, even a liter of intravenous fluids routinely given to the normal intrapartum patient may be excessive because of diminished kidney function. In PIH fluid shifts to the third space. Clinically, the patient's laboratory findings will demonstrate hemoconcentration. Instead of normal postpartum diuresis, a woman with PIH risks the development of pulmonary edema.

In order to minimize the risk of excessive fluid overload, close monitoring is required. A central venous line is placed for accurate fluid assessment and a Foley catheter is placed in order to monitor output. The urine output should be at least 30 ml/hour which indicates minimal kidney function. Oliguria not only indicates kidney compromise, but also may signal acute renal failure. Exogenous oxytocins should be avoided as they possess an antidiuretic effect. Conversely, diuretics offer little protection from excessive fluids since the disease is prerenal, and diuretics act directly on the kidney alone.

An old adage states that PIH is only cured by delivery. However, like many adages, it is only partially true. Although rare, preeclampsia and eclampsia may first appear up to 10 days postpartum (Foster 1981). Close observation of the high-risk patient should continue into the puerperal period, and for a woman with mild PIH, vigilance should not be relaxed postpartum.

Any insult to the maternal-fetal dyad causes concern for the woman. PIH can result in great anxiety for a pregnant woman because of the unseen results to the infant, and the fact that often the woman herself feels well. Patient teaching including the rationale for each intervention, even bedrest, is of utmost importance. Helping a woman understand the importance of the treatment will help her assume some control over the pregnancy and afford her greater psychologic as well as physical health.

EMERGENCY DELIVERY

One of the greatest fears expressed by professionals in an emergency department is not a catastrophic event such as a cardiac arrest but the normal human event of childbirth. An unanticipated delivery in an emergency department can place the staff in a state of therapeutic paralysis. Individual professionals may not be prepared to support and manage the situation. An understanding of the basic physiologic and psychologic components of childbirth will enable the professional to anticipate and safely manage an emergency childbirth.

A primary goal of obstetrical care is safe delivery and therefore avoiding the occurrence of birth in an unprepared environment. As Long (1984, 3) stated, "Prevention begins in the antepartum period, and nursing intervention is embodied in the education of pregnant women. . . . Women need to know how and when to contact their health care providers. They also need permission and encouragement to call and report changes in what they are feeling. Prevention strategies for nurses in emergency or labor settings focus on adequate assessment of labor status and careful monitoring of labor progress."

Clinical Manifestations

To accomplish an accurate assessment of labor status, three parameters are evaluated: (1) behavior of the laboring woman, (2) relevant obstetric history, and (3) physical assessment.

The first component of labor assessment is the pregnant woman's report of her symptoms and feelings. The woman's behavior is an accurate indication of her cervical dilation. With careful observation, the experienced nurse can quickly differentiate the woman in early labor from the woman with an impending delivery. It is important to note that behavior changes often occur a few minutes before cervical change. Nursing observation is a critical tool for early identification of the woman at risk for emergency delivery. A summary of the behavioral changes in labor is given in Table 15 – 3.

The behavioral signs that warn of impending delivery should be well known by all ED nurses. The signs of late transition in labor that indicate impending delivery are

1. Increase in bloody show
2. Rectal pressure and/or passage of feces; woman may request a bedpan or wish to go to the toilet
3. Involuntary and uncontrollable pushing or bearing down
4. Spontaneous rupture of amniotic membranes
5. Perineal and rectal flattening and bulging
6. Woman states, "The baby is coming"

The second component of labor assessment is the obstetrical history. If the behavioral assessment suggests advanced labor, the emergency department nurse should ask questions to elicit information to assist rapid labor evaluation. Standard admission questions should be deferred until a complete assessment of labor is completed. It is inexcusable for an unattended birth to occur while the professional is ignoring clear signs of impending delivery and rigidly following the "routine" triage procedures. If this is a first baby, question the woman about the time of labor onset and frequency and duration of contractions. If the woman is multiparous, ask the woman how long her other labors were and how long after she got to the hospital her other babies were born. Rapid labors tend to repeat — or to be shorter each time. The woman who delivered her last baby in the car, the ED, or elevator is at great risk of repeating emergency delivery. Other important information includes the estimated date of confinement (EDC) to ascertain whether or not this baby is full-term and any obstetric complications that have occurred with this and/or previous pregnancies and deliveries.

The third component of labor assessment is the physical examination. For the woman in active labor, the initial physical assessment includes blood pressure to evaluate risk of preeclampsia-eclampsia, listening to fetal heart tones, and pelvic examination. All other physical assessments can be deferred until labor status is determined. The pelvic examination should be used to confirm the behavioral assessment of labor. On pelvic examination, assess the effacement (thinning), dilation, consistency (softness or firmness), and location of the cervix. The station of the fetal head in relationship to the maternal ischial spines should be noted. In addition, status of the membranes and color of amniotic fluid (if ruptured) should be recorded. It is important to remember that vaginal bleeding is an **Absolute Contraindication** to pelvic examination. Vaginal bleeding may indicate placenta previa. Pelvic examination of a woman with a previa could produce a life-threatening hemorrhage for mother and baby. If there is any difficulty in differentiating bloody show from vaginal bleeding, pelvic examination should be deferred until a qualified obstetric professional (obstetrician or nurse-midwife) evaluates the patient.

Treatment and Nursing Care

Occasionally, the issue of labor diagnosis is moot. The woman arrives in the emergency department in advanced labor with delivery imminent or in progress. On those occasions, seven basic principles should be recognized and followed (Adapted from Long 1984):

1. Never leave the patient alone; call for help, preferably from an experienced birth attendant

2. Use clean technique to decrease the possibility of infection for mother or infant

3. Control expulsion of the newborn in order to avoid infant and maternal birth trauma

4. Clear the neonate's airway to facilitate breathing

5. Avoid neonatal cold stress by quickly drying and wrapping the baby

6. Prevent postpartum blood loss by safe management of third stage

7. Promote early parent-child contact in a safe environment

The woman should be encouraged to assume a position that prevents supine hypotension—i.e., *not* flat on her back. Usually, women will instinctively choose a lateral (on her side with the upper knee drawn toward her chest), hands and knees, or a modified Fowler's position. All of these are safe for mother and baby and permit adequate access for the birth attendant. It is wise not to break the bed into two parts and force a patient into a lithotomy position. The major advantage of the lithotomy position (if stirrups are available and the patient can be placed comfortably in them with her back elevated), is the increased visualization for the birth attendant. The risk of the lithotomy position, as with any broken bed position, is the increased potential for a dropped baby with inexperienced attendants.

It has been suggested that since most emergency deliveries are normal events, the appropriate posture is that of a watchful guardian. However, in order to prevent birth trauma, explusion of the baby must be controlled. The most crucial component is calm, reassuring communication with the mother. She must never be left alone and must always have positive reassurance to enable her to maintain self control. A calm,

TABLE 15–3
Coaching Interventions

Woman's Potential Behaviors/Feelings	Coach's Response
Latent Phase	
Excitement; eagerness to begin work; anticipation	Use of humor, if appropriate
Talkativeness	Movement and ambulation; activity is helpful in stimulating labor
Cheerfulness, contentment	Remind woman to drink clear liquids and to eat no fatty or heavy foods
Perceptual field is broad; focuses on environment	
Comfort—general	Discuss coping tools for use later during labor
Abdominal cramping	Be the partner's advocate; make her wishes known to birth attendants
Mild uterine contractions	Be aware of need to begin use of relaxation and breathing techniques when she can no longer talk or joke her way through the contractions
Active Phase	
Anxiety and apprehension, discomfort and attention to pain, seriousness; ill-defined fears	Give her your undivided attention
Perceptual field narrows; focuses on self in social behavior	Verbal support and encouragement: "This contraction is almost over . . . you're doing great!" "Take one contraction at a time"
Helplessness; tension (grimaces, clenched fists, restlessness, rigidity), dependency; difficulty with concentration	Adapt the environment to provide rest and relaxation:
	• Adjust lights and shades to avoid glare
Desire for companionship; fear of abandonment; isolation	• Use quiet music you and she have selected
Backache; strengthening of contractions	• Arrange focal point for easy viewing
	Encourage use of
	• Attention focal points
	• Relaxation—give periodic feedback: "Feel your body getting heavier"
	• Paced breathing techniques—allow her to establish own rate and assist her with breathing patterns, if necessary
	Use short specific sentences
	Physical measures such as
	• Gentle touch
	• Positioning—assist to a position of comfort such as sitting, standing, leaning on you, leaning forward, side-lying, on hands and knees
	• Cool compresses to her forehead
	• Counter pressure to her lower back—make sure you are in a comfortable position to do this to prevent a backache of your own
	• Apply hot or cold compresses to lower back
	• Effleurage
	• Massage her aching legs
	• Offer ice chips, Chapstick, mouthwash, or toothbrushing
	• Be sure dry pads are kept underneath her
	• Encourage her to urinate regularly to lessen discomfort and promote labor progress
	Be alert for signs of progress and communicate these to her: descent of baby in abdomen; location of fetal heart tones in progressively lower areas
	Remember: do not become discouraged if she does not respond as expected or tell you how much your support means to her; she is very absorbed in labor now
	Take a moment for yourself to consciously relax—take some deep breaths and remember to remain calm; your partner will depend on and benefit from your presence!
	Ask for suggestions, help, or relief from the birth attendant if you find yourself getting discouraged, tired, or impatient
Transitional Phase	
Maximum anxiety and fear:	Realize that she may respond differently now
• Verbalization of desire to give up	Remain with her constantly; reduce environmental stimuli
• Inability to follow breathing routine	Remind of breathing techniques if she loses concentration

TABLE 15–3 *Continued*

Woman's Potential Behaviors/Feelings	Coach's Response
• Emotional outbursts • Loss of ability to evaluate situation	Maintain eye contact — put your face close to hers, tell her to look at you, say "Breathe with me." Use short and simple statements
Narrowed perceptual field; decreased attention span, withdrawal from environment	Be alert for signs of panic
Irritability	Interpret directions and information from birth attendants
Periods of disorientation	Keep in mind that contractions have reached maximum strength, and relief will come with pushing
Irrational statements	Encourage rest between contractions
Dependency; inability to make decisions; coping: "I can't"	Be alert for signs of her urge to bear down: a "catch" in her breath, or a slight grunting sound
Exhaustion, restlessness, discomfort	
Diaphoresis	
Tremors	
Hot or cold flashes	
Nausea, vomiting	
	Birth
Renewed energy	Assist her in finding a good position for pushing (semireclining, side-lying if tired, modified squatting, or hands and knees)
Exhaustion	Be ready to give step-by-step instructions for pushing if necessary
Possible confusion: inability to remember techniques	Give specific verbal encouragement for pushing: "Relax your pelvic floor muscles," "Let the baby out"
Desire to push	Support her shoulders for pushing
	Gentle touch to abdomen to help her focus on pushing
	May need to inform her of contractions if she has had regional anesthesia
	Apply warm perineal compresses if indicated
	Remind her to pant or blow as baby's head crowns

Source: Nichols FH, Humenick SS. 1988. Childbirth Education: Practice, Research, and Theory. WB Saunders, 286–287.

professional approach with gentle repeating of instructions will facilitate controlled birth. Women should not be actively encouraged to push. Expulsive pushing can result in an uncontrolled delivery, predisposing to maternal and fetal trauma. The woman should be encouraged to open her mouth and breathe quickly: "pant like a puppy." As the head emerges, the practitioner should extend the fingers of the dominant hand and place them on the baby's head. Use of all fingers prevents fingertip pressure on a single area. Gentle but firm pressure allows the head to emerge slowly. At no time should the pressure be so pronounced that the head is retarded in its progress. After the head has emerged, a hand should be kept gently in place in order to prevent sudden expulsion of the body. During this time, the head will turn slowly to the side, and the shoulders will rotate to the anterior-posterior position. The rotation occurs spontaneously, usually with the contraction following the contraction that delivered the fetal head. While waiting for rotation, the baby's nose and mouth should be suctioned with a soft bulb and the neck palpated for presence of the umbilical cord. This is accomplished by feeling under the maternal symphysis pubis. If a cord is felt, it can usually be pulled gently over the head or slid back over the shoulders during delivery of the body. It is rare that it must be clamped and cut to allow delivery of the baby's body.

Simple support of the head is all that is required to facilitate delivery of the body. Occasionally, the body may be guided by the professional placing both hands on either side of the baby's head, covering the ears. In this position, gentle downward pressure by the professional assists the anterior shoulder to deliver; gentle pressure upward then facilitates the posterior shoulder. After delivery of the shoulders, the remainder of the baby delivers immediately. It is at this point that the greatest danger of dropping the slippery, wet baby occurs. Placing the baby on the maternal abdomen or on a clean towel between her legs provides a safe immediate resting place. The optimal position is to place the baby on the maternal abdomen so that the mother can be reassured of the baby's condition. Immediate drying and wrapping, even before cord cutting, helps prevent chilling of the newborn. Once the baby is dry, double-clamping and cutting of the umbilical cord can be done (Fig. 15–1) (Varney 1987).

The expulsion of the placenta encompasses the third stage of labor. The length of time between second stage (delivery of the baby) and third stage varies from a few seconds to 30 minutes. Usually, the woman and her baby can be transported to the obstetrical unit prior to placental expulsion. In order to prevent partial separation of the placenta and its accompanying hemorrhage, no uterine massage or manipulation of the umbilical cord should be undertaken. Nipple stimulation by a nursing newborn may be initiated if the mother desires, as it seems to enhance the normal third-stage process. In the event that a brisk gush of blood occurs with simultaneous lengthening of the cord at the introitus, the uterus should be gently palpated abdominally. A firm, globular uterus coupled with the gush of blood and lengthening cord indicates normal placenta will deliver spontaneously. Under no circumstances should the placenta be "pulled" by the cord as this may lead to partial separation, life-threatening inversion of the uterus, or both. All placenta and membranes should be saved for examination by the obstetric professionals.

Complications of Emergency Childbirth

Although most emergency deliveries are simple, normal births occurring in an unusual location, certain emergencies can accompany them. Prominent among birth emergencies are premature births and breech deliveries. Whenever a potentially compromised infant is suspected, not only should a call be made for an experienced birth attendant, neonatology-pediatrics should also be called for neonatal resuscitation and support. Premature infants (less than 37 completed weeks of gestation) are more likely to be the result of an emergency delivery, particularly since they may deliver prior to full dilation of the cervix. Preterm infants are at an increased risk of cold stress that leads to apnea, hypoglycemia, and intracranial hemorrhage from uncontrolled delivery. Careful handling and absolute control at delivery to prevent trauma is of utmost importance. The preterm newborn must be dried immediately and placed in a warmer or other external heat source to prevent hypothermia and its resultant apnea. Small babies require immediate professional attention and should be observed continuously after birth. In the event of an unexpectedly small baby from a term gestation, multiple gestation must be suspected, and the mother must be examined immediately for an additional baby or babies.

A premature infant is more likely than a full-term baby to be in a breech presentation. Breech deliveries have an inherently higher rate of morbidity and mortality. When a breech birth is imminent, the desire to intervene must be controlled. In this situation, nature is a safer attendant than a meddlesome professional. The mother should be verbally encouraged to control the delivery of the body by panting rather than expulsive pushes. This prevents expulsion of the body before the

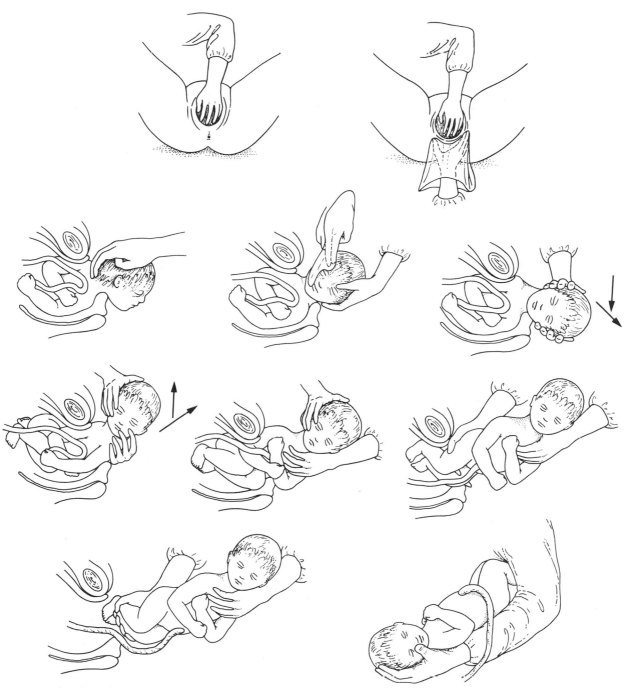

FIGURE 15–1. Hand maneuvers for delivery of the baby in occipital anterior position with the mother in traditional lithotomy position. As noted in the text, other birthing positions are possible. (Redrawn from Varney H. 1987, Nurse-midwifery. Boston, Blackwell Scientific Publications.)

cervix is completely dilated, in which case the smaller body can be forced through the incompletely dilated cervix predisposing to an entrapped head. The fetal body should be supported (by wrapping it with a towel) and held to maintain alignment with the aftercoming head as contractions alone advance the baby. The body will emerge with a slight downward angle until the nape of the neck becomes visible. The mother should be encouraged to pant as the professional holds the body to prevent rapid expulsion of the head. As soon as the mouth and nose are visible, they should be cleared with a suction bulb. The head should be allowed to deliver gently with a contraction.

Immediate Postpartum Nursing Care

Immediately after delivery, the maternal perineum should be inspected for lacerations, unusual bleeding, or both. Bleeding from lacerations can be controlled by applying firm pressure with a sterile dressing until repair can be accomplished. Time of delivery, condition (Apgar score) of the infant, and maternal condition should be documented. If the placenta is expelled before the mother is transferred, the time of expulsion with an approximate blood loss should also be noted. Under no circumstances should the mother and baby be separated until matching identification bands are placed on both mother and child.

Psychologically, it has been noted that a woman needs to discuss the delivery event several times for her to make sense of it and recognize the reality of the event. Alfonso (1977) has referred to this as identifying "missing pieces." Thus, even after the mother has been transferred to an inpatient unit, the professional who was with her during the emergency delivery should see her and help reconstruct the experience for the mother's psychologic health. This is particularly helpful should the mother have feelings of guilt — for example, for waiting at home too long or because she fears her behavior was inappropriate. The individual who cared for the patient can listen and supply the information to help her understand the real situation.

An emergency delivery need not result in therapeutic paralysis if a calm attitude prevails. Attention to basic principles will facilitate optimal care for the woman and child during emergency childbirth. Good communication between the emergency and obstetric departments is of value for emergency staff education to ensure that principles of delivery are well known and clearly remembered for those unexpected emergency deliveries.

CONCLUSION

Women consume more health care than men and are the most frequent clients in the emergency department. Women may seek care for medical, surgical, psychological, gynecologic, or obstetric reasons. All too often, women need care for trauma, domestic violence, rape, or accident. Whatever the precipitating event or condition that brings them to the emergency department, care must be provided in a holistic manner, recognizing the psychologic and physiologic needs unique to women.

REFERENCES

Adkinson C, Frost T, Peterson G. 1986. Evidence collection in sexual assault. Ann Emerg Med 15:878–879.

Alfonso D. 1977. Missing pieces. Birth Fam J 4:159–164.

Alonso B. 1985. Hypertensive disorders of pregnancy. NAACOG Update Ser 3:1–8.

Amadio P, Cummings D. 1986. Nonsteroidal anti-inflammatory agents. Am Fam Physician 34:147–154.

Andolesek K. 1987. Ectopic pregnancy: classic versus common presentations. J Fam Pract 24:481–485.

Baltarowich O, Kurtz A, Pasto M, et al. 1987. The spectrum of sonographic findings in hemorrhagic ovarian cysts. Am J Radiol 148:901–905.

Bayer S, Seibel M. 1986. Endometriosis. Prog Clin Bio Res 225:103–133.

Bisits A, Woodhouse R. 1987. Delayed ectopic pregnancies after sterilization. Med J Aust 147:138–139.

Bobak I, Jensen M. 1987. Essentials of Maternity Nursing. St. Louis, CV Mosby, 818.

Burgess AW, Holmstrom LL. 1974. Crisis and counseling requests of rape victims. Nurs Res 23:196–202.

Byrne J, Blanc W. 1985. Malformation and chromosome anomalies in spontaneously aborted fetuses with single umbilical artery. Am J Obstet Gynecol 151:340–342.

Cardwell M. 1987. Ultrasonic diagnosis of abruptio placentae with fetomaternal hemorrhage. Am J Obstet Gynecol 157:358–359.

Cartwright P. 1987. Factors that correlate with injury sustained by survivors of sexual assault. Obstet Gynecol 70:44–46.

Chesley L. 1985. Hypertensive disorders in pregnancy. J Nurse-Midwife 30:99–104.

Crosby WM, Costiloe MS. 1971. Safety of lap belt restraint for pregnant victims of automobile collisions. N Engl J Med 284:632–636.

Cruikshank DP. 1979. Anatomic and physiologic alterations of pregnancy that modify the response to trauma. In Buchsbaum JJ, ed. Trauma in Pregnancy. Philadelphia, WB Saunders, 21–39.

Diernaes E, Rasmussen J, Soerensen T, Hasch E. 1987. Ovarian cysts: management by puncture? Lancet 1:1084.

Ellish N, Chen H, Jason C, et al. 1986. Pilot study to detect early pregnancy and early fetal loss. J Occupational Med 28:1069–1073.

Eschenbach DA. 1984. Acute pelvic inflammatory disease. Urol Clin North Am 11:65–81.

Filly R. 1987. Ectopic pregnancy: the role of sonography. Radiology 162:661–668.

Fogel CI, Woods NF. 1981. Health Care for Women. St. Louis, CV Mosby.

Foster S. 1981. Magnesium sulfate. MCN6:355.

Giacoia G, Wood B. 1987. Ovarian cyst of the newborn. Am J Dis Child 141:1199–1202.

Gomez-Carrian Y. 1987. Resolving acute pelvic inflammatory disease. Contemp Obstet Gynecol 30 (Suppl):123–144.

Grais FC. 1966. Uterine vascular responses to hemorrhage during pregnancy. Obstet Gynecol 27:549–554.

Hallat J. 1986. Tubal conservation in ectopic pregnancy. Am J Obstet Gynecol 154:1216–1221.

Harlow S. 1986. Function and dysfunction: a historical critique of the literature on menstruation and work. Health Care Women Int 7:39–50.

Heinrich LB. 1987. Care of the female rape victim. Nurse Pract 12:9–29.

Helms J. 1987. Acupuncture for the management of primary dysmenorrhea. Obstet Gynecol 69:51–56.

Hemminki E, Heinonen P. 1987. Time trends of ectopic pregnancies. Br J Obstet Gynecol 94:322–327.

Higgins S, Garite TJ. 1984. Late abruptio placentae in trauma patients. Obstet Gynecol 63 (3 Suppl):10S–12S.

Hill L, Breckle R, Gehrking W. 1985. Abruptio placentae. Am J Obstet Gynecol 148:1144–1145.

Hoffmaster J. 1983. Detecting and treating pregnancy-induced hypertension. MCN 8:398–405.

Kille M. 1986. A sexual assault referral service based on a hospital in a small Australian town. Med J Aust 145:189–194.

Krohn M, Voigt L, McKnight B, et al. 1987. Correlates of placental abruptio. Br J Obstet Gynecol 94:333–340.

Kustin J, Rebar R. 1987. Menstrual disorders in the adolescent age group. Prim Care 14:139–166.

Lavery J, Koontz W, Layman L, et al. 1986. Sonographic evaluation of the adnexa during early pregnancy. Surg Gynecol Obstet 163:319–323.

Lind T, McFayden I. 1986. Human pregnancy failure. Lancet 1:91–92.

Lindbloom B, Hahlin M, Kallfelt B, et al. 1987. Local prostaglandin F_2 alpha injection for termination of ectopic pregnancy. Lancet 1:776–777.

Long PJ. 1984. Emergency delivery. NAACOG Update Ser 1:1–8.

Lumicao GG, Heggi A. 1979. Chlamydial infections. Pediatr Clin North Am 26:269–282.

Martel M, Wacholder S, Lippman A, et al. 1987. Maternal age and primary cesarean section rates. Am J Obstet Gynecol 156:305–308.

Martin L. 1978. Health Care of Women. Philadelphia, JB Lippincott.

McCaffrey M. 1985. Newer uses of NSAIDs. Am J Nurs 85:781–782.

McShane P, Heyl P, Epstein M. 1985. Maternal and perinatal morbidity resulting from placenta previa. Obstet Gynecol 65:176–182.

Mead PB. 1987. PID: best new routes to diagnosis and treatment. Contemp OB/GYN 29:156–176.

Morkovin V. 1986. Trauma in pregnancy. In Farrell RG, ed. OB/GYN Emergencies: The First 60 Minutes. Rockville, Md, Aspen, 71–86.

Nussbaum S, Saunders R, Benator R, et al. 1987. Spontaneous resolution of neonatal ovarian cysts. Am J Radiol 148:175–176.

Nyberg D, Cyr D, Mack L, et al. 1987. Sonographic spectrum of placental abruptio. Am J Radiol 148:161–164.

Ory S, Villaneuva A, Sand P, et al. 1986. Conservative treatment of ectopic pregnancies with methotrexate. Am J Obstet Gynecol 154:1299–1306.

Owen P. 1984. Prostaglandin synthetase inhibitors in the treatment of primary dysmenorrhea. Am J Obstet Gynecol 148:96–103.

Page I. 1987. Aetiological factors in placenta praevia. Br J Obstet Gynecol 94:283.

Pernoll ML, Benson RC. 1987. Current obstetric and gynecologic diagnosis and treatment. San Mateo, Calif, Lange Medical Publishers.

Prepas R. 1984. Pelvic inflammatory disease. NAACOG Update Ser 3:1–8.

Quan M, Rodney WM, Johnson R. 1984. Pelvic inflammatory disease. J Fam Pract 16:131–140.

Queenan JT. 1984. Managing OB/GYN Emergencies. Oradell NJ, Medical Economics Books.

Riesenberg D. 1987. Treating a societal malignancy—rape. JAMA 257:726–727.

Riesenberg D. 1987. Motivations studied and treatments devised in attempt to change rapists' behavior. JAMA 257:899–900.

Rose G, Chapman M. 1986. Aetiological factors in placenta previa. Br J Obstet Gynecol 93:586–588.

Sandelowski M, Pollock C. 1986. Women's experiences of infertility. Image 18:140–144.

Shall J. 1987. Abruptio placenta: clinical management in nonacute cases. Am J Obstet Gynecol 156:40–51.

Sibai B, Taslimi M, el-Nazer A, et al. 1986. Maternal perinatal outcome associated with the syndrome of hemolysis, elevated liver enzymes and low platelets in severe preeclampsia-eclampsia. Am J Obstet Gynecol 155:501–509.

Spellacy W, Miller S, Winegar A. 1986. Pregnancy after 40 years of age. Obstet Gynecol 68:452–454.

Stacey WA, Shupe A. 1983. The Family Secret: Domestic Violence in America. Boston, Beacon Press.

Stark E, Flitcraft A, Zuckerman D, et al. 1981. Wife Abuse in the Medical Setting. Domestic Violence Monograph Ser No. 7. Rockville, Md, National Clearinghouse on Domestic Violence.

Thorton J, Wells M. 1987. Ovarian cysts in pregnancy: does ultrasound make traditional management inappropriate? Obstet Gynecol 69:717–721.

Townsend T, Laing F, Nyberg D, et al. 1986. Technical factors responsible for "placental migration." Radiology 160:105–108.

Vander Veer JB. 1984. Trauma during pregnancy. Top Emerg Med 6:72–77.

Varney H. 1987. Nurse-midwifery. Boston, Blackwell Scientific.

Warner CG. 1983. Emergency care: assessment and intervention. St. Louis, CV Mosby Co.

Wheeler L, Jones M. 1981. Pregnancy-induced hypertension. JOGNN 9:212–232.

Marianne Genge, RN MS

Musculoskeletal Emergencies

All age groups in society have become more mobile and are achieving faster speeds, and more people are involved in sports and fitness activities. As a result, musculoskeletal injuries and surface trauma have become more frequent, acute, and complex. Although these injuries often occur with trauma to other systems, they are seldom viewed as life threatening and are usually the last systems to receive the full attention of the emergency team. Musculoskeletal trauma needs to be treated appropriately in the emergency department (ED), or the residual from these injuries could plague a patient for a lifetime.

Specific diagnosis of an injury may be delayed until after the patient has been assessed and stabilized. Permanent musculoskeletal disability may be avoided by proper positioning, splinting, and bandaging of the injured area in the first stage of emergency nursing care. Injuries may include fractures, dislocations, subluxations, sprains, and strains. The nurse's ability to efficiently assess the patient's injury and intervene appropriately is essential to the successful outcome of musculoskeletal trauma.

There will be no effective method to prevent trauma as long as people are mobile and active. However, injuries can be minimized by encouraging the following interventions: reduce and enforce highway speed limits; enforce seat belt laws; encourage the use of safety equipment (goggles, helmets, and so forth); support sporting safety campaigns; and reinforce drunk driving laws consistently. Accident prevention is vital in minimizing injuries. Nurses have the power to educate the public about accident prevention, to help reduce the number of injuries, and to facilitate the patient's recovery from those injuries already incurred. The emergency nurse there-

363

fore needs to possess skills in the assessment, treatment, and monitoring of musculo-skeletal injuries in persons of all ages.

This chapter reviews musculoskeletal assessment. Musculoskeletal injuries such as fractures, dislocations, subluxations, sprains, and strains are discussed. The following aspects of these injuries also are addressed: mechanism of injury, etiology, clinical manifestations, treatment modalities, and appropriate nursing responsibilities.

MUSCULOSKELETAL ASSESSMENT

History

Assessment is the first and most vital phase of the nursing process. It provides the baseline for subsequent care. The emergency nurse can provide these data by obtaining a thorough history from and conducting a detailed physical examination on the patient who has sustained musculoskeletal trauma.

The history is a vital part of the physical assessment and should include (1) the chief complaint; (2) the mechanism of injury; (3) the past medical history; and (4) the social history (Rodts 1986). All sections should be as complete as possible.

The chief complaint should include, in the patient's words if possible, the primary reason for admission to the ED. The patient should describe what was injured, and what was felt or heard upon injury. Was there pain? If so, when did it begin? What kind of pain was it? Where did the pain radiate? With fractures there is pain on injury that is localized around the fracture site. Was there loss of sensation? If so, when and where was it felt? Was there numbness and tingling anywhere? These questions provide information regarding any possible neurologic damage. Were sounds such as a crack, pop, snap, or crunch heard? Sounds such as these could help determine if there was a fracture, dislocation, or ligament tear. A crack could be a sign of a fracture and the crunching sound, or crepitus, could be the fracture ends rubbing together. By utilizing various communication techniques the nurse should obtain a thorough account of the injury from the patient.

Once it has been established what happened, the mechanism of injury should then be determined. What was the direction and amount of force? When did the injury occur? When was the onset of pain or disability, edema, redness, discoloration, or temperature change? What treatment was done, when was it done, and who assisted? Was first aid such as the application of a dressing, ice, or heat performed? Were any analgesics given? If analgesics were given, was there relief of the pain? Did the interventions alleviate or exacerbate the discomfort? Splinting should relieve the pain of a fracture. How was the patient brought to the ED (Rauscher 1986)? If the patient is unable to communicate effectively, this information should be obtained from companions who were near the patient at the time of trauma, the allied medical personnel who initially treated the patient, or prehospital records. This information should help the nurse determine the type and mechanism of injury.

The mechanism of injury and the degree of force sustained are important aspects of the injury that determine its severity. Certain musculoskeletal injuries occur in patterns, and knowledge of the mechanism of injury could lead to a fairly precise diagnosis (Walt 1982). The severity of the injury is directly related to the force placed on the bone or surrounding soft tissue.

Following an account of the mechanism of injury, the medical and surgical history should be obtained as well as the review of systems once the patient's condition has been stabilized. A surgical history should also be obtained, especially to determine if the patient has had surgery involving the musculoskeletal system. It should be determined if the patient has significant medical problems, such as cardiovascular disease, diabetes, cancer, osteoporosis, arthritis, hemophilia, or other chronic conditions that can affect the musculoskeletal system. For example, if the patient has a compromised cardiovascular status or diabetes mellitus, peripheral pulses may be diminished and difficult to palpate. Comparison of peripheral pulses is necessary. Cancer and osteoporosis may predispose the patient to pathologic fractures related to even the slightest trauma. In both instances, the force impacting on the diseased bone is often minimal as is the displacement of bone fragments (Walt 1982). Patients with hemophilia have the potential for exacerbated hemorrhaging. In addition, they often have evidence of joint deterioration secondary to minor trauma and hemarthrosis.

Arthritis can limit joint range of motion and weaken soft tissue surrounding the joint, leading to a greater potential for dislocation. Joint prostheses are often more prone to injury and infection than are normal joints. If a patient has a prosthesis, prophylactic antibiotics may be ordered by the physician.

The nurse should ask the patient about medications that the patient normally takes. Aspirin, which many persons with arthritis take, can predispose a patient to greater than expected blood loss with fractures. Patients who have had organ transplants and rheumatoid arthritis patients often take corticosteroids, such as prednisone, for their anti-inflammatory properties and may require supplements of these steroids in times of stress. Long-term steroid therapy can contribute to avascular necrosis of such areas as the femoral head. Steroid therapy can also cause osteoporosis and thus the risk of stress fractures.

In addition to a complete list of medications, an allergy and tetanus immunization history should also be obtained from the patient. Tetanus can be prevented as long as people receive the appropriate prophylaxis (Table 16–1).

A thorough social history is obtained from the patient because individuals with musculoskeletal trauma vary in age and pre-existing medical condition and will therefore have different discharge needs. Patients may be young and healthy or elderly with multiple system deterioration, or they may fall midway on the continuum. Although trauma is the leading cause of death in persons under 38 years of age, musculoskeletal trauma can occur at any time over the lifespan. The emergency nurse must be aware of the psychosocial and physiologic impact of the injury on the patient.

Certain musculoskeletal injuries appear to be more common to certain age groups. Congenital hip dislocations obviously occur in infants. Epiphyseal injuries are more significant in children, as are greenstick fractures. Joint sprains and strains are more prone to occur in active young adults. Femoral fractures and hip injuries seem to occur more commonly in the elderly.

Regardless of when a musculoskeletal injury occurs, it always has an impact on a patient's life. The aftermath of musculoskeletal trauma may linger long after the injuries have healed. Thus, the nurse must be aware of the pretrauma lifestyle of the

TABLE 16-1
Short Guide to Tetanus Prophylaxis for Routine Wound Care

History of Adsorbed Tetanus Toxoid	Clean, Minor Wounds		All Other Wounds*	
	Td†	*TIG*	*Td*†	*TIG*
Unknown or <3 doses	Yes	No	Yes	Yes
≥3 doses‡	No§	No	No‖	No

Source: Immunization Practices Advisory Committee. 1985. MMWR *34*:422.

　* Such as, but not limited to, wounds contaminated with dirt, feces, soil, saliva, and so forth; puncture wounds; avulsions; and wounds resulting from missiles, crushing, burns, and frostbite.

　† For children <7 years of age; DPT (DT, if pertussis vaccine is contraindicated) is preferred to tetanus toxoid alone. For persons ≥7 years of age, Td is preferred to tetanus toxoid alone.

　‡ If only 3 doses of *fluid* toxoid have been received, a fourth dose of toxoid, preferably an adsorbed toxoid, should be given.

　§ Yes, if more than 10 years since last dose.

　‖ Yes, if more than 5 years since last dose.

　Td, tetanus-diphtheria toxoid; TIG, tetanus immune globulin; DPT, diphtheria-pertussis-tetanus vaccine; DT, diphtheria-tetanus.

patient and what psychosocial impact the injury may have on the individual. Various patient concerns and questions regarding the injury need to be addressed. Patient education can begin in the ED as appropriate to the patient's physiologic and psychologic status.

　Potential lifestyle changes need to be anticipated and dealt with therapeutically. The belief that discharge planning begins on admission holds true even if the admission is via the ED. To facilitate discharge planning, the patient history should elicit available supports, home environment, and other pertinent data. A referral for either a Public Health Nurse or a Home Health Aide may be required, especially in the case of geriatric patients.

Physical Examination

The initial physical assessment of the injured area may be conducted simultaneously while the preceding information is being obtained. The initial history and assessment provide enough information to allow the nurse to help stabilize the patient's condition and then proceed to obtain a more complete history and physical examination.

　Inspection and palpation are the primary techniques used in assessing the musculoskeletal system. The assessment should be carried out in an organized manner. The skull should be inspected for symmetry. The nurse should then inspect and palpate the spine, upper extremities, lower extremities, and finally the torso. The patient's clothing should be removed to view the torso and extremities. The injured extremity should be compared to the uninjured extremity to better assess the extent of the trauma. To avoid further injury, clothing should be cut away along the seams. Neurovascular assessment, joint range of motion, reflexes, and muscle strength are assessed in relation to the specific injury.

　Following physical assessment, the most definitive diagnostic procedure for

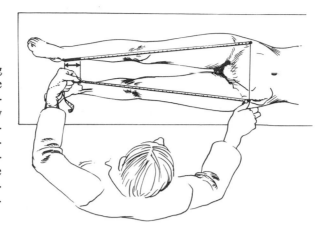

FIGURE 16–1. Determining leg length discrepancy: Measure from one fixed bony point to another. The double-headed arrow shows true leg length discrepancy. (Reproduced with permission from Hoppenfeld S: Physical Examination of the Spine and Extremities, copyright Appleton-Century-Crofts, Norwalk, CT, 1976.)

skeletal injury is the radiograph. Anteroposterior, oblique, and lateral views of the injured area may be done. Computed tomography (CT scans or tomograms) may also be done if more extensive damage is suspected.

Initially, the nurse assesses the patient with specific attention paid to the joints and extremities. The upper extremities should be inspected while the patient is either sitting or standing to allow a clear view of the anatomy. An injured arm should be supported in a comfortable position. The injured extremity should also be elevated to prevent bleeding, edema, and associated complications. Fingers should be identified as thumb, index, middle, ring, and pinkie rather than by number to avoid confusion in referring to them (Chase et al 1986).

Lower extremities are best examined with the patient lying supine and the extremities to be examined exposed. The nurse should inspect for leg length discrepancy and alignment as well as irregularities in the normal contour of the leg (Fig. 16–1). Obvious deformity of a limb is a sign of either dislocation or fracture. However, sprains and strains may produce swelling and pain similar to that of a fracture. Specific fractures and dislocations can be determined only by radiographs. Ligament or tendon injuries and other soft tissue injuries in general are not clearly identified radiographically. Alignment, deformity, length of the opposite extremity, and color of the injured areas should be noted.

Often, injured extremities are immobilized immediately after injury to decrease pain and prevent further injury. The injured area, the joint above the injured site, and the joint below the injured site are all splinted. If the patient is wearing a splint on entry to the ED, the extremity should be reassessed and the area around the splint checked for constriction. The neurovascular status of the extremity should be assessed before and after the splint is applied because splinting may cause neurovascular compromise. It is important to assess neurovascular status, reflexes and muscle strength on the patient's admission to the ED. The information should be re-evaluated periodically and changes noted throughout the patient's stay. Because veins, arteries, and nerves travel in close proximity to one another, the neurovascular assessment is fairly easy to do.

Vascular Assessment

Vascular status is assessed by first checking the color of the injured part. Pallor suggests poor arterial perfusion and cyanosis suggests venous congestion. The temperature of the extremity is assessed with the dorsal aspect of the nurse's hand and compared to the temperature of the uninjured extremity. Capillary refill is checked on both extremities and a refill time of more than 2 seconds (or the time taken to say "capillary refill") usually indicates decreased arterial capillary perfusion. Distal pulses should also be assessed and compared.

Pulses may be described on a scale of 0 to 4, with 0 being no pulse and 4 being a strong bounding pulse. A value of 3 is considered normal. Three major pulses in the upper extremities should be assessed: the radial, the ulnar, and the brachial. The most commonly assessed pulse is the radial, which can be found on the flexor surface of the wrist medially and is palpated when arterial insufficiency is suspected. The brachial pulse is found in the groove between the biceps and triceps muscles and is palpated when arterial insufficiency is suspected (Schoen 1986).

Four major pulses in the lower extremities may be assessed: the femoral, the popliteal, the posterior tibial, and the dorsalis pedis. The femoral pulse is palpable at the inguinal ligament halfway between the pubic tubercle and the anterosuperior iliac spine. With the patient's knee flexed slightly, the popliteal pulse may be felt deep in the popliteal fossa. The posterior tibial pulse is felt behind and below the medial malleolus. The dorsalis pedis pulse is palpable between the first two tendons on the medial side of the dorsum of the foot (Schoen 1986).

Neurologic Assessment

Sensory and motor nerves should be tested to assess for peripheral nerve insult. Sensory (afferent) nerves transport impulses to the central nervous system (CNS) via the posterior horn of the spinal cord. Motor (efferent) nerves carry impulses away from the CNS via the anterior horn of the spinal cord. Peripheral nerves usually combine afferent and efferent pathways. Damage to a peripheral nerve from compression, edema, or direct tauma can result in a nerve deficit distal to the injury. Peripheral nerve injuries usually exhibit generalized sensorimotor signs. A light touch to a dermatome while the patient's eyes are closed is used to assess sensory function (Urbanski 1984). To test motor function the nurse should ask the patient to move the affected limb.

Neurologic assessment should be done in all areas. In the upper extremities, five major nerves should be assessed: the circumflex, the musculocutaneous, the median, the ulnar, and the radial. The sensory portion of the circumflex artery should be tested over the deltoid area. Motor function can be tested by having the patient abduct the arm at the shoulder. The sensory portion of the musculocutaneous nerve can be tested at the radial side of the forearm. The motor function can be tested by having the patient flex at the forearm. The sensory portion of the median nerve is tested at the palmar surface of the thumb, index, and long fingers (Fig. 16–2*A*). Motor function can be tested by having the patient appose the thumb to the little finger (Fig. 16–2*B*) (Schoen 1986).

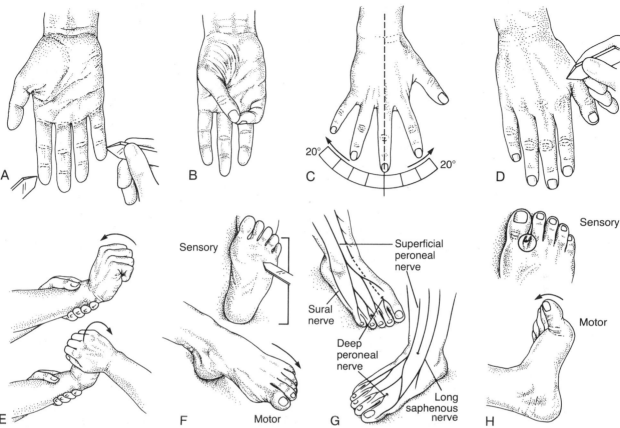

FIGURE 16-2. *A*, The sensory functions of the median and ulnar nerves can be tested at the radial portion of the palm and the ulnar side of the hand respectively. *B*, Motor function of the median nerve is assessed by testing apposition of the thumb and fingertips. *C*, Motor function of the ulnar nerve is assessed by finger abduction. *D*, The sensory function of the radial nerve may be tested at the web space between the thumb and index fingers. *E*, The motor function of the radial nerve may be tested by having the patient extend the wrist. *F*, The sensory function of the tibial nerve may be tested by touching the sole of the foot. The motor function of the tibial nerve may be tested by having the patient plantar flex the toes. (Reprinted with permission from Urbankski P. 1984. The orthopedic patient: identifying neurovascular injury. AORN J, 40:710. Copyright by AORN, Inc, 10170 East Mississippi Avenue, Denver, CO 80231.) *G*, Sensory nerve distribution in the foot and ankle. (Reproduced with permission from Hoppenfeld S: Physical Examination of the Spine and Extremities, copyright Appleton-Century-Crofts, Norwalk, CT, 1976.) *H*, The sensory function of the peroneal nerve may be tested by touching the web space between the great and second toes. The motor function of the peroneal nerve may be tested by asking the patient to dorsiflex the toes. (Redrawn with permission from Urbanski P. 1984. The orthopedic patient: identifying neurovascular injury. AORN J 40:710. Copyright © AORN, Inc, 10170 East Mississippi Avenue, Denver, CO 80231.)

The sensory portion of the ulnar nerve can be tested at the palmar surface of the little finger (Fig. 16-2A). Motor function can be tested by having the patient abduct and adduct all fingers (Fig. 16-2C). The sensory portion of the radial nerve can be tested at the web space between the thumb and forefinger (Fig. 16-2D). Motor function is tested by having the patient extend the wrist and fingers (Fig. 16-2E).

Three major nerves that should be checked in the lower extremities are the femoral, the obturator, and the sciatic. Sensation related to the femoral nerve is felt along the medial side of the foot and leg as low as the medial malleolus. Motor function involves the quadriceps femoris muscle. The obturator nerve has a sensory distribution along the medial side of the thigh. Motor function involves the adductor muscles of the thigh. The sciatic nerve divides into the posterior tibial and common peroneal nerves. The sciatic nerve is responsible for most of the motor and sensory function of the leg supplying the hamstring muscles in the thigh and the muscles below the knee. The motor function of the posterior tibial nerve is tested by having the patient plantar flex the ankle and flex the toes (Fig. 16-2F). Sensory function is checked at the medial and lateral surfaces of the foot (Fig. 16-2G). Motor function of the common peroneal nerve is tested by having the patient dorsiflex and extend the toes (Fig. 16-2H). Sensory function is tested at the lateral surface of the great toe and medial surface of the second toe (Schoen 1986).

Inspection

The nurse observes how a patient actively moves a limb if the patient is able to do so, assessing for guarding of the area or facial grimacing. These signs suggest the presence of pain and should be documented. Abnormal configurations along an otherwise even area of an extremity should be documented because this indicates a possible disruption of bone and soft tissue (Walt 1982). Much information can be obtained from astute observational skills. Precise documentation of these findings is essential.

Palpation

Following inspection, the nurse palpates the extremities proximally to distally, examining the injured area last to avoid painful muscle spasms that might occur when painful areas are palpated. These spasms make further examination difficult. Evaluation for increased pain, crepitus, displacement, edema, and temperature and for decreased or absent pulses, paresthesia, or paralysis can be done while palpating the extremities. The joint above and the joint below a fracture are palpated because twisting or wrenching movements can also injure the soft tissues surrounding the joint. The presence or absence of the active range of motion of a joint should be observed and documented. A joint should not be forced into full range of motion.

Reflexes

Reflexes are graded on a scale of 0 to 4+, with 0 being equal to no response and 4+ equal to a hyperactive response. Normal reflex response is 2+. The examiner should use discretion in assessing deep tendon reflexes in relation to the extremity and severity of the musculoskeletal trauma.

Muscle Strength

The examiner should use care and discretion in assessing the muscle strength of an injured limb. Muscle strength should not be tested when there is an obvious fracture or dislocation. Muscle strength may be graded on a scale of 0 to 5, with 0 being equal to no strength and 5 being equal to a normal contraction. The patient is asked to push against the fixed resistance of the examiner's hand, and the force the examiner feels is compared with that of the opposite extremity and documented.

In summary, assessment and a thorough history and physical examination are a part of the first phase of the nursing process and vital in the nursing care of the musculoskeletal trauma patient. A well-organized approach facilitates the process and helps the nurse obtain a significant amount of data efficiently. These data provide a baseline for future comparison of assessments of the patient.

FRACTURES

Classification of Fractures

A fracture is a partial or a complete disruption in the continuity of bone.

Although there are numerous ways to classify fractures, no single method describes all aspects of a fracture. Radiographs play an essential part in diagnosing fractures and lend the basis for most of the categories. Five general categories of terms can describe a fracture (Simon and Koenigsknecht 1987). The first group, based on *anatomic location,* includes such terms as proximal, distal, head, shaft, and base. These terms describe where the bone is fractured.

The second category describes the *direction of the fracture* (Fig. 16–3). A transverse fracture occurs at 90 degrees to the axis of the bone. An oblique fracture is at 45 degrees to the axis of the bone. A spiral fracture twists around the shaft of the bone. When the bone has more than one fracture line and more than two fragments, it is described as a comminuted fracture. Segmental and butterfly fractures are types of comminuted fractures. A greenstick fracture is an incomplete fracture often seen in children. An impacted fracture is one in which one fragment is driven into another so the fracture line is not quite visible.

A third way to categorize fractures is according to the *relationship of the fracture fragments to each other* (Fig. 16–4). The alignment describes the relationship of the axis of fragments to each other in degrees of angulation. Apposition describes how the fragments contact each other (e.g., "bayonet") (Fig. 16–5).

A fourth way to group fractures is according to their *stability.* Stable fractures are unlikely to be displaced after reduction, whereas unstable fractures are likely to be displaced after reduction.

The fifth category of fractures includes *associated soft tissue injuries.* This group

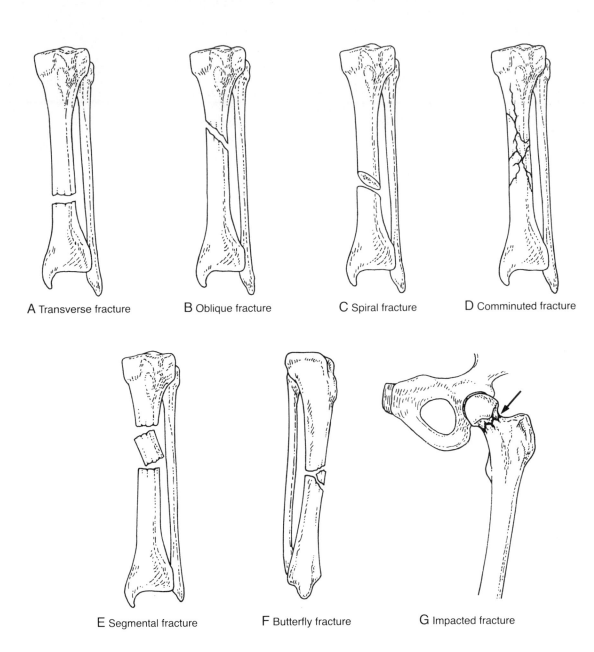

A Transverse fracture   B Oblique fracture   C Spiral fracture   D Comminuted fracture

E Segmental fracture   F Butterfly fracture   G Impacted fracture

FIGURE 16–3. Fractures classified according to the direction of the fracture. (Reprinted with permission, from Koenigsknecht SR: Emergency Orthopaedics: The Extremities, copyright Appleton & Lange, Norwalk, CT, 1987.)

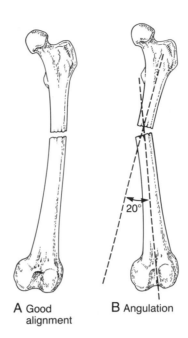

FIGURE 16–4. Fractures can be described by the relation of distal fragments. Angulation is measured by drawing an imaginary line through the long axis of both fragments and measuring the resulting angle. *A*, Fracture with good alignment without angulation. *B*, Fracture with an angulatory deformity of the distal fragment of about 20 degrees. (Reprinted with permission, from Koenigsknecht SR: Emergency Orthopaedics: The Extremities, copyright Appleton & Lange, Norwalk, CT, 1987.)

A Good alignment

B Angulation

includes closed fractures, in which there is no break in the skin; open fractures, in which there is a break in the skin (Fig. 16–6); complicated fractures, in which additional trauma such as neurovascular or ligament injuries is present; and uncomplicated fractures, in which a minimal amount of tissue is injured.

Fractures can also be described according to their mechanism of injury: direct or indirect trauma (Rockwood and Green 1984). Direct trauma can cause tapping,

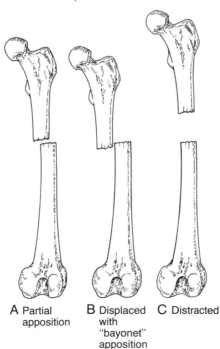

FIGURE 16–5. *A*, A partially apposed fracture. *B*, A displaced fracture in which the two ends also overlap with a shortening of the bone. *C*, Fracture ends are displaced so they are pulled apart. (Reprinted with permission from Koenigsknecht SR: Emergency Orthopaedics: The Extremities, copyright Appleton & Lange, Norwalk, CT, 1987.)

A Partial apposition

B Displaced with "bayonet" apposition

C Distracted

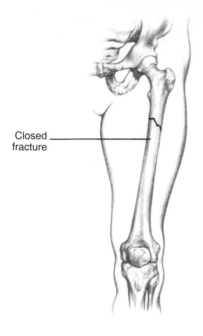

Closed
fracture

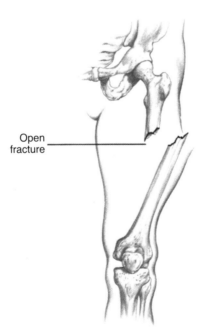

Open
fracture

FIGURE 16–6. Closed and open fractures. (From Stearns C, Brunner, N., 1987. Trauma Fracture Management, 13. Orthopaedic Nursing Care: A Nursing Guide, vol 3. Courtesy of Howmedica, a Division of Pfizer Hospital Product Group, Inc.)

crush, or penetrating (gunshot) fractures. A small force of dying momentum applied to a small area of bone can cause a tapping fracture. This fracture results from frequent hits to a bone with a blunt instrument. Crush fractures are usually comminuted, with much soft tissue damage resulting from a large force on a large area. High-

or low-velocity projectiles such as bullets cause penetrating fractures. These injuries result from a large force on a small area. High-velocity bullets cause much tissue damage and can splinter bone into additional numerous small projectiles, which can lodge in soft tissues or organs (Rockwood and Green 1984).

Indirect trauma can cause traction or tension, angulation, and rotational (twisting) fractures. The pull of a muscle or ligament on bone can be strong enough to cause a traction or tension or avulsion fracture. Angulation fractures can occur as compression force has been placed on the concave portion of the bone and tension placed on the convex portion. Because bone is stronger under compression than under tension, the bone on the convex portion cracks, and bone fibers on the concave portion splinter. Rotational fractures occur when the bone has been twisted (Rockwood and Green 1984).

Etiology and Biomechanics

Extrinsic and intrinsic properties of the bone determine at what point it will fracture. Extrinsic properties include the magnitude, duration, direction, and rate of force applied to the bone. When force is applied to bone, the bone can either deform owing to strain or resist deformation and undergo stress. Force, strain, and stress are experienced as compression, tension, and shear, respectively. Compression is a pressing together, tension is a pulling apart, and shear is a force parallel to the bone (Odling-Smee and Crockard 1981).

Intrinsic properties of bone include the energy-absorbing capacity of bone, its modulus of elasticity (or how it sustains stress), fatigue strength, and density (Rockwood and Green 1984). Energy is absorbed by the surrounding soft tissue when force is applied to bone. The more quickly a bone receives force, the more energy there is to be absorbed. The ratio of muscle mass to bone weight in a healthy average adult is 2:4, but this ratio decreases with age (Odling-Smee and Crockard 1981). This decrease in ratio could, in part, account for the increased incidence of fractures in the elderly. With aging, bone also becomes more porous and thus has less strength, which can also be considered a decrease in density. The modulus of elasticity describes how bone recovers its form once a force is removed. This is analogous to how a rubber band responds after it has been stretched. Fatigue strength describes how long a bone can sustain a repeated stress before it breaks. A good example is a stress fracture. By understanding the properties of bone in relation to the forces that cause fractures, the nurse can better assess and anticipate treatment for the musculoskeletal trauma patient.

Clinical Manifestations

A fracture is a partial or complete disruption of the continuity of the bone. Signs and symptoms of a fracture include (1) pain or tenderness at the injured area; (2) deformity either in alignment, contour, or length; (3) localized ecchymosis; (4) edema; (5) loss of function related to pain, muscle spasm, or bone instability; (6) crepitus on palpation or movement of the injured limb; and (7) visible evidence on radiographs (Chase et al 1986, Schoen 1986). A stress fracture may not be evident on initial radiograph so repeat films should be done in 10 to 15 days on a limb with bone tenderness. Clinical manifestations for upper and lower extremity fractures are similar and will not be discussed in great detail.

Pelvic Fractures

Pelvic fractures can be the most life-threatening of all fractures owing primarily to the large amount of blood loss that can accompany them (2 to 3 L at times). These fractures can be classified according to their mechanism of injury, displacement or anatomic location, and effect on the stability of the pelvis (Fig. 16–7).

Pelvic fractures often have perineal, groin, suprapubic, and flank bruising as presenting features, which implies pelvic disruption. Gentle compression applied to the ischial tuberosities will produce pain in the patient with a pelvic fracture. This is sometimes called the "barrel hoop test" or the "pelvic rock." Likewise, pressure applied over the symphysis pubis will exacerbate pain associated with a pelvic fracture. Urethral, vaginal, and rectal bleeding also may occur and may indicate an open fracture. Pelvic deformity may be obvious, as may a discrepancy in leg length on comparing the limbs.

Nursing Care for Musculoskeletal Injuries

Although treatment of fractures usually takes place during stage II emergency care, appropriate steps to stabilize the patient's cardiovascular system occur during stage I. The interventions discussed in this section reflect the priority of care in appropriate sequence.

Once the patient's condition has been stabilized, the fracture is immobilized. Immobilization prevents further soft tissue injury, limits pain, and limits the release of fat globules from long bone fractures, which can lead to fatal fat emboli. Fat emboli can occur at the time of fracture and can be fatal at the time of trauma if they are massive enough. The specific treatment of a fracture (traction, casting, or splinting) depends on numerous variables: patient age, type and location of fracture, presence of soft tissue damage, and the potential cosmetic effects of the reduction (Chase et al 1986).

Fluid Volume Deficit, Related to

- *Hemorrhage at Fracture Site from Bone, Soft Tissue, and Surrounding Vessels*

Blood loss due to long bone fractures can often be underestimated (Table 16–2). The blood accumulates in the surrounding soft tissue and accounts for much of the increase in size of the extremity. One method of assessing the amount of blood loss from a fracture is to measure the circumference of the injured limb as soon as possible and again periodically throughout the patient's stay in the ED. The bleeding is slow and sometimes difficult to assess. Such bleeding is common with shoulder and pelvic

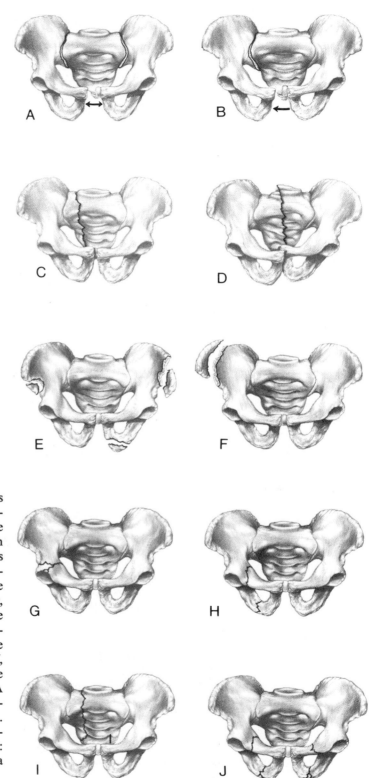

FIGURE 16–7. Classification of pelvic fractures according to their mechanism of injury, displacement, or anatomic location and their effect on the stability of the pelvis. *A, B,* Open book fractures in which there is distraction of two sides of the pelvis anteriorly at the symphysis pubis. *C,* Lateral compression fracture in which two sides of the pelvis are driven into each other anteriorly and posteriorly. *D,* Vertical shear fracture in which two sides of the pelvis are forced in opposite directions. *E, F,* Avulsion fractures. *G,* Acetabular fracture. *H,* Single break in the pelvic ring at the ischiopubic rami. *I,* Fracture at the sacrum. *J,* Unstable saddle fracture or fractures of the bilateral ischial and pubic rami. A Malgaigne fracture is any combination of one anterior and one posterior fracture or joint disruption. (From Stearns C, Brunner N., 1987. Trauma/Fracture Management, 16. Orthopaedic Nursing Care: A Nursing Guide, vol 3. Courtesy of Howmedica, a Division of Pfizer Hospital Product Group, Inc.)

TABLE 16-2
Estimated Blood Loss in
Fractures (Liters)

Humerus	1.0–2.0
Elbow	0.5–1.5
Forearm	0.5–1.0
Pelvis	1.5–4.5
Hip	1.5–2.5
Femur	1.0–2.0
Knee	1.0–1.5
Tibia	0.5–1.5
Ankle	0.5–1.5

Source: Walt AJ, ed. 1982.
Early Care of The Injured Patient.
WB Saunders, 284.

girdle injuries as well as the thigh and multiple extremity injuries (Walt 1982). Death can occur from exsanguination from pelvic and femoral fractures. Blood loss is often greater than expected and can continue up to 48 hours post fracture. Bleeding can be limited by gentle handling of the fracture, prompt reduction, and immobilization (Walt 1982).

To judge the extent of blood loss the nurse should assess the admission hemoglobin and hematocrit values to see if they are within normal limits. Usually they are normal, even if there is hemorrhage, because equal parts of plasma and red blood cells (RBCs) are lost. The initial hemoglobin and hematocrit values should be compared to later values. Dressings should be checked for copious bright red drainage and monitored. Hourly urine output should be monitored to ensure that the kidneys are functioning and fluid volume status is sufficient. A 30-ml per hour urinary output is evidence of adequate renal perfusion. A decreasing urine output, hypotension, and tachycardia indicate fluid volume deficit and impending hypovolemic shock. Fluid resuscitation with crystalloid and colloid may be necessary. (See Chap. 6 on Multiple Trauma.)

Tissue Perfusion, Altered (Peripheral), Related to

- *Vascular Damage*
- *Vessel Compression Due to Edema*
- *Vessel Compression Due to Compartment Syndrome*

Compression in tissue perfusion of an extremity can be due to vascular damage from bone fragments or vessel compression owing to edema or compartment syndrome. Blood loss can be limited by immobilization of a fracture, but major vessel damage often requires surgery to reanastomose severed vessel ends. An emergent problem exists if an extremity is pulseless. The physician should be notified and preparation made for possible immediate realignment of the fracture.

To limit the expected edema that occurs with a fracture, the extremity should be elevated above heart level. Elevation of the limb and application of ice to the area also help decrease the amount of bleeding. When the adequacy of arterial circulation is in question, the limb should be placed at heart level. Elevation, in this case, may further compromise arterial flow.

Compartment syndrome is an increase in the pressure within a muscle sheath following musculoskeletal trauma. It can occur up to 6 days post trauma, but usually occurs between 12 hours and 3 days after the trauma. The increased pressure can compress blood vessels and compromise circulation in the already injured extremity. The nurse should assess for the classic signs of this syndrome, which include (1) paresthesia along the muscle compartment; (2) pallor; (3) pain out of proportion to the injury and not alleviated by narcotics; (4) pain on passive stretch of the muscle; and — an extremely late sign — (5) pulselessness. Diagnosis may be confirmed by insertion of a catheter into the muscle compartment to measure pressure within the muscle. There is controversy regarding the danger values for compartment pressure elevations. The most aggressive recommendation for fasciotomy uses 30 mmHg as the determining level, whereas the most conservative recommendation uses 60 mmHg (Strange and Kelly 1988).

Immediate treatment of compartment syndrome is the splitting of a constrictive cast or removal of constrictive bandages around the involved limb. The limb should not be elevated higher than heart level. Ice is not a treatment of choice in this case. If these interventions fail to relieve the symptoms, treatment is usually an emergency fasciotomy. If numerous limbs have been involved, the nurse should assess for myoglobinuria.

Pain, Related to

- *Fracture*
- *Soft Tissue Injury*

Splinting or immobilization of an injured extremity should decrease pain, as should elevation of the limb and application of ice. Narcotics are administered only after head and abdominal injuries have been thoroughly assessed and stabilized. Pain that cannot be managed adequately could be a sign of compartment syndrome. Extreme gentleness is required when manipulating or repositioning the patient's injured extremity. It is important to explain what will be done prior to any movement. This allays anxiety and helps diminish pain associated with evaluation and treatment.

Skin Integrity, Impaired, Related to

- *Open Fracture*

An open fracture is one in which the bone breaks through the skin. Attempts should not be made to push the exposed bone back beneath the skin, because this can lead to further trauma to surrounding structures and also to infection. A sterile dressing should be placed over the wound until a physician can examine it and decide on a course of treatment. Bacteriostatic agents are sometimes applied and prophylactic broad-spectrum intravenous antibiotics may be administered.

Tissue Integrity, Impaired, Related to

• *Fracture*

Soft tissue can be damaged by a fracture even though the fracture ends do not break the skin. The fracture ends can puncture the soft tissue and cause bleeding. The force that causes the fracture can also traumatize the soft tissue. Ice, cold packs (even on a cast), compression with an elastic wrap, and elevation of the injured extremity are the interventions of choice for soft tissue injury.

Infection, Potential, Related to

• *Open Fracture*
• *Open Wound with Fracture*

Once there is a break in the skin the patient is prone to a wound infection and possibly osteomyelitis. These infections can most often be attributed to *Staphylococcus aureus* with gram-negative bacilli (Simon and Koenigsknecht 1987). Infection that is due to direct contamination is usually localized. Other causes of osteomyelitis include contamination from a skin infection. Peripheral vascular disease can complicate infections.

Although infection will not be obvious in the ED, it is the nurse's role to try to prevent the initiation of infection during this stage of care. This includes monitoring aseptic technique in treating the wound, administering prophylactic antibiotics ordered, and determining if the patient should receive a tetanus vaccination. Cultures of open fractures should be undertaken prior to cleaning and dressing application.

Sensory-Perceptual, Altered (Kinesthetic and Tactile), Related to

• *Peripheral Neurovascular Injury from Extremity Fracture*
• *Peripheral Nerve Compression from Compartment Syndrome*

Nerve injuries can occur in a similar manner as described for vascular injuries. Methods of testing for specific nerve damage are listed in Figure 16–2.

Urinary Elimination, Altered Patterns of, Related to

• *Pelvic Fracture*

Because the major components of the urinary system are housed within the pelvic cavity, injury to the urinary tract should be suspected with all pelvic fractures. The nurse should assess for supraumbilical swelling, which might suggest either a perivesical hematoma or a distended bladder. Blood at the meatus may be a sign of urethral injury. Other signs of possible urinary injury include ecchymosis in the perineum or perianal area (scrotum and thighs). Men are more likely to sustain lower urinary tract injury than women owing to the greater length of the male urethra. If a urinary tract injury is suspected, placement of an indwelling catheter by the nurse is contraindicated. (Genge 1986) (see Chap. 14). Radiographs of the urinary tract assist in diagnosis of specific injuries.

Mobility, Impaired Physical, Related to

• *Lower Extremity Fracture*

The patient should be instructed to actively exercise uninjured limbs at least three times a day. Specific attention should be paid to the upper extremities, which will bear most of the body weight for the injured limb. The triceps muscles will need to be strengthened so the patient can use assistive devices, such as crutches or canes, for ambulating. Exercises that help strengthen the triceps muscles include the following: (1) The patient assumes a sitting position and with a weight in each hand, flexes the arms and extends the hands above the head; (2) the patient pushes down on the bed or floor to lift the buttocks off the bed or floor (Schoen 1986)

The patient should also be encouraged to perform isometric exercises on injured limbs as ordered by the physician, to maintain muscle tone and facilitate recovery.

In the case of lower extremity fractures, the patient may be unable to ambulate without the use of assistive devices, such as crutches or canes. The nurse should instruct the patient how to use such devices. Safe return demonstration should be required prior to discharge from the ED.

First, the patient should practice balancing on the unaffected extremity next to a chair. The patient should be properly fitted for crutches to assure safe ambulation. Adjustable crutches are versatile and can accommodate a patient's progress throughout recovery. Two methods of approximating crutch measurement include the following:

1. While the patient is supine in bed, measure from the anterior fold of the axilla to the sole of the foot and add 5 cm.

2. While the patient is standing, measure from 3.75 to 5.0 cm below the axillary fold to a point on the floor 10 cm in front of the patient and 15 cm laterally from the small toe (Schoen 1986).

Once the patient has been fitted for crutches, have the patient assume a tripod position with the cruches under the arms and the rubber tips 10 cm in front and 10 cm on each side. This tripod position provides the most solid and balanced support. There should be a two finger – width space between the axillary fold and the armpiece on both sides. While the patient is standing erect, with the shoulders and back straight, he or she should be able to flex the elbow at 30 degrees, extend the wrist, and dorsiflex the hand. The hands, not the axilla, should support the weight of the body. Bearing weight at the axilla could damage the brachial plexus even though the armpieces are padded. In addition, the patient should be instructed to wear flat shoes that fit properly.

Selection of a crutch gait depends on variables such as type and severity of

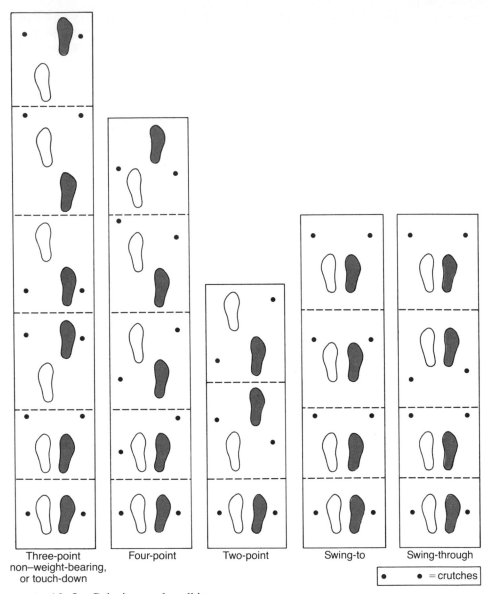

| Three-point non–weight-bearing, or touch-down | Four-point | Two-point | Swing-to | Swing-through |

•   • = crutches

FIGURE 16–8. Gaits in crutch walking.

disability or injury; the patient's physical status; arm, leg, and trunk strength; the patient's sense of coordination and balance; how much weight (nonweight bearing; partial weight bearing; touch-down weight bearing) the affected limb can bear; and whether the crutches are to be utilized for balance or for support. If the patient is taught two gaits, the gaits can be alternated and fatigue reduced by alternating the use of different muscles (Schoen 1986). The five common crutch gaits begin in the tripod position and are as follows (Fig. 16–8).

1. The *three-point gait* requires the most strength and balance because the patient supports all the body weight on the arms. The sequence includes: (a) movement of the weaker leg with both crutches simultaneously; then (b) movement of the stronger leg. This gait is used when one leg is nonweight-bearing (Schoen 1986).

2. The *two-point gait* deals with two points of contact at one time in the following sequence: (a) right crutch and left foot; (b) left crutch and right foot. The gait is quicker than the four-point gait (Schoen 1986).

3. A *four-point gait* is used when both legs can bear weight because three points of contact are maintained with the floor. This is believed to be the safest gait because it provides the most balance. Weight is constantly being shifted in the following seqeunce: (a) right crutch, (b) left foot, (c) left crutch, (d) right foot. (Schoen 1986).

4. The *"swing-to" gait* is utilized by patients with weak leg, abdominal, and back muscles. To move, the patient moves the crutches forward about 30 to 45 cm, lifts the body with the hands on the crutches, and brings the legs to the crutches, regains balance, and continues (Schoen 1986).

5. The *"swing-through" gait* can be used by patients who are stronger and more able to maintain their balance when the body is moved forward. To move, the patient moves the crutches forward, lifts the body with the hands on the crutches, and brings the legs past the crutches, straightens, regains balance, and continues (Schoen 1986).

Besides instructing the patient on ambulation on level ground, the nurse should also instruct the patient on how to get up and down stairs as well as how to get in and out of a chair with crutches.

In going down stairs, the patient should begin from the edge of the stair and lead with the affected weaker limb. With the crutch on the affected side and with weight on

FIGURE 16–9. Correct crutch-walking technique when climbing or descending stairs.

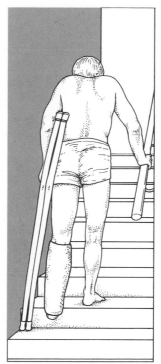
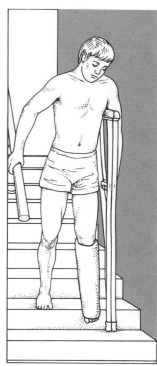

the unaffected leg, the patient should bend at the hip and knee and place the crutch on the next lower step. The stronger leg should then be brought down to share the work of lowering the body with the crutch.

To walk up stairs with crutches, the patient begins with the crutch on the affected side a half-step width from the lowest step. Placing his or her weight on the hands, the patient lifts the stronger leg to the step. An easy way for the patient to remember what limb to lead with is "up with the good and down with the bad" (Fig. 16–9).

To get into a chair, the patient should back up to the chair until it is felt behind the legs. The crutches should be held by hand on the unaffected side. With the hand on the affected side, the patient should reach for the chair seat, bend at the waist, bring the affected leg forward, and sit.

To get out of the chair, the patient does the opposite by pushing off the seat with the hand on the affected side and pulling up on both crutches, which are both on the unaffected side. Or the patient can use one crutch on each side and grasp at the handles to lift out of the chair (Fig. 16–10).

A patient can use a cane instead of crutches for support and balance. To properly fit a patient with a cane, the nurse should have the patient flex the arm on the affected side at the elbow about 25 to 30 degrees and position the cane with the handle even with the level of the greater trochanter.

To ambulate with a cane, the patient should hold the cane close to the body on the unaffected side and move the cane forward just less than one pace in front. The patient should lean on the cane and move the affected leg forward so it is alongside the stick. While the patient is leaning on the cane, the unaffected leg should be moved

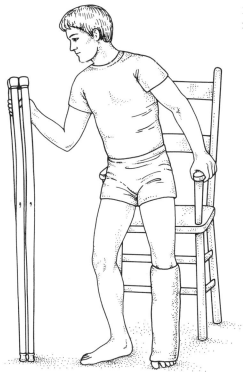

FIGURE 16–10. Correct method of getting into and out of a chair when using crutches.

forward slightly ahead of the cane. The body weight is shifted to the unaffected leg, and the affected leg and cane are then moved forward. Two canes can be used with the four-point and two-point gaits used with crutches.

When the patient goes up stairs with canes, he or she should step up with the unaffected leg and follow with the cane and affected leg. The patient should follow the opposite sequence going down stairs.

Potential Problems Related to Casting

- *Knowledge Deficit of Cast Care*
- *Pressure from Cast on Bony Prominences*
- *Deterioration of Cast*

A cast is often applied to a fractured area to provide temporary immobilization of the fracture. Cast materials vary and include plaster of Paris and synthetic materials, such as polyester-cotton knit, Fiberglas, and Thermoplast. Casts can be applied to various parts of the upper and low extremities as well as to the torso (body spicas). Potential complications following casting include neurovascular compromise, incorrect fracture alignment, cast syndrome or superior mesenteric artery syndrome, or compartment syndrome.

Superior mesenteric artery syndrome can occur with body casts when there is traction placed on the superior mesenteric artery. This causes a decreased blood flow to the bowel. Signs and symptoms include nausea, vomiting, and abdominal pain.

Before applying the cast, the nurse should explain to the patient the purpose of the cast, where it will be placed, the process, the equipment used, and the need to maintain proper position while the cast is being applied.

Plaster and synthetic casts differ in their composition. Plaster casts should be left open to air dry. The cast should be supported with the palms instead of the fingers to avoid indenting the plaster. The cast should be placed on a soft surface, such as a cloth pillow (not plastic) to prevent flattening of the cast and containment of heat. The patient should be repositioned every 2 hours to promote drying of the cast. The patient should not bear weight on the cast until it is completely dry. The cast should be kept dry by covering it with plastic when the patient showers or is in the rain. The cast can be cleansed with a mild powdered soap and damp cloth only when needed.

Synthetic casts dry quickly and patients can bear weight in 30 minutes (depending on their physician's orders). This type of cast can be placed in water. It should be flushed out well with clear water after the patient bathes or swims. It can be dried using a towel and cool hair dryer to thoroughly dry the inside and prevent maceration of the skin.

A stockinette is usually placed on the extremity prior to casting and used as a finishing edge on the cast. Pressure points inside the cast are padded.

The patient should be instructed not to place anything inside the cast. The patient should report any burning sensation or pressure over a bony prominence to the physician immediately. Skin around the edges of the cast should be assessed for redness and for breakdown. Odor or drainage from the cast may suggest a pressure sore (Thompson et al 1986).

Anxiety, Related to

• *Orthopedic Trauma*
• *Alteration in Body Image*

Both trauma and a fracture are anxiety-producing occurrences. Although the trauma episode is short-lived, the effects are long-lasting. The trauma may cause an alteration in body image and in lifestyle.

The nurse should explore with the patient and help identify what coping mechanisms have been utilized in the past in dealing with anxiety and stress. Often the patient will need to replay the incident verbally to work through the anxiety. It is important to take the time to allow the patient to verbalize.

Evaluation

Evaluation of a person who has sustained a fracture requires astute observation. Complications associated with fractures are not as obvious as those related to other systems. Blood loss can be insidious and blood values as well as other signs and symptoms of hypovolemia (decreased urine output, decreased blood pressure (BP), increased pulse) need to be assessed continually. Circulation, sensation, and movement of affected limbs also need to be assessed continually and compared to baseline data. Pain, the most obvious problem, needs to be assessed and monitored more with musculoskeletal trauma because of the potential detrimental effects it may suggest. Tissue and skin integrity need to be examined closely to assess for extensive injury, which may lie hidden beneath the surface. Osteomyelitis needs to be prevented through aseptic techniques. The patient's safety must be anticipated following discharge, so patient instructions regarding the proper use of assistive devices and proper cast care are essential.

FAT EMBOLISM SYNDROME

Fat embolism syndrome is most commonly associated with multiple fractures of the long bones, pelvis, tibia, femur, and ribs and with crush injuries. Two theories attempt to explain the occurrence of fat embolism. The mechanical theory states that bone marrow pressure becomes greater than venous pressure and fat enters the venous circulation. The degree of fat influx is thought to be related to mobility, fracture management, and nearby mechanical factors. The metabolic or biochemical theory states that following trauma, free fatty acids and neutral fats are released, leading to platelet aggregation and fat globule formation. Fat emboli are deposited in lung capillaries and cause an acute pulmonary disorder similar to acute respiratory distress syndrome (VanNoy and Genge 1986)

Clinical Manifestations

Major symptoms of fat embolism are respiratory insufficiency, cyanosis, disorientation, and petechial rash. Minor symptoms include pyrexia, tachycardia, retinal changes, jaundice, and renal problems. Twenty-five per cent of the patients with suspected fat embolism exhibit these symptoms within 12 hours and 75 per cent exhibit them within 36 hours of injury. Sixty to 70 per cent show some degree of hypoxemia (Simon and Koenigsknecht 1987).

Treatment and Nursing Care

Impaired Gas Exchange, Related to

- *Fat Embolism*

Alcohol, heparin, dextran, and corticosteroids are possible medications for treatment. Alcohol can cause vasodilation and inhibit lung lipase. Heparin can clear the plasma of chylomicrons and promote circulation. Dextran is used to promote perfusion and is a volume expander. Corticosteroids reduce interstitial pulmonary edema (Knezevich 1986).

The severity of hypoxemia is assessed by arterial blood gas (ABG) values, which often show a Po_2 value as low as 60 to 70 mmHg (less at higher elevations). Early treatment contributes to a successful outcome, so the patient should be assessed for the earliest symptoms: dyspnea without a change in the level of consciousness, tachycardia, and elevated temperature. Diagnostic data that help confirm the diagnosis include lipuria, elevated serum lipase, thrombocytopenia, a decrease in Po_2, "snowstorm" appearance of lungs on chest radiograph, and EKG changes (Knezevich 1986). The lungs should be auscultated for moist crackles. In many patients the classic petechiae are not visible. Respiratory distress may be managed with supplemental oxygen and intubation with positive end expiratory pressure (PEEP) or continuous positive airway pressure (CPAP) for patients with respiratory compromise. Serial ABGs should be monitored.

Potential for Injury, Related to

- *Fat Embolism*

The frequency of fat embolism can be limited by immobilizing the injured limb as soon as possible; moving the limb as little and as gently as possible; replacing lost blood; and preventing hypotension (Knezevich 1986). Nurses can attempt to control the bleeding, do periodic neurovascular assessment, and splint or immobilize the injury. The most significant factor in identification of fat embolism is early recognition of the onset of respiratory compromise.

TRAUMA TO JOINT: DISLOCATIONS AND SUBLUXATIONS

A dislocation is the displacement of bone from its normal position in a joint to the degree that the articulating surfaces lose contact. Dislocation may be classified as congenital (dislocated hip), pathologic (joint disease), or traumatic (external force) (Schoen 1986). In the instance of a subluxation, the articulating surfaces lose contact only partially (Chase et al 1986). This injury occurs when a joint goes beyond its normal range of motion.

Etiology

No particular age group is prone to dislocation. Dislocation results from either an indirect or a direct force applied to a joint. Upper extremities sustain an indirect force from a fall on an outstretched arm or from a direct blow to the joint. Knees can be dislocated by a twisting motion or a direct hit. Hips dislocate posteriorly when a force is applied along the femur shaft while the hip is flexed and abducted. Hips dislocate anteriorly when they are forced into extension, abduction, and external rotation. Central hip dislocations happen particularly when the hip is abducted and sustains a severe lateral blow (Chase et al 1986).

Clinical Manifestations

To obtain a thorough assessment of the patient who has suffered either a joint dislocation or subluxation, the nurse should first obtain a history of the trauma. Pre-existing joint deformity or compromise should be determined. Although any joint can dislocate, some joints are more apt to do so than others. Signs of joint dislocation vary with location of the joint. Common signs of dislocations include obvious deformity of the joint, pain on range of motion or movement, and change in length of the affected extremity. Because dislocations can cause nerve and blood vessel entrapment, a thorough neurovascular assessment should be done on the involved extremity.

The shoulder, or glenohumeral joint, is the most common upper extremity joint to dislocate and occurs most often with an anterior dislocation of the humerus. The shoulder can also dislocate posteriorly. Recurrent dislocations are common. With shoulder dislocations, the unaffected shoulder may appear higher and more straight (Fig. 16 – 11). The patient may hold the affected arm close to the body (which appears longer in abduction and external rotation). Shoulder dislocation can produce painful, limited range of motion.

An elbow dislocation occurs when the humerus, radius, and ulna shift from their normal anatomic positions. This happens only with great force and often results in soft tissue and neurovascular damage. This injury is more common in young children with falls on an outstretched hand. Wrists rarely dislocate. Fingers can dislocate at the interphalangeal and metacarpophalangeal joints, usually as a result of hyperexten-

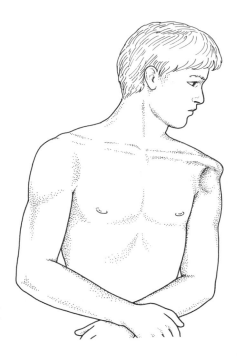

FIGURE 16–11. The dislocated shoulder loses its full lateral contour and appears indented under the point of the shoulder.

sion of the joint. Dislocation of the metacarpophalangeal joint of the thumb is the most common finger dislocation.

The most common lower extremity dislocations occur in the knee. Knees can dislocate in many directions: anteriorly, posteriorly, medially, or laterally, depending on the position of the tibia in relation to the femur, but the most common is the anterior dislocation. Rotational injuries are easy to recognize by the depression over one of the femoral condyles. The patella can dislocate by shifting from the femoral groove. Effusion may or may not occur, and there may be difficulty in attempting to extend the knee. Once the leg is extended, the patella shifts back into place.

Hips are composed of large bones and muscles and normally are stable joints; however, if severe trauma is sustained, they can dislocate either posteriorly or anteriorly. With a central hip dislocation, there is usually a fracture through the acetabulum (Chase et al 1986). These injuries are easily recognized by the description of the trauma. When a leg is held in flexion, abduction, and internal rotation and is shorter than the unaffected leg, a posterior hip dislocation should be suspected (Fig. 16–12). When the leg is held in extension, abduction, and external rotation, an anterior hip dislocation should be suspected. This type of dislocation can cause peroneal nerve injury and, as a result, loss of dorsiflexion of the foot. There may also be decreased sensation on the dorsal aspect of the foot and at the base of the first and second toes (Chase et al 1986). Radiographs once again provide the definitive diagnosis.

Treatment and Nursing Care

In general, initial interventions for dislocations should include gentle palpation of the joint and adequate splinting. Stage I treatment should include rapid reduction for

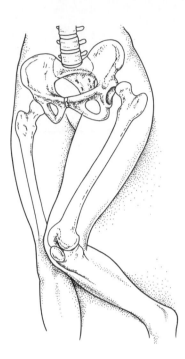

FIGURE 16–12. A posterior dislocation of the left hip.

a neurovascularly compromised limb. The dislocation should ideally be reduced in a hospital setting unless there is obvious neurovascular compromise. Then gentle manipulation and realignment can be attempted in an effort to improve neurovascular status. Reduction should be done under anesthesia or sedation as soon as possible to avoid neurovascular compromise.

Treatment for dislocations following reduction can range from conservative management with slings or traction to surgical interventions. Depending on the severity of the dislocations treatment can range from a sling without reduction, to closed reduction and immobilization for about 3 weeks, to an open reduction with internal fixation with removal of the pin after about 6 weeks. Shoulder dislocations are often reduced manually without surgery and the shoulder immobilized in a sling for 4 to 6 weeks. Elbow dislocations are often reduced under anesthesia and casted at 90 degrees for about a month. Wrist dislocations can be reduced closed and casted from 2 weeks to 3 months. Finger dislocations can often be reduced by manual traction with slight flexion. The finger is then immobilized in slight flexion for about 1 week. Sometimes the end of the dislocating bone goes through the joint capsule with the capsule folding around the bone end ("buttonhole" effect), thus hindering reduction. An open reduction and surgical repair of the capsule is then required (Schoen 1986). Knee dislocations are reduced closed and splinted with posterior support. Patellar dislocations are treated by repairing the surrounding musculature and establishing more stable skeletal support. The knee is allowed to heal for a short period, and then gentle exercises are begun on the joint. Hip dislocations should be reduced in a timely manner to avoid avascular necrosis. The joint can then be casted or supported with a brace to prevent recurrence of the dislocation. If reduction of a dislocation cannot be achieved with closed manipulation, surgery may be required.

Surgery is also suggested if fractures are assumed to have occurred with the dislocation. Radiographs should always be obtained after reduction to look for fracture sites.

Pain, Related to

- *Dislocation or Subluxation*
- *Related Soft Tissue Injury*

As with pain management for fractures, narcotics are not administered for pain until cerebral and abdominal traumas have been assessed and treated. Intravenous diazepam (Valium), midazolam (Versed), or narcotics may be administered to reduce pain and enhance muscle relaxation. Once the dislocation has been reduced, the pain should be alleviated. Ice may then be applied to the area. Supporting the extremity also lessens the stress on the joint and thus the pain.

Anxiety, Related to

- *Pain*
- *Treatment*
- *Decreased Extremity Function*
- *Decreased Joint Mobility*

Once the pain from the dislocation is controlled, anxiety should decrease. The nurse should explain all interventions clearly and allow the patient time for questions to alleviate fear of the unknown in relation to care. The nurse should also explain to the patient why mobility of the joint and decreased extremity function exist. The patient should also be given an anticipated time frame for recovery and told that the joint might be at risk to dislocate more easily in the future than a healthy joint.

Tissue Perfusion, Altered (Peripheral), Related to

- *Dislocation or Subluxation*
- *Soft Tissue Injury*

Stage I care is aimed at preventing increased morbidity with neurovascular compromise. Dislocation of the articulating surfaces of a joint can lead to impairment of the neurovascular status both around the joint and distal to the injury. Edema from trauma to soft tissue around the joint could cause compression on the nerves and vessels. A thorough neurovascular assessment distal to the injured joint should be conducted. Neurovascular assessment was discussed at the beginning of this chapter and will not be covered in detail here. When neurovascular compromise is evident, immediate reduction of the dislocation or subluxation is necessary to restore circulation and neurologic function and prevent overall morbidity.

Tissue Integrity, Impaired, Related to

- *Dislocation or Subluxation*
- *Soft Supports*

Soft tissue trauma may occur not only from injury to the joint but also as a result of treatment. Soft supports, such as bandages, slings, and immobilizers, can compress the injured area. The nurse should assess the patient to make certain that dressings are applied appropriately and are neither irritating the skin nor constricting vessels or nerves.

Evaluation

Most close observation of a patient with a dislocation should take place during the first stage of emergency care prior to reduction. The nurse at this time should be monitoring the patient for any change in neurovascular status of the affected limb. Following reduction, the nurse should assess the neurovascular status of the limb distal to the dislocation for any change or compromise. Early detection could avoid permanent damage.

The patient should be instructed regarding analgesics and care of the extremity. Application of supportive devices, such as slings or braces, should be taught as well as activity restrictions for the affected limb.

TRAUMA TO THE EXTREMITY: AMPUTATIONS

Traumatic amputation of an extremity challenges the ED nurse to both care for the patient and attempt to save the amputated part. Although the patient may not have suffered multiple injuries, the trauma of amputation affects the entire person.

Clinical Manifestations

Although salvage of the amputated limb is important, life-threatening injuries need to be treated first, in all cases. The past medical history, as described at the beginning of the chapter, should be obtained. The following specific information should also be obtained: time and type of amputation, time of warm and cold ischemia, completeness and level of amputation, whether or not the dominant hand was amputated, and previous injuries to the amputated limb (O'Hara 1987).

Treatment and Nursing Care

Treatment of the amputee includes care of the patient physiologically and psychologically as well as care of the amputated body part in anticipation of potential replantation. Successful replants require calm nursing care and keeping the body part cool and dry (O'Hara 1987).

Fluid Volume Deficit, Related to

- *Blood Loss Secondary to Amputation*

Fluid volume deficit is a possibility in the amputee. Severed vessels retract, clamp down, and clot off within moments. Partially lacerated arteries require direct pressure to limit bleeding. To prevent ischemia, the use of tourniquets or clamping or tying of severed vessels is not advised. Elevation of the limb and application of a soft pressure dressing are suggested.

Infection, Potential, Related to

- *Contamination from Trauma Site*

Prophylaxis against infection should include administration of an intravenous antibiotic such as cefazolin, 1 g. Tetanus toxoid should be administered if the patient has not had prophylaxis within the past 5 years. The extremity and amputated part should both be rinsed in normal saline to remove debris. A sterile saline-moistened gauze should cover the stump and then be covered with a dry sterile gauze.

Tissue Perfusion, Altered (Peripheral), Related to

- *Ischemia at Stump*
- *Tissue Maceration of Body Part*
- *Increased Warm and Cold Ischemia Time*

Although the patient may be bleeding, the anticoagulation process essential for the future life of the replanted extremity should begin at this time. With the approval of the microsurgeon, a-600 mg aspirin suppository is administered.

All amputated parts should be saved. The parts should be rinsed with normal saline to remove surface dirt. The parts should then be dried and wrapped in dry gauze, put in a sealable plastic bag, and placed on ice (preferably not Dry Ice, which would be too cold). The part should not be buried in the ice. Moist dressings are avoided because they can macerate the tissues.

In the case of partially amputated parts, time limits for replantation are important. The limb and part cannot be put on ice because blood flow would be further compromised. Interventions should be concerned with limiting "ischemia time." Lack of blood flow, and thus anoxia, leads to cellular edema and fluid loss in the interstitial extracellular spaces. Muscle tissue loses its reactivity within 2 to 4 hours. Digits can tolerate longer ischemic periods than limbs because there is little muscle tissue (O'Hara 1987).

Replantation of an extremity or digit is considered on the basis of function as opposed to aesthetics. Amputated thumbs are usually replanted because the thumb is responsible for 40 to 50 per cent of the hand's function. Because children possess a great ability to regenerate nerves and adapt to sensory and motor changes well, replantations are usually considered for them. If multiple digits are amputated, replantation is considered to restore function. Replantations of amputations at the palm, wrist, or proximal forearm usually result in good functional results (O'Hara 1987). Nursing diagnoses related to pain and anxiety have already been covered. Discussion of rehabilitation of the amputee is beyond the scope of this chapter.

Evaluation

Evaluation of the patient who has experienced a traumatic amputation requires initial assessment of blood loss. Amputees are often alert and oriented, so assessment of their coping ability is important. Explanations regarding interventions should be honest and not foster false hopes of regaining the past integrity of the severed limb. The nurse should stress to the patient that anything that can be done will be done to care for the injury.

TRAUMA TO SOFT TISSUE: SPRAINS AND STRAINS

Etiology and Pathophysiology

A sprain is trauma to the ligaments around a joint. The trauma is usually a sudden twist or hyperextension of the joint. Sprains may be classified as either mild (grade 1), moderate (grade 2), or severe (grade 3). Mild sprains involve only a few ligamentous fibers that are torn or separated. There is a small localized hematoma. Moderate sprains involve about half of the ligament fibers. With a severe sprain, the entire ligament is torn and, at times, can be separated from the bone (Chase et al 1986). The ligament provides stability to the joint and promotes mobility. Thus, when the ligament is torn the joint loses its functional stability.

Sprains are not unique to any age group. Common upper extremity sprains include the wrist, whereas common lower extremity sprains involve the lateral ligaments of the ankle and knee. The cervical spine is prone to extension sprains.

Strains are similar to sprains but involve muscles and tendons. A strain is trauma to the body of a muscle or tendon from overstretching or misuse (Chase et al 1986). As with sprains, strains can be classified as mild, moderate, or severe and occur at any age. A mild strain is due to mild stretching of the muscle or tendon, with some inflammation and disruption of muscle or tendon tissue. With a moderate strain there is a moderate stretch or tear of the muscle or tendon. A severe strain involves severe muscle or tendon stretching. In this case, the muscle or tendon can rupture completely. Muscle can tear away from muscle, muscle can tear away from a tendon, or tendon can tear away from bone (Schoen 1986).

MUSCULOSKELETAL EMERGENCIES

Clinical Manifestations

Signs of a sprain vary with the degree of injury. All sprains show some degree of edema, ecchymosis, and tenderness. Moderate and severe sprains exhibit some degree of loss of function and possibly deformity as well. Radiographs are obtained to assess the presence of avulsion fractures.

Similarly, signs of strains vary with the degree of injury. Tenderness and muscle spasms are present in all strains to some degree. In moderate and severe strains, edema and ecchymosis are also present; however, the ecchymosis is usually delayed. Passive motion of the joint increases discomfort.

Treatment and Nursing Care

Treatment of both sprains and strains follows the mnemonic RICE: rest, ice, compression, and elevation. Cold compresses applied intermittently for 24 hours after the sprain, plus rest and elevation of the injured limb, slow down the extravasation of blood and lymph into surrounding tissues and help reduce pain. After 24 hours, warm applications to the area may be made four times a day to foster reabsorption of the blood and lymph (Schoen 1986). Compression via elastic bandage provides support to the joint. For severe sprains, casts are used as opposed to elastic bandages. In severe strains, surgery is sometimes necessary to suture the muscle and surrounding fascia. Complications after a sprain can include recurrent sprains, an unstable joint, and traumatic arthritis. Complications following strains include recurrent strains, tendinitis, and periostitis of the tendon attachment (Schoen 1986).

Pain, Related to

- *Sprain*
- *Strain*

Analgesics, generally acetaminophen with codeine, may be administered orally to alleviate the discomfort of a sprain or strain. The nurse should again be aware of possible compartment syndrome. Pain should decrease if the RICE method of sprain and strain treatment is followed in the ED and after discharge.

Tissue Integrity, Impaired (Ligament, Muscle, Tendon), Related to

- *Sprains*
- *Strains*

The nurse must be cognizant of the signs and symptoms of sprains and strains to recognize them early in the ED and to initiate appropriate treatment to facilitate the healing process. Resting and elevating the limb limit pressure on vital vessels and nerves. Ice limits hemorrhage into tissue, which can cause more tissue damage.

Compression adds stability to temporarily unstable joints, thus avoiding further injury.

Knowledge Deficit, Related to

- *Sprains and Strains*
- *Care of Sprains and Strains*

Because a patient with a strain or sprain will not remain in the ED for a prolonged period, nor will he or she be likely to be hospitalized, patient education must occur prior to discharge. The patient needs to be cautioned that because a joint has sustained trauma once, it is at risk for injury again owing to a degree of instability. Until the joint is well healed—about 6 weeks if the patient follows RICE therapy—care should be taken by the patient not to place undue stress on the joint.

Evaluation

The nurse needs to intermittently assess the patient who has sustained a strain or sprain for neurovascular compromise. However, if the appropriate interventions are taken, chances for such compromise are minimal. The nurse should evaluate the patient's level of comprehension of instructions. Ambulation with assistive devices should also be assessed.

The RICE method of treatment should be reviewed with the patient. The patient should be instructed on the appropriate use of assistive devices and analgesics. If the patient is athletic, instructions should be given regarding how to decrease the future occurrence of soft tissue injuries, such as sprains and strains.

TRAUMA TO SOFT TISSUE: BURSITIS AND TENDINITIS

Bursitis is an inflammation of one or more of the bursae. A bursa is an enclosed synovial fluid–filled sac that facilitates motion. Tendinitis is the inflammation of a tendon. Bursae are located near tendons and therefore the terms *tendinitis* and *bursitis* are often used interchangeably. Tenosynovitis is an inflammation of a tendon and its sheath.

These problems occur most frequently in adults 40 to 50 years of age, with women being affected more often than men.

Bursitis or tendinitis is due to either direct trauma to the area, strain, systemic disorders, congenital defects, postural malalignment, abnormal body development, or repetitive motion with injury. History of the injury usually includes unusual strain or injury 2 to 3 days prior to onset of pain, localized pain radiating to the extremity, sudden or gradual pain, and pain on motion. Early stage radiographs are usually normal, with later evidence of calcium deposits. Signs and symptoms include the cardinal signs of inflammation: swelling, irritation, tenderness, erythema.

Treatment and Nursing Care

Treatment for bursitis or tendinitis depends on how severe the inflammation is. Anti-inflammatory medications and corticosteroids may be administered. Hydrocortisone injections may be administered to the area. The swollen subcutaneous bursae may also be aspirated. The nurse should instruct the patient to avoid stressing the affected joint and to support it when moving it. The patient should maintain joint mobility with prescribed exercises.

CONCLUSION

Musculoskeletal injuries occur over the entire lifespan. Although often they are not life-threatening injuries, emergency care may be required to avoid long-term complications related to these injuries. Quality emergency nursing care begins with astute assessment skills and a thorough knowledge of the mechanism of injury and the patient's medical and psychosocial history. The plan of care and interventions are continuously assessed while the patient is in the ED. The psychosocial aspect of the patient's care, evident throughout the patient's stay in the ED, should also be addressed.

Discharge from the ED is either to a critical care unit in the hospital, a surgical unit, the operating room, or—if the injuries are minor—home. If the patient is discharged home, nursing care also includes patient teaching regarding care of the injury and activities involved with recovery (e.g., crutch walking, wound care).

REFERENCES

Chase MA, Bolander V, Kasal SE, et al. 1986. Trauma. In Pellino TA, Mooney NE, Salmond, SW, et al, eds. Core Curriculum for Orthopaedic Nursing. Pitman, NJ, Anthony Jannetti, 163–183.

Genge M. 1986. Orthopaedic trauma: Pelvic fractures. Orthop Nurs 5(1):11–19.

Hilt NE, Cogburn SB. 1980. Manual of Orthopedics. St Louis, CV Mosby Co.

Hoppenfeld S. 1977. Orthopaedic Neurology. Philadelphia, JB Lippincott Co.

Key JA, Conwell HE. 1951. Management of Fractures, Dislocations and Sprains. St Louis, CV Mosby Co.

Knezevich BA. 1986. Trauma Nursing: Principles and Practice. Norwalk, CT, Appleton-Century-Crofts.

Odling-Smee W, Crockard A, eds. 1981. Trauma Care. New York, Grune & Stratton.

O'Hara M. 1987. Emergency care of the patient with a traumatic amputation. J Emerg Nurs 13:272–277.

Rauscher N. 1986. Musculoskeletal assessment. In Pellino TA, Mooney KE, Salmond SW, et al. eds. Core Curriculum for Orthopaedic Nursing. Pitman, NJ, Anthony Jannetti, 17–38.

Rockwood CA, Green DP. 1984. Fractures in Adults, vol 1. Philadelphia, JB Lippincott Co.

Rodts M. 1986. Orthopaedic emergencies. In Cahill SB, Balskus M, eds. Intervention in Emergency Nursing: The First Sixty Minutes. Rockville, MD, Aspen Publishers, 269–279.

Schoen DC. 1986. The Nursing Process in Orthopaedics. Norwalk, CT, Appleton-Century-Crofts.

Simon RR, Koenigsknecht RJ. 1987. Emergency Orthopaedics: The extremities, 2nd ed. Norwalk, CT, Appleton-Lange.

Stearns CM, Brunner NA. 1987. Opcare: Orthopaedic Patient Care: A Nursing Guide, vol 3. Trauma/Fracture Management. Bridgewater, NJ, Howmedica (Division of Pfizer Hospital Product Group).

Strange JM, Kelly PM. 1988. Musculoskeletal injuries. In Cardona VD, Hurn PD, Mason PJB, et al (eds). Trauma Nursing from Resuscitation Through Rehabilitation. Philadelphia, WB Saunders, 543.

Thompson D, Blanke K, Fueyo L, et al. 1986. Common concerns: Casts. In Pellino TA,

Mooney NE, Salmond SW, et al, Core Curriculum for Orthopaedic Nursing. Pitman, NJ, Anthony Jannetti, 89–92.

Urbanski P. 1984. The orthopedic patient: identifying neurovascular injury. AORN J 40:707–711.

VanNoy E, Genge M. 1986. Complications. In Pellino TA, Mooney NE, Salmand SW, et al, eds. Core Curriculum for Orthopaedic Nursing. Pitman, NJ, Anthony Jannetti, 111–120.

Walt AJ, ed. 1982. Early Care of the Injured Patient. Philadelphia, WB Saunders Co.

Wolff LW, Weitzel MH, Zarnow RA, et al, eds. 1983. Fundamentals of Nursing. Philadelphia, JB Lippincott Co.

Stephen Adams, MD

Neurologic Emergencies

Persons admitted to the Emergency Department (ED) with alteration in mental status present a challenge to the ED nurse. Nurses must have the knowledge and insight to manage these patients and the foresight to anticipate and react to changes. The central nervous system (CNS) is complex and vital to normal functioning of most organ systems in the body. Causes of neurologic disorders are varied, yet the nursing care required for each is similar. Delivering care and anticipating changes in status require a thorough understanding of the CNS and pathophysiology of specific disorders.

ASSESSMENT

Initial assessment of the neurologically impaired patient begins with the triage interview. Patients with altered mental status may be unable to communicate verbally. The chief complaint may have to be obtained from allied medical personnel, friends, family, or witnesses. Presenting history may include personality change, trauma, seizure activity, the use of pills, empty bottles on the scene, a history of diabetes and insulin usage, or alcohol or drug abuse (or both). Using observation skills and communication techniques, the triage nurse quickly assesses the mental status of the patient and identifies the signs and symptoms leading to the nursing diagnoses associated with different neurologic disorders.

Further history obtained by the triage nurse may help determine the cause of the complaint. For patients who are actively having seizures, is there a known history of seizure disorder? Were there witnesses to the event, and was the seizure typical? Is the patient compliant with anticonvulsant medications, or does the patient have a seizure disorder that is difficult to control? Does the patient have diabetes mellitus and could the seizure be a manifestation of hypoglycemia? Does the patient abuse alcohol? Is there a history of antecedent infection? Was there a history of headache? Was trauma involved before, during, or after the seizure?

If the triage nurse suspects that the patient has had a cerebrovascular accident (CVA), further information is necessary. Does the patient have a history of transient ischemic attacks (TIA) or other neurologic deficits? If so, how long has the patient had the deficits and are they progressing or regressing? Was there any antecedent trauma? Does the patient have a history of cardiac dysrhythmias (such as atrial fibrillation), which may promote mural thrombi and increase the risk of stroke? Are there other risk factors that predispose the patient to ischemic neurologic events, such as hypertension, hypercholesterolemia, triglyceridemia, cigarette smoking, diabetes mellitus, polycythemia, or alcoholism? A medication history may indicate such risk factors as the use of oral contraceptives or anticoagulants.

The triage nurse should be selective in questioning the patient, family, or allied medical personnel. Obtaining the history should take only a few moments. A more complete history can be obtained while medical and nursing care is being carried out to stabilize the patient.

Objective assessment by the triage nurse should include vital signs and a brief assessment focusing on mental status and respiratory and neurologic systems. The rate and regularity of the patient's pulse and respirations should be noted. What is the patient's Glasgow Coma Scale (GCS) score: eye opening, verbal response, motor response? (Refer to Chapter 18 for details concerning the GCS score.) Cardiovascular status and respiratory status are reflected in the color and temperature of the skin. Diaphoresis and clammy skin may suggest hypoglycemia as responsible for change in mental status. Note any obvious signs of trauma. Neurologically, observe for facial droop or extremity paralysis. If seizure activity is occurring, describe the seizure clearly, with respect to onset, location, progression, cessation, and duration. Physical assessment in all neurologically impaired patients begins with evaluation of airway patency, ventilatory rate and pattern, and hemodynamic stability. Stridorous or gurgling respirations may indicate airway obstruction and require immediate suction and placement of an oral or nasopharyngeal airway. An unresponsive and non-breathing patient is a candidate for endotracheal intubation to prevent aspiration and support oxygenation.

Once an effective airway is ensured, the respiratory rate, pattern, depth, and effort are evaluated, noting use of intercostal muscles, abdominal muscles, or supraclavicular retractions. Characteristic breathing patterns have been noted to coincide with various stages of neurologic dysfunction. There are five types of respiratory patterns: the normal respiratory pattern, Cheyne-Stokes breathing, central neurogenic hyperventilation, apneustic breathing, and agonal breathing. Each pattern represents a lesion in a specific area of the brain and aids in defining the cause of or localization of the lesion. Figure 17–1 describes respiratory patterns and site of the lesion.

Blood pressure, pulse, and cardiac rhythm should be evaluated next. Alterations

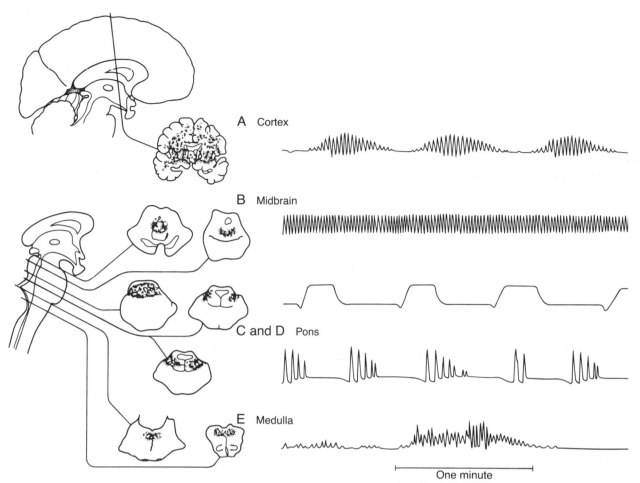

A Cortex

B Midbrain

C and D Pons

E Medulla

One minute

FIGURE 17–1. Abnormal respiratory patterns associated with pathologic lesions (shaded areas) at various levels of the brain. Tracings by chest-abdomen pneumograph, inspiration reads up. *A,* Cheyne-Stokes respiration. *B,* Central neurogenic hyperventilation. *C,* Apneusis. *D,* Cluster breathing. *E,* Ataxic breathing. (Redrawn from Plum F, Posner JB. Diagnosis of Stupor and Coma. FA Davis, 3rd ed, 1980, 34.)

in hemodynamic stability that reduce tissue perfusion may contribute to impaired mental status. Therefore, hemodynamic and cardiac monitoring is important in detecting abnormal vital signs and recognizing variations occurring over time. Intravenous access at this point provides a route for drug administration or fluid resuscitation. If the suspected cause of altered mental status is trauma, or if there is any evidence of head or neck injury, immobilize the cervical spine completely with a hard collar, towel rolls laterally, and tape across the head attached to a long back board. Cervical spine radiographs should be obtained to ascertain injury and rule out fracture, dislocation, or subluxation of vertebrae.

Because hypoglycemia is one of the major causes of altered mental status and is

TABLE 17–1
The Cortical Examination

Cortical Function	Mental Task	Abnormal Response	Suspected Cortical Area
Attention	Spell "earth" backwards. Perform serial sevens test	Improper letter sequence; one or more errors or taking more than 90 seconds to complete	Frontal lobes Frontal lobes
Language Expression	Repeat: "no ifs, ands, or buts," "Methodist Episcopal," "each fight readied the boxer for the championship bout"; listen to spontaneous language for fluency	Dropping words or syllables, repeating syllables, dropping ends of words; nonfluent speech—mostly nouns or verbs, no conjunctions; reading ability usually intact	Dominant frontal lobe (Broca's area)
Reception	Repeat: "Take this book, put it on the window sill, and give me the ashtray"; listen to spontaneous language for fluency	Appreciable difficulty understanding; reacting to isolated words; fluent, effortless speech, often with no nouns; marked reading and writing difficulty; repetition poor	Dominant temporal lobe (Wernicke's area)
Naming	Point to common objects and have patient name them—e.g., pen, stethoscope, book, key	Wrong word (paraphasia): describing function rather than giving name of object	Angular gyrus, dominant temporal lobe
Reading, writing, comprehension	Perform individual tasks of this sentence: "Copy this sentence and read it aloud"	Inability to write in flowing manner; loss of sentence structure	Dominant temporoparietal lobe
Amnestic processes Orientation	Name day of week, month, year, and location	Any error	Frontal lobes if other memory intact; frontal-diencephalon if new learning memory involved
Immediate recall	Remember "brown, honesty, tulip, and eyedropper"; digit recall	One or more errors	Language cortex. Temporal or frontal lobes (hippocampus)
New learning memory	Remember the four words above 3, 10, and 30 minutes after hearing them	One or more errors	Diencephalic structures (hippocampi, mamillary bodies, dorsal medial thalamic nuclei)
Long-term memory	Recite U.S. presidents' names in reverse chronological order; recall historical events	Loss of data; transpositions or loss of proper sequence	Appropriate cortical association area—e.g., language cortex for names
Constructional ability	Copy the outline of a three-dimensional cube, Greek cross, or door key	Loss of symmetry; difficulty with angles; perseveration or closing in on figure	Nondominant parietal lobe if distorted; frontal lobes if perseveration

Source: Granacher RP. 1981. Psychosomatics 22:485–499.

easily correctable, evaluation of the blood glucose level is essential. A blood glucose level of less than 80 mg/dl should be considered hypoglycemic and treated with 50 mEq of dextrose intravenously. If 50% dextrose (D50) was administered to the patient in the prehospital setting, a follow-up blood glucose determination is in order. It may be necessary to repeat the dose. Various products are available for bedside determination of blood glucose levels and are discussed in Chapter 20.

Neurologic Evaluation

Once the patient's condition has been stabilized initially, a thorough evaluation of the CNS is indicated. The evaluation may be modified, depending on the patient's mental status. If the patient is unresponsive, the voluntary response aspects of the examination will be deleted and the examination should focus on reflex or involuntary responses.

Mental status examination partially reflects cerebral function. To participate in a thorough assessment of mental status, the patient must be awake and aware of the environment. The purpose of the mental status examination is to determine if the patient is capable of making appropriate, intelligent responses to the environment and, if not, to identify deficits. Table 17–1 illustrates the specific tests for evaluating cortical function and summarizes the abnormal responses and suspected areas of insult.

Pupillary changes reflect possible causes of coma and may herald the onset of herniation of the brain. Cranial nerve III, located in the midbrain, innervates the ciliary muscles responsible for pupillary reactivity. Pupils should be examined in ambient light, in darkness, and with a directed light source for symmetry of shape, size, and reactivity. They should be round in shape and equal in size. Normal pupillary size in moderate light is approximately 3 mm. A small segment of the

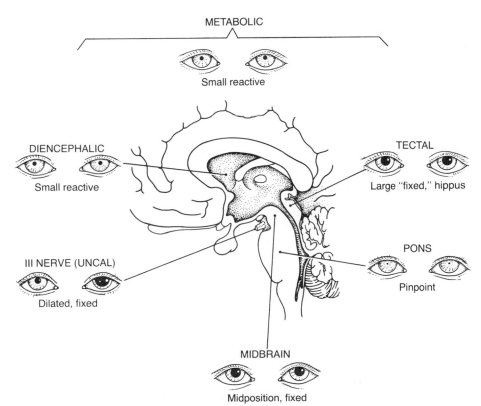

FIGURE 17–2. Pupils in comatose patients according to level of the lesion. (Redrawn from Plum F, Posner JB. Diagnosis of Stupor and Coma. FA Davis, 3rd ed, 1980, 46.)

population (5 to 10 per cent) has anisocoria or unequal pupils. This abnormality does not indicate pathology, and both pupils should react equally to light. It is important to test the reactivity of the pupils with a light strong enough to evoke a response. A magnifying glass may be necessary if the pupil is so constricted that reactivity is barely visible. Figure 17–2 illustrates various pupillary configurations associated with brain lesions.

Obtaining a thorough medication history is essential. Certain drugs will alter pupillary configuration and response and mask presenting symptoms. Table 17–2 describes the effects of selected drugs on pupillary size and reactivity.

The ability to open and close the eyelids depends on intact brain stem sensory pathways. For patients who appear unresponsive and do not open their eyelids upon request, evaluation of eyelid response to tactile stimuli may provide clues to the level of consciousness. In the unresponsive patient, the eyelids are closed by the clonic contraction of the orbicularis oculi muscle. If the nurse lifts the lids and releases them, they should close gradually. A patient who is hysterical cannot mimic this response.

The corneal reflex (CNV) is tested in unconscious patients to determine brain stem function. A corneal response is elicited by gently stimulating the cornea with a fine wisp of cotton using care to avoid causing corneal abrasion. A normal response in the patient with brain stem function is bilateral lid closure and upward deviation of the eye (Bell's phenomenon) (Plum and Posner 1980).

Assessment of extraocular movements (EOMs) (cranial nerves III, IV, and VI) provides an indication of cranial nerve function in the awake patient. Deficits in EOMs indicate a lesion in the CNS. In the unconscious patient, however, when standard examination is not possible the examiner depends on evaluation of reflexes to determine cranial nerve function. Two such reflexes include the oculocephalic and oculovestibular reflexes.

Doll's Eye Phenomenon (Oculocephalic Reflex)

After ensuring that no cervical spine injury is visible on radiographs, the doll's eye phenomenon can be tested in the unconscious patient. The head is rotated to one side

TABLE 17–2
Specific Drug Effects on the Pupils

	Pupillary Response
Drugs	
Atropine or scopolamine	Dilation—fixed
Glutethimide (Doriden)	Moderate dilation—fixed
Barbiturates	Midposition to moderate dilation
Epinephrine	Midpoint fixed—constricted
Opiates	Pinpoint
Conditions	
Anoxia	Dilated—fixed (transient—permanent)
Hypothermia	Fixed
Metabolic encephalopathy	Small
Iridectomy	Asymmetric and nonreactive
Prosthetic eye	Fixed
Cataracts	Nonreactive
Blindness	Nonreactive

while the eyelids are held open and the eyes are observed. A normal response is contraversive conjugate deviation of the eyes — that is, the eyes should deviate to the left with head rotation to the right, and the converse. The presence of this reflex, called the oculocephalic reflex, indicates an intact brain stem. It is mediated by peripheral vestibular inputs to the vestibular nuclei and their interconnections to the nuclei of cranial nerves III, IV, and VI, which control conjugate eye movements. This maneuver tests this system using a physiologic stimulus. The oculocephalic reflex cannot be assessed in the awake patient (Plum and Posner 1980) (Fig. 17–3).

Ice Water Calorics (Oculovestibular Reflex)

If the oculocephalic reflex cannot be elicited in the unresponsive patient, a response to ice water calorics may be evaluated. This procedure evaluates the integrity of the brain between the extraocular muscles and the vestibular nuclei in the brain stem using a supraphysiologic stimulus. The reflex response, also known as the oculovestibular reflex, is caused by excitation of the semicircular canals, which stimulate the vestibular nerve and activate the extraocular muscles (Plum and Posner 1980).

The ears are examined for evidence of tympanic membrane perforation and patency of the canals. If there is no evidence of perforation and injury to the cervical spine has been ruled out, the following procedure is performed. With the patient's head elevated 30 degrees, using a flexible catheter (a butterfly with the needle removed will function well) and a syringe, the tympanic membrane is irrigated through the aural canal with 50 to 100 ml of ice water. After about 30 seconds, the examiner should note tonic and symmetric deviation of both eyes to the side of the irrigation. This indicates the extraocular muscles are intact and no lesions exist from the vestibular nuclei to the extraocular nuclei and their cranial nerves. In the unresponsive patient, the fast component of nystagmus is lost after waiting about 5 minutes. The opposite ear should be tested to determine intactness of the other side. A person in psychogenic coma will exhibit the fast component of nystagmus away from the irrigated side, and may become nauseated and complain of intense ear pain. Figure 17–3 illustrates both reflexes.

If the patient is awake and cooperative, ascertain symmetric movement of the palate and uvula (cranial nerves IX and X) by asking the patient to say "ahh" or to yawn. Stimulation of the back of the throat to elicit the gag reflex should be evaluated in every patient with possible neurologic dysfunction to determine the ability to maintain a patent airway. This can be assessed in a patient who does not respond to verbal commands by applying gentle pressure to the chin and lowering the mandible to open the mouth. A tongue blade can be inserted to stimulate the posterior pharynx.

In the alert, cooperative patient, the motor examination reveals the patient's strength and equality of movement. Muscle groups are evaluated in an effort to discern a generalized weakness or to localize a specific deficit. It is important to note weakness or paralysis and to recognize changes early in the course of illness .

When mental status changes render the patient unable to follow directions, the examiner uses the patient's response to noxious stimuli to assess motor response. Acceptable noxious stimuli used to evoke a response include nailbed, supraorbital, or suprasternal pressure. Three responses may be elicited: appropriate, inappropriate, and absent. These responses depend on the severity of neurogenic dysfunction. An

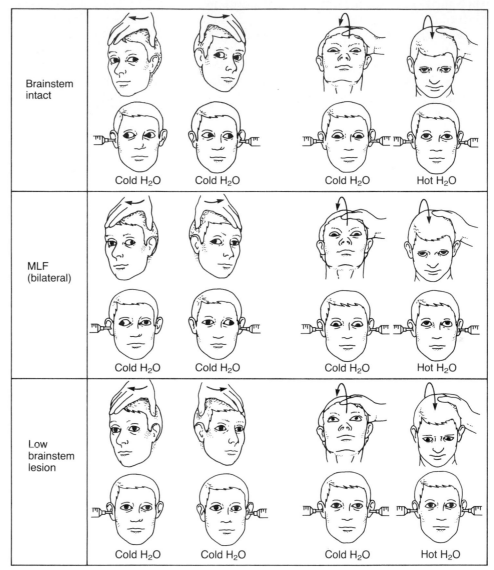

FIGURE 17–3. Ocular reflexes in unconscious patients. The upper section illustrates the oculocephalic (above) and oculovestibular (below) reflexes in an unconscious patient whose brain stem ocular pathways are intact. Horizontal eye movements (upper left) to head turning are full and opposite in direction to the movement of the face. A stronger stimulus to lateral deviation is achieved by douching cold water against the tympanic membrane(s). There is tonic conjugate deviation of both eyes toward the stimulus; the eyes usually remain tonically deviated for 1 minute or more before slowly returning to the midline. Because the patient is unconscious, there is no nystagmus. Extension of the neck in a patient with an intact brain stem produces conjugate deviation of the eyes in the downward direction, and flexion of the neck produces deviation of the eyes upward. Bilateral cold water against the tympanic membrane likewise produces conjugate downward deviation of the eyes, whereas hot water (no warmer than 44°C) causes conjugate upward deviation of the eyes.

appropriate response to noxious stimuli is either withdrawing from the stimulus or purposefully pushing the stimulus away.

If neurologic impairment occurs at the level of diencephalon, midbrain, or pons, the patient may exhibit either decorticate or decerebrate posturing spontaneously or in response to noxious stimuli. A decorticate response is manifested by varying degrees of flexion of the arms at the elbows, the wrists, and the fingers. The shoulder is abducted and flexed. The posturing response may be unilateral or bilateral depending on the location and nature of the lesion. The legs are extended and rotated internally and the feet are plantar flexed. This type of response reflects a lesion that interferes with the internal capsule of the cerebral hemisphere and interrupts the corticospinal pathways.

A decerebrate response is one in which the patient clenches the teeth and adducts, extends, and hyperpronates the arms. The legs are extended and the feet are plantar flexed. This response is seen with a lesion in the midbrain or upper brain stem. Unless it is associated with a metabolic coma, this type of posturing has a poor prognosis (Plum and Posner 1980) (Fig. 17–4).

If the patient is flaccid and does not respond to painful stimuli, the prognosis is generally poor. The pathologic reflexes associated with anatomic lesions are illustrated in Figure 17–4.

Deep tendon reflexes in the comatose patient often yield little valuable information concerning the patient's condition (Scherer 1986). In the patient who is awake, deep tendon reflexes are assessed for symmetry and graded on a scale of 0 to 4+, defined as follows:

0   Absent
1   Diminished
2   Normal
3   Hyperactive
4   Hyperactive with clonus

A screening sensory examination is useful in discerning the patient's perception of light touch, pinprick, and proprioception. In comparing symmetric areas, abnor-

---

In the middle portion of the drawing, the effects of bilateral medial longitudinal fasciculus (MLF) lesions on oculocephalic and oculovestibular reflexes are shown. The left portion of the drawing illustrates that oculocephalic and oculovestibular stimulation deviates the appropriate eye laterally and brings the eye, which would normally deviate medially, only to the midline, because the medial longitudinal fasciculus, with its connections between the abducens and oculomotor nuclei, is interrupted. Vertical eye movements often remain intact.

The lower portion of the drawing illustrates the effects of a low brain stem lesion. On the left, neither oculovestibular nor oculocephalic movements cause lateral deviation of the eyes because the pathways are interrupted between the vestibular nucleus and the abducens area. Likewise, in the right portion of the drawing, neither oculovestibular nor oculocephalic stimulation causes vertical deviation of the eyes. On rare occasions, particularly with low lateral brain stem lesions, oculocephalic responses may be intact even when oculovestibular reflexes are abolished. (From Plum F, Posner JB. Diagnosis of Stupor and Coma. FA Davis, 3rd ed, 1980, 55.)

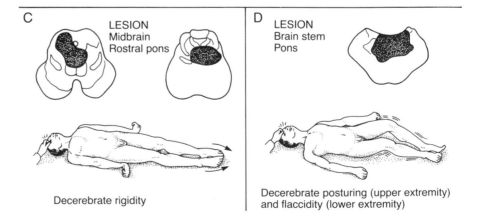

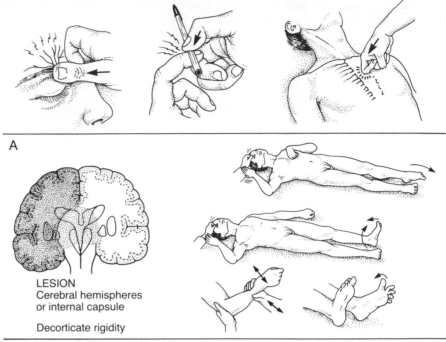

A

LESION
Cerebral hemispheres
or internal capsule

Decorticate rigidity

B

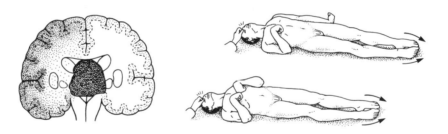

Decorticate or decerebrate rigidity

C   LESION
           Midbrain
           Rostral pons

Decerebrate rigidity

D   LESION
    Brain stem
    Pons

Decerebrate posturing (upper extremity)
and flaccidity (lower extremity)

malities such as numbness may be seen in the patient who has suffered a CVA or has other localized lesions.

ETIOLOGY AND PATHOPHYSIOLOGY

Dysfunction of the CNS is caused by one of three mechanisms: (1) actual disruption of the integrity of the CNS by mass effect, such as from blood, a tumor, or a missile; (2) impairment of the blood supply or of its individual substrates (oxygen and glucose); (3) substances toxic to the CNS, such as poisons and drugs. If the CNS is deprived of oxygen or glucose, neuronal or axonal hypoxemia occurs within 5 minutes. This manifests itself as a depressed level of consciousness or seizure. The following discussion centers on the patient with neurologic dysfunction and the interventions specific for each.

Coma

For a patient to be fully conscious, two distinct areas of the brain must be functional: the reticular activating system (RAS) and the cerebral hemispheres. If the RAS is stimulated experimentally, diffuse activation of both cerebral cortices will occur. The RAS is considered the gateway to consciousness.

If the RAS is damaged, decreased activity will be seen on the EEG and the patient will have a depressed state of consciousness. Altered consciousness indicates dysfunction in both cerebral hemispheres, in the RAS, or in both.

There are essentially three causes of the depressed states of consciousness: (1) mass lesions, (2) metabolic and diffuse cerebral disorders, and (3) psychogenic causes. Mass lesions include epidural, subdural, and intracerebral hematomas, hemorrhages, tumors, and abscesses. The metabolic and diffuse cerebral disorders include anoxia, ischemia, hypoglycemia, concussion, postictal states, infection, subarachnoid hemorrhage, and endogenous and exogenous (e.g., drugs, poisons) toxins. As can be seen from Table 17–3, the most common causes fall into the category of metabolic and diffuse cerebral disorder (Plum and Posner 1980).

FIGURE 17–4. Motor responses to noxious stimulation in patients with acute cerebral dysfunction. Noxious stimuli can be delivered with minimal trauma to the supraorbital ridge, the nail bed, or the sternum, as illustrated at top. Levels of associated brain dysfunction are indicated roughly at left (see text for details). (Redrawn from Plum F, Posner JB: Diagnosis of Stupor and Coma. FA Davis, 3rd ed, 1980, 66.)

TABLE 17-3
Final Diagnosis of 446 Patients Admitted for "Coma of Unknown Etiology"

	No. of Patients	Total
I. Mass lesions		147
Hematoma	74	
epidural		
subdural		
intracerebral		
Infarct	49	
cerebral		
brainstem		
Hemorrhage	11	
Tumor	7	
Abscess	6	
II. Metabolic or diffuse cerebral disorders		295
Anoxia-ischemia	10	
Concussion or postictal state	9	
Exogenous toxins	149	
Infection	14	
Subarachnoid hemorrhage	13	
Endogenous toxins or deficiencies	100	
III. Psychiatric disorders		4

Source: Adapted from Plum F, Posner JB. Diagnosis of Stupor and Coma, 3rd ed. 1980. FA Davis Co, 2.

CLINICAL MANIFESTATIONS

Structural Lesions

A supratentorial lesion is a mass in the cerebral cortices or the diencephalon, or both. When a supratentorial lesion enlarges, it can cause increases in intracranial pressure (ICP). The neurologic examination demonstrates a rostral to caudal involvement. That is, not only are signs of cortical (rostral) involvement evident, as seen in an altered level of consciousness, but also the examination may indicate lower brain area (caudal) involvement with respiratory or hemodynamic changes, or both, as well. Mass lesions causing coma can progress in size and in the amount of pressure exerted within the CNS.

There are two syndromes in the evolution of a mass lesion that should alert the ED nurse to a worsening condition. The central syndrome occurs when a large or diffuse lesion causes compression and pressure in both cortices and then begins to compress the brain stem bilaterally. Fixed and midposition pupils, apnea, and bradycardia occur. The lateral syndrome is caused by an expanding mass in the lateral area of the cortex, which causes compression of specific parts of the brain and initially produces an ipsilateral sluggish reactive pupil that may become progressively dilated as the syndrome progresses. A dilated pupil is apparent prior to peripheral motor paralysis because the fibers causing pupillary dilation are superficial to oculomotor

TABLE 17-4
Syndromes Associated with Structural Lesions

	Area of Compression	Clinical Picture
Central Syndrome	Cerebral cortex	Begins with confusion and drowsiness, progressing to stupor
	Diencephalon	Coma, Cheyne-Stokes respirations; small, reactive pupils; decorticate posturing
	Midbrain	Central hyperventilation; midpoint pupils; positive ice-water calorics; decerebrate posturing
	Brain stem	Shallow, rapid respirations; midpoint pupils, nonreactive; no response to ice-water calorics; flaccid with bilateral extensor plantar response to noxious stimuli
	Medulla	Slow, irregular respirations; dilated pupils; no motor response
Lateral Syndrome	Herniation of uncus of temporal lobe and cranial nerve III compression.	Unilateral dilated pupil; contralateral hemiparesis
	With herniation to midbrain	Impairment progresses rapidly; same presentation as for central syndrome

fibers responsible for motor movement. The patient may have a contralateral hemiparesis initially and develop an ipsilateral paresis as herniation proceeds. Table 17-4 illustrates the rostral to caudal progression of deterioration with these syndromes. Immediate action must be taken with the onset of either of these syndromes.

Metabolic and Diffuse Cerebral Disorders

Metabolic and diffuse cerebral disorders causing loss of consciousness are varied in causation. In general, the patient's clinical manifestations will be similar whatever the cause. Early warning signs may include personality changes, loss of fine motor dexterity, a gait change, or headache. Preceding total loss of consciousness, the patient exhibits confusion or inappropriate verbal responses. Pupils may be constricted but are usually equal and reactive. Motor signs, if present, are variable and symmetric. The doll's eye reflex is preserved until late in the course. Respiratory pattern may be regular, rapid, or slow depending on the cause of unconsciousness. For example, patients with a loss of consciousness related to diabetic ketoacidosis will most likely be hyperventilating to rid the body of excess CO_2, the byproduct of metabolic acidosis. Persons with a depressed level of consciousness related to a narcotic overdose will hypoventilate secondary to respiratory center depression.

Psychogenic Coma

Psychogenic coma is seen uncommonly. Patients have normal pupillary reaction, usually a normal respiratory pattern, normal muscular tone, and nystagmus occurring during ice water calorics.

Table 17-5 summarizes the possible causes of loss of consciousness and the associated clinical presentation.

TABLE 17–5
Causes of Coma, Associated Clinical Signs, and Time Course

Causes of Coma	Clinical Signs	Time Course
Structural	Early: focal signs relative to anatomic location of lesion	Hours (potentially reversible)
Mass lesions		
Supratentorial: Primary lesion enlarges and may induce brain swelling shift compression of RAS herniation	Later: symptoms of transtentorial herniation progressive, rostral-caudal course coma precedes signs of brainstem deterioration; symmetric signs after onset of coma	Minutes (potentially reversible)
• tumor		
• abscess		
• large stroke with edema		
• hematoma: subdural; epidural; parenchymal		
• fulminating meningitis		
Subtentorial: Direct compression and/or destruction of brain stem structures (pons, midbrain, medulla)	Localizing brain stem signs (nystagmus, cranial nerve palsies) precede or accompany changes in level of consciousness	Minutes (rarely reversible)
• stroke		
• hemorrhage	Eye movements, doll's eyes, and caloric responses reflect location of lesion	
• basilar aneurysm		
	Asymmetric	
Metabolic (Diffuse depression of brain function)		
Hemispheral dysfunction (cognitive, purposefulness, wakefulness) usually exceeds motor and sensory impairment.	Delirium, confusion and stupor precede deep coma	Variable (usually reversible)
	Pupils equal and reactive, though often constricted	
	Motor signs variable, usually symmetric with transient or fluctuating asymmetries	
	Doll's eyes preserved until late in course	
	Breathing regular; may hyper- or hypoventilate depending on need and metabolic cause	
Hypoxia: diffuse interference of O_2 supply to brain		Hours to days
• pulmonary disease		
• reduced atmospheric O_2 tension (high altitudes)		
• carbon monoxide poisoning		Minutes to hours
• seizures (brain O_2 needs increase)		Minutes
Global ischemia: diffuse interference of blood supply to brain		Minutes to hours
• cardiac arrest		
• decreased cardiac output (CHF, Stokes-Adams, etc.)		
• orthostatic hypotension		
• low blood volume		
• hypertensive encephalopathy		
Hypoglycemia		Minutes to hours
Vitamin deficiencies		Hours to days
• thiamine, niacin, pyridoxine, B_{12}		
Toxic or enzymatic inhibition		Minutes to hours
• hepatic		
• uremic		
• diabetic		
• other endocrine, thyroid, adrenal, etc.		
• porphyric		
• exogenous poisons, sedatives, acid poisons, cyanide, salicylates		
• meningitis ⎤		
• encephalitis ⎥ producing CNS toxins		
• subarachnoid hemorrhage ⎦		
• fluid and electrolyte imbalance		

TABLE 17-5
Causes of Coma, Associated Clinical Signs, and Time Course *Continued*

Causes of Coma	Clinical Signs	Time Course
Psychiatric		
Hysteria	Normal respirations	Erratic (usually reversible)
Catatonia	Doll's eyes present	
	Pupils normal-sized, equal, reactive	
	Nystagmus present during cold caloric testing (nystagmus is not present in coma of organic cause)	

Source: Scherer P. 1986. Am J Nurs 86:549.

TREATMENT AND NURSING CARE

During assessment and initial stabilization of the unresponsive patient, medical and nursing diagnoses are formulated. These diagnoses guide the implementation of appropriate interventions for each patient. Goals of stage I care involve accurate identification of changes in neurologic status and application of interventions to prevent further complications.

Stage I care begins with establishment and scrupulous maintenance of an airway to ensure optimal oxygenation of brain tissue. Intravenous access provides a route for administering medications and fluid to restore fluid and electrolyte balance. Electrocardiographic monitoring should be standard. Altered mental status may be due to hypoperfusion secondary to a dysrhythmia, such as ventricular tachycardia.

Exogenous toxins are responsible in a large percentage of patients with changes in mental status. A serum or urine toxicology screen and intravenous administration of naloxone (Narcan) and 50% dextrose (D50) may be necessary. Narcan may be given as both a diagnostic and a therapeutic trial. The patient who has overdosed on narcotics should respond with an increased level of consciousness to administration of this antidote. If not obtained in the prehospital phase of care, a blood glucose level should be determined. Because hypoglycemia is a highly probable and easily correctable cause of altered mental status, D50 should always be administered by intravenous (IV) push. Thiamine should be given prior to or with glucose in the patient suspected of being a chronic alcohol abuser to avoid precipitation of Wernicke's encephalopathy.

Mental Status, Impaired, Related To

• *Mass Lesion or Metabolic Disorder as Manifested by GCS Score of Less Than 8*

Nursing assessment includes accurate identification of the patient's level of responsiveness and prompt recognition of changes. The GCS, discussed in Chapter

18, is a useful tool in quickly identifying changes in responsiveness. This scale includes the patient's spontaneous motor activity, response to painful stimulation, and verbal response. Although the patient may seem unable to comprehend what is occurring, the nurse should explain all procedures as though the patient is awake. It is well documented that hearing is the final sense to disappear.

Once baseline level of consciousness has been established, identification of neurologic changes associated with decreased level of consciousness should be determined. Evaluate pupillary size and equality every 15 minutes to ascertain any impending deterioration. A unilateral sluggish and dilated pupil may indicate cranial nerve III compression. If this is found, consider impending medial herniation of the uncus. As herniation develops, the pupil progresses to full dilation and becomes fixed. Patients with lesions in the diencephalon may have small reactive pupils. Midbrain lesions will yield fixed and midposition pupils. Lesions in the pons will produce pinpoint pupils. Patients in metabolic coma may have preserved light reflex until the terminal stages of coma (Plum and Posner 1980) (Fig. 17–2 and Table 17–1).

Ocular movement must be determined and monitored closely. With increased ICP, the cranial nerves III and VI may be compressed, limiting movement of the eye medially or laterally. Testing of eye movements by evaluating oculocephalic or oculovestibular response is necessary once cervical spine integrity is ensured.

Once there is evidence of stabilization, other diagnostic modalities may be anticipated. A computed tomographic (CT) scan to evaluate mass lesions and lumbar puncture to diagnose meningitis are given consideration here. Note that if a mass lesion is suspected, a CT scan should be done to assess midline shift before a lumbar puncture is attempted. Lumbar puncture may alleviate pressure and cause rapid expansion of the lesion, inducing deterioration and even causing death.

Breathing Patterns, Ineffective

Persons with alteration in respiratory function require close monitoring of breathing patterns and assistance with airway clearance or mechanics of breathing as necessary. Hypoxia or hypoventilation must be avoided. Supplemental oxygen should be administered. Stage I care involves assessing and establishing an airway and monitoring the patient's respiratory status. The gag reflex must be assessed to anticipate possible difficulty in managing secretions. Patients in a coma may need assistance with airway control or mechanical ventilation. Because CO_2 retention causes cerebral vasodilation, hyperventilation to maintain the patient's CO_2 at 25 torr is beneficial in reducing ICP.

Stage II care involves scrupulous monitoring of respiratory status and prevention of complications such as aspiration and respiratory infections. Auscultate breath sounds on a regular basis for symmetry of air movement and adventitious sounds. Baseline blood gas values should be obtained, and if changes in respiratory status are noted, repeat determinations of ABGs are indicated. Use suctioning as needed but limit the duration to 15 seconds to avoid hypoxia and resultant increased intracranial pressure.

Family Processes, Altered, Related To

• *Ill Family Member*

Involving family members in the patient's care is important. Providing ongoing updates and anticipatory guidance should alleviate some anxiety. The family should see the patient as soon as feasible and be reassured of the importance of their support. They may ask the nurse whether the patient can hear them or feel their touch. Encouraging exchanges such as talking and touching are important, even when the patient may seem unresponsive. Assure families that their loved one may have some sense of their presence. The family may experience both grief and the impact of the illness simultaneously. Offering other family support systems available to the family in the hospital, religious or otherwise, is an important aspect of care.

EVALUATION

Further evaluation and disposition of the patient depend on response to emergency management. Continued close monitoring of neurologic status and patient response to treatment is essential. Table 17–6 illustrates a summary of nursing care for the patient with altered mental status.

TABLE 17–6
Summary of Nursing Care for Patients in Coma

Goal	Desired Patient Outcome	Nursing Measures
Prompt recognition of changes in state of responsiveness	No clinical signs of decreased LOC	Utilize Glasgow Coma Score to measure and record mental status
Prevent further increase in ICP	No clinical signs of increased ICP; no change in LOC, pupils equal and reactive to light, HR > 60 and < 100 bpm	Elevate head of bed 30 degrees; avoid flexion, extension, or rotation of head; monitor pupillary response every 15–30 min
Avoid hypoxia and hypercapnia	Arterial pH 7.35–7.48 $PaCO_2$ 32–45 PaO_2 80–100	Limit suctioning duration to 15 seconds; hyperoxygenate and hyperventilate patient before and after suctioning; auscultate breath sounds; administer supplemental oxygen if needed; obtain ABGs if RR > 24 min or < 12; LOCs.

Prevent fluid-electrolyte imbalance	SBP > 100 and < 150 mmHg
	NSR on cardiac monitor
	Normal serum electrolytes:
	   Na 135–145 mEq/L
	   K 3.5–5.5 mEqL
	   BS 60–100 mg/dl
	   BUN 5–20 mg/dl
	Urine output ≥ 30 ml/hr
		Monitor I & O; observe for signs of dehydration or overhydration; monitor vital signs; obtain serum electrolyte values on admission

Family support available	Family interaction with patient	Allow family to stay with patient when possible; explain status and therapies; respond to concerns; refer to other support services if needed

ICP, intracranial pressure; LOC, level of consciousness; HR, heart rate; NSR, normal sinus rhythm; RR, respiratory rate; SBP, systolic blood pressure; I & O, intake and output.

SEIZURES

Etiology

The causes of seizures may be divided into two general categories: idiopathic and acquired. Idiopathic seizures have no identifiable cause, although some patients may have a genetic predisposition. The acquired causes of seizures are myriad and include head trauma, infection (e.g., meningitis, encephalitis), tumor, cerebrovascular accident, collagen vascular diseases, toxemia of pregnancy, congenital malformations, toxins, metabolic disorders, and alcohol withdrawal (Glaser 1982). Patients with known controlled seizure disorders may have breakthrough seizures. There are four major causes for breakthrough seizure: noncompliance, infection or illness, drug or drug interaction (ethyl alcohol being the predominant offender), and an increase or decrease in amounts of sleep.

Pathophysiology

Seizures are produced by paroxysmal abnormal neuronal discharge in various parts of the brain. The manifestations of the seizure depend upon the location of the neurons that fire. Seizures are classified into two broad categories: partial seizures and generalized seizures. Partial seizures result from abnormal neuronal discharge in focal areas of the cortex. Generalized seizures occur with abnormal electrical discharge by neurons scattered throughout the brain. Table 17–7 outlines the international classification of seizures used currently (Snyder 1983).

Clinical Manifestations

The clinical manifestations of the seizure depend upon the type. A generalized tonic-clonic seizure, previously called grand mal seizure, is probably the most familiar and generally the most disconcerting in the ED. It may begin with a prodrome or aura lasting several minutes or more. The aura may be a taste, smell, sound, unusual tactile or visual experience, or emotional change. The patient with recurrent seizures may be aware of the impending seizure. The seizure is usually manifested by a loss of consciousness, tonic extensor rigidity of the trunk and extremities, and then repetitive tonic-clonic movements. The patient may cease respirations and become cyanotic during this episode. He or she may have urinary incontinence, and there is often evidence of trauma, such as from falling, tongue-biting, or flailing of the extremities.

Once the seizure stops, the patient becomes quiet and breathing returns to normal, although respirations may be noisy from accumulated oral secretions. The patient gradually awakens and may complain of a range of symptoms, from generalized confusion and headache to neurologic signs mimicking paralysis and sensory deficits. The confusion and neurologic deficits are referred to as the postictal state and may persist for minutes to hours after the cessation of the seizure.

A focal seizure involves only specific parts of the body—for example, the arm. The seizure activity may be manifested as repetitive movement of the finger. It may

TABLE 17–7
International Classification of Epileptic Seizures

I. Partial Seizures (seizures beginning locally)
   A. Partial seizures with elementary symptoms (generally without impairment of consciousness)
      1. With motor symptoms (includes jacksonian seizures)
      2. With special sensory or somatosensory symptoms
      3. With autonomic symptoms
      4. Compound forms
   B. Partial seizures with complex symptoms (generally with impairment of consciousness)
      (temporal lobe or psychomotor seizures)
      1. With impairment of consciousness only
      2. With cognitive symptoms
      3. With affective symptoms
      4. With "psychosensory" symptoms
      5. With "psychomotor" symptoms (automatisms)
      6. Compound forms
   C. Partial seizures secondarily generalized
II. Generalized Seizures (bilaterally symmetric and without local onset)
      1. Absences (petit mal)
      2. Bilateral massive epileptic myoclonus
      3. Infantile spasms
      4. Clonic seizures
      5. Tonic seizures
      6. Tonic-clonic seizures (grand mal)
      7. Atonic seizures
      8. Akinetic seizures
III. Unilateral Seizures (or predominantly)
IV. Unclassified Epileptic Seizures (due to incomplete data)

Source: Adapted from Gastaut H. 1970. Epilepsia 11: 102–113.

progress to involve the rest of the extremity, which is known as a *jacksonian march.* Focal seizures can progress to a generalized seizure called a secondary generalized seizure.

Absence seizures, formerly called petit mal seizures, are brief episodes of loss of consciousness lasting from a few seconds to 30 seconds. The patient usually stops all motor activity abruptly and stares blankly into space. He or she may blink or exhibit minor motor activity. These patients usually have a history of seizures beginning in childhood and experience no postictal state.

Akinetic seizures are those associated with a complete loss of motor tone and an interruption in consciousness. The patient is usually alert after the episode but may have sustained an injury during a fall.

Partial seizures with complex symptoms (psychomotor seizures) are due to excessive neuronal activity in the temporal lobe. Varying from patient to patient, they begin with a distinct aura, often a smell or peculiar feeling. Motor activity stops and simple movements such as smacking of the lips, sucking, or chewing occur. Abdominal symptoms such as hunger pains may be described (Glaser 1982). Consciousness is interrupted but not totally lost.

Status epilepticus is one continual seizure or multiple intermittent seizures without recovery between seizures. All classifications of seizure activity can occur as status epilepticus; however, only generalized tonic-clonic status epilepticus is considered life threatening. Consciousness is not regained and respiratory status is compromised (Snyder 1983). A generalized status epilepticus must be treated immediately, as the longer it continues, the more difficult it may be to control and the higher the morbidity and mortality (Delgado-Escueta et al 1982). Neuronal damage can ensue with prolonged seizures. Metabolic abnormalities may develop, including lactic acidosis. Autonomic disturbances such as hyperthermia occur along with excessive sweating; both can result in dehydration. Hypertension may be followed by hypotension and shock. Excessive muscle activity caused by a prolonged convulsion results in myelosis, myoglobinuria, and subsequent renal failure (Delgado-Escueta et al 1982).

Not all patients coming to the ED with symptoms of a seizure have a seizure disorder as the underlying cause. Patients experiencing a syncopal episode from any number of causes may manifest minimal tonic-clonic activity as they lose consciousness (Martin et al 1984). Do not let the description of a seizure cause the label of "epilepsy" to be given to a patient without further evaluation of the cause.

There are variations of seizure activity too numerous to discuss here. The reader is referred to a textbook of neurology for further information.

Treatment and Nursing Care

The patient experiencing a seizure must be cared for immediately. Most commonly, patients in the ED whose presenting feature is seizure activity have a diagnosed seizure disorder and have not taken their medication. Despite this, it is important to recognize and treat any underlying disorders causing the seizure.

Interventions for generalized tonic-clonic status epilepticus involve activities similar to those discussed under coma. Establish intravenous access for administration of antiepileptic medications. Electrocardiographic (EKG) monitoring is indicated. Seizures may be due to dysrhythmia, such as ventricular tachycardia. If phenytoin is used to manage status epilepticus, cardiac monitoring is essential as the drug can cause dysrhythmias during administration. Monitor vital signs frequently, including temperature, because of the possibility of hyperthermia. Carefully observe and record seizure activity according to type of behavior observed.

Patients exhibiting generalized tonic-clonic status epilepticus should be treated with anticonvulsants. Indicated anticonvulsants may include diazepam (Valium), phenytoin (Dilantin), and phenobarbital. There are multiple regimens available for the patient with active seizures (Delgado-Escueta et al 1982). Serum levels of anticonvulsants the patient is currently taking should be determined before medication is administered. Valium is the medication of choice for treatment of status epilepticus. It should be given at an intravenous rate of no more than 2 mg/minute until seizure activity ceases or a total of 20 mg has been given. Seizures may recur within 20 to 30 minutes of initial control because of redistribution of the drug. A contraindication to the use of diazepam to control seizure activity is allergy to the drug.

Phenytoin should be administered at a rate no faster than 50 mg/minute and to a total of 18 mg/kg. Because phenytoin crystallizes very rapidly in dextrose solutions, it must be given in normal saline and administered slowly and preferably near the intravenous injection site. The patient should be monitored for hypotension and dysrhythmias, and ventilatory supportive equipment should be available (Delgado-Escueta et al 1982).

Although phenobarbital may be administered in conjunction with diazepam, the possibility of respiratory depression exists. Laboratory diagnostic tests, such as a complete blood count (CBC), electrolytes, and anticonvulsant levels, may be indicated in specific patients.

Airway Clearance, Ineffective, Related to

• *Seizure Activity*

As discussed previously, airway control is a difficult problem in the patient with active seizures. Never insert fingers into a patient's mouth during seizure activity. Use of a nasopharyngeal airway may be indicated. Forcing a tongue blade into the mouth of a patient who is having a seizure may cause damage to teeth and mouth and promote the potential for aspiration and airway compromise. Restrictive clothing may require loosening. If possible, position the patient on his or her side to facilitate breathing. If this is not possible, tilt the head backward and lift the mandible up and forward. The head of the bed should be elevated slightly when the patient's condition allows. Prevent aspiration by clearing secretions from the mouth with suction.

Potential for Injury, Related to

• *Seizure Activity*

Provide padded side rails to prevent injury during seizure activity. Although the patient may not be having active seizures when admitted, the risk of another seizure is always present. Never leave the patient unattended. Side rails should be up at all times and the patient encouraged to remain in bed to prevent injury from a fall during another seizure. Special precautions should always be taken to prevent movement to the head or the foot of the bed during violent seizure activity.

Once the seizure has stopped and the acute phase has passed, vital signs and neurologic status should be reassessed. When the patient awakens from the postictal state, attempt to ascertain information pertinent to the etiologic basis of the seizure. Inquire if a prodrome or aura was present. This may indicate whether the seizure was typical for this patient or not. Often, status epilepticus results from the patient's discontinuation of anticonvulsant medications. Ascertain if noncompliance is a problem for the patient (Snyder 1983).

Noncompliance

Noncompliance with prescribed medical regimens can be the result of many factors. The side effects of the medications used for seizure control may be contributing to a lack of compliance. Often cost prohibits the patient from obtaining medications or results in rationing dosages to make the prescription last longer. The patient or family, or both, may have other financial priorities or responsibilities. Ascertain the causative or contributing factors in noncompliance with prescribed regimens of medication. Discuss them with the patient and the physician to determine alternatives. Sometimes just simplifying the regimen will facilitate compliance. If the patient needs financial support or community support, referral to social service or other support services may be of some assistance.

Knowledge Deficit

The patient may have recently begun taking seizure medication and not fully understand the importance of maintaining therapeutic blood levels of antiepileptic medication. On the other hand, the patient may have never experienced a seizure prior to admission to the ED. This patient may know little about the medication, the disorder, or the prescribed management. The patient may be an elderly person living at home with memory or sensory deficits interfering with his or her ability to adhere to the prescribed medical regimen. Whatever the reason, once stabilization has occurred, it is the ED nurse's role to ascertain the patient's level of knowledge regarding the disease and to explain or clarify information about seizures, medications, and management. If the seizure was due to another disease process, such as the poor control of diabetes, providing the patient with a good knowledge base will perhaps prevent future seizures and minimize the patient's anxiety.

Anxiety

Alleviation of anxiety and stress is an important aspect of total patient care. Generalized tonic-clonic seizures are especially frightening to patients and family members. The family needs support and information concerning the status of the patient. Stress has been recognized as a contributing factor in seizure activity (Snyder 1983). Information from patient or family concerning stress level and stress factors prior to admission may help to indicate areas in which patient teaching in methods of stress reduction may be helpful. Of course, referrals to community agencies for follow-up are necessary to ensure optimal attention to these areas.

Evaluation

Evaluation and disposition of patients with seizures depend on response to medication, etiologic basis for the seizure, and the need for further medical management. First-time seizure patients may require an in-patient evaluation. Refer to Table 17 – 8 for a summary of important aspects of discharge instruction.

TABLE 17-8
Nursing Measures and Discharge Instructions for Patients with Seizures

Goal	Desired Patient Outcome	Nursing Measures
Avoid recurrence of seizures	No further seizure activity	Encourage patient follow-up with private physician or clinic; reinforce importance of periodic evaluations to monitor blood levels of antiepileptic medications to ensure that levels are achieved.
Compliance with drug regimen	Understands medication's actions, dosage; importance of compliance and adverse effects	Validate compliance; provide information on actions, dosage, importance of compliance and adverse effects; evaluate effectiveness of teaching through return demonstration of knowledge; determine concurrent prescriptions and interactions with antiepileptic medications
Prevent injury	No concomitant injury from seizure or postictal state	Assess mental status prior to discharge to assure orientation; provide information to patient and family about care after seizure; emphasize importance of reducing stressors; assure patient is accompanied by family at discharge in case seizure recurs

CEREBROVASCULAR ACCIDENTS

Etiology

A cerebrovascular accident (CVA) results from an injury to part of the brain. The extent of injury, manifestations, and prognosis depend on the location and size of the insult and its duration. Ischemia due to inadequate blood flow to the brain can be the result of arteriosclerotic disease, emboli of cardiac origin in the patient with atrial fibrillation, mural thrombi, bacterial endocarditis, intracranial hemorrhage, or an episode of hypoperfusion caused by myocardial dysfunction.

Pathophysiology

Ischemia of the brain may be classified in one of the following categories:

transient ischemic attack (TIA): The loss of neurologic function owing to ischemia that persists for less than 24 hours. Symptoms usually last only minutes and may be considered precursors of further neurologic insult.
reversible ischemic neurologic deficit (RIND): Symptoms persist for longer than 24 hours but resolve, leaving the patient without neurologic sequelae.
stroke in progress: The neurologic deficits continue to occur or worsen after time of presentation.
completed stroke: This usually results in permanent neurologic damage, and the deficit is maximal at the time of presentation.

TABLE 17-9
Symptoms of CVA Classified According to Cerebral Artery Occluded

Artery	Symptoms Displayed
Middle Cerebral	Aphasia, dysphasia, visual field cuts, hemiparesis, and sensory changes of the face and arm
Carotid	Decreased level of responsiveness; aphasia if left carotid; weakness, numbness, or paralysis of contralateral side; visual field cuts and ptosis; carotid bruits may be found on examination
Vertebrobasilar	Poor coordination and ataxia; weakness of lower extremities; dizziness; diplopia and visual field cuts; numbness around mouth and weakness of the affected side of the face; dysphasia; nausea and vomiting; dysarthria; contralateral motor or sensory loss
Anterior cerebral	Confusion and changes in personality; weakness of lower extremities; impaired sensory functions; incontinence
Posterior cerebral	Normal motor examination (no paralysis) but sensory impairment; cortical blindness; dyslexia

Clinical Manifestations

The clinical presentation of a patient who has suffered a CVA varies with the cerebral artery affected, the severity of the damage, and the extent of collateral circulation that later may develop. A CVA occurring in the left hemisphere produces symptoms on the right side of the body; a CVA that damages the right hemisphere will affect the left side of the body. If cranial nerves are damaged, the symptoms will occur on the same side of the body as the nerve affected. Table 17-9 summarizes the symptoms and physical findings that may be present when a specific cerebral artery is affected. Figure 17-5 illustrates cerebral artery anatomy.

Examination of patients experiencing a CVA focuses on the neurologic and vascular structures. History of risk factors that predispose the patient to CVAs should be ascertained. Vital signs are evaluated for hypertension. The cardiac examination focuses on determining the presence of murmurs and atrial fibrillation. Neurologic deficits should be carefully noted.

Bell's Palsy

Bell's palsy is often mistaken for a CVA. The peripheral facial nerve (cranial nerve VII) is affected in Bell's palsy. This peripheral nerve deficit is of unknown cause, although a viral basis has been suggested. Presenting symptoms are similar to those of a CVA: rapid onset of facial paralysis and a facial droop are seen. Symptoms are retraction on the angle of the mouth and impairment of eye closure. Taste perception may also be impaired. Bell's palsy may be differentiated from a central lesion (CVA) by the involvement of the motor aspect of the forehead and lack of other associated symptoms. In Bell's palsy, the patient will not be able to wrinkle the forehead; in the CVA patient, forehead movement is possible (DeGowin and DeGowin 1976; Weiner and Levitt 1978). This lack of motor control in Bell's palsy occurs because of a defect that results in loss of innervation to muscles of the forehead. Motor control of the forehead remains following a CVA because of crossed motor innervation from the other hemisphere.

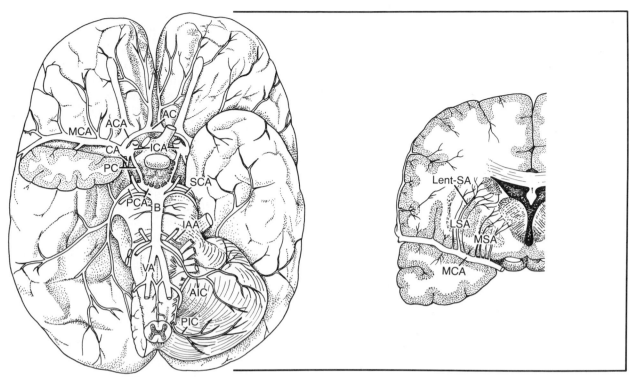

FIGURE 17–5. Cerebral blood supply. AC = anterior communicating artery, ACA = anterior cerebral artery, AIC = anterior inferior cerebellar artery, B = basilar artery, CA = choroidal artery, IAA = internal auditory artery, ICA = internal carotid artery, Lent-SA = lateral lenticular striate artery, LSA = lenticular striate artery, MCA = middle cerebral artery, MSA = medial striate artery, PC = posterior communicating artery, PCA = posterior cerebellar artery, PIC = posterior inferior cerebellar artery, VA = vertebral artery, SCA = superior cerebellar artery.

Recovery from Bell's palsy usually begins within 3 weeks and approximately 70 per cent of patients recover fully within 3 months (Parry 1977). Some investigators have suggested the use of steroids in treatment of this disorder. Appropriate diagnosis, treatment, and reassurance are necessary. Patients have much anxiety about the possibility that they have had a stroke.

Treatment and Nursing Care

Tissue Perfusion, Altered (Cerebral), Related to

- *Cerebrovascular Accident*
- *Transient Ischemic Attack*

Stage I care for the patient who has suffered a CVA or TIA involves keen observation of the patient and careful neurologic assessment. Often patients may be lethargic or unresponsive to all stimuli, and nursing measures are similar to those discussed under coma. Maintenance of a patent airway and adequate oxygenation are essential. Observe for "ballooning" of the cheek with respirations; the side on which ballooning occurs is the affected side. Position the patient to prevent aspiration and use suction if necessary to remove secretions. Supplemental oxygen may be needed. Insert an artificial airway or, if needed, begin mechanical ventilation. Blood gases should be monitored and the lungs auscultated frequently.

Intravenous access should be established at a "keep open" rate for the administration of medications. Level of consciousness, pupillary changes, and voluntary and involuntary motor function should be monitored and changes noted. Observe the patient closely for signs of increased intracranial pressure: increasing blood pressure (BP), increasing pulse pressure, and decreasing heart rate. Electrocardiographic monitoring is essential to monitor for dysrhythmias. A 12-lead EKG is necessary to rule out myocardial infarction as the precipitating event.

Anxiety, Related to

- ### *Actual Threat to Biologic Integrity and Self-Concept, Secondary to CVA*

A CVA is often perceived as one of the most devastating illnesses. The patient, if awake, may not be able to communicate, his or her mobility may be compromised, and he or she may be unable to perform even the simplest activities of daily living. Overwhelming fear and anxiety may ensue, as well as feelings of confinement, helplessness, and hopelessness. The ED nurse should establish rapport with the patient and provide a means of communication for the patient. Use simple questions that require "yes" and "no" answers whenever possible. Touch is an excellent means of communication and reassurance. The family's role is essential in providing comfort to the patient. Inform them of the situation and encourage them to participate in the patient's care by assisting with basic care, such as turning, positioning, and communicating with their loved one.

Mobility, Impaired (Physical), Related to

- ### *Motor Dysfunction*

Although the patient who has suffered a CVA may not remain in the ED for long, rehabilitation of the patient should begin here. Careful turning of the patient and positioning of extremities at least every 2 hours will help to prevent foot drop and contractures. Place the patient's hands in functional position. Assess lungs frequently and turn the patient every 2 hours to prevent development of pneumonia. Observe for edema, especially dependent edema that could warn of fluid overload.

Evaluation

Disposition and further evaluation of the patient depend on physical findings and how the patient responds to emergency treatment. As stated previously, astute and continuous monitoring of the patient who has suffered a CVA is a nursing priority. Careful neurologic assessment, including mental status, continuous monitoring of vital signs and fluid-electrolyte status, careful positioning, and pulmonary toilet are essential if early changes indicating deterioration or complications are to be noted.

CONCLUSION

From a nursing perspective, the approach to the neurologically impaired patient is dynamic and challenging. Although initial management of all neurologically impaired persons may be similar, the presentation and complications are varied and require the ED nurse to be an astute observer, possess excellent assessment and documentation skills, and have a thorough knowledge of pathophysiology to provide optimal nursing care during the emergency phase of care.

REFERENCES

Barnett HJM. 1979. The pathophysiology of transient cerebral ischemic attacks. Therapy with platelet antiaggregants. Med Clin North Am 63:649–679.

DeGowin EL, DeGowin RL. 1976. Bedside Diagnostic Examination, 3rd ed. New York, Macmillan, 764–765.

Delgado-Escueta AV, Wasterlain C, Treiman DM, et al. 1982. Management of status epilepticus. N Engl J Med 306:1337–1340.

Diseases: Nurses' Reference Library. 1983. Nursing 83 Books. Springhouse, PA, Intermed Communications, 608–611.

Glaser GH. 1982. The epilepsies. In Wyngaarden JB, Smith LH, eds. Cecil Textbook of Medicine, 16th ed. Philadelphia, WB Saunders Co, 2114–2124.

Martin GJ, Adams SL, Martin HG. 1984. Prospective evaluation of syncope. Ann Emerg Med 13:499–504.

Parry CBW, King PF. 1977. Results of treatment in peripheral facial paralysis: A 25-year study. J Laryngol Otol 91:551–563.

Plum F, Posner JB. 1980. Diagnosis of Stupor and Coma, 3rd ed. Philadelphia, FA Davis Co, 1–86.

Posner JB. 1975. The comatose patient. JAMA 233:1313–1314.

Scherer P. 1986. Assessment: The logic of coma. Am J Nurs 86:542–549.

Snyder M. 1983. A Guide to Neurological and Neurosurgical Nursing. New York, John Wiley & Sons, 128–137, 172–177.

Weiner HL, Levitt LP. 1978. Neurology for the House Officer, 2nd ed. Baltimore, Williams & Wilkins Co, 117–119.

Judith Zoellner-Hunter, RN MS

Head Trauma

Head injuries constitute a significant percentage of annual patient visits to emergency departments. Jennett and Teasdale (1981, 5) estimated the incidence of fatal head injuries in the United States at approximately 2.4 per 100,000 individuals. Other sources (Caveness 1979); (Kalsbeek, McLaurin, and Harris 1980) estimate the total number of head injuries of all severities as between 422,000 and 644,000 cases per year.

Head trauma is difficult to define, is quantified differently in different countries, arises from a multitude of events, and produces a wide range of effects—from a slight headache to permanent disability or death. Head trauma can be categorized according to the severity of injury. Minor head injuries were described by Langfitt (1969) as producing a period of unconsciousness of less than 20 to 30 minutes, eliciting a Glasgow Coma Scale (GCS) score of 13 to 15, and requiring a stay in the hospital of 24 to 48 hours. These patients can also be said to have sustained concussion, but *minor head injury* is a more descriptive term.

Jennett and Galbrath (1983, 216) discuss grading of head trauma and use a combination of the GCS (discussed later in this chapter) and posttraumatic amnesia (PTA) to describe severity. The end of PTA, with its implications for the patient of being able to remember or "learn" new things, signals a return to normal function. If recovery does not occur or the patient remains in a chronic vegetative state, his or her potential for recovery is obviously severely impaired. In the emergency setting, the patient's GCS score, combined with pupil assessment, is the best guide to severity of injury.

Jennett and Teasdale (1981, 13) describe three stages related to management of head trauma: (1) forestalling the accident, (2) minimizing the injuries sustained on impact, and (3) ensuring that the risk of subsequent brain damage is reduced. The first stage relates to accident prevention. Countries concentrating on accident prevention show a decreased morbidity and mortality related to head trauma. Strict law enforcement against drinking and driving, reduction of speed limits on highways, and mandatory use of seat belts have significantly lowered morbidity and mortality associated with motor vehicle accidents. The use of helmets for motorcycle riders and contact sport participants has also been effective in reducing the incidence of head injuries (Jennett and Teasdale 1981, 1–17). Since home falls contribute significantly to the incidence of head trauma, particularly in the elderly, the use of safety devices such as rubber mats for the bathtub and safety "grab bars" should be encouraged.

The second stage, minimizing injuries sustained on impact, concerns the management of the victim at the scene of the accident and in the emergency department. The injuries sustained at the scene may be skull fractures, shearing of white and grey matter, brain contusion, or laceration. Injuries that emerge by the time the patient arrives in an emergency department include space-occupying lesions and bleeding, which can be epidural, subdural, intraparenchymal, or a combination of these.

Assessment and management of these injuries blend into the third stage, which involves ensuring that risk of subsequent brain damage is reduced. Management of the head injury must be concomitant with cardiovascular and respiratory stabilization to promote the best possible outcome for the head-injured patient. These therapies begin in the emergency department and continue in the intensive care setting.

ASSESSMENT OF INDIVIDUALS WITH HEAD INJURY

Ascertaining from the trauma victim or witnesses details of an accident is critical in identification of individuals with actual or potential head injuries. Primary assessment and treatment of life-threatening conditions should be performed as discussed in Chapter 6.

Victims with head trauma severe enough to cause a loss of consciousness are presumed to have an associated spinal cord injury. Initial assessment and stabilization include complete cervical spine immobilization. The patient should have a firm cervical collar, towel rolls around the head, and tape across the forehead and should be secured on a long backboard. A cross-table lateral cervical spine x-ray film that includes all seven cervical vertebrae is necessary in the initial assessment to rule out cervical spine injury.

If the patient has lost consciousness, the duration of unconsciousness should be determined. In many instances, patients are unable to remember if they lost consciousness or not. Thus it is important to ask the patient what he or she last remembers. A lack of memory surrounding events of the accident may signify loss of consciousness. It is important to try to determine chronology—i.e., did the patient lose consciousness and then have an accident or did the accident occur first?

Once airway, breathing, and circulation (ABCs) have been assessed and stabilized, a careful examination of the head and neck can be performed. Assess the scalp for lacerations, foreign bodies, skull deformities, or any source of bleeding. Note ecchymosis or contusions of the head and face. "Battle's sign," which is bruising over the mastoid process (often associated with cerebrospinal fluid [CSF] leaks from the ear [CSF otorrhea]), is a classic pattern of ecchymosis and is often associated with posterior basilar skull fracture. "Raccoon" or "panda" eyes is periorbital bruising from anterior fossa basilar skull fractures and is often associated with CSF leaks from the nose (CSF rhinorrhea). These patterns of bruising are not generally evident in the emergent phase as they take several hours to develop.

In order to determine if the patient has a CSF leak, the drainage can be tested for the presence of glucose. However, CSF drainage is often mixed with blood; therefore, glucose-strip testing is not useful, since blood also contains glucose. The halo sign refers to the presence of a xanthochromic, or yellow, "halo" that appears on the dressing if CSF is mixed with blood. The halo appears as the blood dries and confirms the presence of CSF. It is important to allow the CSF to drain unimpeded: a loosely applied 4 × 4 gauze can be taped over the ear, or a mustache dressing can be placed under the nose. Obstructing the CSF flow with an occlusive dressing could potentiate the development of an ascending infection or meningitis. Frequent changes of dressings, with appropriate documentation, should be done.

Level of consciousness is a major component of assessment of head-injured patients. The GCS, published in 1974 by Jennett and Teasdale, provides a means to objectively rate a patient's level of consciousness, the best guide to neurologic status. The scale is based on three parameters: eye opening and verbal and motor responses (Table 18–1). The patient is given a score in each category and the categories are totaled to obtain a total score. The best score that a patient can obtain is 15, the worst 3. Morbidity and mortality sharply increase for patients with scores of 8 and below. The GCS and all observations must be performed on a continuum to identify trends.

PATHOPHYSIOLOGY

The pathophysiology of head trauma can be divided into two phases. The *initial phase* occurs at the scene and is a fixed anatomic fact. Clinicians cannot reverse this damage but will direct therapy toward preventing the complications related to the second phase, which will evolve during the hospital stay. The second phase can be called *evolving,* or secondary, injuries.

Initial Phase

The initial trauma can cause skull fractures or rotational shear injuries to the grey and white matter of the brain and to blood vessels. Skull fractures can be simple linear fractures of the cranial vault and seldom produce significant pathology with the exception of temporal or parietal bone fractures (discussed under epidural hematomas). Fractures of the base of the skull correlate with high morbidity and mortality

TABLE 18–1
Glasgow Coma Scale

Eye Opening		
Spontaneous	4	The patient's eyes open when you come to the bedside
To voice	3	The patient's eyes open to command
To pain	2	The patient's eyes open on suctioning, starting an IV, drawing blood gases, sternal rubbing, or finger nailbed pressure
None	1	The patient's eyes do not open
Best Verbal Response*		
Oriented	5	The patients can give name, address, and day of the week
Confused	4	The patients give name but are less likely to know the day of the week or address. Most patients at this level can name the president of the United States or the mayor of their city. Names seem to be retained better than numbers.
Inappropriate words	3	Inconsistent answers; patients can give you their name only occasionally. Profanity is often retained, and frequently the patient perseverates, or repeats the same word over and over.
Incomprehensible sounds	2	These patients may have deteriorated to the point that intubation has been done. Intoxicated patients are most likely to be at this level, with mumbling and inarticulate sounds, with no apparent meaning.
None	1	No verbal response
Best Motor Response		
Obeys commands	6	Commands can be complex, as in a cranial nerve assessment, or "Touch your right ear with your left thumb" or "Squeeze my hand." A positive response from the patient is only meaningful for a reasonable level of function if the second part of the command, "Now let go" is also performed. The squeeze is reflex, the release is purposeful.
Localizes pain	5	The patient is able to localize the source of the pain and will grab at the offender, and withdraw his extremity from the needle or cause of pain. (See section on eye opening.)
Withdraw (pain)	4	The individual knows there is pain but cannot localize it, and the whole body withdraws from the pain.
Flexion (pain)	3	Sometimes called decortication, this stereotyped response is better termed abnormal flexion. The patient flexes his arms tightly on his chest and extends the lower extremities.
Extension (pain)	2	Sometimes called decerebration, this stereotyped response is better termed abnormal extension. The upper extremities extend and internally rotate, the lower extremities extend on stimulation or as the situation worsens, spontaneously.
None	1	No response: the patient is flaccid. Occasionally, as the situation worsens, a weak flexor response develops in the lower extremities. This is a spinal reflex and is a grim prognostic sign.

Source: Adapted from Jennett B, Teasdale F. 1981. Management of Head Injuries. FA Davis.

* The non–English speaking patient presents a dilemma; families can be helpful. The intoxicated patient or the patient who has used recreational drugs also presents a dilemma. Drug and alcohol screen tests should be done on most head-injured patients.

(Jennett and Teasdale 1981, 23). Open, comminuted skull fractures, with the possibility of spicules of bone lacerating the brain, will worsen the initial injury and may introduce infection.

Rotational shear injuries to the gray and white matter and the blood vessels include cortex contusion, lacerations, or both—in other words, brain tissue disruptions. The mechanisms are deceleration and rotational forces, which may be direct (coup), or the result of the brain impacting on the side opposite the blow (contrecoup); in most cases, differentiation is impossible and management modalities address the injuries, regardless of mechanism. The most vulnerable areas of the cortex are the tips of the temporal lobes and the bases of the frontal lobes (Fig. 18–1). They lie adjacent to the irregular ridges of the skull, and the custard-like consistency of the brain is afforded little protection by the meninges. Contusions and lacerations occur as the brain impacts on these rough surfaces. The white matter of the brain is made up

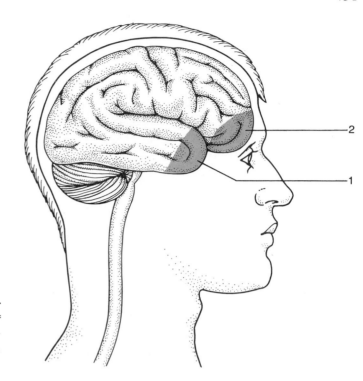

FIGURE 18–1. Common sites of cerebral contusions and lacerations. 1 = tip of temporal lobe; 2 = base of frontal lobe. (Redrawn from Abeloff D. Medical Art: Graphics for Use. © Williams & Wilkins, 1982, p 5.8.)

of axons, and their myelin sheaths can be stretched and disrupted, resulting in neurologic dysfunction. Jennett and Teasdale (1981, 26–29) discuss these injuries and their implications.

Evolving Injuries: Phase II

The second phase of head injury involves the sequelae of the primary injury. It can be worsened by events occurring below the neck and demands precise assessment and appropriate, aggressive management. These secondary events or evolving injuries can be understood in the context of the Monro-Kellie principle. This 150 year old principle states that the skull is an unyielding container, and since the contents of the skull are essentially liquid (which is incompressible), any increase in the contents of one of the compartments will be at the expense of one of the other compartments. The compartments are brain substance (80%), cerebrospinal fluid (10%) and blood (10%). The percentages given above are approximate, and will vary with different authors, but the concept is significant in understanding the pathophysiology and management of head injuries. Evolving injuries are space-occupying lesions and include epidural, subdural and intraparenchymal bleeds. They can occur singly or in combination, and will be discussed in the following section. Cerebral edema within a broadened definition is also a space-occupying lesion, and will be present in and compound all the more tangible lesions.

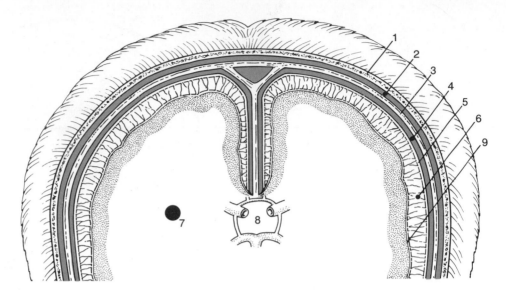

FIGURE 18-2. Potential sites for space-occupying lesions. All spaces are potential and are exaggerated for purposes of drawing. 1 = skull (with hair); 2 = epidural space or bleeding; 3 = dura; 4 = subdural space or bleeding; 5 = arachnoid; 6 = subarachnoid space or bleeding; 7 = brain; 8 = circle of Willis (subarachnoid space).

Epidural Hematoma

> **epidural hematoma:** A collection of blood between the dura and the skull (Fig. 18-2 [2]).

Patients with a bleeding disorder (i.e., hemophilia) or patients on anticoagulants (including aspirin) are more likely to develop epidural hematomas or any of the following intracerebral hemorrhages. They are usually arterial in origin but may be venous, particularly in children. Most result from a fracture across the thin parietal or temporal bone that lacerates a branch of the middle meningeal artery. (Baseball helmets were specifically designed to prevent this injury.) The arterial bleeding "peels" the dura from the cranial vault, and the rapidly expanding clot produces a midline shift or uncal herniation. The computed tomographic (CT) scan will show a typical lens-shaped, or lenticular, clot. Time from impact to death may be as short as two to six hours.

Clinical Manifestations

The "classic" signs occur in about 40% of patients. The patient presents with a history of a direct blow to the side of the head and a short period of unconsciousness. There is usually evidence of soft tissue trauma to the area involved, and there may be crepitus. This is followed by a lucid interval. Within a few hours, the patient becomes increasingly lethargic and develops a decreased level of consciousness (LOC). If admission to the emergency department (ED) does not occur quickly after the accident, the ipsilateral pupil (on the same side as the injury) will have a sluggish light reaction or may be fixed or dilated. Motor changes may be ipsilateral or contralateral, and a major motor seizure can occur. The patient's GCS score rapidly deteriorates. The diagnosis is usually made from clinical signs and symptoms. Deterioration may be so sudden that there may be only time for one quick CT "slice" before the patient must go to surgery for evacuation of the hematoma.

Subdural Hematoma

> **subdural hematoma:** A collection of blood, fluid, or both in the subdural space (above the arachnoid, below the dura) (Fig. 18–2[4]).

Since this space is normally only a potential space, either the trauma was severe or cortical atrophy is present. With cortical atrophy, the dura remains attached to the skull, and the shrinking brain has made this potential space an actual one.

Acute Massive Subdural Hematoma

Acute massive subdural hematomas occur in major head trauma: severe motor vehicle accidents (MVAs) or falls. This injury causes tissue disruption in the cortex and underlying structures. The collection of blood in the subdural space from the primary injury then forms a secondary space-occupying lesion. At surgery the brain is often swollen, discolored, and massively edematous. Postoperative management of intracranial hypertension is difficult.

Clinical Manifestations

These patients usually present with a significant decrease in their level of consciousness and a low GCS score. They are almost surely to have been brought in by ambulance. Pupils are often sluggish or nonreactive. A CT shows lesions, often very large, or substantial bleeding and significant cerebral edema. Even with prompt diagnosis and appropriate intervention (evacuation of the hematoma), the prognosis in general is poor. The real pathology is not the clot but the underlying damage that produced it.

Acute Subdural Hematoma

Acute subdural hematoma can occur in relatively minor head trauma; the patient frequently does not remember the injury. The hematoma often occurs in the elderly and in alcoholics who have some degree of cerebral atrophy. This results in the shrinking of brain substance, leaving space between the brain and the dura, which remains attached to the skull (Fig. 18–2[4]). The bridging veins between the dura and the cortex are thereby put under tension. A minor trauma, such as bumping into a wall or even sitting down quickly, may tear these veins, producing an accumulation of subdural blood.

Clinical Manifestations

Symptoms occur over 12 to 24 hours and primarily involve a deteriorating GCS score. If the clot is unilateral, the patient will develop pupillary changes on the involved side and motor changes on the opposite side. Not infrequently, they are bilateral, in which case diagnosis is more difficult until a CT scan reveals the presence of hematoma. Even when the hematoma is surgically evacuated, the patient's ultimate return to normal functioning is in jeopardy. Damage from the clot, a space-occupying lesion, destroys the little cortical reserve in some instances.

Chronic Subdural Hematoma

The history of chronic subdural hematoma is often difficult to ascertain, since the original incident may have occurred 2 to 4 weeks before the emergency visit. The mechanism involves a small subdural collection of clotted blood. The initial bleeding has stopped but may recur intermittently. The clot is hyperosmotic to the brain, and its protein-rich fluid attracts more fluid from the surrounding tissue, enlarging in size over a period of time. The fluid in the hematoma is less dense than brain. On CT the clot is hypodense to the brain and appears similar to CSF, which is dark gray. Because this lesion enlarges slowly and these patients are often (as in acute subdural hematoma) victims of cerebral atrophy, the clot may reach a significant size before the patient becomes symptomatic. These clots can also occur bilaterally.

Clinical Manifestations

Symptoms center around a changing or decreasing level of consciousness. These patients may display personality changes, slurred speech, decreased judgment, decreased fine motor control, ataxia, or incontinence. They may be diagnosed as psychotic, drug or alcohol intoxicated, or suffering from dementia until an astute examiner notices papilledema and orders a CT scan. An ED clinician needs to consider the possibility of both acute and chronic subdural hematoma in an inebriated patient or in fact in any patient with alcohol on his or her breath. Since head trauma occurs more often in those who drink alcohol, organic causes for changes in mental status should be considered. A history may be difficult to obtain, and it is difficult to distinguish between intoxication and a space-occupying lesion as causes of a decreased level of consciousness. CT can save a patient's life.

Intraparenchymal Hemorrhage (Intracerebral Bleeding)

intraparenchymal hemorrhage: Bleeding into the substance of the brain (Fig. 18–2[7]).

Intracerebral bleeding can occur with head trauma. It is more common in patients with bleeding disorders or those on anticoagulant drugs. CT differentiation from a tumor that has bled or a hemorrhagic stroke may be difficult. The pathology may occur alone or in combination with the other bleeding. The expanding lesion may be due to disrupted blood vessels or contusion of the brain. The hemorrhage distorts anatomic relationships, stretches blood vessels, leads to shifts in brain compartments, and causes cerebral edema. The hemorrhage and its resulting edema may obstruct CSF outflow tracts and produce hydrocephalus, another space-occupying lesion.

Clinical Manifestations

The patient usually presents with an altered level of consciousness and a deteriorating GCS score. Pupillary changes are related to the size and location of the hemorrhage. As in all physiologic systems, a slowly developing mass allows time for compensatory mechanisms to develop, whereas one that develops rapidly causes much more rapid deterioration.

Cerebral Edema

Just as the presence of blood jeopardizes the intracranial compartments, intracerebral edema can also form a space-occupying lesion or cause mass effect (refer to the Monro-Kellie principle). Intracerebral edema may be *vasogenic* (caused by a breakdown in the blood-brain barrier and an interstitial capillary leak with fluid accumulation) or it may be *cytotoxic* (caused by increased intracellular fluid in the brain tissues). Cytotoxic edema is the result of a breakdown in the sodium-potassium pump, most likely because of severe hypoxemia. Both types occur in head trauma and during the emergency phase of care are best monitored with the GCS.

The formation of edema can be drastically worsened by hypotension. Cerebral perfusion pressure (CPP) is a derived figure representing the difference between mean arterial pressure (MAP) and intracranial pressure (ICP). In the normal individual, MAP is approximately 70 to 80 mmHg, and ICP is approximately 0 to 15 mmHg— CPP (70) = MAP (80) − ICP (10) (Table 18–2).

Although ICP measurements may not be possible in the emergency department, one can see how the MAP affects the CPP and that hypotension has the potential to further damage an injured brain. Hypercarbia, or an increased Pco_2, will cause

TABLE 18–2
CPP Equals MAP Minus ICP

	CPP (mmHg)	MAP (mmHg)	ICP (mmHg)	ICP (cm H_2O)*
Normal	70	80	10	147
Brain starvation	40	60	20	294

*Remember that each mmHg must be multiplied by 14.7 to translate this figure into centimeters of water, which is how a spinal tap is measured.

cerebral vasodilation and increase vasogenic cerebral edema. Hypoxia will potentiate cytotoxic edema.

Clinical Manifestations

Clinical manifestations of cerebral edema will be the signs and symptoms of increased intracranial pressure. The deteriorating level of consciousness is best described with the GCS. Vital sign changes in increased intracranial pressure are very unreliable and occur late. Tachycardia and hypotension are usually from systemic causes and will worsen cerebral damage as it worsens CPP. In a situation in which ICP is monitored, the Cushing reflex of an elevated systolic blood pressure and bradycardia is rarely seen. As final events, blood pressure may fall, pulse may rise, and pupils may fix and dilate, but therapy should have been instituted well before this, and is unlikely to affect outcome at this point.

Postconcussive Syndrome

The preferred term for concussions is *minor head injury*. The mechanism is a blow to the head with resulting rotational force. The period of unconsciousness is less than 20 to 30 minutes, the GCS is 13 to 15 after regaining consciousness, and hospitalization (if any) of less than 48 hours is required. Gennerelli, Thibault, and Adams, et al. (1982) discuss concussion, which was previously assumed to have no anatomic basis. However, sophisticated staining techniques in an animal model show evidence of white matter "shear injuries," and the "postconcussive syndrome" appears to have an anatomic basis. Although these injuries are classified as minor, patients may suffer significant morbidity and lost work days.

Clinical Manifestations

Hinkle (1988) summarizes the findings associated with the postconcussive syndrome as follows:

- Generalized mild to moderate headache
- Dizziness
- Irritability
- Short-term memory loss with retrograde or anterograde amnesia
- Visual changes
- Weakness
- Tinnitus
- Nausea

The duration of these symptoms may vary from a week to six months or longer. Referral of these patients and their families to a support group or the National Head Injury Foundation can provide support during this trying time.

Treatment and Nursing Care

Clinicians in the emergency department and, later, those in the ICU will focus their attention and management on the secondary lesions of head trauma. A conceptual approach with an integration of the Monro-Kellie principle is important. Understanding that all intracranial problems will involve too much volume in too little space and that all management modalities are directed to decreasing volume is necessary. Management may involve removal of a clot or drainage of CSF but will always involve control and management of cerebral edema. Clinical manifestations of neurologic trauma almost always imply decreased level of consciousness and a worsening of the GCS score, but a careful history and ongoing neurologic assessment are imperative.

During initial stabilization of the head-injured patient, medical and nursing diagnoses are formulated. These diagnoses guide the implementation of appropriate interventions for each patient. Goals of stage I nursing care involve accurate identification of changes in neurologic status and interventions to prevent further injury. Initially, the ABCs are secured, an IV established, and the patient placed on the cardiac monitor.

Tissue Perfusion, Altered (Cerebral), Related to Increased Intracranial Pressure Secondary to

- **Cerebral Edema**
- **Hypotension**
- **Breathing Pattern, Ineffective**
- **Occluded/Obstructed Venous Drainage**
- **Seizures**
- **Agitation**

Attempts to lower intracranial pressure are aimed at reducing cerebral edema, securing cardiovascular stabilization, and controlling the variables that decrease cerebral perfusion pressure. Each category is discussed separately.

Cerebral Edema

Cerebral edema may be lessened by avoiding hypoosmolar fluids and administering osmotic agents. Hypoosmolar fluids such as D5W should be avoided in the head-injured patient. The brain metabolizes dextrose, leaving free water to be absorbed by brain cells. This contributes to cerebral edema. Isotonic agents such as 0.9 normal saline solution (NSS) or Ringer's lactate are suggested solutions for resuscitation. Keep-open infusion rates are acceptable when hypovolemia is not suspected.

Mannitol, a hyperosmotic agent with large glucose molecules, is a diuretic that works primarily by pulling fluid from the interstitial space and drawing it into the vascular space. This allows the damaged brain cells more room to swell. Mannitol is often used to "buy time" to get to CT. It has the potential to worsen an intracerebral hemorrhage by giving it more room to expand, but it may be life-saving. The usual dose is 0.25 to 1 g/kg given as a bolus or a drip. Monitoring for potential dehydration and increased serum osmolarity caused by fluid diuresis is an important aspect of care for the patient who is receiving an osmotic agent. The so-called rebound effect of mannitol is more likely a result of the continued presence of cerebral edema that remanifests itself as the effect of the mannitol is dissipated. Lasix may also be used in the acute situation, but blood pressure should be closely monitored to avoid hypotension.

Steroids are still used in some situations. The basis for their use is that in high doses for a short period of time they may protect cell wall stability and treat cytotoxic edema. Some clinicians have questioned their efficacy. The complications from this therapy will not be seen in the ED but can occur in the intensive care unit and include delayed wound healing, disturbances in electrolyte balance, and gastrointestinal bleeding.

Hypotension Secondary to Blood or Fluid Loss

Monitor the patient's blood pressure and try to ascertain baseline, or normal, blood pressure from previous medical records or family. Administer fluids as ordered, both crystalloids (avoiding D5W) and colloids, to maintain blood pressure within physiologically normal ranges. A low blood pressure contributes significantly to cerebral disaster, because oxygenation to the already damaged brain diminishes. Be aware that a decreased blood pressure is hardly ever cerebral in origin and a search for other causes of hypotension is necessary. Observe the patient for signs of fluid overload: pulmonary edema, diminished oxygenation, an S_3, heart sound, or crackles on auscultation of the lungs.

Breathing Pattern, Ineffective, Secondary to Airway Obstruction Caused by

- *Decreased level of consciousness*

- *Soft tissue injury*

Monitoring of blood gases and respiratory patterns on a continuum is necessary. (Although Plum and Posner [1980] discuss correlation of breathing patterns with neurologic deterioration, in acute head injury when there is a variety of potential problems below the neck, breathing patterns are not as useful.) In severe head injury, suction should be readily available and a controlled, pharmacologically assisted endotracheal intubation is usually necessary. Patients with neurologic injuries may stop breathing with little warning, and their blood gases often show a poor correlation with their observed ventilatory pattern and breath sounds.

Maintain the P_{CO_2} between 25 and 30 mmHg. Many spontaneously breathing head trauma patients will hyperventilate to this level at least for a *short period of time*. Hypercarbia causes significant cerebral vasodilation, thus increasing intracranial pressure, and is to be avoided. If a patient shows signs and symptoms of CNS deterioration — pupils become less reactive or the GCS score deteriorates — manual hyperventilation at a fast rate and small tidal volume with a mask and bag-valve device can often improve the situation until more definitive therapy can be instituted. This maneuver effectively lowers P_{CO_2} without increasing intrathoracic volume and its concomitant, decreased venous return from the head. A patient with significant head injury may have soft tissue injuries to the face that may mandate immediate intubation or, if severe enough, a cricothyroid airway or emergency tracheostomy.

Maintain oxygenation within normal levels, usually above 80 mmHg. Hypoxemia will contribute to cerebral edema. Development of adult respiratory distress syndrome (ARDS) can occur in head injury for reasons that are somewhat unclear. Oxygenation abnormalities in the head-injured patient are often related to aspiration, and intubation for both pulmonary toilet and oxygenation may be necessary. Concomitant lung injuries frequently compound ventilation and oxygenation problems.

Occluded Venous Drainage, Secondary to Positioning

Decreased cerebral venous drainage can potentially increase cerebral edema. Some of these interventions will be difficult to achieve in the emergent phase of the injury, but should be addressed as soon as possible. Maintain the head of the bed at a 30-degree angle to enhance venous drainage. This therapy along with manual hyperventilation is often successful in the immediate treatment of a deteriorating LOC. Obviously, this therapy can only be carried out when the integrity of the spinal cord has been determined and fractures have been appropriately immobilized. Elevation of the head of the bed may also unmask hypovolemia and produce orthostatic vital signs. Even if the head of the bed cannot be elevated, maintain the patient in a neutral midline position; avoid hip flexion and head turns. Ideally, the nose should be in line with the xyphoid process to facilitate venous outflow drainage.

Seizures

In both the acute and chronic stages of head injury, seizures, which increase brain metabolic demands by 300% while the patient is not breathing, are unacceptable. If the patient has a major motor seizure, nursing care during the seizure is to do nothing except watch and time the seizure carefully. Tongue blades are to be avoided at all times; insertion during a seizure is impossible, and leaving a tongue blade or an oral airway — which is often difficult to insert properly — in place has the potential to obstruct the airway and produce gagging and vomiting. If the patient bites such an object, breakage that can obstruct the airway may result.

After the seizure, the clinician should prevent aspiration, ideally by turning the patient to one side if the cervical spine is intact. Oral suctioning is often necessary, since in the postictal stage, the patient may lose the ability to protect the airway. If the patient is not breathing adequately, supplemental oxygen and/or manually assisted bag-valve breaths may be necessary. Acute treatment of a seizure often involves 5 to 10 mg of a diazepam (e.g., Valium), which should be injected directly into a vein or given in a small volume of normal saline: these drugs may precipitate in D5W. At this dosage range, the patient can stop breathing and may require ventilatory support.

Prevention, a much better therapy, usually involves phenytoin (Dilantin). A loading dose must be administered and is generally 1 g. Most hospitals have a protocol for this therapy. One gram is administered in 250 ml of NSS with the use of a volumetric pump, over a period of 30 minutes. Administration should not exceed 50 mg/minute. The nurse must monitor the patient closely for dysrhythmias and hypotension. Phenytoin is extremely irritating to veins because of its high pH, and care must be taken to choose a patent vein of a reasonable size. The antecubital vein is ideal, since it is not useful for maintenance IV therapy. Administration through a vein in a distal extremity is to be avoided.

Patient Agitation, Secondary to

- *Head injury*
- *Pain*
- *Anxiety*
- *Increased intracranial pressure*

Patient agitation due to head injury, pain, or increased intracranial pressure is common. A few years ago, sedation for a head-injured patient would have been viewed with alarm. However, with monitoring and with the availability of frequent neurologic assessment and blood gas analyses, allowing a patient with an already increased intracranial pressure to struggle seems at odds with good management.

Analgesia or sedation is usually accomplished with morphine, 1 to 4 mg/hour, IV push. At this dosage, pupils can still be assessed, and pharmacologic reversal can be accomplished easily. The clinician must monitor the patient closely for hypotension and hypercarbia. Hypotension is usually not an issue if the patient's volume repletion is adequate. The opiates tend to cause patients to breathe more slowly but also more deeply. Although analgesics may cause confusion and interfere with accurate neurologic evaluations, the benefits in reducing patient agitation are clear. Patient agitation not only increases intracranial pressure but can be dangerous (should the patient become violent) to both patient and clinicians.

Knowledge Deficit, Patient and Family

Discharge instructions for the patient with minor head injury should be given to family or significant others (Table 18–3). Whether the patient has suffered a minor

---

TABLE 18–3
Head Injury: Important Points in Treatment

Activities
  Limit your activity as directed

Diet
  There is no special diet to follow; however, it is best not to eat heavy
    meals or drink alcoholic beverages for 24 hours

Medications
  Take only aspirin or acetaminophen (Tylenol) for headache
  Avoid other over-the-counter medications unless approved by your
    doctor

Seek Medical Attention Immediately If Any of the Following Occurs
  Oral temperature over 101°F
  Severe headache not relieved by aspirin or Tylenol
  Dizziness or blurred vision
  Vomiting
  Stiff neck
  Unusual sleepiness
  Convulsions
  Stumbling or weakness in your arms or legs
  Numbness of any part of the body
  Confusion, memory loss

---

head injury with no sequelae, posttraumatic concussive syndrome, or a severe head injury, families will need support and teaching.

Emergency department nurses should be actively involved in promoting and practicing ways to prevent head injuries — e.g., restraints for drivers and passengers, legislative support for significant penalties for drinking and driving, and the use of helmets for contact sports. There is no panacea for head injuries, but prevention can help.

Subarachnoid Hemorrhage

Subarachnoid hemorrhage (SAH) is another form of intracerebral bleeding. Jennett and Galbrath (1983) and Kistler and Heros (1983) discuss this difficult problem. The mechanism is not traumatic, although the patient may have suffered SAH and subsequently sustained a fall or MVA. The cause of SAH in the adult population is usually a ruptured aneurysm in the circle of Willis (Fig. 18 – 2[8]). The circle of Willis provides the blood supply to the brain, lies at the base of the skull in the subarachnoid space, and is bathed in the CSF.

An aneurysm is usually less than 10 mm in diameter; when it ruptures, it bleeds approximately 15 to 30 ml before the procoagulant substances of the brain and CSF stop the hemorrhage (Fig. 18 – 2[6]). However, since the normal volume of CSF is approximately 100 ml, the hemorrhage represents a substantial volume increase. Not only does the volume of CSF increase, blood in the CSF can decrease normal CSF reabsorption mechanisms.

According to Jane and colleagues (1985) SAH occurs at the rate of approximately 12 per 100,000, or about 25,000 per year in the United States. Peak incidence occurs between ages of 35 and 55, with a slight increase in women who smoke.

Clinical Manifestations

Approximately 40% of these patients have had a severe headache in the previous few days to four weeks. The headache symptoms were different from those of their normal headaches but did not prompt them to seek medical attention. When these patients do present in the ED they complain of the acute onset of the "worst headache of my life," which is unrelenting. Associated findings include a stiff neck, or nuchal rigidity, and photophobia, caused by the presence of blood in the subarachnoid space. Hypertension even in the previously normotensive patient is common in acute SAH. Nausea and vomiting and a period of unconsciousness, the length of which may vary, are also common. The patient often does not know of the period of unconsciousness; the family should be questioned. The patient may also have a major motor seizure. The GCS score can vary from 15 to 3. Diagnosis is made from the history and confirmed with a CT, which shows blood in the subarachnoid space and often in the ventricles. Jane and associates state that approximately 33% of these patients will be dead on arrival at the ED or will die shortly afterward.

Treatment and Nursing Care

Pain, Related to

- **Blood in the Subarachnoid Space**

These patients have a severe, unremitting headache. Many neurosurgeons feel that adequate analgesia is important. Codeine not infrequently worsens nausea. Small doses of hydromorphine hydrochloride (Dilaudid; 1 to 2 mg IV) or morphine sulfate (1 to 4 mg IV) will lessen the headache, but will not obscure pupillary reaction or diminish level of consciousness.

Nausea and vomiting are both common in these patients and can raise intracranial pressure and potentiate rebleeding. Prochlorperazine maleate (Compazine; 10 mg IV or IM) is usually necessary to control these symptoms. Milder antiemetics do not seem useful.

Knowledge Deficit (Patient and Significant Others), Related to

- **Subarachnoid Hemorrhage (Etiology, Treatment, Prognosis)**

The sudden onset of this event, usually in a patient who is a healthy, middle-aged individual, produces severe anxiety in both family and patient. Families frequently express feelings of guilt ("It's my fault, I should have insisted she see the doctor," or "He's been under stress, and I just made it worse.") that need to be addressed. The only sure way to diagnose this condition is with a four-vessel cerebral angiogram, an expensive and potentially hazardous invasive test. Families need to be reassured that the SAH was not the result of interpersonal interactions and that an aneurysm, prehemorrhage, is too small to have caused any symptoms that would have warranted an angiogram.

These patients should be transferred to an appropriate environment, preferably a neuroscience intensive care unit, and to the care of a skilled neurosurgeon as soon as possible. The patient will need a four-vessel angiogram to locate the site of the aneurysm. Patients with a subarachnoid hemorrhage are graded according to the Hunt-Hess scale (1968) ranging from Grade I, awake and alert with a mild headache, to Grade V, moribund. Both the potential outcome and the timing for surgery are controversial. Most neurosurgeons now feel that a patient who is a Grade I or II should have an angiogram immediately and should undergo surgery within 24 to 36 hours posthemorrhage. The management of patients with other grades is difficult and varies from institution to institution. Complications include rebleeding, most likely within the first 2 to 3 days, with a mortality rate of over 30%. Vasospasm due to the presence of blood in the subarachnoid space causes blood vessel narrowing and progressive strokes. Vasospasm occurs in over 50% of the patients who have survived to this point and begins on approximately day 3 or 4 posthemorrhage and usually lasts to day 14 but may extend to day 21.

CONCLUSION

This chapter has addressed the etiology, pathophysiology, clinical manifestations, and management of head trauma and subarachnoid hemorrhage. Management modalities are directed at identifying mass lesions and treating them and the cerebral edema they cause. Maintenance of systemic vascular and ventilation/oxygenation homeostasis is imperative. Providing neurosurgical patients with an accurate and ongoing neurologic assessment and interventions that maintain a well-perfused brain maximizes the ability of the neurosurgical staff and intensive care personnel to help these patients to recover.

REFERENCES

The American Association of Neuroscience Nurses. 1984. Core Curriculum for Neuroscience Nursing, vols 1 & 2. Chicago. American Assoc. Neuroscience Nurses.

Bruce D, Gennarelli T, Langfitt T. 1978. Resuscitation from coma due to head injury. Crit Care Med 6:254.

Carpenter MB. 1985. Core Text of Neuroanatomy. Baltimore, Williams & Wilkins.

Caveness WJ. 1979. Incidence of Craniocerebral Trauma in the United States in 1976, with Trends from 1970. Thompson RT, Green JR, eds. Advances in Neurology, 22. New York, Raven Press, 1–3.

Gennarelli T, Thibault LE, Adams JH, et al. 1982. Diffuse axonal injury and traumatic coma in the primate. Ann Neurol 12:564.

Gennarelli T, Spielmun GM, Langfitt TW, et al. 1982. Influence of the type of intracranial lesion on outcome from severe head injury. J Neurosurg 56:26–32.

Gillies DA, Alyn IB. 1976. Patient Assessment and Management by the Nurse Practitioner. Philadelphia, WB Saunders.

Hayward R. 1980. Essentials of Neurosurgery. London, Blackwell Scientific Publications.

Henning R, Jackson DL. 1985. Handbook of Critical Care Neurology and Neurosurgery. New York, Praeger.

Hinkle J. 1988. Nursing care of patients with minor head injury. J Neurosci Nurs 30:8–14.

Hoyt DB, Shackford SR, Marshall LF. 1985. Initial resuscitation. In Initial resuscitation: the trauma surgeon and neurosurgeon—a combined perspective. Trauma Q 2:8–19.

Hunt WE, Hess RM. 1968. Surgical risk as related to time of intervention in the repair of intercranial aneurysm. J Neurosurg 28:14–20.

Jane JA, Kassell NF, Torner JC, et al. 1985. The natural history of aneurysms and arteriovenous malformation. J Neurosurg 62:321–323.

Jennett B, Galbrath S. 1983. An Introduction to Neurosurgery. Chicago, William Heinemann Medical Books.

Jennett B, Teasdale F. 1981. Management of Head Injuries. Philadelphia, FA Davis.

Kalsbeek WD, McLaurin RL, Harris BS, et al. 1980. The national head and spinal cord injury survey: major findings. J Neurosurg 53:819–831.

Kistler JP, Heros RC. 1988. Management of subarachnoid hemorrhage from ruptured saccular aneurysm. In Ropper AH, Kennedy SK, Zervas NT, eds. Neurological and Neurosurgical Intensive Care. 2nd ed. Rockville, Md, Aspen, 219–232.

Langfitt T. 1969. Increased intracranial pressure. Clin Neurosurg 16:436.

Mancall EL. 1981. Essentials of the Neurologic Examination. Philadelphia, FA Davis, 13–20.

Mitchell PH. 1986. Decreased adaptive capacity, intracranial: a proposal for nursing diagnosis. J Neurosci Nurs 19:183–190.

Nelson PB. 1987. Fluid and electrolyte physiology, pathophysiology, and management. In Wirth EP, Racheson RA, eds. Neurosurgical Critical Care. Baltimore, Williams & Wilkins, 69–80.

Pitts LH, Trunkey DD, 1987. The multiple trauma patient in the NICU. In Wirth EP, Racheson RA, eds. Neurosurgical Critical Care. Baltimore, Williams & Wilkins, 215–230.

Nikas DL. 1982. The Critical Ill Neurosurgical Patient. New York, Churchill Livingstone.

Plum F, Posner JB. 1980. The Diagnosis of Stupor and Coma, 3rd ed. Philadelphia, FA Davis, 13–14.

Purchese G, Allen D. 1984. Neuromedical and Neurosurgical Nursing. London, Bailliere-Tindall, 59–90.

Rauch Rhodes P. 1982. Nurses' Guide to Neurosurgical Patient Care. Oradell, NJ, Medical Economics Books.

Rimel R, Jane J, Edlich R. 1979. Assessment of recovery following head trauma. Crit Care Q 2:97.

Ropper AH, Kennedy SK. 1988. Neurological and Neurosurgical Intensive Care. 2nd ed. Rockville, MD, Aspen, 9–17, 165–171.

Rowlands BJ, Litofsky NS, Kaufman HH. 1987. Metabolic physiology, pathophysiology, and management. In Wirth EP, Racheson RA, eds. Neurosurgical Critical Care. Baltimore, Williams & Wilkins, 81–108.

Seelig JM, Becker DP, Miller DJ, et al. 1981. Traumatic acute subdural hematoma: major mortality reduction in comatose patients treated within four hours. N Engl J Med 304:1511–1518.

Stevens M. 1983. Proconcussion syndrome. J Ncurosurg Nurs 14:239.

Taylor JW, Ballenger S. 1980. Neurological Dysfunctions and Nursing Intervention. New York, McGraw-Hill Book Co. 399–411.

Teasdale G, Jennett B. 1974. Assessment of coma and impaired consciousness. Lancet 2:81–84.

Mary Wlasowicz, RN MS

Spinal Cord Injuries

EPIDEMIOLOGY

Traumatic spinal cord injury (SCI) in the United States has an annual incidence of nearly 8000 cases/year. The prevalence of persons living with an SCI is estimated as between 150,000 and 200,000 (Young et al 1982). SCI is primarily a disease of the young, with the majority of injuries occurring in boys and men (80 per cent) in their second or third decade of life. Nevertheless, Figure 19–1 confirms that all ages are susceptible to this devastating injury (MRSCICS 1986; Young et al 1982). There are differences in the causes of injury between men and women. Women tend to have a higher percentage of injuries caused by motor vehicle accidents (MVA), in comparison to a higher rate of sports injuries for males (Young et al 1982). MVAs account for the largest factor (38 per cent) contributing to the incidence of spinal cord injuries (Fig. 19–2). Data from the Midwest Regional Spinal Cord Injury Care System (MRSCICS, 1986), however, demonstrate a gradual decrease in motor vehicle–related injuries, with a noticeable increase in falls (Fig. 19–3).

The steady decline of MVA-related SCI can be partially explained by speed limit controls on freeways, stringent laws for drunk drivers, and seat belt usage. Mandatory seat belt and child restraint laws have reduced the incidence, morbidity, and mortality associated with SCI. There is an inverse relationship between seat belt use and incidence of spinal cord injury resulting from MVAs; persons who wear seat belts are less likely to sustain this severe and irreversible disability (Huelke et al 1979).

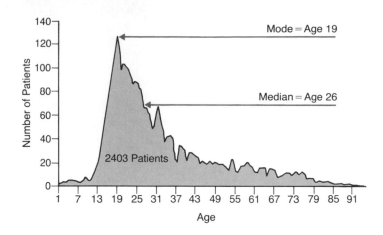

FIGURE 19–1. The median age of all patients admitted to the Acute Unit between 1972 and 1985 is 26 years; 19 is the mode. Although the mode has remained the same over the past few years, the median age has been continually rising. This finding supports the observation that although the acute unit still treats a large percentage of young trauma victims, the number of elderly (76 years and older), medically based spinal cord admissions is rising (carcinoma, stenosis, rheumatoid arthritis, osteoporosis). (Redrawn by permission from Midwest Regional Spinal Cord Injury Care Systems, 1986.)

Spinal cord injury resulting from falls has increased dramatically over previous years (Fig. 19–3). Construction workers fall from scaffolding, ladders, or other elevated platforms. Persons who attempt suicide fall from windows, balconies, or bridges. Elderly persons are prone to falls from lower heights, such as a chair or stairs. Arthritic changes in the cervical spine predispose the elderly to injuries that may seem disproportionate to the mechanism. For example, a simple fall may cause acute hyperextension of the neck as the chin strikes a hard surface (Dudas and Stevens 1984).

Gunshot wounds (13 per cent) and knife stabbings are the third largest factor contributing to spinal cord injury. Major metropolitan cities show that these injuries are almost as frequent a cause of spinal injury as MVAs (Green and Eismont 1984).

Surprisingly swimming, diving, and athletic injuries account for 9 to 15 per cent of all spinal cord injuries, depending on site of the trauma (Young et al 1982). There

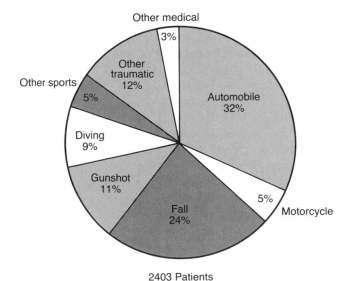

FIGURE 19–2. Overall causes of spinal injury. (Modified by permission from Midwest Regional Spinal Cord Injury Care Systems, 1986.)

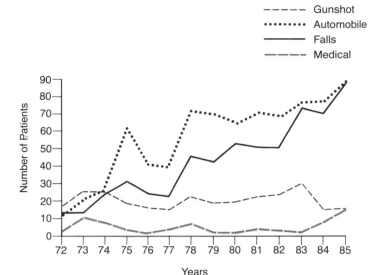

FIGURE 19–3. Annual causes of injury. (Modified with permission from Midwest Regional Spinal Cord Injury Care Systems, 1986.)

is alarming evidence that 94 per cent of patients who sustain injuries while diving become quadriplegic. Most often these victims have dived head first and struck the head on the bottom in water less than three feet deep. Most sports-related spinal cord injuries occur during the summer months when people are most active and engage in activities that put them at risk for injury.

Case histories indicate that injuries tend to occur during an episode of acting out, risk taking, or impulsive behavior. There is a direct relationship between drug and alcohol use (8 to 10 per cent) and mental health problems (3 to 8 per cent) with victims who sustain spinal cord injury (Athelstan and Crewe 1979; Young et al 1982).

The prevalence of spinal cord injuries varies both by season and by day of week. The summer season, particularly the month of July, is the most prevalent period, and Saturday and Sunday are by far the days with highest risk statistically (Young et al 1982).

MODEL SPINAL CORD INJURY CARE SYSTEMS

Historical interest in spinal cord injuries dates back to 2500 BC. At that time the philosophy on management of victims with spinal cord injuries was "an ailment not to be treated" (Guttmann 1974). Since then, evolution of spinal injury management systems has reduced mortality and morbidity.

Guttmann (1974), of Stoke Mandeville, England, demonstrated a decrease in the morbidity and mortality associated with SCI using his model system care approach to spinal cord–injured victims. The system approach introduced by Guttmann was adopted by the United States Rehabilitation Services Administration in 1970. The Model Systems concept embodies the following objectives:

> To establish a multidisciplinary system so as to provide (1) comprehensive rehabilitation services from point of injury (emergency treatment and transportation) through acute care; (2) rehabilitation, including vocational and educational preparation; (3) community and job placement; and (4) long-term follow-up to a specified catchment area.

Additional objectives include arrangement and acceleration of appropriate transport, prehospital, and in-transit care to a Regional Spinal Cord Injury Care System (RSCICS); gaining knowledge through research aimed at preventing and reducing the impact of disability; and improving management of SCI and its associated complications through all phases of recovery. Emphasis on curative research on spinal cord injury, such as cord regeneration and functional electrical stimulation, is an objective of RSCICS centers but is yet in its infancy.

The key to system care lies in the development of a multidisciplinary team of physicians, nurses, and allied health professionals dedicated to and specializing in the treatment of this disease. RSCICS centers have been successful in achieving the objectives of saving lives, preventing and reducing the extent of neurologic trauma, and ultimately increasing functional abilities of the SCI victim. The dramatic impact of the SCI programs is shown in expeditious transfer of patients to a RSCICS (median time from injury to admission is 8 hours, mode 4 hours) and a decrease in the percentage of patients with complete neurologic injuries from 90 per cent in 1972 to 33 per cent in 1986 (Fig. 19–4) (MRSCICS 1986).

Considering all forms of trauma, the societal impact of spinal cord injury is disproportionate to the numbers of patients injured. The cost in terms of hospitalization and disability is astronomical and the highest for all illnesses. The initial months

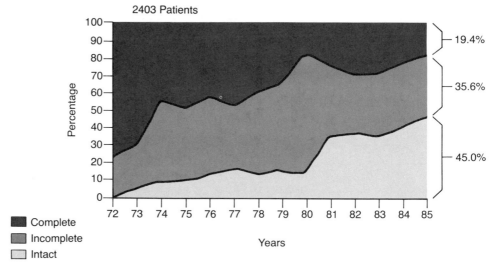

FIGURE 19–4. Neurologic changes in ten years. (Modified with permission from Midwest Regional Spinal Cord Injury Care Systems, 1986.)

of hospital care can cost from $56,000 to $80,000 and lifetime costs are conservatively estimated to be from $300,000 to $600,000 (Young et al 1982).

The Model Systems approach to management of SCI demonstrates reduction in hospital length of stay, costs, incidence of complications, and morbidity and mortality resulting from post-traumatic complications. Most importantly there is evidence that patients who are managed at a RSCICS demonstrate better neurologic recovery than those patients managed at other institutions (Young et al 1979).

ANATOMY AND PHYSIOLOGY

Spine

The spinal column is composed of 33 vertebrae; seven cervical, 12 thoracic, five lumbar, five fused sacral, and, usually, four rudimentary coccygeal vertebrae (Fig. 19-5).

With the exception of the atlas (C1) and the axis (C2) all vertebrae are anatomically alike but differ in size and function. Each vertebra consists of a body anteriorly and a vertebral arch posteriorly. Each arch is composed of two paired pedicles connecting the arch to the body, two paired laminae, and seven spinal processes (Fig. 19-5).

The human vertebral column allows people to assume an upright position. It provides a base for muscle attachments, protects the spinal cord and vital organs in the thorax, supports the head, and allows for body movements. Flexion, extension, and rotational movements vary according to vertebral segments.

The cervical spinal column has maximal flexibility. It supports the entire weight of the skull and brain and allows flexion, extension, and rotation movements to occur. Flexibility of the cervical spine makes it extremely vulnerable to fractures and dislocations. The C5-C6 area of the spine is most commonly injured (Adelstein and Watson 1983; MRSCICS 1986; Young et al 1982). The thoracic region is relatively fixed, as it is attached to the thoracic rib cage. The thoracolumbar junction (T12-L1) is the second most common site for injury, owing to the normal curvature of the spine at this level. Vertebrae in the lumbar sacral region are heavily constructed and supported by paraspinal musculature, requiring a great deal of force to cause disruption.

Disks and Ligaments

Intervertebral cartilaginous disks provide cushioning and shock absorption between vertebral segments. Vertebral bodies are joined throughout the length of the spine by longitudinal ligaments anteriorly and posteriorly. These ligaments protect the spine against severe hyperextension or extreme flexion.

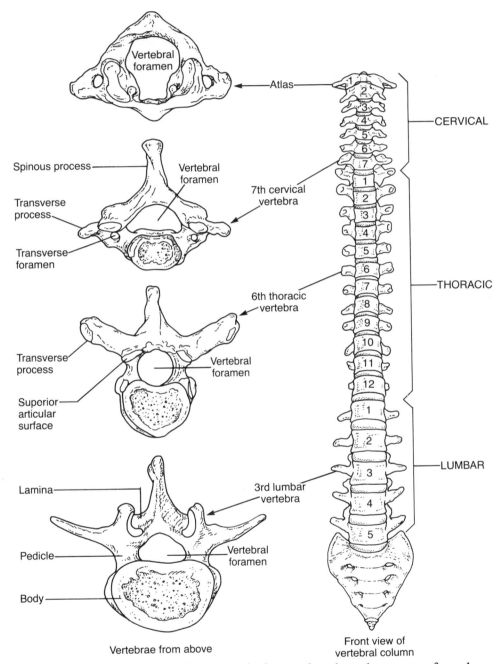

FIGURE 19–5. Anterior view of the vertebral column; selected vertebrae are seen from above.

Spinal Cord

The spinal cord (Fig. 19–6), as part of the central nervous system, lies protected within the spinal canal, which is a hollow tunnel extending the length of the vertebral column. The spinal cord descends from the medulla oblongata near the atlas to the level of the second lumbar vertebra. The distal portion of the cord, termed the conus medullaris, tapers to the level of the second lumbar vertebra. A non-neural filament called the filium terminale continues caudally and attaches to the back of the coccyx.

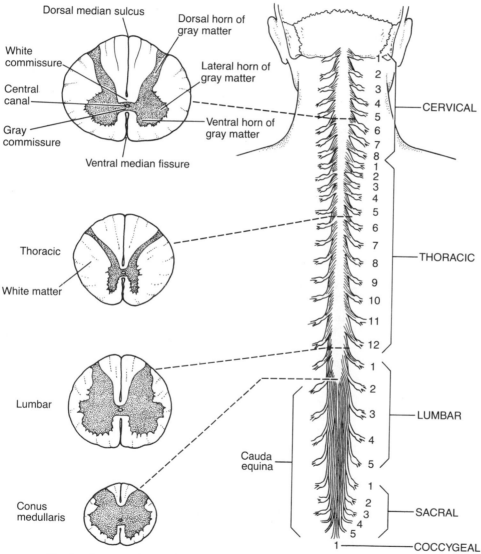

FIGURE 19–6. Cross-sectional views of the spinal cord, showing regional variations in the gray matter.

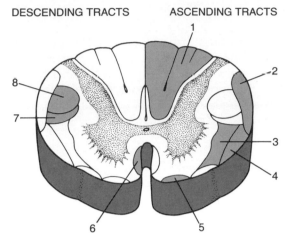

DESCENDING TRACTS   ASCENDING TRACTS

All tracts are bilateral

1 Dorsal columns:
   conscious muscle sense, touch, vibration

2 Dorsal spinocerebellar tract:
   unconscious muscle sense

3 Lateral spinothalamic tract:
   pain and temperature

4 Ventral spinocerebellar tract:
   unconscious muscle sense

5 Ventral spinothalamic tract:
   light touch

6 Ventral pyramidal tract:
   voluntary control of skeletal muscle

7 Extrapyramidal tract:
   automatic control of skeletal muscle

8 Lateral pyramidal tract:
   voluntary control of skeletal muscle

FIGURE 19–7. Cross section of the spinal cord showing principal conduction pathways. These tracts are bilateral, but in this diagram ascending tracts are numbered on the right only, and descending on the left only. Redrawn from Chaffee EE, Lytle IM. 1980. Basic Physiology and Anatomy, 4th ed. JB Lippincott, 241.

The spinal cord is nearly circular in section and about 1 cm in diameter with two enlargements. On cross section the spinal cord has gray matter, appearing in the form of the letter H. The gray matter consists of nerve cells that act as relay stations for nerve impulses transmitted up and down the spinal cord. White matter surrounds the gray matter. The white matter contains longitudinal myelinated fibers organized in tracts or bundles to carry information to and from the brain. Ascending tracts are sensory and descending tracts are motor.

Spinal Cord Tracts

Assessment and diagnosis of spinal cord injuries depend principally on the integrity of the following prominent spinal cord tracts (Fig. 19–7).

1. The spinothalamic tract, located anterolaterally, is an ascending tract carrying information regarding pain, touch, and temperature sensation to the cortex.

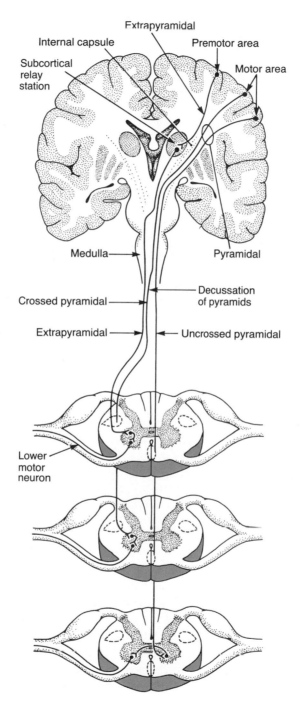

FIGURE 19-8. Diagram of motor pathways between the cerebral cortex, one of the subcortical relay centers, and lower motor neurons in the spinal cord. Decussation (crossing) of fibers means that each side of the brain controls skeletal muscles on the opposite side of the body.

2. The posterior column spinal tract, also an ascending sensory tract, provides information regarding deep touch, vibration, and proprioception.

3. The corticospinal tract is located anterolaterally and is a descending tract. Voluntary motor activity from the cortex to the spinal column is accomplished via the corticospinal (pyramidal) tract.

Pathways of communication to and from the brain depend on the manner in which the tracts cross. The corticospinal tract crosses in the medulla, so that the opposite side of the brain controls motor activity. Sensory information of proprioception, vibration, and deep touch (posterior column) ascends along the same side of the cord and crosses at the level of the medulla. Fibers for pain and temperature sensation (spinothalamic) cross when entering the cord and ascend (Fig. 19–8).

Spinal Nerves

There are 31 pairs of spinal nerves originating from the spinal cord. Each has a ventral (anterior) root and a dorsal (posterior) root. The anterior root is motor, and the posterior root is sensory. There are eight cervical, 12 thoracic, five lumbar, five sacral, and one coccygeal pairs of spinal nerves. Each pair of spinal nerves corresponds to a spinal cord segment. The group of nerve rootlets and fibers resembling a horse's tail extends beyond the end of the cord and is termed the cauda equina.

Spinal nerve roots exiting from the cord at each segmental level are numbered in relation to the level from which they exit. Cervical nerves exit above each vertebral

TABLE 19–1
Spinal Nerves, Associated Muscles Innervated, and
Patient Response

Nerve Level	Muscles Innervated	Patient Response
C4	Diaphragm	
C5	Deltoid	Shrug shoulders
	Biceps	Flex elbows
	Brachioradialis	
C6	Wrist extensors	Extend wrist
	Extensor carpi radialis longus	
C7	Triceps	Extend elbow
	Extensor digitorum communis	Extend fingers
	Flexor carpi radialis	
C8	Flexor digitorum profundus	Flex fingers
	Flexor digitorum superficialis	
T1	Hand intrinsic muscles	Spread fingers
T2-L1	Intercostals	Evaluate vital capacity
	Abdominals	Abdominal reflexes
L2	Iliopsoas	Hip flexion
L3	Quadriceps	Knee extension
L4	Tibialis anterior	Ankle dorsiflexion
L5	Extensor hallucis longus	Ankle eversion
S1	Gastrocnemius	Ankle plantar flexion
		Big toe extension
S2-S5	Perineal sphincter	Sphincter control

SENSORY DERMATOMES

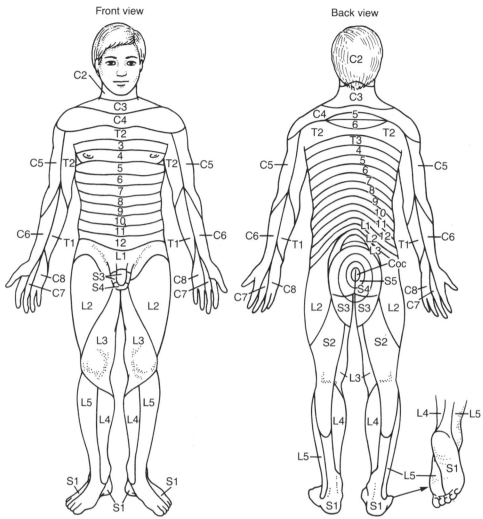

FIGURE 19-9. Sensory dermatomes, anterior and posterior views. (Redrawn from Standards for Neurological Classification of Spinal Injury Patients, American Spinal Injury Association, 1982.)

level whereas thoracic and lumbar nerves exit below the vertebrae. This explains why there are eight cervical nerve roots. A key assessment of injuries to the spinal cord or nerve root lies in the segmental pattern of alteration of motor, sensory, and reflex activity in the extremities. The dorsal root of each nerve supplies sensory innervation of a body segment known as a dermatome. Arrangement of dermatomes is illustrated in Figure 19-9.

Distribution of motor activity is in segments known as myotomes. Table 19-1 details the muscles innervated at each level and the muscle actions to be tested for spinal cord integrity of the corticospinal tracts.

Vascular Supply to the Cord

Vascular supply to the spinal cord originates from two main sources: from anterior and posterior spinal arteries, and from a series of spinal rami that enter the intervertebral foramina at successive levels. The anterior spinal artery lies in the median fissure throughout the length of the spinal cord. The two posterior spinal arteries descend toward the emerging spinal roots. Typically, the anterior artery distributes to the ventral two thirds of the spinal cord, while the dorsal one third is supplied by the posterior arteries.

Disruption of vascular supply to the cord results in deprivation of oxygen and nutrients and subsequent necrosis of neural tissue. Compromised arterial supply may give rise to clinical evidence of ischemia at a level above the actual site of the lesion owing to proximal loss of blood flow. This is particularly noted in the segmental area between T1 and T4 where perfusion is normally thought to be diminished. Spinal cord arteries are unable to develop collateral circulation to preserve neurologic function.

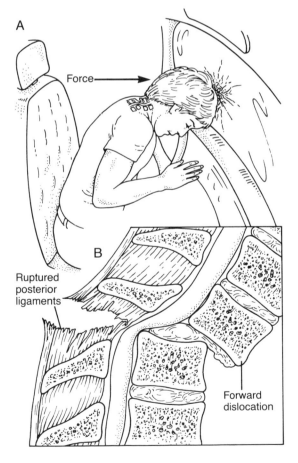

FIGURE 19–10. Posterior ligament rupture resulting from forward dislocation of the vertebrae.

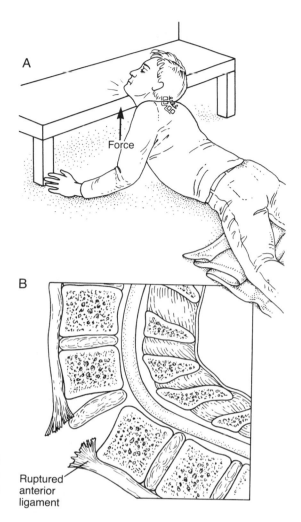

FIGURE 19-11. Anterior ligament rupture resulting from hyperextension and posterior dislocation of the vertebrae.

Ruptured anterior ligament

MECHANISMS OF INJURY

The majority of injuries to the spine are closed. The four vectors of force applied to the spinal column are flexion, extension, compression and rotation. The amount of force required to injure the spine depends, in part, on the level of the spinal column affected. The cervical and lumbar areas are designed for mobility. Injuries are easier to produce in these regions, especially in the cervical spine where the musculature to support the neck is not as strong as in the lumbar spine. More force is required to produce an injury to the thoracic region than to any other portion of the spine because of its rigidity.

By far the major mechanism of injury is flexion motion. This commonly occurs with MVAs in which the victim strikes the head against the steering wheel or windshield and the spine is forced into acute hyperflexion with the chin thrown forward to the chest. Rupture of the posterior ligaments results in forward dislocation of the spine (Fig. 19-10).

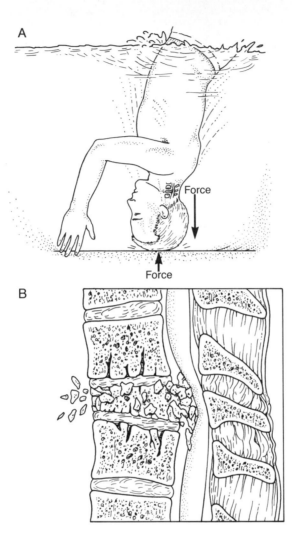

FIGURE 19–12. Compression force causing wedging and crush type injury of the vertebrae.

Extension injuries result after a fall where the chin hits an object and the head is thrown back. The anterior ligament is ruptured with a fracture of posterior elements of the vertebral body (Fig. 19–11).

Axial load injuries, commonly known as compression type injuries (Fig. 19–12), occur most frequently with falls. Vertebral bodies are wedged and compressed. The burst vertebral fragments enter the spinal canal, piercing the cord.

Rotational injuries can occur as a result of a variety of accidents. Disruption of the entire ligamentous structure, fracture, and fracture-dislocation of the facets occur. Flexion-rotational injuries are highly unstable fractures.

Penetrating cord injuries result from either gunshot wounds or knife wounds. The lacerated neural tissue causes disruption of blood flow to the cord. Generally, there is no ligamentous instability or damage to the vertebral bodies.

Pathophysiology

The spinal cord may be injured by a number of mechanisms that compress or impair its blood supply and disrupt tissue integrity. The level of injury is determined by the lowest (most caudal) spinal cord segment with intact sensory and motor function. MRSCICS (1986) reports a steady rise (45 per cent) of neurologically intact patients at admission despite the presence of vertebral column fractures. These gains are attributed to the improved emergency care and spinal cord management.

Spinal Cord Injury

Neurologic injuries to the spinal cord can be either complete or incomplete. A complete injury is loss of all voluntary motor, reflex, and sensory function below the level of the lesion. An incomplete injury results in partially preserved motor or sensory function, or both, below the level of the lesion. The presence of rectal sensation indicating preservation of some sensory function at the sacral level confirms the clinical diagnosis of an incomplete injury. Presence of rectal tone alone is not an indication of an incomplete injury. Positive rectal tone often indicates return of spinal reflexes and resolution of spinal cord shock.

SPINAL SHOCK

The term "spinal shock" was coined in the early nineteenth century and is still used despite its various definitions and applications. Spinal shock signifies absence of reflexes and of motor and sensory functioning below the level of the lesion following a severe spinal cord injury.

This areflexive state is due to the sudden withdrawal of the many excitatory and inhibitory influences that occur within the spinal cord. Spinal shock is accompanied by other autonomic deviations from normal in the patient with high cervical spine injury. These deviations produce symptoms of hypotension, bradycardia, and hypothermia owing to the loss of sympathetic control and tone.

The areflexive state of spinal shock may last from several hours to several weeks. Emergence from spinal shock is evident with the return of reflex functioning (e.g., bulbocavernosus reflex). The bulbocavernosus reflex is tested by squeezing the glans penis, tapping the clitoris, or tugging on the uretheral catheter. This causes a reflex contracture of the anal sphincter.

INCOMPLETE SPINAL CORD INJURIES

Spinal cord injuries may be complete with no neural function below the level of injury or may be incomplete. Persons with incomplete spinal cord injuries exhibit

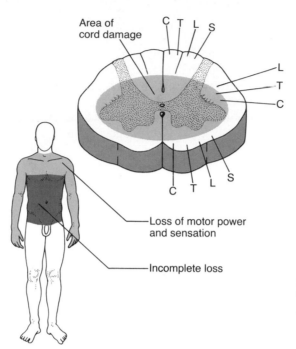

Area of
cord damage

Loss of motor power
and sensation

Incomplete loss

FIGURE 19–13. A cross section of the spinal cord showing area damaged and associated motor and sensory loss. C, Cervical; T, thoracic; L, lumbar; S, sacral.

some motor or sensory function below the level of the injury. Sacral sparing, represented by sensation in the perineum or voluntary anal sphincter contraction, may be the only early evidence that an injury is incomplete (Green et al 1982; Meyer 1982). Some patients with incomplete injuries demonstrate distinct patterns of neurologic deficits classified as syndromes.

Central Cord Syndromes

A central cord syndrome is caused by a hyperextension injury to the central area of the spinal cord (Fig. 19–13). The tracts of the cord are organized such that cervical fibers are central, and lumbar and sacral fibers are on the outermost portion of the cord. Clinically, the patient demonstrates motor and sensory impairment that is more marked in the upper extremities. Prognosis of recovery from central cord syndrome is relatively good (Dudas and Stevens 1984; Green et al 1982). This injury, generally occurring as a result of a fall, is easily overlooked in the elderly because no radiologic signs of trauma are present apart from cervical spondylolysis. The elderly are most prone to this type of syndrome owing to pre-existing weakness of the intervertebral disks, which are fragmented and fissured as a result of degeneration (Scher 1983).

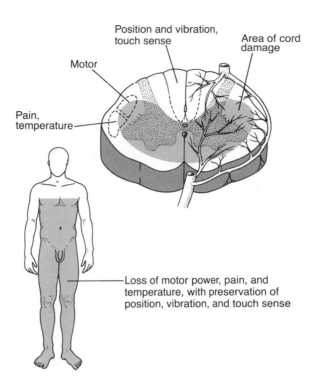

Position and vibration, touch sense

Motor

Area of cord damage

Pain, temperature

Loss of motor power, pain, and temperature, with preservation of position, vibration, and touch sense

FIGURE 19–14. Anterior cord syndrome; cord damage and associated motor and sensory loss.

Anterior Cord Syndromes

Damage to the anterior aspect of the cord, where the corticospinal (motor fibers) and spinothalamic (pain, temperature) tracts lie, results in loss of both voluntary motor activity and pain and temperature sensation. This anterior cord syndrome is commonly produced by flexion or rotational forces occurring in MVAs and diving accidents. Disruption of the anterior spinal artery results in vascular insufficiency to the anterior two thirds of the cord. Preservation of deep touch and vibration senses is typical because the posterior column tract remains intact (Fig. 19–14).

Posterior Column Syndrome

Posterior cord syndrome, although rare, is associated with cervical hyperextension injuries. The posterior column tract is damaged. Clinically, voluntary motor function and pain perception are preserved. Because the posterior tracts carry sensory fibers providing information on deep touch and proprioception, these functions are typically absent.

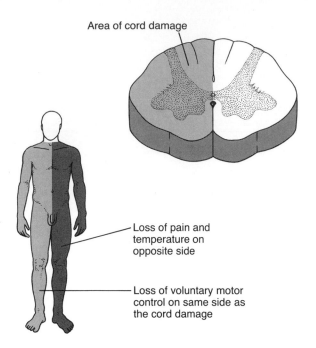

Area of cord damage

Loss of pain and
temperature on
opposite side

Loss of voluntary motor
control on same side as
the cord damage

FIGURE 19–15. Brown-Séquard
syndrome; cord damage and associated motor and sensory loss.

Brown-Séquard Syndrome

Brown-Séquard syndrome (Fig. 19–15) is most often associated with penetrating
knife or gunshot wounds or rotational type forces. The result is a transverse hemisec-
tion of the cord. Clinical findings relate directly to where each major tract decussates.
The corticospinal tract decussates in the brain and then descends. Therefore, the right
side of the brain controls left side motor activity. The spinothalamic tract crosses at
the same level of the cord it enters and ascends on the opposite side of the cord. The
posterior column tract ascends on the side on which it enters the cord and crosses at
the level of the medulla to be interpreted on the other side of the brain.

 Clinical presentation of Brown-Séquard syndrome demonstrates motor paralysis, loss of deep touch, vibration, and proprioception, with preservation of pain and
temperature sensations on the same side of injury below the level of lesion. Pain and
temperature sensations are lost on the opposite side of the injury. This syndrome has
a good prognosis for improved functional recovery.

Conus Medullaris and Cauda Equina Injuries

Damage to this portion of the spinal cord and its nerves causes the following effects:
asymmetric loss of motor function and no remarkable impairment in sensory function. Disturbance in bowel, bladder, and sexual function occurs. Lesions of the cauda
equina show a greater propensity to improvement and recovery than other spinal
cord lesions.

CLINICAL MANIFESTATIONS

Ascertaining from the trauma victim or witnesses details of an accident is key in identifying actual or potential spine injuries. Primary assessment and treatment of life-threatening conditions should be performed with an orientation toward the possibility of spinal cord injury. Victims with head trauma severe enough to cause a loss of consciousness are presumed to have an associated spinal cord injury.

Unconscious patients who are thrown from a car or sustain a fall may well have concomitant injuries. Forty per cent of SCI victims have at least one associated injury other than a spine or spinal cord injury (Fig. 19–16) (MRSCICS 1986). Damage to the spinal cord will mask the painful sensations of associated injuries. The patient will require close observation and diagnostic evaluation.

Initially, the patient's primary focus is on pain relief, chances of surviving, and the safety of others involved in the accident. Once these issues are addressed, the victim may begin to appraise the severity of his or her injuries.

Conscious patients may complain of pain at the level of the bony (vertebral) injury and may have blatant complaints of paralysis or paresthesia. If paralysis occurs the patient may recall the point at which he or she could not move.

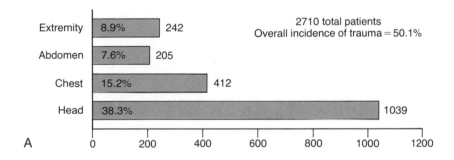

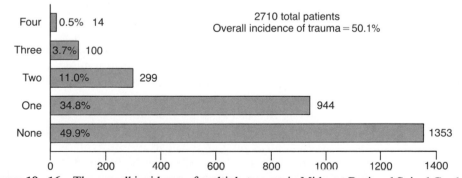

FIGURE 19–16. The overall incidence of multiple trauma in Midwest Regional Spinal Cord Injury Care System acutely spine-injured patients is 50.1%. *A*, Incidence of trauma by system. Incidence of head trauma is 38.3%. *B*, Incidence of multitrauma by number of traumatized systems. Many patients (15.2%) have trauma at more than one anatomic region. (Modified from Midwest Regional Spinal Cord Injury Care Systems, 1986.)

Physical assessment in the emergency department often reveals an awake patient. It is important to assess for evidence of head injury and whether the patient experienced any period of unconsciousness. Investigations have reported that 25 to 50 per cent of SCI victims sustain some form of head trauma (Wilmont et al 1985). A small percentage of these individuals demonstrate severe signs of head trauma; 57 per cent demonstrate higher level cognitive dysfunction (Davidoff et al 1985; Schueneman and Morris 1982). Such cognitive abnormalities will affect their safety needs, psychologic state, rehabilitation outcomes, and ability to comprehend patient teaching for the acquisition of new skills.

Respiratory assessment includes the presence, rate, and depth of ventilations. Breath sounds, symmetry of chest movement, ability to cough and mobilize secretions, and the color of skin are important parameters to assess.

Although respiratory compromise may be due to associated injuries, such as flail chest or a hemothorax or pneumothorax, most ventilatory insufficiency associated with SCI is a result of ventilatory nerve dysfunction. Nerve fibers responsible for respiratory function include C3-C5 innervating the diaphragm; C5-T1, the pectoralis muscles for upper chest expansion; T1-T12, the intercostal muscles; and T5-T12, the abdominal musculature.

Complete injuries above C3-C5 result in total loss of spontaneous respirations and will require mechanical ventilation for survival. Incomplete injuries are monitored closely for sudden ventilatory failure due to an ascending lesion. Persons with thoracic and cervical injuries below C5 commonly exhibit respiratory compromise demonstrated by shallow ventilations, decreased chest expansion, paradoxic or abdominal breathing, and the use of accessory muscles of breathing. Effective ventilation, chest expansion, and mobilization of secretions may be altered.

Respiratory parameters, including vital capacity, tidal volume, and arterial blood gases, are assessed, especially with cervical injuries. Serial vital capacity measurements provide a good predictor of impending pulmonary failure due to muscular fatigue. A vital capacity less than 15 ml/kg is cause for grave concern. With less than 12 ml/kg, intubation and mechanical ventilation frequently are warranted (Shapiro 1985).

Cardiovascular dysfunction in the spinal cord patient is generally due to disruption of sympathetic outflow tracts at the cervical and upper thoracic regions. Hypotension, bradycardia, and hypothermia are classic signs of spinal cord shock that occur immediately after injury. Spinal cord shock is the result of sudden loss of continuity between the spinal cord and higher nerve centers. In addition to loss of autonomic nervous system function below the level of the lesion, spinal cord shock is manifested by complete motor and sensory loss, sphincter paralysis, and absence of reflexes below the level of the lesion.

Disruption of sympathetic nervous system innervation results in loss of vasomotor tone causing vasodilation and decreased cardiac return. Unopposed parasympathetic innervation to the sinoatrial node in the heart results in bradycardia. Cool, dry skin is also a classic sign of spinal shock. Effective perfusion of vital organs is determined by level of consciousness, urinary output, and peripheral pulses. Blood studies, including hemoglobin, hematocrit, and electrolyte determinations, are performed to evaluate homeostasis and response to trauma or detect abnormalities, such as blood loss from hemorrhage.

Palpation of the spine may reveal point tenderness or deformity. A thorough neurologic examination of the patient's motor, sensory, and reflex functions is imperative. One of the most important aspects of the neurologic assessment is the rectal examination. Any evidence of motor (voluntary sphincter contraction) or sensory function classifies the injury as incomplete. Sensory examination must identify any deficit of pain, temperature, and fine touch (spinothalamic tract function) as well as of proprioception, deep touch, and vibration (posterior tract function). Level of sensory deficit is correlated with motor deficit. Symmetry of responses to both sides of the body is also assessed.

Use of standardized neurologic assessment forms (Fig. 19–17) in the emergency department augments evaluation of the spinal cord patient and facilitates communication of neurologic assessments to other practitioners.

Autonomic dysfunction, as a result of spinal shock, may be assessed by checking for diminished sweating, piloerection, vasomotor instability, loss of bladder and rectal control, and priapism.

Continued diagnostic evaluation focuses on determining the presence and extent of spine injury. Motor and sensory evaluations are significant in determining level, extent, and type of injury. With the spine in proper anatomic alignment, anteroposterior and lateral radiographic views of the entire spine are obtained in the emergency department. Twenty per cent of all patients with a spine injury have lesions at multiple levels (Green 1982).

Supplemental radiologic projections that may be obtained include open mouth (odontoid) and swimmer's (one arm raised) views. Flexion and extension maneuvers should not be performed in patients with neurologic deficit but reserved for persons without neurologic deficit in whom a question of stability exists. The extent to which diagnostic procedures are performed in the emergency department depends on the institutional protocols for spine management, availability of personnel and equipment, and the patient's ability to tolerate such procedures. Table 19–2 outlines the various diagnostic procedures that spine-injured victims may require for further evaluation and management of their injuries.

Continued assessment of other organ systems demonstrates any impairment of neural control of gastrointestinal and urinary function. The abdomen is distended and taut. There is absence of peristalsis and an accumulation of fluid and gas in the bowel. Although a paralytic ileus is a likely consequence of SCI, when there is hypotension or decreased hematocrit, acute abdominal trauma should be ruled out via a peritoneal tap. Unchecked ileus can lead to aspiration of vomitus and compromised ventilations.

A major risk immediately after injury is the possibility of overdistention and rupture of the bladder. Spinal shock prevents the involuntary reflex emptying of the bladder in a person who has lost sensation and voluntary control. Hypotension, secondary to neurogenic or hypovolemic shock, compromises urinary output. In addition to assessing renal perfusion, urine should be tested for hematuria, which may indicate urinary system trauma. Evidence of priapism in SCI victims is considered a poor prognostic sign for neurologic recovery.

The impact of spinal cord injury on the patient's and family's psychosocial well-being is manifested in a variety of ways. Although many psychologists and social workers report a variety of responses to spinal cord injury, most concur with Wright (1960) that there is no direct relationship between a patient's reaction to disability and the type or severity of injury (Athelstan and Crewe 1979; Cleveland 1979).

SPINAL CORD NEUROLOGIC ASSESSMENT

LEVEL OF CONSCIOUSNESS

A = Alert
C = Confused

PUPIL REACTION

PERL, L > R or R > L

MUSCLE GRADING

0 = Absent
1 = Trace
2 = Poor
3 = Fair
4 = Good
5 = Normal

DATE/TIME															
SIGNATURE															
LEVEL OF CONSCIOUSNESS															
PUPIL REACTION															
KEY MUSCLE FUNCTIONS		RT	LT	RT	LT	RT	LT	RT	LT	RT	LT	RT	LT	RT	LT
Shoulder elevators	C-4														
Elbow flexion	C-5														
Wrist dorsiflexion	C-6														
Elbow extension	C-7														
Finger abducters, adducters	C-8														
Hip flexion	L-2														
Knee extension	L-3														
Ankle dorsiflexion	L-4														
Great toe extension	L-5														
Ankle plantar flexion	S-1														
Voluntary rectal tone	S-2, 3														

DEEP TOUCH
+ = Present
− = Absent

PAIN SENSATION
S = Sharp to pinprick
D = Dull to pinprick
A = Absent to pinprick

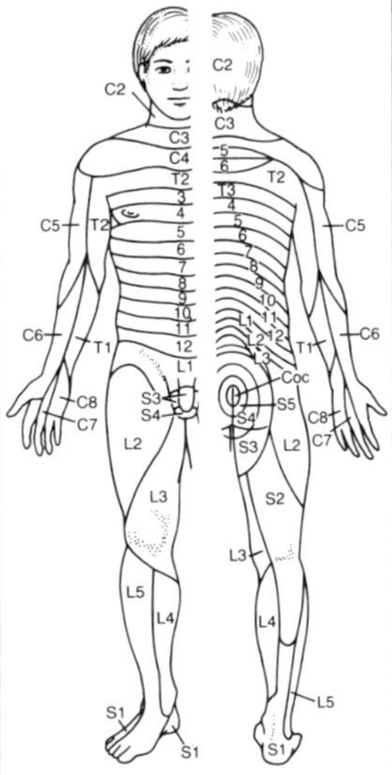

SENSORY LEVELS		RT		LT		RT		LT		RT		LT		RT		LT		RT		LT		RT		LT		RT		LT	
		Pain	D T	Pain	D T	Pain	D T	Pain	D T	Pain	D T	Pain	D T	Pain	D T	Pain	D T	Pain	D T	Pain	D T	Pain	D T	Pain	D T	Pain	D T	Pain	D T
CERVICAL	2																												
	3																												
	4																												
	5																												
	6																												
	7																												
	8																												
THORACIC	1																												
	2																												
	3																												
	4																												
	5																												
	6																												
	7																												
	8																												
	9																												
	10																												
	11																												
	12																												
LUMBAR	1																												
	2																												
	3																												
	4																												
	5																												
SACRAL	1																												
	2																												
	3																												
	4																												
	5																												
Complete (C) Incomplete (Inc.)																													

FIGURE 19–17. Spinal cord neurologic assessment form. (Modified courtesy of Northwestern Memorial Hospital.)

TABLE 19-2.
Diagnostic Procedures for Spinal Cord Evaluation

Procedure	Comments
Radiography	Visualizes the entire spine to delineate exact site and nature of bony injuries
Anteroposterior (AP)-lateral views	Radiographs should be viewed for
	Contour and alignment of vertebral bodies according to normal curvature of the spine
	Presence of all cervical vertebrae
	Displacement of bone fragments into the spinal canal
	Fracture of the laminae, pedicles, spinous processes to determine ligamentous stability
	Spinous process distances
	Degree of soft tissue damage especially when no fracture is present
Swimmer's view	Perform when all cervical vertebrae are not visualized with AP films
Open-mouth series	Evaluates integrity of odontoid body and C1 and C2 vertebrae
Tomography	
Conventional	Provides longitudinal visualization of the spine
	Increases accuracy of diagnosis and evaluation of fractures of the spine
	Requires movement of the patient by certified personnel to obtain adequate films
Computed (CT)	Imaging that provides transverse views through the spine and body
	Assists in assessing the patency of the neural canal
	Most often used for C1, C2, or lumbar fractures
Myelography	Use in the immediate diagnostic work-up of spinal cord injury is controversial
	Rules out surgically correctable lesion, herniated disk, or hematoma that is compressing or impinging on the cord
	Common indications for myelography:
	Preoperative evaluation of incomplete injuries
	Changing neurological condition, either deterioration or improvement
	Recovery plateau unanticipated
	Inconsistent finding between bony and neurologic injury
	Inconsistent findings between somatosensory evoked potentials (SSEP) and neurologic findings
Magnetic Resonance Imaging (MRI)	Noninvasive technique
	Utilizes radiofrequency radiation in presence of strong magnetic field to provide cross-sectional display of various anatomic structures, including soft tissue
	Role of MRI during acute care management has yet to be elucidated
	This technique may afford greater advantages over other diagnostic methods
Somatosensory Evoked Potentials (SSEP)	Assists in establishing the extent of injury to the nervous system; often performed within 24-48 hr after admission
	Used to monitor intraoperative neural function during surgical reduction or instrumentation of the spine

Assessment of psychoemotional and social needs includes determining pre-injury coping strategies, current developmental tasks, strengths, past experiences with acute crises, and available support systems. The emergency department nurse can draw upon other available resources, such as clergy or social workers, to assist in psychoemotional assessment and intervention.

TREATMENT AND NURSING CARE

Impaired Gas Exchange, Related to

- *Muscular Fatigue and Retained Secretions*

Breathing Patterns, Ineffective, Related to

- *Diaphragmatic Paralysis and Muscular Fatigue*

Airway Clearance, Ineffective, Related to

- *Loss of Innervation to Respiratory Musculature Responsible for Respiration*

Establishment of airway patency and breathing is paramount for the patient with an ineffective breathing pattern, even to the extent that other injuries may be initially neglected or untreated. The unconscious patient poses a more difficult problem in management, because the need to prevent further cervical spine injury is a priority. Care to establish an airway and breathing must be adapted to the possibility of spinal cord injury.

An airway is established utilizing the modified jaw thrust or chin lift. The neck is maintained in proper alignment, establishing only mild hyperextension and straight traction to secure a patent airway. Because 90 per cent of all spinal cord injuries are flexion related, extension with mild traction applied to the head and neck is more likely to improve cervical spine alignment than to produce deleterious effects (Meyer 1982).

Nasotracheal intubation is the preferred method for airway control. It requires the least amount of manipulation to the neck. Elective intubation must include preoxygenation and administration of atropine, because intubation stimulates vagal tone. Unopposed vagal activity may result in severe bradycardia or cardiac arrest. Pancuronium or thiopental is sufficient for induction. Succinylcholine should *not* be used as a muscle relaxant; cardiac arrest from severe hyperkalemia has been described after use of this drug during intubation (Snow et al 1973). If an airway cannot be established by intubation, a cricothyrotomy may be performed by certified personnel.

Nursing interventions include the ongoing assessment of respiratory rate and depth and the possibility of an ascending lesion. An ascending lesion of the cord may result in life-threatening respiratory compromise. Treatment focuses on maintaining a clear airway and promoting adequate ventilation.

Once an airway has been established, the nurse will need to assure that the endotracheal or cricothyrotomy tube is securely fastened. Suctioning, using sterile technique, is performed as needed to eliminate secretions. Ventilatory assistance with a bag-valve device and supplemental oxygen may be necessary to minimize the effects of dominant parasympathetic innervation that will increase the likelihood of bradycardia.

Patients not requiring an artificial airway will require nursing interventions directed toward preventing respiratory failure. As for all traumatized individuals, supplemental oxygen is in order. The awake patient with no obvious difficulties in breathing is a candidate for oxygen by nasal cannula or face mask at approximately 4 to 6 or 6 to 10 L, respectively.

Patients with injuries above T12 may lose abdominal (T6-T12) or intercostal (T1-L5) muscle function, or both. Ability to cough effectively is altered, requiring the introduction of assistive cough. Braun and colleagues (1984) demonstrated that when assisted cough was used, there was an 13.8 per cent improved peak expiratory flow and cough than with unassisted cough. Assisted cough requires a coordinated effort between the nurse and the patient. By pushing the abdomen inward and forward during a full expiratory phase, the diaphragm rises sharply and secretions are forced into lower airways, producing maximal expiratory effort. Aggressive pulmonary toileting, coupled with incentive spirometry, position changes, and assisted cough and breathing will prevent retained secretions.

Decreased Cardiac Output, Related to

• *Loss of Sympathetic Tone*

The patient with an alteration in cardiac output related to loss of sympathetic tone will generally have stabilization of systolic blood pressure at 100 mmHg. Bradycardia is common. Patients with a heart rate below 40 beats per minute and demonstrated diminished cardiac return should be treated with an anticholinergic (atropine) or adrenergic (norepinephrine) drug. Urinary output should remain at least 30 ml/hour, and the patient should exhibit normal mental status.

Extreme caution is taken in performing activities that trigger vasovagal responses, as loss of the sympathetic tone reduces the patient's ability to compensate for dominant vagal activity. Tracheal suctioning should be preceded with oxygenation and if necessary by administration of atropine. The patient's response to suctioning should be noted and documented. Turning and positioning patients may precipitate bradycardia. Assessment of the patient's response to immobilizing beds such as the Wedge-Stryker Turning Frame or the Roto-Rest Kinetic Turning Table should be noted.

Ongoing monitoring of the patient's thermal status is necessary to avoid excessive hypothermia, which will contribute to decreased cardiac functioning or hyperthermia when appropriate bodily responses of shivering and sweating to control temperature are absent.

Fluid Volume Deficit, Related to

• *Hypovolemia and Massive Vasodilation Secondary to Loss of Sympathetic Tone*

If the mean blood pressure falls below 70 mmHg, volume replacement with 0.45 normal saline, 5% dextrose in lactated Ringer's solution (D5LR), or blood products under cardiac and venous pressure monitoring is in order. In the presence of profound shock, military antishock trousers (MAST) may be applied by allied medical personnel for initial treatment and during transport. Fluid therapy is implemented with care not to overhydrate the patient and create pulmonary edema or additional edema surrounding the area of spinal cord injury. Continued spinal cord edema leads to diminished cord oxygenation and perpetuates traumatic necrosis of spinal nerve tissue.

Nursing interventions are directed toward ongoing assessment of cardiopulmonary function, including heart rate, rhythm, cardiac output, and perfusion. Intake and output are closely monitored.

Potential for Injury, Related to

• *Vertebral Injury and Manipulation*

Whether or not neurologic deficit is present, the goal of acute management is to immobilize and align the spine with the least amount of movement and to prevent further injury until the danger to the spinal cord has been eliminated. Radiographic evaluation determines the presence of unstable spine fractures.

At the scene of the accident, the victim should be moved only with sufficient help and immobilization devices. The neck should be stabilized in a neutral position without flexion or extension motion until a fixed immobilizing device can be applied. Many different cervical spine immobilization devices are available to accomplish this goal.

The simplest and most effective means of cervical spine immobilization remains the combination of the spine board, hard collar, towel or foam rolls, and adhesive tape. Podolsky (1983) and McCabe (1986) found the Philadelphia brand of hard collars provided the best support, limiting flexion, extension, and lateral movements of the cervical spine.

Special devices to extricate, immobilize, and transport patients may include the Kedrick Extrication Device (KED) (Fig. 19–18). This device provides cervicothoracic stabilization. The KED board is extremely useful in extrication of victims in confined spaces. Cervical traction should not be used at the scene of the accident or during transport because of the potential for exacerbating spinal deformity without radiographic control, thereby increasing neurologic deficit (Meyer 1978; Zejdlik 1983).

The goal of acute care is to furnish the spinal cord with the best possible conditions for improvement. This can be accomplished through traction, decompressive laminectomy, or fusion. One or all may be prescribed in certain circumstances and the judgment of the physician is crucial. The role of surgical intervention is minimal during the initial emergency treatment stages. Instead, alignment and immobilization of the spine with traction is the preferred method.

Unstable or dislocated spinal fractures must be reduced and the space realigned anatomically. Cervical and high thoracic (C1-T6) spinal dislocations are treated using cranial traction. In many RSCICS, Gardner Wells tongs are replacing Crutchfield and Vinke tongs for better fixation, ease of application, and reduction of meningitis resulting from infected tong sites. Halo Ring application is advocated by some

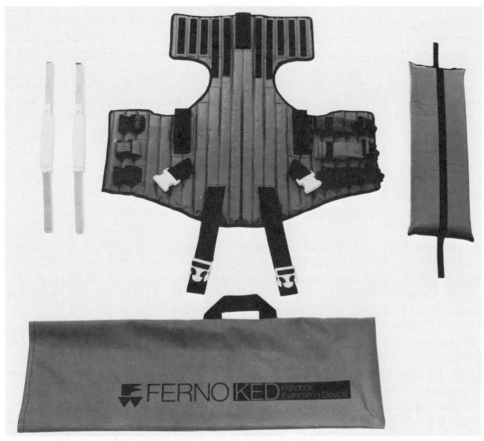

FIGURE 19–18. Kedrick extrication device. (Courtesy of Ferno Division.)

who anticipate Halo Ring immobilization later in the patient's course of rehabilitation. The area for tong insertion is shaved and prepared with a local anesthetic.

Traction is applied in the direction of the axis of the spine. Traction is added slowly in 5-pound increments under close radiographic monitoring. The goal is to produce distraction of the spine without causing extensive tension to the spinal arteries that may result in an ascending lesion. Sedation and pain relief with intravenous narcotics or sedatives are required during tong insertion and initial reduction procedures.

Patients with fractures of the spine are placed on either a Stryker frame or a Roto-Rest bed depending on the scope of associated injuries and preferred method of management. The Stryker frame is widely used and is most suitable for uncomplicated low cervical and thoracic and lumbar injuries. It provides immediate and maximal spine immobilization. Patients are easily managed and turned to prone or supine positions. Roto-Rest beds facilitate maintenance of correct alignment and traction of the spine and other long bone injuries. This type of bed promotes cardiovascular and respiratory function and prevents pressure sores while patients are continuously rotated from side to side (Adelstein and Watson 1983). Circular electrical beds are no longer utilized because of demonstrated effects on cardiovascular stability and axial loading on the spine, thereby complicating neurologic and spine recovery. Turning or rotation of patients commences once bony alignment is established and documented radiographically, and the patient is appropriately secured in the bed to assure safety.

In addition to establishing alignment of the spine, many RSCICS advocate approaches to minimize edema formation and necrosis of injured spinal cord tissue. Use of diuretics or high-dose steroids is a commonly accepted practice. Management of spinal edema is complicated when cardiovascular instability is present. Corticosteroids, such as dexamethasone (Decadron), are potent anti-inflammatory drugs that reduce edema and provide protection to cells at the site of trauma. Initial dosage of Decadron is 50 mg by intravenous push and followed by titrated doses over several days. It is believed that Decadron acts directly by stabilizing the cell membrane.

Other approaches include use of neuropeptides — thyrotropin releasing hormones (TRH) and naloxone — which show reversal of some lesions by interrupting the post-traumatic ischemia and tissue damage thought to be caused by endogenous opioids (endorphins) (Geisler 1988). Use of hyperbaric oxygen in acute injuries has been found not to change neurologic outcome but does accelerate the recovery rate. Future focus on spinal cord regeneration involves fetal tissue transplants, bypass grafts of peripheral nerves, and protein tissue nerve bridges.

Focus of nursing management includes continual assessment and maintenance of vertebral column stability. Neurologic assessments are performed every hour. As the patient's condition stabilizes, it may be done less frequently. Rationale for frequent assessments is to determine the possibility of an ascending lesion that may require emergency interventions, such as surgery to decompress the spine.

Patients on Stryker frames should never be transported in a prone position. Principles of traction need to be maintained. The weights hang freely except during transportation, when taping of the weights to the frame becomes necessary to prevent movement of the spine. The knot is free from the pulley to ensure maintenance of adequate traction.

Gastrointestinal Dysfunction, Related to

• *Paralytic Ileus*

Initial management of spinal cord victims with evidence of paralytic ileus is withholding any oral intake and insertion of a nasogastric tube for low intermittent suction. The goal is to decompress the stomach and prevent aspiration of stomach contents.

Prevention of Stress Ulcers

An antacid program is initiated to decrease stress ulcer formation secondary to trauma and high-dose steroid therapy. With the lack of rectal emptying reflexes, the patient should be placed on a bowel program once he or she arrives on the nursing unit. Cimetidine is advocated as a prophylaxis against acid peptic disease. Primary nursing interventions include maintenance of patent tube to intermittent suction, monitoring intake and output, and administration of medications.

Urinary Elimination, Altered Patterns of

• *Related to Spinal Shock*

Spinal shock prevents the involuntary reflex emptying of the bladder in the SCI patient. The bladder may remain areflexic for weeks or months. Utilizing strict sterile technique, an indwelling Foley catheter is inserted for continuous drainage. An indwelling catheter is maintained for the first 24 to 72 hours, depending on the patient's medical stability, to monitor fluid balance and avoid overdistention of the bladder. As soon as the patient begins taking oral fluids, an intermittent catheterization program is initiated to reduce the sequelae of urinary tract infections that are associated with long-term catheter use.

Taping of the catheter is important to prevent ischemia of the urethra or accidental dislodging. Taping the catheter to the abdomen of men and the inside leg of women is the preferred method.

Coping, Ineffective Individual

Knowledge Deficit, Related to

• *Acute Injury*

Spiritual Distress

The newly injured SCI victim will face many unusual stimuli during the acute care, during rehabilitation, and through the remainder of his or her life, which may lead to special problems with self-concept, body image, frustration, anger, dependency, and motivation.

Management of anxiety for the patient and family during acute care is complex but of the utmost importance, regardless of how much physical care is required.

Bouman (1980) suggests that assessments and interventions of patients' and families' psychoemotional needs can be provided on the basis of the following framework. This framework leads to rapid evaluation and intervention for the emergency department nurse. These categories consist of cognitive or informational needs, emotional needs, and physical needs.

Cognitive or Informational Needs

The need to have information during an acute crisis takes higher precedence for the patient and family than physical or emotional needs. The cognitive needs are fulfilled by providing specific and complete information in understood terms. The information SCI victims and their families require includes rationale for tests and procedures, extent and degree of disability, and plans for medical and nursing management. The rationales for the use of unfamiliar hospital beds (Stryker, Roto-Rest) and tongs are of particular importance to patients and their families. It is important to remember that during acute crisis, the patient may seem to understand, but information and instructions may need to be repeated.

Physical Needs

Physical needs are identified as those providing for a measure of comfort to the patient or family. Concrete interventions that will afford some relief of physical needs include careful control and management of pain or discomfort by administering analgesics and muscle relaxants.

The family's physical needs may include the need for a private waiting area, assistance with finances, arrangement for temporary housing, and food, coffee, and telephone and restroom facilities.

Emotional Needs

As information and physical needs have been met, both patients and families begin identifying emotional needs. Interventions that will meet emotional needs include the assurance that medical personnel care about the patient and family and are sensitive to their needs. They need honest and open communication about the injury, the consequences, and rehabilitation potential. Provide encouragement that displays hope for the best, yet prepares the patient and family for the worst.

Social workers or clergy can provide early supportive care, detect misconceptions, and help the family and patient to express their grief and concerns.

SUMMARY

Spinal cord injury is the most complex form of serious trauma that causes disruption in function in almost every organ in the body. SCI requires the emergency department nurse to have astute assessment skills of actual and potential problems, a solid understanding of the pathophysiology, and the ability to intervene with both physical and psychosocial care.

Goals of treatment include management of life-threatening conditions, with orientation to protect the spine from further neurologic injury. Once the patient's condition has been stabilized, he or she should be transported to an RSCICS that is dedicated to the management of the acute and rehabilitative needs of this patient. Studies have demonstrated unequivocally that a coordinated approach to the management of SCI is the most effective and efficient alternative to achieving the goal of improved neurologic recovery, rehabilitation, and reintegration in the community.

REFERENCES

Adelstein W, Watson P. 1983. Cervical spine injuries. Neurosurg Nurs 15(2):65–71.

Athelstan GT, Crewe NM. 1979. Psychological adjustment to spinal cord injury as related to manner of onset of disability. Rehabil Counsel Bull 4:311–319.

Bouman CC. 1980. Self-perceived needs of family members of critically ill patients. Master's Thesis, University of Rochester, New York.

Braun SR, Giovanni R, O'Connor M. 1984. Improving the cough in patient's with spinal cord injury. Am J Phys Med 63:1–16.

Chaffee EE, Lytle IM. 1980. Basic Physiology and Anatomy, 4th ed. Philadelphia, JB Lippincott Co.

Cleveland M. 1979. Family adaptation to the traumatic spinal cord injury of a son or daughter. Soc Work Health Care 4:459–471.

Davidoff G, Roth E, Morris J, et al. 1986. Assessment of closed head injury in trauma-related spinal cord injury. Paraplegia 24, 97–104.

Dudas S, Stevens KA. 1984. Cervical cord injury: Implications for nursing. J Neurosurg Nurs 16:84–88.

Geisler FH. 1988. Acute management of cervical spinal cord injury. Trauma Q, 4:14.

Green BA, Eismont FJ. 1984. Acute spinal cord injury: A system approach. Central Nervous System Trauma 1(2):173–195.

Green BA, Marshall LF, Gallagher TJ. 1982. Intensive Care for Neurological Trauma and Disease. New York, Academic Press.

Guttmann L. 1974. Spinal Cord Injuries: Comprehensive Management and Research. Oxford, Blackwell Scientific Publications, 1–42.

Huelke DF, Lawson TE, Scott R, et al. 1979. The effectiveness of belt systems in frontal and rollover crashes. Warrendale, PA, Society of Automobile Engineers, SAE #770148.

McCabe JB, Nolan DJ. 1986. Comparison of the effectiveness of different cervical immobilization collars. Ann Emerg Med 15:93–96.

Meyer PR. 1978. The Illinois emergency medical service. Emergency medical services, Model Systems Conference, National Spinal Cord Injury, Care Systems, Chicago.

Meyer PR. 1982. The spinal cord injury patient. In Beal JM, ed. Critical Care for Surgical Patients. New York, Macmillan.

MRSCICS. 1986. Annual Progress Report. Chicago Midwest Regional Spinal Cord Injury Care System.

Podolsky H, Baraff LJ, Simon RR, et al. 1983. Efficacy of cervical spine immobilization devices. J Trauma 23:461–465.

Scher AT. 1983. Hyperextension trauma in the elderly: An easily overlooked spinal injury. J Trauma 23:1066–1068.

Schueneman A, Morris J. 1982. Neuropsychological deficits associated with spinal cord injury. SCI Digest 4:35–36, 64.

Shapiro BA. 1985. Clinical Application of Respiratory Care, 3rd ed. Chicago, Year Book Medical Publishers.

Snow JC, Kriphe BS, Sessions GP, et al. 1973. Cardiovascular collapse following succinylcholine in a paraplegic patient. Paraplegia 11:199–204.

Wilmont CB, Cope DD, Hall KM, et al. 1985. Incidence of occult head injury in those with a primary diagnosis of spinal cord injury. Houston, Proceedings from the American Spinal Injury Association, 105–108.

Wright BA. 1960. Physical Disability — A Psychological Approach. New York, Harper & Row.

Young JS. 1979. Hospital study report. Model Systems SCI Digest 1:3, 11–32. National Spinal Cord Injury Data Research Center. Phoenix, Good Samaritan Medical Center.

Young JS, Burns PE, Bowen AM, et al. 1982. Spinal Cord Injury Statistics. Phoenix, Good Samaritan Medical Center.

Zejdlik CM. 1983. Management of Spinal Cord Injury. Monterey, CA, Wadsworth Health Sciences Division.

Cheryl Jenkins, RN MS

Endocrine Emergencies

The endocrine system is composed of a variety of glands located throughout the body. Via hormones (substances secreted by these glands directly into the blood stream), the endocrine system regulates metabolism and maintains body homeostasis.

A carefully regulated system, the endocrine system relies on specific levels of hormones to maintain its regulatory and homeostatic function. Elaborate feedback mechanisms regulate the level of each hormone. These feedback mechanisms may be controlled either directly by the level of the hormone itself or indirectly by other substance levels, such as the relationship between insulin, a hormone, and blood glucose. Often it is an interaction of various feedback systems that interplay to regulate metabolism and maintain homeostasis.

ANATOMY AND PHYSIOLOGY

The glands of the endocrine system consist of the pituitary, thyroid, parathyroids, pancreas (islet of Langerhans), adrenals, testes, and ovaries (Fig. 20–1). This chapter focuses on some of the more frequently encountered emergencies associated with the thyroid, pancreas, and adrenal glands.

Before describing specific emergency situations involving the endocrine system, each gland (discussed in this chapter), the hormone(s) secreted by it, the specific

477

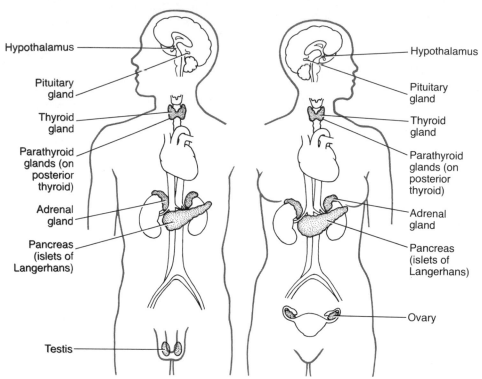

FIGURE 20–1. Glands of the endocrine system.

function of the hormone(s), and the feedback mechanisms are reviewed. In this way, it will be easier to discuss and understand endocrine-related problems that may arise.

THYROID

The thyroid is a butterfly-shaped gland composed of two lobes connected by an isthmus. It is located below the cricoid cartilage and partially encircles the trachea. The thyroid gland alters metabolic activity of the body by increasing or decreasing the level of thyroid hormones.

Two substances, thyroxine (T_4) and triiodothyronine (T_3) are released by the thyroid gland. Although 90 per cent of thyroid secretion consists of T_4, some T_4 is converted to T_3 in the circulation. At the cellular level, T_4's duration of activity is four times that of T_3, whereas T_3 is four times more potent than T_4 (Guyton 1981). The combined action of these hormones enables the body to maintain its metabolic activity. Thyroid hormones increase heart rate, cardiac output, motility of the gastrointestinal tract, and muscle activity. An excess or a deficit of thyroid hormones will result in these activities being exaggerated or diminished, respectively.

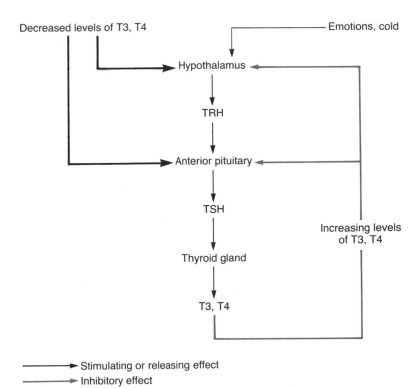

FIGURE 20-2. Feedback mechanism for regulation of thyroid hormones. (Thyroid hormone levels are the major determinant of TRH and TSH release.) T3 = triiodothyronine; T4 = thyroxine; TRH = thyrotropin releasing hormone; TSH = thyroid-stimulating hormone.

The release of thyroid hormones is controlled through a specific feedback mechanism via the hypothalamus and the anterior pituitary gland. The hypothalamus releases thyrotropin releasing hormone (TRH), which stimulates the anterior pituitary gland to release thyroid stimulating hormone (TSH). TSH stimulates the thyroid itself, thereby increasing the amount of thyroid hormones released. Emotion and exposure to the cold have some effect on TRH release and thus may affect TSH levels. However, probably the most important feedback control for release of TRH and TSH is the actual level of the thyroid hormones themselves. An increased blood level of the thyroid hormones has a negative (inhibitory) effect on the anterior pituitary, leading to a decrease in TSH release. The hypothalamus is only minimally affected by this method. Conversely, a decrease in the blood level of thyroid hormones will have a stimulating effect on the hypothalamus and the anterior pituitary (Fig. 20-2).

ADRENALS

The adrenal glands are located above the upper pole of each kidney. The adrenals consist of two separate parts: the medulla or inner aspect of the gland and the cortex, the outer aspect of the gland. Each segment has distinct functions and secretes separate substances. The adrenal medulla is related functionally to the nervous system as it secretes epinephrine and norepinephrine. The adrenal cortex secretes corticosteroids (mineralocorticoids and glucocorticoids), which are synthesized from cholesterol. The cortex also secretes a small amount of sex (androgenic) hormones.

The mineralocorticoids (mainly aldosterone) are released from the zona glomerulosa of the adrenal cortex and affect the level of extracellular electrolytes. Aldosterone causes the kidney to reabsorb sodium ions in exchange for potassium ions and, to a lesser degree, hydrogen ions. Water is also absorbed with the sodium, thereby allowing the sodium concentration to remain fairly stable even though the extracellular fluid volume may fluctuate. Aldosterone has a similar effect on sodium reabsorption in the salivary glands, sweat glands, and intestines. Without aldosterone, a person would excrete up to one fifth of the body's sodium while retaining potassium, leading to hyperkalemia (Guyton 1981; Muthe 1981).

Aldosterone secretion is interrelated to the various mechanisms that regulate extracellular fluid volume, extracellular fluid electrolyte concentrations, and renal function. However, there are four factors that are important in the regulation of aldosterone secretion. First is the potassium level in the extracellular fluid. As the potassium level increases, there is an increase in aldosterone secretion. This leads to an increase in the renal excretion of potassium ions thereby reducing the extracellular potassium level. The stimulus for aldosterone secretion is then diminished. This is probably the strongest of the feedback mechanisms for aldosterone secretion (Guyton 1981).

Other controls over aldosterone secretion include blood renin and angiotensin levels, total body sodium, and adrenocorticotropic hormone (ACTH). As renin and angiotensin levels increase, so does the level of aldosterone secretion. A decrease in extracellular sodium will also increase aldosterone secretion in an effort to restore and maintain normal sodium levels. Adrenocorticotropic hormone is released from the anterior pituitary gland and stimulates the adrenal cortex's release of glucocorticoids. Although the effect is only minimal, ACTH release does result in increased aldosterone secretion (Guyton 1981). Without ACTH, parts of the zona glomerulosa will atrophy and thereby decrease the amount of aldosterone that can be secreted (Fig. 20–3).

Cortisol, also referred to as hydrocortisone, is the most important of the glucocorticoids. Although corticosterone and cortisone (also glucocorticoids) do have a minor effect in people, cortisol exerts the most profound effect. The name *glucocorticoids* implies that their function involves glucose regulation, and although they do have an effect on blood glucose levels, they also play a part in both protein and fat metabolism.

Cortisol increases gluconeogenesis in the liver by increasing the availability of amino acids (which results from the catabolic effects of cortisol on protein) for conversion to glucose. Cortisol also enhances the activity of the enzymes needed for this conversion. Cellular glucose utilization is also decreased by cortisol (Guyton 1981; Muthe 1981). This decrease may be due to a decrease in glucose transport across the cell membrane as well as a decrease in NADH oxidation, which is needed for glycolysis.

Cortisol decreases the protein stores in the body by decreasing protein synthesis and increasing protein catabolism. This is seen in all body tissues except the liver, where cortisol increases amino acid use by enhancing the secretion of liver enzymes needed for protein synthesis. The result is an increase in plasma proteins.

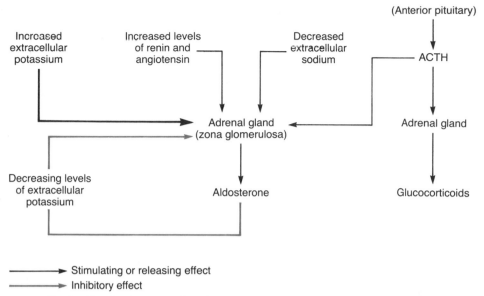

FIGURE 20-3. Feedback mechanism for regulation of aldosterone secretion. (Extracellular potassium levels are the major determinant of aldosterone secretion.) ACTH, Adrenocorticotropic hormone.

Fat metabolism is also affected by the glucocorticoids. Cortisol promotes lipolysis, enhancing fatty acid mobilization from adipose stores, and increases the cellular utilization of fatty acids for energy by increasing fat oxidation.

The glucocorticoids also have an anti-inflammatory effect. Briefly, cortisol stabilizes the membrane of lysosomes, thereby decreasing the release of substances responsible for inflammation, such as histamine. Cortisol also reduces the permeability of capillary walls, which reduces plasma leakage responsible for edema at injury sites. The phagocytic ability of white blood cells is also decreased, causing a further reduction in the release of inflammatory substances. Cortisol in essence suppresses the immune system, leading to a reduction in local tissue reactions.

Glucocorticoid secretion is controlled by a feedback mechanism similar to that of the thyroid hormones. The hypothalamus stimulates the anterior pituitary via corticotropin releasing hormone (CRH) to release ACTH. It is ACTH that stimulates the adrenal cortex to secrete the glucocorticoids and also to a lesser degree enhances the production of adrenal androgens. The hypothalamus and anterior pituitary respond to stressors such as infection, trauma, surgery, pain,, and intense heat or cold by releasing CRH and ACTH, thus leading to an increase in glucocorticoid release. The increased levels of glucocorticoids then have a negative (inhibitory) effect on the release of more CRH and ACTH, thereby controlling glucocorticoid levels (Fig. 20-4). There is also a circadian rhythm to the release of glucocorticoids regardless of presence of stressors. Glucocorticoids are present in highest concentration in the morning and lowest in the evening (Guyton 1981; Muthe 1981).

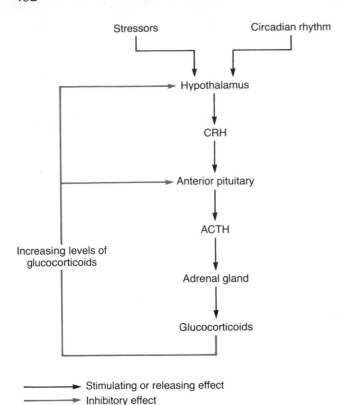

FIGURE 20–4. Feedback mechanism for glucocorticoid secretion. CRH, corticotropin releasing hormone; ACTH, adrenocorticotropin hormone.

PANCREAS

The pancreas is located adjacent to and below the stomach. It consists of two types of tissue: the acini, which play a role in the digestion of food, and the islets of Langerhans, which play a role in glucose, protein, and fat metabolism. The islets of Langerhans are discussed here.

The islets of Langerhans consist of three types of cells, beta, alpha, and delta, each secreting a separate hormone. The beta cells secrete insulin, a protein that exerts many effects on glucose, fat, and protein metabolism. By binding with a receptor on or in the cell membrane, insulin regulates the blood glucose level by allowing glucose to enter the cell. Insulin facilitates glucose uptake by the liver while decreasing glycogen breakdown. It also increases glycogen formation by enhancing the liver enzymes responsible for this process (Felig 1983).

All tissues and cells, except the brain, require insulin for glucose uptake. Glucose uptake, in these tissues, is facilitated in a similar fashion to that of the liver uptake of glucose.

Insulin also has an effect on fat metabolism. Once liver glycogen formation has reached a certain point (approximately 5 to 6 per cent of total liver mass), the liver is no longer able to form glycogen and will convert its glucose to fatty acids (Guyton 1981). These fatty acids are converted into fat and stored as adipose tissue. Insulin

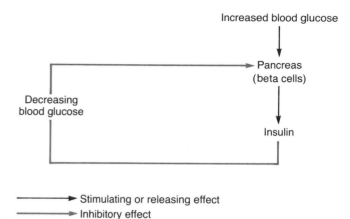

FIGURE 20–5. Feedback mechanism for insulin secretion.

will also inhibit the activity of lipase, thus preventing the breakdown of adipose tissue and the release of fatty acids. In a similar fashion, but to a lesser degree than in the liver, glucose transport into the fat cells themselves is also facilitated by the presence of insulin.

The effect of insulin on protein metabolism is that of inhibition of gluconeogenesis. Amino acids that would have been used in this process are now available for protein synthesis. Additionally, insulin also has an inhibitory effect on the enzymes that mediate protein catabolism.

In summary, insulin is necessary for the proper use of glucose by all tissues of the body except the brain. It also plays an important role in glucose, fat, and protein metabolism.

The level of glucose in the blood is the stimulus for insulin secretion. A basal rate of insulin secretion is always maintained, even during fasting states. However, an increase in blood glucose (as commonly occurs after a meal) causes the beta cells to respond by increasing the rate of insulin secretion. This, in turn, causes the blood glucose to decrease and thereby reduces the need for insulin secretion. Thus, insulin secretion is a finely regulated system which allows for normalization (80 to 120 mg/dl) of blood glucose levels quickly (Fig. 20–5).

The alpha cells of the islets of Langerhans secrete glucagon, which has an exactly opposite effect of insulin. Glucagon raises the blood glucose level by increasing gluconeogenesis and liver glycogenolysis.

Secretion of glucagon is carefully regulated by the blood glucose level. When the blood glucose level decreases (to approximately 70 mg/dl), glucagon is secreted to raise the blood glucose to normal. Exercise, with its blood glucose–lowering effect, is also a stimulus for glucagon secretion (Fig. 20–6).

The delta cells of the islets of Langerhans secrete somatostatin. The role of somatostatin is not fully understood, but it is known to inhibit insulin and glucagon secretion.

As has been discussed, the endocrine system is a finely tuned system that controls the metabolic activity of the body. This activity is regulated by specific hormones. As will be seen, an endocrine emergency can develop when there is either too much or too little of any given hormone.

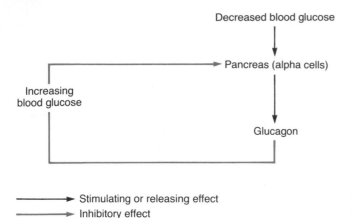

———————► Stimulating or releasing effect

———————► Inhibitory effect

FIGURE 20–6. Feedback mechanism for glucagon secretion.

EMERGENCIES OF THE THYROID

Approximately one fifth of the United States population is affected by disorders of the thyroid gland (Bailey and Baker 1984). These disorders may be manifested as either hyperthyroidism (a clinical condition characterized by hyperfunction of the thyroid gland, elevation of T_4 and T_3 levels, and increased metabolic activity), or hypothyroidism (a clinical condition characterized by hypofunction of the thyroid gland, decreased levels of T_4 and T_3, and decreased metabolic activity).

Thyroid disorders can develop from many causes. An excess amount of TSH or TRH (as seen with pituitary tumors) will result in an excess amount of T_4 and T_3 (or hyperthyroidism). Likewise, in Graves' disease (the most common form of hyperthyroidism), in which there is an excess amount of thyroid stimulating immunoglobulin (TSI), there is also an excess of T_4 and T_3. Thyroid stimulating immunoglobulin acts similarly to TSH; however, it does not respond to increasing levels of T_4 and T_3. As such, there is no "shut-off" point, and thyroid hormone levels continue to rise.

Alternatively, hypothyroidism develops from a deficiency of T_4 and T_3. Two common causes of this deficiency are iatrogenic and occur as the result of treatment modalities for persons with hyperthyroidism: radioactive iodine and surgery (both of which destroy cells of the thyroid gland). Hypothyroidism may also develop from a deficit of iodine in the diet. (Iodine is necessary for the synthesis of T_4.) Additionally, many patients treated with lithium develop hypothyroidism as a side effect of treatment because lithium may block thyroid hormone synthesis. In other instances, hypothyroidism may develop from a lack of TSH or TRH stimulation.

Emergencies relating to the thyroid gland are the result of a significant exacerbation or worsening of the hyper- or hypothyroid state. In general, 60 per cent of them are related to recent surgery, trauma, or infection (Bailey and Baker 1984). Thyroid storm (an extreme exacerbation of hyperthyroidism) may be precipitated not only by recent surgery, trauma, or infection, but also by diabetic ketoacidosis (DKA), embolism, or failure to continue antithyroid medications. Myxedema coma (a severe worsening of hypothyroidism) may be precipitated by trauma, infection, exposure to the cold, cessation of thyroid replacement therapy, or the use of central nervous system (CNS) depressants. (Hypothyroid individuals become hypersensitive to almost all CNS depressants, whereby therapeutic doses may be toxic to them.) Thyroid storm, even with treatment, has a 20 per cent mortality rate, and myxedema coma has a 50 per cent mortality rate (Hamburger et al 1984).

Thyroid Storm

With thyroid emergencies, the patient's presentation depends on whether he or she is suffering from thyroid storm (hyperthyroidism) or myxedema coma (hypothyroidism). Both conditions have the potential to affect nearly all body systems, and symptoms therefore will reflect either a hyper- or a hypometabolic state.

Clinical Manifestations

Fever (due to hypermetabolism and heat intolerance) is the classic presenting sign of a patient in thyroid storm. It is not unusual for the patient to have a temperature of 106°F. Other classic signs and symptoms of thyroid storm (all of the result of a hypermetabolic state) include restlessness, irritability, delirium, and weakness. Tachycardia is present and dysrhythmias are common: particularly atrial fibrillation, premature ventricular contractions, and paroxysmal atrial tachycardia (Bailey and Baker 1984). A widened pulse pressure is also commonly seen, as is an elevated blood pressure. Patients may be dyspneic as the result of a decrease in pulmonary compliance and vital capacity in response to weakened respiratory muscles. Increased gastrointestinal motility causes vomiting and diarrhea. Central nervous system hyperexcitability may trigger seizures. Deep tendon reflexes are brisk and hyperkinesis is usually present. Patients may have difficulty concentrating, and emotions may be very labile. Exophthalmos is not uncommon. History may reveal recent trauma, neck surgery, or infection, although 40 per cent of patients will have no such history.

Treatment and Nursing Care

Because of the high mortality rate for persons who experience thyroid storm, stage I care for these persons often needs to be instituted prior to beginning definitive treatment of its underlying cause. Airway, breathing, and circulation may need to be supported and should be scrupulously monitored throughout the patient's ED stay.

Decreased Cardiac Output, Related to

- **Tachycardia, Dysrhythmias, Elevated Blood Pressure, or Congestive Heart Failure (CHF) Secondary to a Hypermetabolic State Owing to an Increased Level of Thyroid Hormones**

Alterations in cardiac output as the result of an increased level of thyroid hormones in patients experiencing thyroid storm are not uncommon. For this reason, cardiac function (e.g., vital signs, cardiac rhythm) must be monitored at all times. As discussed, the patient will be tachycardic and may have dysrhythmias; this could precipitate heart failure or angina, or both. Propranolol (Inderal) may be given either intravenously or orally, depending on the patient's condition, to alleviate this problem provided that the patient does not have a previous history of CHF or asthma. If propranolol is contraindicated, reserpine or guanethidine may be used (Hamburger et al 1984). If there is no improvement and CHF ensues, digoxin, oxygen, and diuretics would be the next course of therapy. Short-term use of glucocorticoids may also be considered if there is any evidence that the patient is suffering from adrenal insufficiency.

Thermoregulation, Ineffective, Related to

- **Hypermetabolic State Secondary to an Increased Level of Thyroid Hormones**

Patients with alterations in temperature regulation secondary to an increased level of thyroid hormones owing to thyroid storm have extreme elevations in temperature (at times exceeding 106°F) and require continuous temperature monitoring with a rectal probe. It is extremely important to reduce their fever as this will reduce the workload of the heart and the metabolic rate of the body. To reduce the body temperature, hypothermia blankets, ice packs, or sponge baths may be used. Shivering must be avoided as this will only increase the metabolic rate and workload of the heart. If shivering does occur, antipyretics should be given and acetaminophen, rather than salicylates, should be employed. Salicylates will cause further release of thyroid hormones by displacing them from their binding proteins. Avoid using rubber sheets and maintain a calm, cool environment to reduce patient stressors.

Fluid Volume Deficit, Related to

- **Hyperpyrexia, Profuse Diaphoresis, Vomiting, or Diarrhea Secondary to a Hypermetabolic State Owing to an Increased Level of Thyroid Hormones**

Hyperpyrexia, profuse diaphoresis, vomiting, and diarrhea as the result of a hypermetabolic state all contribute to the individual's potential for, or actual, fluid volume deficit. Intravenous fluids will be ordered to correct dehydration and electrolyte abnormalities. The patient may be hypokalemic from gastrointestinal losses and may have hypercalcemia as the result of increased bone metabolism. The type of solution administered will depend on the degree and type of loss. Astute assessment of the patient's cardiovascular and respiratory status in addition to monitoring intake and output must be done as these patients are at an increased risk for congestive heart failure. Patients in thyroid storm also exhibit insulin resistance and may be hyperglycemic. Therefore, a blood glucose level in addition to electrolyte levels should be obtained.

Potential for Injury, Related to

- **CNS Excitability, Osteoporosis, or Exophthalmos Secondary to a Hypermetabolic State Owing to an Increased Level of Thyroid Hormones**

The potential for injury in persons experiencing a hypermetabolic state is primarily the result of (1) central nervous system excitability, (2) osteoporosis promoted by hyperthyroidism, and (3) exophthalmos. Owing to CNS excitability, seizure precautions should be instituted. Side rails should be padded and left up at all times. Additionally, the patient should not be allowed to ambulate in the emergency services center as osteoporosis increases a patient's susceptibility to fractures should he or she stumble and fall in the weakened state. Shielding the patient's eyes from bright lights and instilling isotonic eye drops in an effort to minimize discomfort and prevent corneal abrasion may also be necessary.

*Mental Status, Altered, Related to**

- **Hypermetabolic State Secondary to an Increased Level of Thyroid Hormones**

Alterations in mental status as the result of an increased level of thyroid hormones necessitate frequent reassurance to the patient (and his or her significant others) and explanations of all procedures which will be done to minimize anxiety. The patient with increased emotional lability and sensitivity will respond best to a quiet environment. The nurse should ensure that the patient is minimally disturbed, both physically and emotionally. Family members need to be reassured that the patient's irritability will be reduced as his or her condition improves.

Once life-threatening conditions are treated or are no longer in danger of occurring, investigation of and definitive treatment for the underlying precipitating factor or cause of the thyroid storm, along with stage II care, can begin. For patients experiencing thyroid storm, it is necessary to prevent both thyroid hormogenesis and further release of thyroid hormones. To prevent further synthesis of thyroid hormones, the patient should receive propythiouracil (PTU), a thyroid antagonist, which blocks the organic binding and coupling of iodine required for synthesis of thyroid hormones (Bailey and Baker 1984; Hamburger et al 1984; Sheehy 1985). This is given orally as it is unavailable in parenteral form. The patient may also receive saturated solution of potassium iodide (SSKI). This should be administered approximately 1 hour after the PTU to allow blockage of thyroid hormone synthesis to begin. Iodide therapy temporarily acts to prevent the release of thyroid hormone into the circulation by increasing the amount of stored thyroid hormone in the thyroid gland.

It is extremely important that blood studies be done on all patients experiencing thyroid storm. Routine laboratory tests should be performed, and thyroid hormone levels should be determined. Arterial blood gas values should also be obtained from those persons who experience difficulty breathing. Blood, urine, and sputum should be evaluated for infections to rule these out as a precipitating cause of the emergency. Additionally, a blood glucose level should be obtained to rule out diabetic ketoacidosis as a precipitant. Electrolyte concentrations should also be determined to monitor the patient's hydration status.

---

* Non – NANDA-approved nursing diagnosis.

The underlying cause of thyroid storm must be treated. If the patient has an infection, antibiotic therapy should be begun. If the cause is acidosis, the acidosis will need to be treated in addition to the thyroid storm. Lastly, if the thyroid storm resulted from a knowledge deficit or to noncompliance with anti-thyroid medications, patient education will need to be provided.

Myxedema Coma

In contrast to the patient with thyroid storm, the patient with myxedema coma will be stuporous or comatose. Myxedema coma should therefore be considered in the differential diagnosis of all unexplained cases of coma. Myxedema coma can develop quickly (within hours) in hypothyroid persons following exposure to one of its common precipitants.

Clinical Manifestations

Clinical manifestations of myxedema coma reflect the physiologic effects caused by a deficiency of thyroid hormones. A lowered metabolic rate and a generalized decrease in muscle tone (the most pronounced of these effects) have the potential to cause problems in nearly every body system. Consequently patients with myxedema coma commonly have a temperature that is below normal owing to their lowered metabolic rate and intolerance to cold. Problems with ventilation and maintenance of a patent airway are not uncommon. Bradycardia, hypotension, and a narrow pulse pressure are usually noted. Bradycardia in addition to a decrease in cardiac contractility may precipitate congestive heart failure. Generalized nonpitting interstitial edema occurs and is responsible for the facial puffiness, periorbital edema, and masklike facies commonly seen in individuals with myxedema coma. Neurologically, a decrease in cerebral blood (resulting from a decreased cardiac output) causes changes in mental status, which may range from lethargy and mental sluggishness to pronounced personality changes with florid psychosis.

Treatment and Nursing Care

Patients with myxedema coma, like those experiencing thyroid storm, have extremely high mortality rates and usually require stage I care prior to the initiation of definitive treatment of the underlying precipitating factor or cause.

Breathing Pattern Ineffective, Related to

- **Decreased Muscle Tone Secondary to a Hypometabolic State Owing to a Decreased Level of Thyroid Hormones**

  Patients with thyroid hormone deficits may experience ineffective breathing patterns as the result of decreased muscle tone. Mechanical ventilation via intubation or tracheostomy may be indicated. Assisted ventilation along with oxygen therapy will usually take care of any respiratory acidosis which may be present.

Thermoregulation, Ineffective, Related to

• Hypometabolic State Secondary to a Decreased Level of Thyroid Hormones

In direct contrast to patients experiencing thyroid storm, patients in myxedema coma will be hypothermic. Their body temperatures should be monitored carefully and continuously and they will need assistance in maintaining body warmth. Extra blankets are needed. When using a glass thermometer, it is important to shake the mercury all the way down because the body temperature may be very low. Use of a hypothermic thermometer is recommended when available.

Mental Status, Altered, Related to*

• Decreased Level of Thyroid Hormones, Hyponatremia, or Hypoglycemia Secondary to a Hypometabolic State Owing to a Decreased Level of Thyroid Hormones

Patients with thyroid hormone deficits (e.g., myxedema coma) experience alterations in their mental status and usually are in a stuporous or comatose state. Contributing to the alteration in mental status (in addition to the thyroid hormone deficits) are hypoglycemia and hyponatremia.

Twenty five per cent of patients with myxedema coma experience hypoglycemia from an unknown cause. This hypoglycemia will usually respond to intravenous infusions of 50 per cent dextrose. Glucocorticoids may also be used in the treatment of hypoglycemia.

Hyponatremia may also be seen and may be due to a dilutional factor or to inadequate water excretion. This may occur as the result of inappropriate secretion of antidiuretic hormone (ADH) (Hamburger et al 1984). Thyroid replacement therapy and restricting the amount of fluids should treat the hyponatremia. In replacing the thyroid hormones, one half to one third of the calculated deficit will be given intravenously. It is given in the form of T_4 (Guyton 1981; Hamburger et al 1984). If there is no response to this treatment or the patient has severe hyponatremia, an infusion of a hypertonic saline solution may be indicated.

Tissue Perfusion, Altered, Related to

• Hypotension Secondary to a Hypometabolic State Owing to a Decreased Level of Thyroid Hormones

Vasopressors may be ordered if the patient is hypotensive and should be instituted with care. Hydrocortisone may be ordered as a precautionary measure to prevent an adrenal crisis owing to a decreased blood supply to the adrenals.

---

* Non–NANDA-approved nursing diagnosis.

Infection, Potential for, Related to

- **Hypometabolic State Secondary to a Decreased Level of Thyroid Hormones**

Infection may precipitate myxedema coma or occur as the result of it. Patients with myxedema coma do not respond adequately to infection. Any invasive procedure should be done with strict sterile technique. It is important to institute antibiotic therapy as soon as possible. However, with myxedema coma, the patient does not metabolize drugs efficiently (Muthe 1981). Thus, it is extremely important to assess the patient for signs of drug toxicity for all drugs administered.

Once the patient's condition is stabilized, stage II care may begin. Continuous monitoring of the patient's vital functions, along with constant assessment, evaluation, and re-evaluation of his or her status, must follow. It is extremely important to review the cause of the emergency with the patient and his or her significant other(s). If the cause of the crisis was the result of noncompliance or a knowledge deficit related to the importance of adherence to a prescribed treatment regimen, education must also be given. Close contact with the patient's physician during illnesses should be encouraged, and the patient with hypothyroidism should be told to avoid prolonged exposure to the cold.

EMERGENCIES ASSOCIATED WITH THE ADRENAL GLANDS

An adrenal emergency, otherwise known as addisonian crisis, may have a multitude of causes. The result of adrenal insufficiency, addisonian crisis may occur from either an idiopathic cause (in which the adrenals atrophy and cease secreting steroids) or an inadequate secretion of ACTH (possibly owing to a pituitary tumor) with resultant adrenal atrophy. Precipitating factors of addisonian crisis include the abrupt cessation of steroid medications or failure of the patient to increase glucocorticoid medication during stress or illness. Other, less common causes may be removal of an adenoma of one adrenal, with resultant contralateral adrenal suppression, or adrenal hemorrhage due to sepsis or anticoagulant therapy. Regardless of the cause, the patient will experience a deficiency of glucocorticoids and mineralocorticoids.

Clinical Manifestations

A patient suffering from addisonian crisis will have a variety of complaints, all related to inadequate adrenal secretion of corticosteroids. A decrease in cortisol secretion results in slowed gluconeogenesis with resultant hypoglycemia, weakness, and generalized malaise. Hyposecretion of mineralocorticoids results in increased excretion of salt and water with consequent hypovolemia and dehydration. Blood urea nitrogen (BUN) levels subsequently rise, causing anorexia, nausea, and vomiting and serving to further worsen the patient's hydration status. Laboratory data most commonly reveal hemoconcentration with hypoglycemia, hyponatremia, hyperkalemia, and an elevated BUN.

Treatment and Nursing Care

Fluid Volume Deficit, Related to

- *Hyponatremia, Anorexia, Nausea, Vomiting, or Diarrhea Secondary to Adrenal Insufficiency*

A fluid volume deficit as the result of adrenal insufficiency necessitates immediate intervention to maintain or correct renal function, blood pressure, and cardiac output. Glucocorticoid replacement therapy should begin as soon as possible. Hydrocortisone acetate (approximately 200 to 300 mg) should be given as an intravenous bolus with a continuous infusion of a lesser dose of hydrocortisone for the next 24 hours. Often, an intramuscular injection of 50 mg will be given concurrently as a precaution in case of problems with the intravenous infusion (Adams 1983; Hamburger et al 1984).

Mineralocorticoid replacement therapy (for hyponatremia) is not necessarily instituted because hydrocortisone does lead to sodium retention. However, if the patient is severely hypotensive, hyponatremic or hyperkalemic, desoxycorticosterone acetate (5 to 10 mg) may be given intramuscularly (Adams 1983; Hamburger et al 1984). (Desoxycorticosterone is a mineralocorticoid that promotes sodium reabsorption and potassium and hydrogen excretion in the renal tubule.)

Actual fluid replacement therapy may be of 1 L of 5% dextrose in normal saline (NS) given over approximately 2 hours to correct hypoglycemia and fluid volume depletion, with a slower rate thereafter. If hypoglycemia is severe enough, more dextrose may be needed. The intravenous fluids should be infused rapidly enough to maintain blood pressure and may be based upon CVP readings. Often, the patient will receive from 3 to 5 L of fluid within the first 24 hours (Adams 1983; Hamburger et al 1984).

Decreased Cardiac Output, Related to

- *Fluid Volume Deficit or Hyperkalemia Secondary to Adrenal Insufficiency*

Fluid volume deficits resulting in hypotension (secondary to a decrease in aldosterone secretion with resultant sodium and water loss) and hyperkalemia (with its potential for causing dysrhythmias) both contribute to a potential or actual decrease in cardiac output. These patients should be monitored continuously. Hypotension in them usually requires additional treatment besides fluid replacement. To prevent severe circulatory collapse and coma, vasopressors are usually indicated during the first few hours of treatment. The hyperkalemia will usually respond to both the steroid therapy and rehydration, and there is generally no need for further measures. The patient should, however, be monitored frequently for the development of hypokalemia and supplemental therapy should be initiated, if it occurs.

Infection, Possible, Related to

- *Development of Adrenal Insufficiency*

Because infection is a common precipitating factor in the development of adrenal insufficiency, blood, sputum, and urine samples should be obtained and evaluated for infection. A course of broad-spectrum antibiotics may then be initiated. The patient's temperature should be monitored frequently.

It is extremely important to respond to the patient's other symptoms, and prochlorperazine (Compazine) may be used to decrease the nausea and vomiting associated with addisonian crisis. Patients should not be moved, nor should they be allowed to care for themselves during the acute phase of addisonian crisis, as these persons cannot cope with even minimal stress. Therefore, all forms of external stimuli (e.g., loud noises, lights) should be eliminated. It is extremely important to address the patient's and family's questions and concerns as this will also decrease stress.

Knowledge Deficit, Related to

- *Importance of Compliance with Steroid Medication Regimen*

On stabilization of the patient's condition, it is important for the patient and family to understand the need for taking prescribed medications as scheduled. It must be pointed out to them that abrupt cessation of steroids may trigger addisonian crisis. They should also be aware that during periods of increased stress and illness, there is an increased need for glucocorticoids. Education on how to adjust the dose appropriately during these times will need to be given. Patients taking steroids should be informed of the availability and importance of wearing a Medic Alert bracelet.

EMERGENCIES ASSOCIATED WITH THE PANCREAS

Emergencies associated with the pancreas are related to diabetes mellitus. These emergencies are caused by either a deficit or an excess of insulin. Insulin deficiency is seen in insulin-dependent diabetes mellitus (IDDM), in which the beta cells are destroyed, and from an unknown cause cease to release insulin. Without insulin, the body is unable to use the available glucose for energy, and hyperglycemia ensues. Insulin excess, also seen in patients with IDDM, results when there is too much exogenous insulin in relation to available glucose. This is most likely to occur when persons with IDDM skip meals or engage in excessive physical activity.

Insulin deficiency may lead to diabetic ketoacidosis (DKA), which has a mortality rate of 6 to 10 per cent (Johnson 1985). Insulin excess (which results in hypoglycemia) may lead to a hypoglycemic coma or hypoglycemic seizures. Complications related to either an insulin deficit or excess necessitate rapid identification (via astute assessment skills) and prompt treatment to effect a positive outcome. Symptoms and treatment depend on whether an insulin deficit or excess is present.

Diabetic Ketoacidosis

Clinical Manifestations

Diabetic ketoacidosis, a complication of inadequately treated IDDM, may develop quickly or over several days to weeks. Although most persons who come to EDs in DKA have a history of IDDM, it is not uncommon for a patient to be diagnosed for the first time as having diabetes mellitus following presentation to an ED in diabetic coma. The clinical manifestations displayed by persons with DKA are related to the metabolic chain of events that occur in response to an insulin deficit: hyperglycemia, lipolysis, and protein catabolism.

Insufficient insulin prevents the entry of glucose into cells, which results in an accumulation of glucose in the blood (hyperglycemia). Hyperglycemia, which has an osmotic diuretic effect, results in glucosuria and polyuria with subsequent dehydration and polydipsia.

Concurrently, fat and protein stores are being broken down in an attempt to provide energy to glucose-starved cells. Ketones (which are end products of fat metabolism) accumulate in the blood stream (ketonemia), causing acidosis. As the body tries to rid itself of these acids, ketonuria (ketones in the urine) and further dehydration result. Protein catabolism, which ultimately results in amino acid breakdown to glucose and nitrogen, additionally serves to worsen the patient's dehydrated status by further elevating his or her blood sugar concentration. Anorexia, nausea, and vomiting in response to rising blood urea nitrogen (BUN) levels (and acidosis) also contribute to the patient's dehydration.

When the pathophysiologic processes that occur in response to an insulin deficiency (as described above) are understood, the presenting signs and symptoms of patients in DKA come as no surprise. These persons (or their significant others) may relate a history of any one or all of the following: polyuria, polydipsia, anorexia, nausea, vomiting, weight loss, lethargy, fatigue, and even an altered mental status. Upon questioning, it is not uncommon to discover that the patient has experienced one of DKA's common precipitating factors: recent illness or infection, increased stress, or noncompliance with insulin administration or diet, or both.

Objective assessment of the patient will usually demonstrate a Kussmaul breathing pattern as a result of metabolic acidosis as the body tries to rid itself of carbonic acid by rapidly exhaling carbon dioxide (CO_2). If the pH is at least 7.30, the respiratory drive is generally enhanced, although a pH of less than that will lead to respiratory center depression. An acetone odor to the breath is commonly noted.

Hypotension with a rapid, thready pulse is also commonly noted in patients with DKA. This is due partly to the acidosis, but largely the result of the patient's dehydrated status.

Laboratory analysis may reveal a blood glucose level greater than 300 mg/dl. The urine specimen will be positive for glucose and ketones; protein may be seen if there is renal ischemia. The pH is decreased and is usually less than 7.30. Bicarbonate

(HCO_3^-) is decreased due to renal excretion of chloride ions and pulmonary excretion of CO_2. Due to dehydration and resultant hemoconcentration, the hemoglobin and hematocrit values are often increased. The white blood cell count also may be increased with concurrent infections. Other electrolyte concentrations vary according to the degree of dehydration.

Treatment and Nursing Care

Diabetic ketoacidosis (DKA) is a medical emergency that requires multiple stage I interventions to be implemented expediently and concurrently. Priority goals of therapy for individuals experiencing DKA include the correction of hyperglycemia with simultaneous restoration of normal fluid, electrolyte, and acid-base status.

Fluid Volume Deficit, Related to

- **Osmotic Diuresis, Anorexia, Nausea, or Vomiting Secondary to Hyperglycemia**

The initial line of therapy for patients experiencing a fluid volume deficit as the result of hyperglycemia is to begin rehydration. Generally, infusion of a solution of 0.9% normal saline (NS) is begun at a rate of 10 to 20 ml/kg over the first 1 to 2 hours (Johnson 1985; Kreisberg 1983). Although the patient is generally hypertonic, 0.9% NS is used to prevent the problems that result from too rapid a correction of hypertonicity. After initial replacement, the solution usually will be changed to 0.45% NS at a rate to correct the remaining fluid deficit and supply fluid maintenance. This rate will vary according to the ongoing fluid losses. Rapid rehydration may result in cerebral edema, and nurses must therefore continually assess for signs of it (decreased pulse rate, widened pulse pressure, increased blood pressure, pupils that fail to react to light, Cheyne-Stokes respirations). If noted, a hypertonic solution or mannitol may be indicated to reverse the process (Hamburger et al 1984).

When the blood glucose decreases to 250 mg/dl, dextrose should be added to the intravenous fluids. If the blood glucose level at the start is 250 mg/dl or less, initial fluids should contain dextrose.

Although it is important to monitor the patient's intake and output, an indwelling catheter should be avoided in an effort to decrease the risk of infection. A nasogastric tube may aid in decreasing stomach dilation, allow for accurate measurement of stomach losses, and prevent aspiration of the stomach contents.

Because the cause of DKA is a relative deficit of insulin, insulin replacement therapy must also be initiated. It is only with insulin therapy that the ketogenesis can be reversed and metabolism returned to normal. The quick-acting form of insulin (regular) should be used. Continuous intravenous infusion of insulin is the method of choice because insulin has a relatively short half-life and therapeutic blood levels are easy to achieve. It also allows for easy dose adjustments. The usual dose is approximately 10 units/hour (for adults). This should be diluted in 0.45% NS and administered via a pump. The goal is to reduce the blood glucose approximately 75 mg/dl per hour (Johnson 1985; Kreisberg 1983).

Intramuscular and subcutaneous injections of insulin should be avoided because absorption will be erratic while the patient is dehydrated. However, if an intravenous line is not or cannot be started, a priming dose of insulin may be given intramuscularly followed by hourly injections. Insulin therapy should not be stopped until the blood and urine are free from ketones. Once this occurs, subcutaneous injections may be started or restarted. Subcutaneous insulin (regular) should be given 15 minutes to one half hour prior to discontinuation of the intravenous insulin to prevent rebound ketosis.

The patient with DKA will generally be either hyperkalemic or normokalemic as a result of acidosis, dehydration, and insulin deficit. With correction of the acidosis, rehydration, and insulin therapy, potassium (K^+) will re-enter the cells and the serum K^+ will decrease. Hypokalemia and its ensuing problems may then develop. Because of this, it is important to monitor the patient by EKG. If the patient is hyperkalemic, K^+ replacement therapy is not initiated until the serum K^+ decreases to normal (it will usually continue to decrease) and urine output is established. If the patient has a normal serum K^+, supplements will begin after fluid therapy has been initiated and urine output is established. The person with hypokalemia at presentation needs replacement therapy immediately and K^+ should be added to the intravenous fluids. In general, K^+ supplements are given when the patient is able to tolerate oral feedings. Serum K^+ levels should be checked every 1 to 2 hours to assess the efficacy of the supplements (Johnson 1985; Kreisberg 1983).

Sodium bicarbonate ($NaHCO_3$) therapy is not necessarily needed, and studies have shown DKA to improve at the same rate with or without it (Johnson 1985). Owing to the potential problems associated with $NaHCO_3$ administration (hypokalemia and CSF acidosis), most institutions do not use supplements unless the person's pH is less than 7.10. Arterial blood gas values should be determined to assist with dosing of $NaHCO_3$ therapy when it is utilized. Sodium bicarbonate therapy should be instituted only to raise the pH to 7.20, and blood pH should be checked approximately 30 minutes after it is initiated. Because $NaHCO_3$ therapy may cause hypokalemia, do not start it if the patient is hypokalemic and not receiving K^+ supplements.

Knowledge Deficit, Related to

- **Etiology, Pathophysiology, and Treatment of Diabetes**

Upon stabilization, it is important to begin diabetes education. If the patient is a newly diagnosed diabetic all facets of diabetic education will need to be addressed beginning in the ED and continuing throughout the patient's hospital stay. If an illness was the precipitating cause of the DKA, sick day rules should be reviewed. If the cause of the DKA is stopping insulin injections, the reasons for this should be explored.

Hypoglycemia

Clinical Manifestations

A patient with hypoglycemia may have a multitude of symptoms. Because of a decrease in the amount of glucose available to the brain, he or she commonly exhibits a change in behavior, often being emotionally labile. The person may also complain of headaches and blurred vision. Confusion is not uncommon. As the glucose supply to the brain diminishes, the patient may become unresponsive or comatose or have hypoglycemic seizures. It is not uncommon for the person to be pale and diaphoretic, to have an increased pulse, to complain of an upset stomach, and to feel dizzy, shaky, or faint. These symptoms may be due to the release of the counterregulatory hormones (glucagon, epinephrine, cortisol, and growth hormone) as the body tries to correct the low blood glucose by converting glycogen to glucose (Sklarin and Sklarin 1985).

Treatment and Nursing Care

Mental Status, Altered, Related to*

- **Hypoglycemia**

When a person with known diabetes appears with an alteration in his or her mental status, it is imperative to obtain a blood glucose measurement as soon as possible. There are a variety of methods available for obtaining a blood glucose level immediately at the bedside, and one of these should be employed. It is imperative that the person doing the measurement be knowledgeable on the method employed. A meter will give a more accurate measurement than visual strips, but either one may be considered reliable if the person's technique is accurate. (Bedside blood glucose determinations should be verified with serum glucose determinations by the laboratory.) If a patient has a blood glucose level of 60 mg/dl or lower (usually it will be lower if the cause of unresponsiveness is hypoglycemia), treatment should be initiated immediately to raise the blood glucose concentration. A solution of 50% dextrose given intravenously is the treatment of choice.

If it is impossible to start an intravenous line, 100 units (1 ml) of glucagon should be given subcutaneously (Gever 1985; Lefebvre and Luyckx, 1983). If glucagon is given, turn the patient's head to the side because vomiting commonly occurs after glucagon injections. Rubbing honey or a glucose solution on the gums, or placing it under the tongue, should be avoided as this increases the risk of aspiration. (Alert persons who are able to tolerate oral intake may be given quick acting carbohydrates to eat or drink [e.g., orange juice, sugar packets].)

Frequent monitoring of blood glucose level to ensure that it is rising is imperative. Once the patient regains consciousness and is able to swallow, oral feedings of longer acting carbohydrates (e.g., bread, milk) should be given to maintain the blood glucose level, restore liver glycogen supplies, and prevent further hypoglycemia.

Potential for Injury, Related to

- **Alteration in Mental Status, Possible Seizure Activity, Dizziness, or Blurred Vision Secondary to Hypoglycemia**

It is imperative that the blood glucose level be raised as soon as possible to avoid

---

* Non – NANDA-approved nursing diagnosis.

hypoglycemic seizures. The patient should be placed on seizure precautions while treatment is being initiated and until the blood glucose level increases. He or she should not be allowed to ambulate in the ED as chances for injury are increased.

Knowledge Deficit, Related to

• **Causes, Prevention, and Treatment of Hypoglycemia**

Once the blood glucose level has increased, it is important to assess the cause of the hypoglycemia. If the patient takes insulin, he or she and the family should understand the importance of eating meals as scheduled. Exercise and its effect on blood glucose levels should be reviewed and exercise precautions given. The use of glucagon in hypoglycemic emergencies should be reviewed with responsible significant others, and all learning needs of both the patient and the significant others should be assessed prior to the patient's discharge. Appropriate referrals (e.g., dietician, diabetic clinical nurse specialist) on the basis of learning needs of the patient and the significant others can then be made.

Occasionally, the patient on oral hypoglycemic agents, commonly chlorpropamide (Diabenese), will develop hypoglycemia. Initial treatment is the same as described earlier, but because of the long duration of the hypoglycemic effect of the oral agents, the patient should not be discharged immediately (Hamburger et al 1984; Lefebvre and Luyckx 1983). He or she may need to be maintained on a dextrose solution for a day until the blood glucose level stabilizes. This will decrease the risk of developing hypoglycemia again that day.

CONCLUSION

In conclusion, the emergencies associated with the endocrine glands are a result of either an excess or a deficit of a specific hormone. These excesses and deficits have a major impact on all body systems and unless the patient is treated promptly they can lead to death.

REFERENCES

Adams CE. 1983. Pulling your patient through an adrenal crisis. RN 46(10):38, 75.

Bailey I, Baker W. 1984. Disorders of the thyroid and parathyroid glands. In Hamilton H, ed. Endocrine Disorders. Springhouse, PA, Springhouse Corp, 72–89.

Felig P. 1983. Physiologic action of insulin. In Ellenberg M, Rifkin H, eds. Diabetes Mellitus: Theory and Practice, 3rd ed. New Hyde Park, NY, Medical Examination Publications, 77–78.

Gerich J. 1983. Somatostatine and analogues. In Ellenberg M, Rifkin H, eds. Diabetes Mellitus: Theory and Practice, 3rd ed. New Hyde Park, NY, Medical Examination Publications, 225–254.

Gever L. 1985. Administering glucagon in an emergency. Nursing 15(1):66.

Guyton A, ed. 1981. Textbook of Medical Physiology, 6th ed. Philadelphia, WB Saunders Co.

Hamburger S, Rush D, Bosker G. 1984. Endocrine Metabolic Emergencies. Bowie, MD: Robert J. Brady.

Johnson J. 1985. Management of diabetic ketoacidosis. Clin Diabetes 3:121–30.

Kreisberg R. 1983. Diabetic ketoacidosis, alcoholic acidosis, lactic acidosis and hyporeninemic hypoaldosteronism. In Ellenberg M, Rifkin H, eds. Diabetes Mellitus: Theory and Practice, 3rd ed. New Hyde Park, NY, Medical Examination Publications, 621–653.

Lefebvre P, Luyckx A. 1983. Hypoglycemia. In Ellenberg M, Rifkin H. eds. Diabetes Mellitus: Theory and Practice, 3rd ed. New Hyde Park, NY, Medical Examination Publications, 987–1004.

Muthe N. 1981. Endocrinology: A Nursing Approach. Boston, Little, Brown and Co.

Sheehy S. 1985. Metabolic and endocrine emergencies. J Emerg Nurs 11:49–52.

Sklarin B, Sklarin L. 1985. Brittle diabetes. Diabetes Self-Management, Winter, 18–23.

June Kaiser, RN MS

Hematologic Emergencies

Disorders of the blood and blood-forming organs have the potential to offset the normal functioning of virtually every organ system in an individual's body. Typically, these disorders are the result of an alteration in the production, function, or both of blood components: erythrocytes, leukocytes, platelets, and coagulation factors.

Frequently, individuals presenting to emergency services with hematologic emergencies have previously been diagnosed as having a chronic blood disorder and are seeking treatment for an acute exacerbation or a complication of it. However, it is not uncommon for an individual to present with seemingly benign complaints but after examination and evaluation to be identified for the first time as having a chronic hematologic disease. Hematologic emergencies, whether an acute event or an exacerbation of a chronic disorder, may have severe and potentially fatal consequences. Because of the diversity of presenting symptomatology, emergency nurses must possess excellent assessment skills and must be aware of hematologic disease processes.

This chapter begins with an overview of a hematologic assessment and then discusses the etiologies, pathophysiology, clinical manifestations, treatment modalities, and nursing responsibilities for a variety of specific hematologic disorders.

HEMATOLOGIC ASSESSMENT

The chief complaint of individuals with hematologic disorders may vary widely, depending on underlying pathology and organ system involvement. Frequently, presenting symptomatology is easily identifiable and characteristic of a previously diagnosed blood disorder (e.g., the bone pain of sickle cell crisis, the bleeding of hemophilia, and so forth), allowing the triage nurse's assignment of an acuity rating for these individuals to be determined with little difficulty. There are, however, a host of symptoms that are nonspecific and are found not only in most hematologic disorders but also in many disorders not included in the hematopoietic system. These complaints may involve weakness, dizziness, fatigue, fever, syncope, dyspnea on exertion, or a combination of these. When these vague, generalized and sometimes seemingly benign complaints are offered, the triage nurse may have more difficulty in determining patient acuity. Decision making must take into account a strong likelihood that individuals who present with these complaints may be experiencing a hematologic emergency.

At triage obvious physical findings should also be noted. The skin is the largest organ system of the body that may reflect hematologic problems. Its color, turgor, and surface characteristics should be noted. Is there cyanosis, pallor, jaundice, or ruddiness? Are signs and symptoms of dehydration evident? Are there any rashes, areas of ecchymosis, or petechiae? The temperature and moisture of the patient's skin should also be noted. Is it warm or cool? Is it dry or clammy and diaphoretic?

Other data that the triage nurse should attempt to obtain includes the patient's vital signs and medication and allergy history. The use of anticoagulants and other drugs that can impair the production or function or both of any blood components must be ascertained.

Following this brief but thorough history and cursory physical assessment, the triage nurse must determine the patient's acuity. Most if not all hematologic emergencies will be either urgent and stable or emergent and unstable. Those individuals who are stable at the moment may be able to wait a short period of time prior to treatment without any untoward effects. However, when determining the acuity of these patients, the triage nurse must also consider the potential complications that may be imminent and life-threatening. Therefore, all patients experiencing hematologic emergencies should be brought to the treatment area as quickly as possible.

Once inside the treatment area, further details of the chief complaint should be elicited from either the patient or significant others. Even if the patient has a known, previously diagnosed hematologic disorder, this does not substitute for or negate the importance of a full assessment. The onset, nature, severity, and duration of the chief complaint; the setting in which it occurred; and the aggravating and alleviating factors should be elicited. If patients have had similar episodes in the past, the similarities and differences and the frequency of attacks or episodes should be investigated. Old records that may assist in obtaining such data should be retrieved when available.

Depending on the condition of the patient, the nature of the problem, and the baseline data already known to the emergency services staff, more details of the individual's past medical and family history may be investigated. Previous hospitalizations, reasons for them, diagnostic findings, treatments, responses to treatments, and the patient's drug history or exposures to toxic substances or both should be obtained. Underlying pathology that may be indicative of uremia, liver disease or malignancy must be sought. The occurrence of blood disorders in any family members is particularly helpful when the initial diagnosis of a chronic hematologic disorder is entertained.

A final aspect in gathering the patient's subjective history is the review of systems. Special attention may be focused on those systems most likely to manifest symptoms reflective of hematologic disorders: the skin and the hematopoietic, gastrointestinal, and neuromuscular systems. The occurrence of rashes, lumps, itching, skin color changes, spontaneous or prolonged bleeding, gastrointestinal or genitourinary bleeding, and easy bruising; past histories of anemia, blood transfusions, or both; and episodes of syncope, joint pain, stiffness, and limitation of mobility should all be ascertained. Although attention is focused on the systems just described, a complete review of all body systems helps to ensure that more subtle symptoms of other organ system involvement are not missed.

Objective evaluation of the patient's status includes a physical examination and laboratory analysis. Again, special attention should be focused on target organs most likely to be reflective of hematologic disorders: skin, abdomen, and the neuromuscular systems. The color, turgor, and surface characteristics of the patient's skin should be examined and described. Areas of petechiae, ecchymosis, or both should be noted. The abdomen should be examined for tenderness and organomegaly (especially the spleen and liver) and the bones and joints should be examined for effusions, hemarthrosis, and range of motion. In addition, all body systems must be examined to ensure that the assessment is complete and that diagnosis and treatment are accurate.

Laboratory tests commonly obtained for individuals with hematologic disorders include a complete blood count with differential, reticulocyte count, platelet count, sickle cell preparation, serum electrolytes, prothrombin time (PT), partial thromboplastin time (PTT), and urinalysis. The indications for these tests are discussed in detail under specific hematologic disorders.

Last, while gathering data for assessment (which is all too often focused on the patient's physiologic status), the emergency services nurse must not lose sight of the fact that patients with hematologic disorders may suffer considerable psychologic and emotional discomfort as the result of their often chronic and ultimately fatal disease. The nurse should elicit the patient's feelings about the illness, perception and outlook toward the future, and the impact of the illness on the patient's life. This assessment may assist the nurse in determining the patient's level of coping and in identifying the need for psychologic and emotional support.

DISORDERS OF RED BLOOD CELLS

Sickle Cell Anemia

Sickle cell anemia or disease is a chronic, inherited, autosomal recessive, hemolytic disorder characterized by the presence of abnormal hemoglobin within the erythrocytes. It occurs predominantly in the black population; however, it has also been identified in individuals of Mediterranean descent. The prevalence of African Americans with sickle cell disease is estimated to be approximately 50,000 with an incidence rate of one in 400 births (Forget 1985). Sickle cell trait (discussed later) is found in 8% to 10% of African Americans (Forget 1985).

Etiology

Hemoglobin, the major constituent of RBCs, is normally present in three major forms: hemoglobin A (HbA), hemoglobin A_2 (HbA$_2$), and fetal hemoglobin (HbF). Each molecule of hemoglobin is composed of four iron-porphyrin molecules, called heme, and one protein molecule, called globulin. The globulin molecule is composed of four polypeptide chains that contain a total of 574 amino acids. The substitution of two of these amino acids gives rise to hemoglobin S (HbS), an abnormal variant of HbA that is responsible for the severe and ultimately fatal consequences of sickle cell disease.

Hemoglobin S can be found in either a heterozygous (HbSA) or a homozygous (HbSS) state. When it occurs in a heterozygous state, approximately 24% to 45% of an individual's hemoglobin is HbS (Whaley and Wong 1983, 1346); the remainder consists of HbA and HbF. Such an individual is said to have sickle cell trait and will generally remain asymptomatic throughout his or her life. Sickle cell trait is differentiated from sickle cell disease, in which HbS is present in its homozygous state and composes nearly all of the individual's hemoglobin; only a small percentage of the hemoglobin is HbF. Persons with sickle cell disease manifest varying degrees of symptomatology throughout their lives and eventually suffer disabling long-term complications.

Whether an individual has sickle cell disease or sickle cell trait depends on the genes inherited from each parent. Sickle cell trait is the result of one parent passing along the sickle cell gene to offspring, whereas sickle cell disease is the result of both parents passing along the sickle cell gene to offspring (Fig. 21–1).

Pathophysiology

Sickle cell crises are episodic manifestations of sickle cell disease. There are four types of sickle cell crises: vaso-occlusive (thrombotic), aplastic, sequestrative, and hemolytic. Vaso-occlusive crisis is the most common.

Vaso-occlusive crisis occurs when the RBCs of an individual with sickle cell disease are exposed to hypoxic or acidotic conditions or both. HbS within the RBCs undergo polymerization, a process in which the intracellular contents of the RBCs are transformed from a fluid state to a viscous gel. The membranes of the RBCs subsequently take on the typical crescent, or sickle, shape of the intracellular polymerized hemoglobin. These sickle cells are less flexible, less soluble, and more fragile than normal erythrocytes and are responsible for the clinical manifestations of the disease.

Events that may cause or exacerbate a vaso-occlusive crisis include any activity that increases the body's need for oxygen (e.g., strenuous activity, climbing at high altitudes, flying in nonpressurized planes, and the like), fever, infection, dehydration, exposure to cold, pregnancy, trauma, and emotional upsets.

The rate and degree of RBC polymerization is primarily dependent on the concentration of HbS in the individual's blood and the length of time the erythrocytes are exposed to hypoxic or acidotic conditions or both (Forget 1985). In general, the greater the concentration of HbS and the longer the exposure to hypoxic or

FIGURE 21–1. Inheritance pattern of sickle cell disease.

	S	S
S	SS	SS
S	SS	SS

(row/column label: AFFECTED PARENT)

Offspring of 2 affected parents
• all children will be affected

HETEROZYGOUS PARENT

	S	A
S	SS	SA
A	SA	AA

(row label: HETEROZYGOUS PARENT)

Offspring of 2 heterozygous parents
• one fourth of all children will be affected
• one fourth of all children will be unaffected
• one half of all children will be heterozygous

NORMAL PARENT

	A	A
S	SA	SA
A	AA	AA

(row label: HETEROZYGOUS PARENT)

Offspring of a normal parent and a heterozygous parent
• one half of all children will be unaffected
• one half of all children will be heterozygous

HETEROZYGOUS PARENT

	S	A
S	SS	SA
S	SS	SA

(row label: AFFECTED PARENT)

Offspring of a heterozygous parent and an affected parent
• one half of all children will be affected
• one half of all children will be heterozygous

NORMAL PARENT

	A	A
S	SA	SA
S	SA	SA

(row label: AFFECTED PARENT)

Offspring of a normal parent and an affected parent
• all children will be heterozygous

Affected individuals have sickle cell disease; heterozygous individuals have sickle cell trait; unaffected individuals will not transmit the disorder; males and females are equally affected acidotic conditions, the greater the degree of sickling. For this reason, individuals with sickle cell trait and a relatively low concentration of HbS remain asymptomatic under conditions that would cause individuals with sickle cell disease, who thus have a high concentration of HbS, to experience crisis.

During vaso-occlusive crisis, the increased rigidity of sickled RBCs hampers their ability to traverse the microcirculation. The poor solubility of these RBCs causes an increase in blood viscosity and sluggish circulation. Frequent sickling and unsickling of RBCs leads to an increase in RBC fragility. The resulting accelerated rate of hemolysis and shortened RBC life span causes a significant amount of debris to be deposited in the vascular system. This triad of events leads to vascular occlusion, ischemia, and infarction of vital organs. The tissue hypoxia and subsequent acidosis perpetuate more sickling, vaso-occlusion, ischemia, and infarction. Without treatment, this vicious cycle continues. With treatment, it is possible to reverse the sickling process and arrest the cycle.

Clinical Manifestations

The primary basis for symptoms in individuals with sickle cell disease is the chronic compensated hemolytic anemia (with resultant elevation of bilirubin) that they experience secondary to a shortened RBC life span and the cycle of thrombosis, ischemia, and infarction of organs in response to occlusion of the microcirculation.

Sickle cell disease manifests early in life, but usually not before 5 or 6 months of age, when greater amounts of HbS begin to replace HbF (Price and Wilson 1986, 194). Sickle cell crisis in children under 2 years of age is commonly characterized by painful swelling of the hands and feet (dactylitis) as the result of ischemia and the infarction of metacarpal and metatarsal bones. Definitive diagnosis is made on the basis of hemoglobin electrophoresis.

Older children and young adults who present to emergency services during a sickle cell crisis are typically known to have the disease. In them, vaso-occlusive crises are characterized by the acute onset of excruciating pain owing to vaso-occlusion of the microvasculature of one organ or another, most commonly the bones of the trunk and extremities (Forget 1985). These individuals typically experience a significant amount of pain, usually in the chest, abdomen, back, and extremities. Pain in other areas reflects the organs occluded. Episodes may vary in severity and may last anywhere from hours to days.

Physical examination reveals a chronically ill–appearing individual experiencing moderate to severe discomfort. The person may demonstrate pallor, jaundice, or both caused by chronic anemia and elevated bilirubin. Signs of dehydration, organomegaly (e.g., spleen and liver), or infection may or may not be evident. Fever may or may not be present.

Laboratory data of an individual with sickle cell disease will demonstrate a lower than normal hematocrit, usually in the range of 18% to 30%, hemoglobin between 6.0-10.0 g/dl, and an elevated reticulocyte count that usually ranges between 4% and 30% (Vichinsky and Lubin 1980). The anemia of sickle cell disease remains relatively stable during a vaso-occlusive crisis. Therefore, if there is an acute change or rapid worsening of an individual's anemia, other pathologic processes need to be ruled out (e.g., aplastic, hemolytic, or sequestrative crisis). Serum electrolytes may be normal or may reflect dehydration. White blood cell counts may be normal or may reflect an infectious process. Coagulation times, clotting tests, and platelet counts remain within normal limits. A sickle cell preparation will yield positive results.

The chronic complications that individuals with sickle cell disease may experience are many. Leg ulcers, renal failure, and aseptic necrosis of bones as the result of poor circulation and vaso-occlusion in these areas may be present. Osteoporosis owing to bone marrow proliferation may also occur. Cholelithiasis may result from increased bilirubin secondary to RBC breakdown. Osteomyelitis and frequent infections, possibly resulting from splenic autoinfarction (and subsequent functional asplenia), are not uncommon. Priapism may also occur. Cardiac involvement owing to chronic anemia may manifest as tachycardia, cardiomegaly, and eventual congestive heart failure.

As a result of their chronic illness, individuals with sickle cell disease may exhibit difficult behavior patterns. Most commonly, they are manipulative or dependent, and often feel helpless and hopeless, at times influenced by drug abuse. Parents may also experience a sense of remorse and guilt for having produced a child with a chronic illness.

Other types of sickle cell crises are aplastic, sequestrative, and hemolytic crises. Aplastic crisis, which is most often triggered by infection, occurs when an individual's bone marrow stops functioning. There is cessation of erythropoiesis, anemia rapidly worsens, and the usually elevated reticulocyte count drastically falls. Sequestrative crisis results from the sudden trapping and pooling of large volumes of blood in the spleen and is typically characterized by weakness, pallor, and severe abdominal pain. This pain must be differentiated from the abdominal pain of vaso-occlusive crisis or from an acute abdomen. There is a precipitous drop in blood volume with subsequent shock-like symptomatology. Hemolytic crisis is the least common occurring crisis and usually occurs in patients with glucose-6-phosphate dehydrogenase (G6PD) deficiency. It is characterized by the rapid destruction of RBCs as a result of infection or in response to certain medications (e.g., phenothiazines, large quantities of aspirin, and so forth). Its manifestations include anemia, pallor, jaundice, and reticulocytosis.

During and upon completion of a thorough patient assessment, medical and nursing diagnoses can be formulated. These diagnoses guide the subsequent planning and implementation of therapeutic interventions most appropriate for each individual patient.

Treatment and Nursing Care

Although research regarding sickle cell disease has accelerated in recent years, there presently is no cure. Treatment is symptomatic and supportive.

Stage I care may need to be initiated when individuals with sickle cell disease present with its life-threatening complications. These complications include cardiac and renal failure; major organ infarcts (primarily of the brain, kidneys, and lungs); aplastic, hemolytic, or sequestrative crisis; infection and sepsis, severe dehydration, or a combination of these. Airway, breathing, and circulatory status must be scrupulously monitored and supported. Intravenous access must be established for possible administration of any or all of the following: blood (and/or blood components), antibiotics, or emergency drugs. Emergency resuscitation equipment should also be readily available. Specific treatment will be dictated by the patient's presenting condition.

Tissue Perfusion, Altered (Cerebral, Cardiopulmonary, Renal, Gastrointestinal, and/or Peripheral), Related to

- **Vaso-occlusion Secondary to Sickling of RBCs**
- **Anemia Secondary to Increased Rate of Hemolysis**

Once life-threatening conditions are ruled out, treated, or no longer imminent, stage II care can be initiated and will probably dominate the remainder of the patient's emergency stay. Hydration and pain management are the mainstays of treatment for persons experiencing alterations in tissue perfusion resulting from vaso-occlusive sickle cell crisis. Initial interventions should include blood specimen collection for a CBC, reticulocyte count, electrolytes, and arterial blood gases (ABGs). If not already done, intravenous access should be established. Hydration (IV, oral, or both) is imperative to decrease blood viscosity and improve circulation. Intravenous dehydration is guided by the individual's electrolyte status and fluid requirements for body weight and usually consists of alternating maintenance solutions of D5/0.45 NaCl and D5/0.2 NaCl. Exchange transfusions to decrease the concentration of sickled cells or the administration of packed RBCs (PRBCs) to correct severe anemia may also be indicated.

Supplemental oxygen at flow rates of 2 to 3 L/minute per nasal cannula has traditionally been administered. However, its use has come under scrutiny in recent years (O'Boyle, Davis, Russo, et al 1985, 446). Although somewhat beneficial in the prevention of further sickling, oxygen administration has not been proved to be effective in reversing the sickling process that already exists during crisis. In fact, it is believed that hyperoxygenation may lead to RBC suppression (Solanki 1983). Its use is therefore reserved for those individuals who are actually hypoxic.

Acidosis, when present, should be corrected. However, alkalinization in the absence of acidosis is not recommended (Vichinsky and Lubin 1980).

Pain, Related to

- **Alteration in Tissue Perfusion Secondary to Vaso-occlusive Crisis**

Intramuscular narcotics (e.g., Demerol) are usually required to control the pain associated with alterations in tissue perfusion in vaso-occlusive crisis since the patient has probably already tried oral analgesic pain management without success before coming to the emergency department (ED). Although narcotic dependency is a real possibility in individuals with sickle cell disease, they should not be denied pain management. Reluctance to administer parenteral narcotics in therapeutic doses results in inadequate pain relief, serving only to exacerbate the pain and anxiety the patient is already experiencing. Rest is encouraged and painful joints should be supported and positioned to provide optimal comfort.

Infection, Possible, Related to

- **Functional Asplenia Secondary to Splenic Autoinfarction**
- **Unknown Cause**

Often, infection related to functional asplenia resulting from splenic autoinfarction (and other unknown causes) may trigger sickle cell crisis. It is therefore imperative to determine if any underlying infection is present. The patient's temperature should be monitored and a CBC should be obtained to aid in this determination. Fever or leukocytosis (or both) is suggestive of infection. Blood cultures and a spinal tap (especially in infants and young children) may be required if either sepsis or meningitis is suspected. Radiographs of the chest and extremities are also commonly needed to identify underlying pneumonia (or cardiomegaly), aseptic necrosis, osteomyelitis or osteoporosis, and joint effusions. Additionally, joint effusions may need to be tapped to rule out septic arthritis. A urinalysis may also be helpful in demonstrating if renal system infection is present or if there is renal involvement. Depending on the nature and severity of suspected infection along with other practical considerations (e.g., how long the patient will remain in emergency services, if the person will be sent home or if she or he will be admitted, and so forth), antibiotics (IV or oral) may be initiated in the ED.

Coping, Ineffective (Potential), Individual or Family, Related to

- **Frequent Hospitalizations Secondary to Chronic Illness**
- **Frequent Separation from Family Secondary to Chronic Illness**
- **Interruption of Lifestyle Secondary to Frequent Hospitalizations**
- **Imposed Adaptations of Lifestyle Secondary to Chronic Illness**
- **Sense of Helplessness Related to Chronic Illness**
- **Parental Guilt Because Offspring Has a Genetic Disorder**

The potential for ineffective coping related to chronic illness and frequent hospitalizations for individuals with sickle cell disease (or their family or both) is a continuing, real concern. Allowing these individuals to express their feelings, fears, and concerns is often beneficial and should be encouraged. Additionally, support to encourage as independent a life as possible for patients with sickle cell disease should be conveyed by the ED nurse to both the patient and significant others. Normal activities (within patient capabilities) and relationships should be promoted and encouraged. When indicated, referrals for genetic screening and counseling should also be offered.

Knowledge Deficit, Potential, Related to

- **Etiology, Pathophysiology, Treatments, Complications, and Prognosis of Illness**

The ED nurse also has the responsibility to ensure that patients with sickle cell disease are educated regarding it. Patients should be aware of precipitating events that lead to crises and what to do when one occurs. All too often, individuals with sickle cell disease receive only crisis-triggered, episodic emergency care. Principles of health promotion and health maintenance and the importance of receiving continuous, coordinated health care to decrease the incidence of complications must be stressed.

Individuals experiencing aplastic, sequestrative, or hemolytic sickle cell crises require blood transfusions (e.g., PRBCs, whole blood, or both) in addition to the other treatment outlined thus far. For sequestrative crisis treatment similar to that for hypovolemic shock is also used.

Evaluation

Close patient monitoring and astute evaluation of the responsiveness of the symptoms to treatment is a critical nursing function. Vital signs should be checked frequently, and identification of signs and symptoms suggestive of worsening anemia and shock must be noted and reported to the physician at once. If the pain episode can be arrested and treated in the ED (and no other complications are evident), the patient may be able to go home. However, adherence to a treatment plan that includes rest, oral hydration, and oral pain management for the next several days must be encouraged (in addition to any treatment the patient has received for underlying problems). If pain is not able to be controlled after 4 to 6 hours in the ED, plans for hospital admission should be made. Rest, IV hydration, and IM analgesics, together with treatment for underlying problems, will then continue to be administered in the hospital.

DISORDERS OF COAGULATION

Hemostasis

The etiology, pathophysiology, and treatment modalities for individuals with coagulation abnormalities can only be appreciated when normal hemostasis is understood. Therefore, before discussion of specific clotting disorders, normal hemostasis is reviewed.

Hemostasis refers to the cessation of bleeding. This may occur naturally (e.g., clot formation) or artificially (e.g., by compression or ligation of a vessel). Only the natural process is discussed here.

There are three main processes involved in the natural occurrence of hemostasis following vascular injury. They are (1) local vasoconstriction; (2) platelet aggregation, adhesion, and release of chemical agents; and (3) the activation of clotting factors.

When vessel trauma and bleeding occur, the injured and surrounding vessels at the damaged site immediately constrict. The flow of blood to the area is thereby decreased and blood loss is lessened.

Vasoconstriction alone, however, usually is not adequate to stop bleeding. Aggregation and adherence of platelets (i.e., formation of a platelet plug) to exposed collagen of traumatized vessel walls must ensue. Exposure of platelet factor 3, a lipoprotein surface on the cell membrane of platelets, plays a vital role in strengthening the platelet plug by ultimately assisting in the formation of fibrin. Fibrin transforms blood surrounding the original platelet plug into a solid gel acting to further reinforce, strengthen, and support it. Platelet factor 3 is therefore essential for coagulation to occur. (For further details regarding the structure, function, and action of platelets and all chemical agents secreted by them, the reader is referred to any hematology textbook.)

When minor injuries occur, hemostasis may be effected by local vasoconstriction and platelet adhesion and aggregation alone. When more severe injuries occur, however, the activation of clotting factors (with resultant fibrin clot formation) is essential to arrest bleeding.

Most clotting factors are plasma proteins that circulate in blood as inactive molecules. Once activated, they initiate a complex series of chain reactions that lead to fibrin clot formation at the site of injury. There are two main pathways by which blood clotting is initiated and fibrin is formed: the intrinsic and extrinsic.

The intrinsic pathway is stimulated when the inactive form of Factor XII (which normally circulates in blood) comes in contact with exposed skin or collagen of a damaged vessel. Factor XII is then activated and a "cascade effect," which employs a multitude of reactions, each dependent upon the activation of a precursor factor (and the presence of other substances—e.g., calcium, platelet factor 3), follows (Fig. 21–2). The intrinsic pathway derives its name from the fact that all the substances and factors required for the events occurring in it are contained within the blood.

The extrinsic pathway is stimulated when tissue thromboplastin (or tissue factor) is released from damaged cells or vascular endothelium at the site of injury into the blood. Because tissue factor may be released from damaged cells (tissue) outside the vascular system this clotting pathway is referred to as the extrinsic clotting pathway. Both the intrinsic and extrinsic systems ultimately lead to the activation of Factor X, which, in the presence of calcium, Factor V, and platelet factor 3, converts prothrombin to thrombin. Thrombin in turn converts fibrinogen in the presence of calcium and Factor XIII to fibrin (Fig. 21–2). As fibrin is laid, the platelet plug is strengthened and stabilized. If any one of the substances or factors required for either the intrinsic or extrinsic pathway is lacking, problems with clotting will occur.

Simultaneous with the activation of factor XII (and subsequent clot formation), plasminogen is converted to plasmin (Vander et al 1985, 377). Plasmin is responsible for the degradation of fibrin (i.e., clot lysis) and the formation of fibrin split products which act as powerful anticoagulants. Thus, both the clotting and anticlotting systems are triggered simultaneously by the activation of factor XII. It is for this reason that prolonged, continuous, and widespread clotting throughout the vascular system does not normally occur.

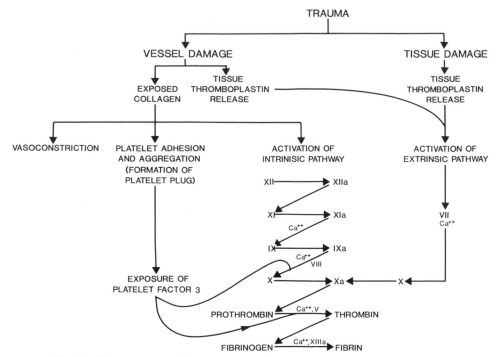

FIGURE 21-2. Components of hemostasis, which is caused by vasoconstriction, platelet aggregation and adhesion, and activation of clotting pathways. (IXa, Xa, XIa, and XIIa are activated factors.)

Hemophilia

Hemophilia is a sex-linked, recessive hereditary coagulation disorder that is transmitted by females and occurs almost exclusively in males. It is characterized by prolonged bleeding that may occur spontaneously or in response to varying degrees of physical injury or insult. Two types of hemophilia constitute the majority of inherited coagulation disorders: Hemophilia A (classic hemophilia) and hemophilia B (Christmas disease) result from a deficiency of Factors VIII and IX, respectively. A third type of inherited coagulation disorder is von Willebrand's disease (an autosomal dominant coagulation disorder affecting males and females), in which there is both a deficiency of Factor VIII and defective platelet function. The incidence of hemophilia A is approximately 1 in 10,000 male births, and the incidence for hemophilia B is approximately 1 in 40,000 male births (Hilgartner 1982).

Etiology

Hemophilia is an X-linked recessive disease. Females (who have two X chromosomes) become carriers of hemophilia when they inherit the defective gene on the X chromosome from either a carrier mother or hemophiliac father. Males (who have

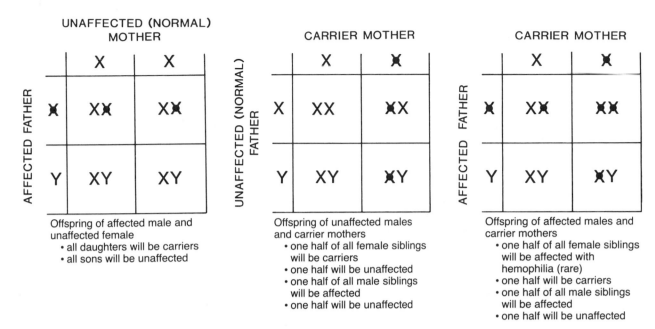

FIGURE 21–3. Inheritance pattern of hemophilia.

one X and one Y chromosome) inherit hemophilia if they receive the defective X chromosome from a carrier mother or a hemophiliac father (Fig. 21–3 illustrates the inheritance pattern for hemophilia).

Pathophysiology

In individuals with hemophilia A or hemophilia B, either Factor VIII or Factor IX activity, respectively, is defective, deficient, or absent. Factors VIII and IX are plasma proteins (clotting factors) required by the intrinsic pathway for fibrin clot formation. When either is defective, absent, or deficient, the normal sequence of reactions (cascade) that ultimately leads to fibrin clot formation is interrupted. Bleeding is then prolonged and difficult to control. Platelets and blood vessels are usually normal.

Clinical Manifestations

Hemophilia is characterized by excessive, prolonged, and persistent internal or external bleeding or both that may occur spontaneously or following injury. It is usually diagnosed early in infancy (often at the time of circumcision) or during early childhood. A history of spontaneous or prolonged bleeding following minor injuries or procedures (e.g., dental extractions) is usually present. Common sites for bleeding include joints and muscles; pain, warmth, and swelling result at the area of bleeding. Definitive diagnosis is made on the basis of assays of Factors VIII and IX. PTT, which reflects the intrinsic clotting pathway, is prolonged, whereas PT, which reflects the extrinsic clotting pathway, remains normal. Platelet count is also normal.

The degree and severity of bleeding experienced by individuals with hemophilia is inversely related to the existing factor activity present and is directly related to the severity of the injury. If factor activity level assay (of either Factor VIII or Factor IX) is less than 1% of normal (normal equals 100% activity), spontaneous bleeding without trauma frequently occurs (Buchanan 1980). Individuals with factor activity level assays between 1% and 5% of normal experience significant bleeding following only minor trauma, while those with factor activity level assays between 5% and 25% can lead relatively normal lives with severe bleeding occurring only after major surgery or trauma (Buchanan 1980).

Long-term complications that may occur as a direct result of this bleeding disorder include joint deformities and muscle contractures (from frequent bleeding into joints and muscles) severely limiting the patient's mobility. Nerve compression (from muscle hemorrhage) may also occur. Individuals who require frequent transfusions and blood components additionally run the increased risk of contracting hepatitis, acquired immune deficiency syndrome (AIDS), or both.

Treatment and Nursing Care

Fluid Volume Deficit, Related to

- **Hemorrhage Secondary to Defective, Absent, or Deficient Clotting Factors**

Stage I care will need to be initiated when life-threatening complications of hemophilia occur. These may result from massive blood loss in response to an acute injury or a spontaneous bleed. Significant blood loss may even follow as a delayed response days after an injury. Bleeding that is most life-threatening for hemophiliacs is retroperitoneal, intracranial, and peritracheal soft tissue hemorrhages. In these instances, intravenous access must immediately be established for the administration of blood, blood components, fluids, emergency drugs, or all of these. The individual's airway, breathing, and circulation must be supported and emergency resuscitation equipment (including a tracheostomy tray) must be readily available.

Infusion of the deficient, absent, or nonfunctional clotting factor must occur at the earliest indication of bleeding, regardless of severity. Delays in treatment contribute to a slower rate of recovery, prolongation of therapy, and greater likelihood of chronic complications (Buchanan 1980).

The dose and frequency of factor replacement is dependent upon the location and severity of hemorrhage. Additional considerations are the patient's weight and existing factor activity level. Accordingly, the practitioner determines the factor activity level necessary to arrest bleeding (Table 21 – 1). Once this factor activity level is known, the practitioner can calculate the actual number of Factor VIII or Factor IX units necessary to achieve that level (Table 21 – 2). Additionally, the expected per-

TABLE 21-1

Management of Specific Bleeding Episodes in Patients with Hemophilia A and B

| Type of Hemorrhage | Minimal Factor Activity Level (% of Normal) | | Other Therapy |
	To Be Achieved by Initial Infusion	Subsequent Infusions	
Early spontaneous joint or muscle bleed (pain but no swelling)	10%–15%	Usually not necessary	
Joint or muscle bleed after trauma or inadequate early treatment (pain, swelling, and muscle spasm present)	40%–50%	Often required daily for 2 or 3 days	Decrease weight bearing Wrapping or splinting sometimes useful
Soft tissue bleeding	No treatment necessary if small 25%–30% if hemorrhage is large and expanding	Usually not required	
Oral mucous membrane bleeding (following small lacerations or tooth extractions)	50%–75%	Usually not required if Amicar is given	Aminocaproic acid (Amicar) (see PDR or drug formulary for dose) Liquid and then soft diet for 3–4 days
Hematuria	None if mild or lasting <24 hours 50 per cent for severe, prolonged, or painful hemorrhage	Variable; usually not required	Vigorous hydration (as tolerated by patient) Short course of steroids is advised by some
Suspected or proven intracranial hemorrhage*	100%	Daily for 7 to 14 days to maintain level over 40%–50% at all times†	CT scan and other diagnostic tests to ascertain extent of hemorrhage
Surgery or major lacerations‡	100%	Daily for 7 to 14 days to maintain level over 40 to 50% at all times†	

Source: Adapted from Buchanan GR. 1980. Pediatr Clin North Am 2: p.317.

* Minor head trauma requires single dose to 100% and careful outpatient observation for signs and symptoms of increased intracranial pressure.

† Laboratory monitoring of factor level is required on daily or every other day basis.

‡ Minor superficial lacerations are sometimes managed with single dose or no replacement therapy at all.

centage increase in factor activity level that will result from the administration of a given number of Factor VIII or Factor IX units can be estimated (Table 21–2).

The formulas outlined in Table 21–2 are guidelines only. Their use should not preclude the evaluation of individual clinical responses and laboratory analysis. Furthermore, the factor activity levels of hemophiliacs who present to the emergency department with acute bleeding episodes are oftentimes not known. In these instances, factor replacement therapy may be initiated prior to this determination. If the bleeding episode is minor (e.g., small, limited area of soft tissue bleeding) and ceases after the initial infusion of replacement factor, further therapy and factor activity level determination may not be necessary. If subsequent therapy is required, factor analysis must then be done to guide ongoing treatment.

In the past, bleeding in hemophiliacs was controlled by the administration of whole blood or fresh frozen plasma (which contains all clotting factors). Circulatory overload became a problem, however, when large quantities of plasma and blood were required. Currently, most individuals with hemophilia receive cryoprecipitate,

TABLE 21-2
Formulas Used in Determining Factor Unit Requirements and Approximate Factor Level Activity Increases

Factor VIII

$$\text{Units required} = \frac{\text{body weight}}{\text{(kg)}} \times 0.5 \times \frac{\text{desired Factor VIII increase}}{\text{(\% of normal)}}$$

$$\frac{\text{Expected Factor VIII increase}}{\text{(\% of normal)}} = \frac{\text{units administered}}{\text{body weight (kg)}} \times 2$$

Infusion of 1 unit/kg of Factor VIII raises the factor level by 2% with a subsequent half-life of 12 hours

Factor IX

$$\text{Units required} = \frac{\text{body weight}}{\text{(kg)}} \times 0.8 - 1.0 \times \frac{\text{desired factor IX increase}}{\text{(\% of normal)}}$$

$$\frac{\text{Expected Factor IX increase}}{\text{(\% of normal)}} = \frac{\text{units administered}}{\text{body weight (kg)}} \times 1.0 - 1.3$$

Infusion of 1 unit/kg of Factor IX raises the factor level by 1% with a subsequent half-life of 24 hours

a concentrated form of Factor VIII that is produced from a single donor unit of fresh plasma. Other commercially prepared forms of concentrated Factor VIII or Factor IX, produced from large pools of plasma utilizing multiple donors, are also available.* Products in this latter category are listed in Table 21-3.

Once factor replacement therapy is under way and life-threatening hemorrhage is not imminent, stage II nursing care may be initiated. Local treatment, which consists of ice, elevation, and immobilization of the affected extremity, may be instituted. Treatment for oral bleeding resulting from dental procedures or small lacerations from local trauma may include direct pressure along with the use of antifibrinolytic agents such as epsilon aminocaproic acid (Amicar). Intramuscular injections and repeated venipunctures should be avoided if at all possible.

The threat of spontaneous bleeding and fear of accidental trauma are very real and consistent sources of stress for hemophiliacs and their significant others. Referrals for psychologic or genetic counseling or both should be offered. Reinforcing principles of prevention along with educating patients and their significant others about hemophilia is also a nursing responsibility.

Pain, Related to

• Hemorrhage into Joints, Muscles

Pain usually diminishes shortly after the cessation of bleeding. If short-term pain management is required, acetaminophen is preferred over aspirin (ASA), which may interfere with platelet aggregation. Comfort measures such as the application of ice to an injured extremity or immobilization and support of the affected extremity (e.g., Ace wrap, knee immobilizer) may be beneficial.

---

* Recommended rates of infusion may vary among commercially prepared Factors VIII and IX concentrates. Therefore, nurses are referred to the PDR, drug formulary, or hospital policy for this determination.

TABLE 21-3
Concentrated Factor Products

Factor VIII	Manufacturer	Heat-Treated
HT Factorate	Armour	Yes
HT Factorate Generation II	Armour	Yes
Hemofil T	Hyland Therapeutic	Yes
Koate H.T.	Cutter Biological	Yes
HT Profilate	Alpha Therapeutic	Yes (dry method)
Profilate Heat-Treated	Alpha Therapeutic	Yes (wet method)
Factor IX		
Konyne H.T.	Cutter Biological	Yes
Profilnine Heat-Treated	Alpha Therapeutic	Yes (wet method)
Proplex SX-T	Hyland	Yes

Source: Compiled from data in McEvoy GK. 1987. American Hospital Formulary Service: Drug Information, 1987. Bethesda, Md, American Society of Hospital Pharmacists.

Potential for Injury, Related to

- **Iatrogenic-Induced Complications Secondary to Multiple Blood or Blood Component Transfusions**

Circulatory overload with the use of concentrated preparations of Factor VIII and Factor IX are no longer a problem because only 10 to 30 ml are contained in each bag or vial. Other problems with their use do however exist and include the increased risk of contracting hepatitis, AIDS, or both. The incidence of these complications are less likely with the use of cryoprecipitate than with the use of other commercially prepared concentrates, because cryoprecipitate is produced from the plasma of a single donor. A heat treatment process, however, is now employed during the manufacturing of Factors VIII and IX concentrates. This process is believed to reduce the risk of transmission of human immunodeficiency virus. Further studies to determine the efficacy of this treatment are needed, however.

A disadvantage of using cryoprecipitate is that wide variations exist in the number of units of Factor VIII in each bag. Commercially prepared concentrated forms of Factors VIII and IX contain a known number of factor units per bag or vial. See Table 21–4 for a summary of recommendations for the treatment of patients with hemophilia.

Evaluation

Evaluation of individuals with acute bleeding episodes involves astute observation of the patient's responsiveness to treatment. This includes watching for any signs and symptoms of continued bleeding. The patient's subjective symptoms (e.g., pain), vital signs, hematocrit (Hct) and Hb, and skin observations are the best parameters in

TABLE 21–4
Summary of Recommendations for Treating Patients with Hemophilia[1] from the National Hemophilia Foundation

---

1. The risks of withholding factor treatment far outweigh the risks of treatment.
2. Desmopressin (DDAVP), a synthetic analog of vasopressin that markedly increases Factor VIII activity in patients with mild to moderate hemophilia, should be used whenever possible: when feasible, an alternative to concentrates may be the use of cryoprecipitate prepared from one well-screened and repeatedly tested donor or from a small number of such donors
   a. Products that are heated in aqueous solution (pasteurized), treated with solvent/detergent, purified with monoclonal antibody, heated in suspension in organic media, or dry heated at high temperatures for long periods are preferred; these products are at substantially reduced risk of transmitting HIV
   b. Preliminary data suggest that products that are heated in aqueous solution (pasteurized), solvent/detergent treated, or monoclonal-antibody purified are at reduced risk of transmitting hepatitis viruses: uninfected patients with hemophilia should receive HB vaccination

---

Source: Centers for Disease Control. 1988. MMWR 37:903.

gauging a patient's status. Additionally, when blood or blood components is being transfused, signs and symptoms of transfusion reactions must be watched for.

DISSEMINATED INTRAVASCULAR COAGULATION

Disseminated intravascular coagulation (DIC) is a complex, potentially fatal coagulation disorder characterized initially by hypercoagulability of blood and secondarily by hemorrhage. An imbalance exists between the states of coagulation and anticoagulation in which diffuse clotting occurs throughout the entire vascular system, followed by clot dissolution and subsequent exhaustion of clotting factors and platelets.

Etiology

Pathologic disease processes underlie nearly all cases of DIC. Any condition that causes vessel damage or aberrant release of thromboplastin serving to activate the clotting pathways may be causative. The flow of blood over damaged vascular endothelium resultant from traumatic injuries, sepsis, or shock stimulates the intrinsic clotting pathway. Obstetric complications (because of the placenta's rich source of

TABLE 21-5
Common Causes of DIC

Obstetrical Complications
    Abruptio placentae
    Intrauterine fetal death
    Toxemia of pregnancy
Malignancies
Sepsis
    Bacteria (e.g., urinary, gastrointestinal, pulmonary)
    Viruses
    Parasites
Trauma
Shock
Liver disease
Transfusion reactions
Snakebites
Heatstroke

tissue thromboplastin) such as abruptio placentae and intrauterine fetal death stimulate the extrinsic clotting pathway and are frequent causes of DIC. See Table 21 – 5 for a listing of common causes of DIC.

Pathophysiology

Once the clotting mechanism is initiated (as previously described), widespread, diffuse clotting occurs throughout the individual's circulation. This results in a hypercoagulable state with concomitant stimulation of the normal fibrinolytic mechanism to begin clot lysis. During these two adverse processes, coagulation factors are consumed, clotting is inhibited, and clot lysis is occurring. A vicious cycle of clotting and bleeding results.

Clinical Manifestations

DIC may occur with varying degrees of severity. It may be acute with severe symptomatology or chronic with more subtle manifestations of the disease. In either case, unless nurses are astute in their observations, the diagnosis may easily be missed, especially in the face of major trauma with significant blood loss. The presentation of individuals with severe symptomatology may be that of a hypovolemic, shock-like state. Peripheral cyanosis, gangrene of the digits, and major organ infarcts (e.g., cerebral vascular accidents) caused by circulatory obstruction resulting from microthrombi may also be present. Oral, vaginal, genitourinary, gastrointestinal, or central nervous system bleeding are not uncommon. Diffuse areas of ecchymosis, petechiae and prolonged bleeding following procedures or treatments may be evident. The first clue may be bleeding from an injection site or surgical incision.

    Laboratory results reveal thrombocytopenia and prolonged PT and PTT. Fibrinogen levels are also reduced, with a concomitant elevation of fibrin-split products.

Treatment and Nursing Care

The priority in treatment for individuals with DIC is focused on the underlying pathologic disease process (Lamb 1985). This treatment may include the administration of antibiotics, chemotherapeutic agents, and/or surgery to empty uterine contents if obstetric abnormalities are contributory. Once the underlying pathology is corrected, DIC usually resolves.

Fluid Volume Deficit, Related to

- *Hemorrhage Secondary to Ongoing Cycle of Coagulation and Anticoagulation*

The unstable patient with DIC who presents to the emergency department with imminent life-threatening complications of the disorder (e.g., hemorrhage), requires immediate stage I care. Airway, breathing, and circulatory status must be supported. Emergency resuscitation equipment should be readily available, and intravenous access should be established. Blood specimens for a CBC, reticulocyte and platelet count, PT, PTT, typing, and cross-matching should be obtained. The primary goal of management is to restore fluid-volume status by administering blood, blood components, and specific clotting factors. Whole blood, PRBCs, fresh frozen plasma, platelets and cryoprecipitate may all be used. These may need to be administered even before hemostasis is achieved. Heparin therapy, which is aimed at blocking the ultimate formation of fibrin by interfering with the intrinsic coagulation pathway, may also be initiated. Although the use of heparin may seem paradoxic, control of intravascular coagulation by heparin therapy often results in the cessation of concurrent fibrinolysis (Rooney and Haviley 1985).

More often than not (especially in EDs), individuals who present with DIC are critically ill. The potential clinical problems they may experience are many. As a result, nursing care should be dynamic and often must alternate between stage I and stage II. Ongoing assessment of the patient's responsiveness to treatment, prevention of further complications, and the continued administration of drugs or blood and blood components (or all three) comprise stage II nursing care. The patient is assessed for new sources of bleeding (especially if heparin is being administered) and any increase or decrease in the amount of bleeding. Care must be taken when cleaning and shaving wounds, giving injections, starting IVs, and obtaining blood samples. To prevent injury and further bleeding, siderails may need to be padded if there is seizure activity, combative behavior, or a changed level of consciousness. Signs and symptoms of anaphylaxis and transfusion reactions must be assessed. Additionally, because DIC is frequently a sudden and dramatic occurrence requiring long-term therapeutic interventions, patients and their significant others are often frightened. Offering explanations at their level of understanding in accordance with their readiness to accept information is helpful in alleviating anxiety. Patients and their families need much emotional support during an extremely stressful and often uncertain time.

Evaluation

Ongoing and vigilant monitoring of patients experiencing DIC is a critical nursing responsibility. Often, the nurse is the first to notice signs and symptoms indicative of DIC and of improvement or worsening of the patient's condition. Vital signs, laboratory data (CBC, PT, PTT, platelet count, and electrolytes), fluid-volume status, and the patient's level of consciousness and subjective complaints are critical in assisting the nurse to evaluate the patient's status.

CONCLUSION

The nursing care of patients experiencing hematologic emergencies is both demanding and challenging. Presenting symptomatology is often emergent in nature and varied in etiology. Therapeutic interventions must be initiated expediently to decrease the morbidity and mortality of these individuals. For this reason, nurses need to possess excellent assessment skills and a sound scientific knowledge base relating to the pathophysiology of disease.

REFERENCES

Buchanan GR. 1980. Hemophilia. Pediatr Clin North Am 2:309–326.

Forget BG. 1985. Sickle cell anemia and associated hemoglobinopathies. In Wyngaarden JB, Smith LH, eds. Cecil Textbook of Medicine. Philadelphia, WB Saunders, 927–932.

Hilgartner MW. 1982. Hemophilia in the Child and Adult. New York, Masson.

Lamb C, ed. 1985. When you suspect DIC. Patient Care 19:84–105.

McEvoy GK. 1987. American Hospital Formulary Service: Drug Information 1987. Bethesda, American Society of Hospital Pharmacists.

O'Boyle C, Davis DK, Russo BA, et al. 1985. Emergency Care: The First 24 Hours. Norwalk, Conn. Appleton-Century-Crofts.

Price SA, Wilson LM. 1986. Pathophysiology: Clinical Concepts of Disease Processes, 3rd ed. New York, McGraw-Hill Book Co.

Rooney A, Haviley C. 1985. Nursing management of disseminated intravascular coagulation. Oncol Nurs Forum 12:15–22.

Solanki DL. 1983. Sickle cell anemia, oxygen treatment, and anaemic crisis. Br Med J 287:725–726.

Vander AJ, Sherman JH, Luciano DS. 1985. Human Physiology: The Mechanisms of Body Function, 4th ed. New York, McGraw-Hill Book Co.

Vichinsky EP, Lubin BH. 1980. Sickle cell anemia and related hemoglobinopathies. Pediatr Clin North Am 2:429–447.

Whaley LF, Wong DL. 1983. Nursing Care of Infants and Children, 2nd ed. St. Louis, CV Mosby.

Selected Topics in
Emergency Nursing

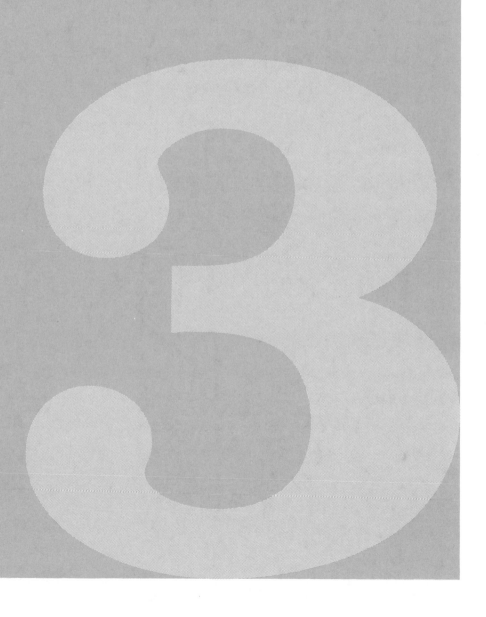

Mary Beth Carrier Goldman, RN MS CCRN

Pediatric Medical Emergencies

It is well recognized that children are not "little adults." In providing care to children in emergent situations, it is critical to be aware of how children differ from adults. Therefore, this chapter begins with an overview of the pediatric assessment, noting concepts unique to children. Problems (described by nursing diagnoses) commonly experienced by children and their families who require emergency services and related interventions are then addressed. A discussion of specific illnesses and injuries common to children follows.

PEDIATRIC ASSESSMENT

Vital sign ranges change with age and are reviewed in Table 22–1. Apical pulse is auscultated, especially in infants, as peripheral pulses may be difficult to palpate. Although not uncommon, sinus dysrhythmias and functional murmurs in children should be investigated. The child's heart is unable to significantly increase stroke volume, so the need for increased cardiac output is met by increasing heart rate. The circulating blood volume ranges from 90 ml per kilogram body weight in the neonate to 75 ml per kilogram body weight in the child. The absolute quantity of blood is small and must be considered when multiple blood specimens are requested.

A blood pressure should be recorded on all children admitted to the emergency

TABLE 22–1
Pediatric Vital Signs

Age Group	Heart Rate	Respirations	Blood Pressure
Infant	120–160	30–60	74–100/50–70
Toddler	90–140	24–40	80–112/50–80
Preschool	80–110	22–34	82–110/50–78
Schoolage	75–100	18–30	84–120/54–80
Adolescent	60–90	12–16	94–140/62–88

Source: Reproduced by permission from Hazinski MF. Nursing Care of the Critically Ill Child, 2–3. St. Louis, 1984, The C.V. Mosby Co.

department (ED). An appropriately sized cuff covers one half to two thirds of the upper arm. Because values may be difficult to auscultate, an ultrasonic blood flow detector (Doppler) or automatic blood pressure monitor (Dinamap) may be used. The automatic devices are very useful in emergency situations, as they provide accurate determination of blood pressure and can be set to cycle, freeing the nurse to perform other duties (Park and Menard 1987).

In infancy the chest wall is cartilaginous with horizontal ribs and poorly developed musculature. By adolescence the structure is rigid with oblique ribs and well developed intercostal muscles. The child depends on the diaphragm for adequate chest expansion. This is demonstrated by abdominal breathing. Softness of the chest wall causes it to move inward with inspiration resulting in retractions. Airways of children will grow in size and firmness as the number of alveoli increases. Anything that decreases airway radius, such as edema or mucus plugs, increases the resistance in these small airways. Neonates are obligate nose-breathers and must maintain open nasal passages. Careful auscultation for changes in intensity or pitch of breath sounds is necessary as sound is easily transmitted through the thin chest wall.

Young children have a high surface area : volume ratio and can lose heat rapidly. Infants have immature temperature control mechanisms. They are unable to shiver and must use chemical thermogenesis to produce heat through the breakdown of brown fat. Oxygen and calorie demands are increased during the breakdown and regeneration of this special fat. A neutral thermal environment allowing for a rectal temperature of 37°C must be maintained.* Rectal temperature may be taken in infants. Axillary temperatures are used in young children, as they are less threatening. A schoolage child can be expected to cooperate with the oral route.

The higher surface area : volume ratio and greater metabolic rate increases the child's fluid and calorie requirements. Maintenance fluid requirements are outlined in Table 22–2. Intravenous (IV) fluid should contain dextrose, except in instances of major trauma requiring rapid fluid resuscitation or when the child has diabetes. An adequately hydrated child averages 0.5 to 1.0 ml per kilogram body weight per hour of urine output. Intravenous access can be difficult to obtain and maintain. Commonly used sites are the dorsal aspects of the hands and feet and the scalp veins in infants. Plastic cannulas are more stable than metal ones (butterflies) and come in sizes as small as 27-gauge. A T-connector may be placed on the catheter to provide direct access for administration of medication without requiring large fluid flushes.

---

* A neutral thermal environment is one in which the infant expends the least amount of energy to maintain temperature.

TABLE 22–2
Pediatric Maintenance Fluid Requirements

Weight	Amount of Daily Fluid
0–10 kg	100 ml/kg
11–20 kg	1000 ml + 50 ml for each kg > 10
21–30 kg	1500 ml + 20 ml for each kg > 20

Continuous IV fluid administration devices are important in maintaining IV patency and regulation of fluid amount given. Intravenous sites should be secured carefully and covered with a clear cup to avoid dislodgement by movement or an inquisitive child. Soft restraints may be necessary.

Psychosocial development influences how the child reacts to illness, which in turn affects caregivers' responses. An understanding of developmental stages and sensitivity to nonverbal cues by ED nurses is vital.

Infancy is a time of trust development. Early in infancy, provision of physical needs is essential. Later, attachment to parent figures occurs, and separation causes great protest. Whenever possible, parents should be allowed to stay with their infant. Infants feel pain and initially respond with generalized body movements and crying. Older infants are able to localize pain and direct body movement to that area. They are also attuned to their parents' emotions. Parents may prefer to leave until painful procedures are completed. The performance of painful procedures should be done skillfully and quickly.

Toddlers are developing autonomy and are characterized by their poor understanding of body boundaries and fear of mutilation. Intrusive procedures (ear examination) can be as threatening as painful ones. Their reactions are also physically aggressive but are much more goal directed. Screaming, hitting, pushing, and running away are typical.

Preschoolers have a sense of omnipotence. They are egocentric, seeing events only from their point of view. Magical thinking provides fantasy explanations for events. Because they feel they can control the world, they are vulnerable to suggestions that their "bad" thoughts or deeds have caused illness or injury. They are able to utilize some self control during pain and may feel shame when unable to maintain it. Explanations are taken literally and poor understanding of body function and integrity exists. They may fear that the nurse will "take" all their blood or that it will all leak out unless covered by a bandage.

Schoolagers are industrious and are challenged by their physical and cognitive abilities. Disability and death can be of greater concern than pain. They are increasingly able to understand body anatomy and function and seek information about their illness. Maintenance of privacy and control are important. Passive methods of dealing with pain have been developed. Pain can be localized and described. They appreciate preparation and being allowed choices. Pride in independence can inhibit schoolage children from seeking support, although they will accept it if offered.

Adolescence can be a stage of conflict. Independence, sense of self, and peer relationships are paramount. Teens are especially concerned with functional and visible changes that will alter their place within the group. Privacy during examinations and opportunities for and encouragement of their questions should be provided.

COMMON PROBLEMS EXPERIENCED BY CHILDREN AND THEIR FAMILIES WHO REQUIRE EMERGENCY CARE

The act of bringing a child to the ED is threatening to the family regardless of how minor the illness or injury. Therefore, prior to discussing specific disorders of or traumatic events for children, common problems (nursing diagnoses) experienced by children (and their families) who require emergency services and their related interventions are discussed. These problems and their related interventions should be considered, adapted, and individualized for the conditions subsequently discussed in this chapter.

Family Processes, Altered (Potential), Related to

- *Illness of a Member*

Parents should be allowed to stay with their children (although this may not be possible if a child is critically ill or the ED busy). Time drags for the worried family in the waiting area. A hospital chaplain or social worker can be helpful to the family during this time.

Provision of information can ease fear of the unknown. As soon as possible, a staff member, preferably the primary nurse or physician, should meet with the family to discuss the child's condition and the therapies initiated. Technical explanations should be clear and concise, especially if the family will be asked to make treatment decisions.

Limiting the number of staff members who interact with the family can lessen their confusion and anxiety and can encourage the development of a trusting relationship with the staff and the institution. Parents should be encouraged to stay at the hospital and should frequently be updated concerning the child's progress and whether discharge will be to home, a general pediatric unit, or intensive care.

Admission of the child to an inpatient unit should be handled as smoothly as possible. The family is given the name of the inpatient nurse if it is known. When a delay is anticipated, the family should be informed and allowed to remain with the child. If the child is admitted to the Pediatric Intensive Care Unit (PICU), the family should be informed that they may not be with their child immediately; stabilization measures often need to be done.

Fear (Children and Family Members), Related to

- *Illness, Separation, and/or Hospitalization*

The ED is an area of fear, anxiety, and change for children and their families. With an understanding of the physiologic and psychosocial development of childhood, an astute ED nurse can provide care to these families in crisis.

Children should receive a careful assessment of growth and development with a history of attainment of developmental milestones from the family. These are compared to age norms and serve as a basis for interacting with the child. A determination of the child's understanding of his condition is made. Questions can be clarified and support can be given.

Separation from the family is to be minimized when possible. It should be noted that for the schoolager and adolescent, the opposite may be true. Privacy and freedom to ask and respond to questions concerning sexuality and substance use may be crucial.

The child is prepared according to his or her developmental level for pain, procedures, and examinations. When they exist, choices are given to allow for control. When appropriate, the child is informed of the diagnosis and treatment plan.

ILLNESSES AND INJURIES COMMON TO CHILDREN

Croup

The severity of laryngotracheitis, or viral croup, can be highly variable. It occurs primarily during the winter months, affecting children 3 months to 5 years of age.

Etiology and Pathophysiology

Invasion of the tissues of the subglottic area by parainfluenza viruses causes edema and inflammation of the larynx, trachea, and, possibly, even the bronchial tree (Hen 1986). The resultant airway narrowing produces respiratory distress and hypoxemia.

Clinical Manifestations

Croup develops slowly, over about two weeks. The child presents with a prodromal illness of mild upper respiratory symptoms and low-grade temperature. Classically, there is a "barking" cough. Edema and mucoid plugging of the small airways and larynx produce hoarseness and stridor. Nasal flaring and retractions indicate increasing respiratory distress. Agitation and crying worsen the symptoms. The white blood cell count is normal or slightly elevated, and blood cultures are negative. Arterial blood gas analyses reveal the degree to which edema and atelectasis have caused carbon dioxide retention and hypoxemia. Differentiation of severe croup from epiglottitis is essential, as care is disease-specific (Table 22-3).

TABLE 22–3
Comparison of Epiglottitis and Viral Croup

	Epiglottitis	Croup
Age	2–7 years	3 months–5 years
Sex	M, F equally	M > F (2 : 1)
Duration before hospitalization	2–48 hours	12–78 hours
Progression	Rapid	Slow
Prodromal illness	None	Viral URI
Manifestations		
Appearance	Toxic	Nontoxic
Barking cough	Uncommon	>60%
Cyanosis	20%	10%
Drooling	10%	None
Dysphagia	10%	None
Hoarseness	Uncommon	20%
Position	Sitting up	Lying down
Retractions	Uncommon	Common
Stridor	Uncommon	Common
Temperature	38.6°C	37.8°C
Wheezing	None	5%

Source: Adapted from Hen J. 1986. Pediatr Ann 15:276, by permission of Slack, Inc.

Treatment and Nursing Care

Airway Clearance, Ineffective, Related to

- **Airway Narrowing Secondary to Edema and Inflammation**

Whether stage I or stage II care needs to be initiated is determined by the severity of the child's respiratory distress on presentation to the ED. Resuscitation equipment should be readily available.

Respiratory assessment, ongoing during treatment, includes color, respiratory effort, flaring, retractions, ability to swallow, aeration, and whether wheezing and cough are present. A croup score may be used (Table 22–4).

TABLE 22–4
Clinical Croup Score

	0	1	2
Inspiratory breath sounds	Normal	Harsh, with rhonchi	Delayed
Stridor	None	Inspiratory	Inspiratory and expiratory
Cough	None	Hoarse cry	Barking cough
Retractions/flaring	None	Flaring, suprasternal retractions	As in 1 plus subcostal/ intercostal retractions
Cyanosis or	None	In room air	In 40% O_2
Pao_2 (mmHg)	70–100	>70	<70
CNS Function	Normal	Depressed/agitated	Coma

Source: Adapted from Downes JJ, Raphaely R. 1975. Anesthesiology 43:242–250, by permission.

If needed, cool mist with oxygen is administered to decrease subglottic edema. Failure of this therapy to ease the patient's stridor or presentation of more severe respiratory distress warrants the administration of racemic epinephrine (Vaponefrin) by nebulizer or mask.

Because there can be a rebound effect from racemic epinephrine, the child receiving this treatment is admitted to the hospital. Though rarely needed, intubation is necessary for a child with severe respiratory distress who is unresponsive to treatment. The endotracheal tube should be one size smaller than usual because of edema.

Intravenous access should be established, with the fluid rate dependent upon the degree of dehydration with which the child presents. Steroids may be ordered. Unless needed to treat a concurrent infection, antibiotics are not used.

Evaluation

The child with viral croup requires close monitoring of his or her respiratory status and response to treatment modalities. The vast majority of cases are mild and the child is discharged home. Gradual improvement to recovery usually occurs over a period of three to seven days. More severe cases require hospitalization and respiratory support.

Epiglottitis

A potentially life-threatening form of upper airway obstruction, epiglottitis requires assertive and vigilant nursing care. Although reported in all age groups, it is primarily found in children from ages 2 to 7 years. There is no seasonal variation.

Etiology and Pathophysiology

Swelling occurs from bacterial invasion of the epiglottis and epiglottic folds. This swelling is life-threatening, since it increases dramatically with minimal stimulation and can completely occlude the opening to the trachea. *Haemophilus influenzae* is the most common agent, with rare cases of *Streptococcus pneumoniae, Staphylococcus aureus,* and group A streptococci reported.

Clinical Manifestations

The onset of epiglottitis is rapid and highly characteristic. The patient presents acutely ill with high fever, tachypnea, sore throat, drooling, dysphagia, muffled voice, and inspiratory stridor. An upright, forward leaning position with the neck extended (tripod position) is frequently assumed by the child. The epiglottis is swollen and bright, cherry red. This cluster of signs is highly suggestive of epiglottitis. The diagnosis can be confirmed by lateral neck radiogram showing a large, swollen epiglottis, if clinical manifestations are questionable.

Treatment and Nursing Care

Airway Clearance, Ineffective, Related to

- **Airway Swelling Secondary to Bacterial Infection of Epiglottis and Surrounding Areas**

Stage I care is initiated for all patients with an epiglottitis-like presentation. The major nursing focus in the ED is to assure maintenance of a calm, protective environment for the distressed child. Allowing the child's parents to stay with him or her is usually conducive to promoting this sort of environment. Because any stimulation of the oropharynx can precipitate airway obstruction, all examinations, including vital signs, are to be avoided. Resuscitation equipment including a tracheotomy tray should be immediately available. If needed, the lateral neck radiography is performed and evaluated immediately.

Intubation is required for all patients with epiglottitis regardless of the amount of distress in which they present. Nasotracheal intubation is performed in the controlled environment of the operating room. Securing intravenous access, blood specimen and culture collection, and the initiation of antibiotic therapy is done after the airway is secured. Should the airway be obstructed before transfer to the operating room, bag-valve-mask ventilation is attempted. If this is unsuccessful, an emergency tracheotomy is performed. Following intubation, the child is transferred to the PICU.

Evaluation

All children with confirmed or suspected epiglottitis are admitted to the hospital. Ongoing respiratory assessment until admission to the operating room is crucial. Because the potential for death from airway obstruction exists, only the most experienced nurses and physicians should care for this child.

Shunt Malfunction

Hydrocephalus results from an accumulation of cerebrospinal fluid (CSF) within the ventricular system. Pressure from this accumulation is relieved by placement of a shunting device. Shunts may drain from the ventricles, cysts, or spine to the peritoneum or right atrium.

Etiology and Pathophysiology

Build-up of CSF may result from increased production, obstruction, or inadequate reabsorption. Production of CSF beyond the capacity for reabsorption is rare and when present, usually results from a tumor in the choroid plexus. Obstruction in one of the CSF pathways resulting from congenital narrowing of the aqueduct of Sylvius, Chiari II malformation in spina bifida, or pressure from a space-occupying lesion is more common. Scarring of the subarachnoid space from meningitis, encephalitis, or hemorrhage may interfere with CSF absorption.

Malfunction of a shunt causes a build-up of CSF and increases intracranial pressure. Causes include infection, kinking, clogging, or displacement of the shunt with growth.

Clinical Manifestations

The child with a malfunctioning shunt can present with a wide variety of manifestations reflective of increase intracranial pressure. Infants may show increased head circumference, bulging fontanels, sunsetting eyes, separated sutures, irritability, lethargy, poor feeding, and vomiting. The older child may present with behavioral, sensory, or gait changes; headache; irritability; anorexia; and vomiting. Parental assessment should be heeded as many children show a characteristic pattern. Initial work-up includes differentiation of shunt malfunction from other neurologic and infectious processes. Computed tomography (CT) scan may show ventricular enlargement or shunt displacement.

Treatment and Nursing Care

Neurologic status, Impaired, Related to*

- **Increased Intracranial Pressure Secondary to Increased Production, Obstruction, or Inadequate Reabsorption of CSF in the Ventricular System**
- **Shunt Malfunction**

Unless the child presents with severely increased intracranial pressure, apnea, or bradycardia, stage II care will dominate the ED stay.

Frequent neurologic assessments should be performed and will include level of consciousness, pupillary reaction and sunsetting, response to stimuli, movement of extremities, quality of cry, condition of fontanels, seizure activity, and sensory disturbances. Baseline head circumference is measured in children under two years of age. Vital sign changes (apnea, bradycardia, increasing blood pressure) are late signs of worsening neurologic status. A pediatric coma scale can be useful in objectively assessing neurologic changes (Table 22–5). An elevated temperature may indicate shunt infection.

The head of the bed should be elevated 30 degrees, and the head should be kept midline. Intravenous access is obtained and fluids are administered if dehydration has resulted from vomiting. The patient should be placed on nothing by mouth (NPO) orders. Blood should be obtained for CBC, electrolytes, and cultures. A blood specimen for typing and cross-matching should also be obtained in the event the patient needs to go to the operating room (OR).

The shunt reservoir is pumped and may be tapped with a butterfly valve. Pressure may then be read on a manometer to determine the degree of the obstruction. CT scan may reveal dilated ventricles and is especially useful when compared with previous scans. Plain radiograms and shunt studies may show damage, migration, or cyst formation to the shunt system. Surgery is indicated to relieve the pressure and to repair or replace the shunt.

---

* Non–NANDA-approved nursing diagnosis.

TABLE 22-5
Pediatric Coma Scale*

	Score	Age Over 1 Year	Less Than 1 Year
Eye opening	4	Spontaneously	Spontaneously
	3	To verbal command	To shout
	2	To pain	To pain
	1	No response	No response
Best motor response	6	Obeys	
	5	Localizes pain	Localizes pain
	4	Flexion withdrawal	Flexion withdrawal
	3	Flexion—abnormal (decorticate rigidity)	Flexion—abnormal (decorticate rigidity)
	2	Extension (decerebrate rigidity)	Extension (decerebrate rigidity)
	1	No response	No response
		Age Over 5 Years	Age 2-5 Years	Age 0-23 Months
Best verbal response	5	Oriented and converses	Appropriate words and phrases	Smiles, coos
	4	Disoriented and converses	Inappropriate words and phrases	Cries appropriately
	3	Inappropriate words	Cries and/or screams	Cries, screams
	2	Incomprehensible sounds	Grunts	Grunts
	1	No response	No response	No response
Total	3-15		

Source: Reproduced by permission from Whaley L, Wong D. Essentials of Pediatric Nursing, St. Louis, 1985, The C.V. Mosby Co.
* Modification of Glasgow coma scale.

Evaluation

Careful monitoring and identification of worsening neurologic status are necessary. Deterioration is reported to the physician. A child with a shunt malfunction may be admitted for observation before surgery. Patients with greatly increased pressure or infection may be transferred directly from the ED to the operating room.

Bacterial Meningitis

An inflammatory condition of the meninges covering the brain and spinal cord, bacterial (purulent) meningitis is a potentially fatal disease that can leave the surviving child with lifelong sequelae, including seizures, brain damage, and sensory impairment.

Etiology and Pathophysiology

Bacteria most often gain access to the meninges through hematogenous spread from a distant site. Direct contamination may occur during surgery or trauma to the head. Organisms involved are generally characteristic for a particular age group. *Escherichia coli* and group B streptococci are common in neonates, *H. influenzae* is found in infants and young children, *Neisseria meningitidis* in older children. *S. aureus* is commonly isolated in cases of direct contamination.

These organisms and their toxic products cause inflammation within CSF pathways and adjoining structures. Areas of fibrosis, infarction, and effusion can occur, causing signs of meningeal irritation and long-term sequelae.

Clinical Manifestations

Infants and young children present nonspecifically with fever, poor feeding, irritability, and lethargy. The open anterior fontanel in infants may be bulging and firm. Older children show fever, severe headache, nuchal rigidity, and positive Kernig's and Brudzinski's signs. Seizures may be present in all age groups.

Cerebrospinal fluid analysis typically shows cloudy fluid with an increased protein and cell count, a decreased glucose level, and the specific organism on culture. Blood cultures may or may not reveal bacteremia. Complete blood count (CBC) may show a white cell count of more than $10,000/\mu l$.

Treatment and Nursing Care

Neurologic Status, Impaired, Related to*

- **Inflammation of the Meninges, Brain, and Spinal Cord Secondary to Bacterial Meningitis**

Stage I care is indicated, since rapid institution of interventions is crucial in diminishing the potential for death and disability.

Initial interventions will include a complete neurologic assessment, including level of consciousness, pupillary reaction, response to stimuli, movement of extremities, quality of cry, head circumference, and condition of the fontanels. Neurologic checks should be recorded every 15 minutes. The skin, especially on the chest, is carefully examined for petechiae, which are often associated with meningococcemia, a particularly devastating form of meningitis. Once bacterial meningitis is suspected, implementation of respiratory isolation should ensue.

Blood specimens are collected for CBC, glucose, and electrolytes. Blood, urine, and other cultures are obtained. A chest radiogram is obtained. A lumbar puncture is performed unless intracranial pressure is greatly increased and the risk of herniation is present.

Intravenous access is obtained. A dilemma in treating bacterial meningitis is that shock and cerebral edema can occur concurrently. Intravenous fluids are administered in quantities sufficient to stabilize cardiovascular status and then restricted to reduce cerebral edema and the risk of syndrome of inappropriate antidiuretic hormone (SIADH) secretion.

Once cultures are obtained, antibiotics are started. Initial drug therapy in neonates is ampicillin and an aminoglycoside. Ampicillin and chloramphenicol are given for suspected *H. influenzae* infections. Third-generation cephalosporins may be used, although their superiority to traditional therapy has not been demonstrated (Stuttman and Marks 1987).

---

* Non-NANDA-approved nursing diagnosis.

The critical nature of bacterial meningitis requires that resuscitative equipment be readily available. These patients frequently require intubation and ventilatory management.

Evaluation

Ongoing assessments of neurologic and cardiovascular status are necessary to evaluate the efficacy of therapy. Subtle changes in level of consciousness can indicate improvement or deterioration. Vigilant attention to vital signs, fluid-volume status, and laboratory data is crucial in stabilizing a child with bacterial meningitis.

Fever

Elevated body temperature is one of the most common reasons for children presenting to the ED. Although not a disease, it is a significant manifestation of underlying pathology.

Etiology and Pathophysiology

Fever most often results from viral or bacterial invasion. The release of pyrogens from macrophagic activity is thought to alter temperature control in the hypothalamus, causing temperature elevation. A slight increase in body temperature may also be caused by any activity (exercise, crying) that raises the metabolic rate.

Clinical Manifestations

Initial assessment includes determination of current temperature and its deviation from the norm. Fever is considered significant when temperature exceeds age-based

TABLE 22-6
Significant Temperatures by Age*

Age	Temperature
Birth to 8 weeks	100.6°F
8 weeks to 6 months	101°F
6 to 24 months	103°F
over 24 months	102°F

Source: Data from Crain E, Gershel J. 1986. A Clinical Manual of Emergency Pediatrics, 283–284. Appleton-Century-Crofts.
    * Significant temperatures related to age are only guidelines to be utilized in determining the extent of diagnostic work-up and therapeutic interventions that should be implemented for febrile children. The clinical condition of each patient must always be taken into consideration in making such determinations.

levels (Table 22-6). Damage to the central nervous system can occur when body temperature exceeds 106°F.

The child may present with changes in mood and behavior, tachypnea, tachycardia, lethargy, pallor, and dehydration. Obvious signs of a particular infection (such as meningeal irritation) may be present. It should be considered that the immature temperature regulation system of prematures and neonates can cause hypothermia with sepsis. A detailed history of the fever and related signs and symptoms should be elicited from the parents.

Treatment and Nursing Care

Hyperthermia, Related to

- **Increased metabolic rate**
- **Pathology**

Keeping in mind that fever is a sign, not a disease entity, nursing care will focus on the determination of cause and alleviation of related discomfort.

Every attempt is made to determine the focus of the infectious process. A complete septic work-up may be necessary and is most commonly indicated in infants under 8 weeks old with significant fevers. A septic work-up includes blood specimens for CBC, electrolytes, and culture; urine for analysis and culture; lumbar puncture for pressure, culture, and analysis; chest radiography; and culture of any suspected focal site. After obtaining laboratory specimens, a broad-spectrum antibiotic may be administered and continued pending test results.

Antipyretics may be administered. Salicylates (aspirin) are rarely used, as they have been associated with the development of Reye's syndrome. Acetaminophen can be given orally or rectally in a dose of 10 to 15 mg/kg.

Excess clothing should be removed. A cooling blanket or lukewarm sponge bath can be used. Attempts to lower temperature too rapidly can cause shivering and raise temperature.

Fluid Volume Deficit, Related to

- **Hyperthermia**

Hyperthermia causes an increase in the metabolic rate and results in fluid and electrolyte loss through diaphoresis, increased respiration, and evaporation. Losses may also occur through vomiting and diarrhea.

Three types of dehydration can occur, differentiated by the relationship of fluid and electrolyte (sodium) levels. Table 22-7 reviews signs of dehydration and their severity based on percent.

Isotonic dehydration results when fluid and electrolyte losses are proportional to normal serum concentrations. Serum sodium is normal. A common cause is vomiting, diarrhea, or both.

A rare occurrence, hypotonic dehydration is characterized by electrolyte loss

TABLE 22-7
Estimation of Dehydration

	5%	5%-7%	10%	15%
Heart rate	Nl*	Moderate↑	Marked↑	Marked↑
Respiratory rate	Nl	Nl	Hyperpnea	Hyperpnea
Blood pressure	Nl	Orthostatic drop	Narrowed pulse	Hypotensive
Skin turgor	Nl	Nl to slight↓	Decreased	Decreased
Eyeballs	Nl	Nl	Sunken	Sunken
Mucous membranes	Nl to dry	Dry	Dry	Dry
Fontanel	Nl	Slightly depressed	Sunken	Sunken
Mental status	Nl	Nl to irritable	Lethargic	Comatose
Urine output	Nl to slight↓	↓to none	None	None
Urine specific gravity	>1.020	>1.030		

Source: Adapted from Crain E, Gershel J: *A Clinical Manual of Emergency Pediatrics,* 189. Copyright Appleton-Century-Crofts, 1986.
   * Nl = normal limits.

exceeding water loss and subnormal serum sodium (<130 mEq/L). It results from use of a nonelectrolyte solution (such as water) to treat diarrhea.

Hypertonic dehydration results when water loss exceeds electrolyte loss, as in severe, watery diarrhea. Serum sodium is elevated (>150 mEq/L) in such instances.

Treatment of dehydration depends on the type, degree, and cause of fluid and electrolyte loss. In general, therapy includes rehydration (oral or parenteral) with an appropriate solution.

The child with mild dehydration, fever, or both may be discharged home with instructions concerning temperature-relieving modalities and rehydration. More severe cases require hospitalization for detection and treatment of the underlying cause.

Evaluation

Assessment for determination of temperature resolution and hydration status is ongoing. Clinical assessment for such determinations includes the monitoring of vital signs and urine output and specific gravity. Fontanels, mucous membranes, and skin turgor should be assessed.

Near-Drowning

Near-drowning means survival, however temporary, after asphyxia caused by submersion in liquid. Drowning is the second most common cause of accidental death in children under 14 years. Fresh water accounts for the overwhelming majority of drowning accidents, most of which take place in swimming pools or natural bodies of water. However, any receptacle containing fluid is a potential hazard.

Etiology and Pathophysiology

Factors contributing to the pathology of near-drowning include water temperature, salinity, aspiration of water and gastric contents, and level of consciousness before submersion. Although the physiologic explanation is not understood, some cases of submersion in freezing water have demonstrated protection of the brain from anoxic damage. Salt water is hypertonic, and its aspiration causes intraalveolar fluid accumulation via osmosis from isotonic pulmonary capillary fluid. Pulmonary edema with subsequent hypoxemia and vascular hemoconcentration ensues. Aspiration of fresh water causes an increase in intravascular volume and vascular hemodilution as hypotonic fluid shifts from the alveoli to the pulmonary capillaries. An altered level of consciousness secondary to intoxication, head trauma, and so forth contributes to a poor prognosis.

Clinical Manifestations

Cardiopulmonary resuscitation should be initiated by primary responders and should be continued as needed through transfer and admission to the ED. The child may present in any condition from alert and oriented to comatose and pulseless. Arterial blood gases reveal the degree of respiratory and circulatory compromise. Serum CBC and electrolytes rarely show an initial derangement unless underlying pathology is present.

A complete history of the accident and previous health status should be obtained. Although uncommon in young children, spinal cord injury should always be considered as a cause of or concurrent with near-drowning incidents. Toxicology screens are requested if alcohol or drug use is suspected.

Treatment and Nursing Care

Tissue Perfusion, Altered (cerebral), Related to

• **Severe Anoxia**

Stage I care dominates the severely affected near-drowning victim's ED stay. Resuscitation measures that likely began at the scene are continued as needed. A victim who is spontaneously breathing may only need supplemental oxygen, whereas one who is not requires intubation and mechanical ventilation. Peripheral and central venous access should be obtained. Specimens are taken for CBC, electrolytes, and arterial blood gas analysis.

Thorough and ongoing assessment of neurologic and respiratory function, including serial ABGs, is imperative. A coma scale score can be useful in detecting deterioration. Adequate oxygenation and perfusion are essential in the prevention of further damage.

A nasogastric tube should be inserted to decompress the stomach and avoid aspiration of gastric contents. Antibiotics are not routinely administered, although the type of submersion should be considered for bacterial contaminants (bathtub or pond).

Stage II care is implemented for children who arrive without deficits and for those who respond to therapy. Neurologic and respiratory assessment remains important as cerebral and pulmonary edema can develop over a period of hours.

Ice water submersion presents additional challenges. Heart and respiratory rate may be extremely slowed. Their presence or absence must be carefully assessed over at least one full minute as the patient is placed on an EKG monitor. Until the patient has been rewarmed, resuscitative measures are continued despite lack of response. Warming with blankets, warmed IV and lavage fluid, and warmed humidified oxygen are used. In the most severe cases, warming with peritoneal dialysis and cardiopulmonary bypass have been used.

Evaluation

All patients submerged for more than one minute or for an unknown period of time and those who were apneic or cyanotic should be admitted for observation. The severely compromised child should receive aggressive pulmonary care and cerebral monitoring in the PICU. Various prognostic indicators have been employed to predict outcome (Orlowski 1987). However, institution of aggressive initial intervention and ongoing assessment by the ED nurse is essential in saving those patients who will benefit from further aggressive care.

Sudden Infant Death Syndrome

Sudden infant death syndrome (SIDS), the most common cause of death in infants between one month and one year of age, peaks at two to three months. Typically, the infant was considered healthy and is found dead sometime after being put down to sleep. Males are affected more often than females, blacks more often than whites.

Etiology and Pathophysiology

The etiology of SIDS is unclear but may be multifactorial and may involve an abnormality in cardiorespiratory control (Hunt and Brouillette 1987). A variety of risk factors exist, including low birth weight, prematurity, previous apneic episodes, a young mother, and low socioeconomic status.

A second group of infants experience "near-miss" episodes. These infants are found limp, cyanotic or pale, and apneic. They can be revived with mouth-to-mouth resuscitation. Whether these are truly interrupted cases of SIDS or another entity is unclear.

Clinical Manifestations

The victim of SIDS or a near-SIDS event presents to the ED either receiving or having received resuscitative measures. These measures continue until the outcome is clear. The near-SIDS infant usually arrives with a pulse and some respiratory effort.

In either case, a careful history is obtained of the circumstances surrounding the event; prenatal, perinatal, and postnatal complications; and growth and development. A sample form is shown in Table 22–8.

Treatment and Nursing Care

Breathing Pattern, Ineffective, Related to

- **Unknown Cause**

    Stage I care is implemented for an infant requiring continued resuscitative measures, including cardiopulmonary resuscitation (CPR), intubation, line placement, and administration of medication. A near-SIDS patient will receive stage II care, consisting of ongoing assessment of respiratory, cardiovascular, and neurologic function.

    Intravenous access should be obtained. Blood specimens for CBC, electrolytes, glucose, and calcium assays and for culture are obtained. Lumbar puncture, electrocardiography (EKG), and chest radiography are performed to rule out metabolic and infectious causes of the episode.

    The infant is transferred to the inpatient unit for further diagnostic studies, including electroencephalography (EEG), apnea monitoring, pneumogram, and reflux studies.

Grieving, Related to

- **Death of an Infant**

    When resuscitative measures are unsuccessful, care will focus on the family. Parents should be informed as soon as possible in an area of privacy. The chaplain is called, and the nurse remains with the family. The nurse should be prepared for a wide variety of emotions from the family including shock, anger, denial, and guilt. It should be stressed that everything possible was done and that the parents are not at fault. In this time of crisis, families may have a difficult time comprehending what is said and can misinterpret comments. Comforting words can be impossible to find, but presence and touch can communicate concern effectively.

    The nurse can make calls to members of the family's support system. All resuscitative equipment should be removed from the infant (unless the state medical examiner requires that it not be). The infant is dressed in a clean gown and wrapped in a blanket. After a brief explanation of what to expect, the family is allowed to see the infant. They are encouraged to hold the infant and unwrap the gown if desired. Private time for the family is encouraged.

TABLE 22–8
Assessment of SIDS and Near SIDS

Patient Information

Name _____ Age ____ Sex: M ____ F ____
Birthdate: _____
Last seen alive: Date _____ Time _____
Found dead: Date _____ Time _____
            By whom: _____
            Place: crib, parents' bed, other _____
            Position _____
Appearance of infant: Body temperature _____
            Color of skin _____
            Nasopharyngeal discharge: Yes ____ No ____

Resuscitative Efforts

CPR: Yes ____ No ____
Intracardiac medication: Yes ____ No ____
Other medication (please specify) _____

Birth and Medical History

Birth weight ____ Gestational age ____ Birthplace _____
Source of medical care _____
Well-baby visits: Yes _____ No _____ Unknown _____
            Most recent visit _____
            Most recent weight _____
            Immunizations: Yes ____ No ____ Date _____
Type of feeding: Breast _____ Bottle _____ Both _____
Illness in last 2 weeks: Yes _____ No _____
            Cold, sniffles, stuffy nose _____
            GI symptoms _____
            Other minor/major _____
            Describe _____

Medical examiner

_____

Autopsy: Yes _____ No _____ By whom _____

Parental data

Mother _____ Age ____ Father _____ Age ____
Address _____
Telephone _____ Emergency phone _____
Pregnancy complications _____
Type of delivery _____ Anesthesia _____
Complications during labor, delivery, or neonatal period _____
_____
_____

Previous infant deaths: Yes ____ No ____ Cause _____
Numbers of siblings _____
            Report filed by _____
            Date _____

Source: From SIDS: A Guide for Emergency Department Personnel, Boston, 1984. Massachusetts Center for Sudden Infant Death Syndrome. Reprinted by permission.
CPR = Cardiopulmonary resuscitation; GI = gastrointestinal.

The necessity of autopsy to confirm the diagnosis of SIDS is explained and consent is obtained. The physical effects of autopsy and the fact that an open casket can be used are explained. Information concerning funeral arrangements is offered. A list of resources for parent support should be made available. Some health care providers may offer a sedative medication to the family. However, this is not helpful, as it only serves to delay the grief process and can cloud a family member's understanding of the event.

Evaluation

The death of an infant is stressful for the staff as well as the family. Nurses may be uncomfortable dealing with intense grief. It should be realized that families will remember thoughtless comments and that frequently the best action is to offer "I'm sorry." Follow-up contact with the family can provide an opportunity for parents to clarify events surrounding the death of their child.

Cardiopulmonary Arrest

Cardiopulmonary arrest occurs when there is a sudden cessation of functional ventilation and circulation. In infants and children, this can occur when pulse and respiratory effort are present but tissue oxygenation and perfusion is inadequate.

Etiology and Pathophysiology

Common precipitating factors for nonhospitalized children include trauma or injury, suffocation, smoke inhalation, SIDS, and infection. Children may also present in the ED with unstable cardiovascular status (congenital heart defects), with progressive pulmonary disease (asthma, croup, pneumonia), and with a permanent artificial airway.

It is important to recognize that 90% to 95% of children who suffer arrest have a primary respiratory, not a cardiac, event. This causes hypoxia, leading to bradycardia and asystole. Early intervention for a respiratory problem may prevent deterioration to a cardiac arrest.

Treatment and Nursing Care

Basic life support (BLS) for infants and children differs significantly from that for adults in several ways. Guidelines for pediatric BLS are reviewed in Table 22–9.

Following establishment of BLS, pediatric advanced life support (PALS) should be instituted. An oral airway can be inserted to depress the tongue to avoid obstruction of the pharynx. Unlike insertion of oral airways in adults, insertion of oral airways in children is best accomplished via direct insertion with the aid of a tongue depressor as opposed to the rotating technique. Insertion in a conscious patient can cause gagging, vomiting, and aspiration.

TABLE 22–9
Pediatric Basic Life Support

	Infant	Child	Adolescent
Respiratory rate	20	15	12
Pulse check	Brachial	Carotid	Carotid
Hand placement	2–3 fingers 1 finger below line between the nipples	Heel of hand 1 finger above rib/breast bone notch	Two hands Same as child
Depth (inches)	1/2–1	1–1 1/2	1 1/2–2
Compression/ ventilation ratio	5:1	5:1	15:2
Compression rate	100	80–100	80–100
Airway obstruction	Back blow chest thrust	Abdominal thrust	Abdominal thrust

Source: Data from Standards and Guidelines for Cardiopulmonary Resuscitation (CPR) and Emergency Cardiac Care (ECC) by the American Medical Association, 1986. JAMA, 255:2905–2984.

In an arrest situation, an Fio_2 of 100% should be delivered, preferably with a self-inflating bag. The mask should be small enough to maintain a tight seal. When the need for artificial ventilation will be prolonged, endotracheal intubation will be performed. In children less than 8 years of age, the cricoid cartilage will form a seal around the tube to prevent air leak. In older children, a cuffed tube will be needed.

TABLE 22–10
Medications Used During Pediatric Advanced Life Support

Drug	Dose	How Supplied	Remarks
Atropine sulfate	0.02 mg/kg/dose	0.1 mg/ml	Minimum dose of 0.1 mg (1.0 ml)
Calcium chloride	20 mg/kg/dose	100 mg/ml (10%)	Give slowly
Dobutamine hydrochloride	5–20 μg/kg/min	250 mg/vial lyophilized	Titrate to desired effect
Dopamine hydrochloride	2–20 μg/kg/min	40 mg/ml	α-Adrenergic action dominates at 15–20 μg/kg/min
Epinephrine hydrochloride	0.1 ml/kg (0.01 mg/kg)	1:10,000 (0.1 mg/ml)	1:1,000 must be diluted
Epinephrine infusion	Start at 0.1 μg/kg/min	1:1,000 (1 mg/ml)	Titrate to desired effect (0.1–1.0 μg/kg/min)
Isoproterenol hydrochloride	Start at 0.1 μg/kg/min	1 mg/5 ml	Titrate to desired effect (0.1–1.0 μg/kg/min)
Lidocaine	1 mg/kg/dose	10 mg/ml (1%), 20 mg/ml (2%)	. . .
Lidocaine infusion	20–50 μg/kg/min	40 mg/ml (4%)	. . .
Norepinephrine infusion	Start at 0.1 μg/kg/min	1 mg/ml	Titrate to desired effect (0.1–1.0 μg/kg/min)
Sodium bicarbonate	1 mEq/kg/dose or 0.3 × kg × base deficit	1 mEq/ml (8.4%)	Infuse slowly and only if ventilation is adequate

Source: Data from Standards and Guidelines for Cardiopulmonary Resuscitation (CPR) and Emergency Cardiac Care (ECC) by the American Medical Association, 1986. JAMA 255:2905–2984.

TABLE 22-11
Average Weight in Kilograms by Age

Age	Females	Males
Newborn	3.2	3.1
3 months	5.4	6.0
6 months	7.2	7.8
9 months	8.6	9.2
1 year	9.5	10.2
18 months	10.8	11.4
2 years	11.9	13.6
4 years	16.0	17.0
6 years	19.5	20.5
8 years	25.0	25.0
10 years	33.0	31.5
12 years	41.5	40.0
14 years	50.0	51.0
16 years	56.0	62.0
18 years	57.0	69.0

Source: Data from Whaley L, Wong D. 1985. *Essentials of Pediatric Nursing.* St. Louis: C.V. Mosby, 1022-1027.

The tube size can be selected by the following formula:

$$\frac{\text{Age in years}}{4} + 4 = \text{approximate size in mm}$$

The child's little finger or nostril size can also be used as a guide.

At least one secure IV line is needed for administration of fluids and medications. A central line is best; however, if unable to insert one, the largest line closest to the heart is preferred (e.g., an 18-gauge angiocatheter in the antecubital space is preferred over a 23-gauge butterfly in the foot). Whether or not the line is supra or infra diaphragmatic is only important in older children, as young children are more equally proportioned. If venous access is unobtainable, the intraosseous route using an intraosseous bone marrow or cardiac needle in the anterior tibia should be considered. Atropine, epinephrine, and lidocaine may be mixed with 1 to 2 ml of normal saline and given through the endotracheal tube. Medications most often used in arrest situations are listed in Table 22-10. For administration of medication, a child is considered to weigh 40 kg or less. Adult dosages are used for those weighing more than 40 kg. Average weights by age for children are found in Table 22-11. Prepared sheets, kept on the crash cart, indicating dosages for various weights can be useful. Infants and children should receive IV fluid containing both dextrose and saline. Adolescents and adults may receive normal saline.

Rhythm disturbances in children are rare. Those occurring are 90% bradydysrhythmias or asystole and 10% ventricular dysrhythmias. Because primary cardiac disturbances are uncommon, when they do occur, metabolic derangements involving glucose, potassium, calcium, and temperature should be investigated. For documented ventricular fibrillation, defibrillation with 2 watt sec/kg is used. This can be doubled and repeated twice. Cardioversion with 0.2 to 1.0 watt sec/kg is used for symptomatic supraventricular or ventricular tachycardia.

In an arrest situation, tension can run high. The nurse has a vital role not only in coordinating the actions of other team members but in maintaining a calm, professional atmosphere.

CONCLUSION

Caring for children and their families in emergency situations presents a variety of challenges to the ED nurse. Remaining aware of the uniqueness of each child not only in physiology but also in growth and development allows for the individualization of competent, compassionate care.

REFERENCES

American Medical Association. Standards and guidelines for cardiopulmonary resuscitation and emergency cardiac care. JAMA 255:2905–2989.

Hazinski M. 1984. Nursing Care of the Critically Ill Child. St. Louis, CV Mosby.

Hen J. 1986. Current management of upper airway obstruction. Pediatric Annals 15:274–294.

Hunt C, Brouillette R. 1987. Sudden infant death syndrome: a 1987 perspective. J Pediatr 110:669–678.

McClain M. 1985. Sudden infant death syndrome: An update. J Emerg Nurs 11:227–233.

Orlowski J. 1987. Drowning, near-drowning and ice-water submersion. Pediatr Clin North Am 34:75–92.

Park M, Menard S. 1987. Accuracy of blood pressure measurement by the Dinamap monitor in infants and children. Pediatr 79:907–914.

Stuttman H, Marks M. 1987. Bacterial meningitis in children: diagnosis and therapy. Clin Pediatr 26:431–438.

Whaley L, Wong D. 1985. Essentials of Pediatric Nursing. St. Louis, CV Mosby.

William Donnellan, MD

Pediatric Trauma

Injuries to children have reached epidemic proportions in the United States. Each year from 12,000 to 13,000 children die from trauma, a figure that is perhaps nearer 25,000 when all types of injury are considered. Fifty-five percent of all childhood deaths result from injuries, exceeding cancer, congenital anomalies, and infections by a large margin. A further 50,000 children will remain permanently disabled following recovery from their initial injuries (Fig. 23–1).

The costs associated with pediatric trauma are staggering, yet only recently has the problem been fully addressed either medically or socially. Although most major childhood injuries are caused by motor vehicles, few states have passed seat-belt laws, and there is no national campaign to instruct parents concerning accident prevention in general. Nursing organizations can play a large role in bringing these matters to the attention of the public.

SCOPE OF THE PROBLEM

Table 23–1 lists the injuries seen at a major pediatric trauma center during the period 1979–1981. The Cook County Children's Hospital and Trauma Center is located in Chicago and serves a population of seven million. During this time, 719 patients were treated, of whom 344, or 47.8 per cent, suffered head injury alone or in combination with other injuries (Reyes 1985). Nearly 50% of all injuries are caused, in one way or another, by motor vehicles. The majority of injuries occur in the summer months when the children are more likely to be out of doors.

545

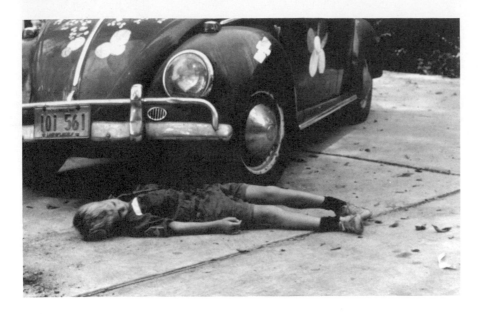

FIGURE 23–1. The clinical problem: child struck by a car.

TRAUMA MANAGEMENT IN THE EMERGENCY DEPARTMENT

When major injuries occur, the adequacy of the first few minutes of care may make the difference between prompt recovery, an extended and costly hospital stay, and an increased need for long-term rehabilitation (Haller 1983). Therefore, hospital emergency rooms and their associated transport systems have great responsibility for the development of efficient methods of handling injured children and for early resuscitative care after the injury.

TABLE 23–1
Pediatric Trauma Injuries

Head trauma	344	47.84%
(70 with multiple injuries)		
Extremity injury	330	45.9 %
Gunshot wounds	16	2.23%
Straddle injuries	11	1.53%
Stab wounds	8	1.11%
Miscellaneous injuries	8	1.11%
(3 drownings)		
Blunt chest injuries	2	0.28%
	719	100%

Source: Reyes HM. 1985. Management of trauma in the pediatric patient. In: Vidyasagar D, Sarnaik AP, eds. *Neonatal and Pediatric Intensive Care.* Littleton, MA, PSG Publishing Co. Inc, 204.

Evaluation of the pediatric patient must be completed quickly, efficiently, and with as little added pain and psychologic derangement as possible under the trying conditions in an emergency department (ED). The best care of injured patients is provided by the team approach. The nurses and paramedics who first see these children need the immediate assistance of respiratory therapists, experienced physicians, radiology and laboratory departments, and eventually, efficient operating room personnel. Most of the injuries of childhood, of course, are relatively minor. Ordinary lacerations, fractures, or sprains can be handled expeditiously in the ED, and the patients can be sent home. On the other hand, serious crushing damage or head injuries resulting from automobile accidents, falls from open windows, sports accidents, and child abuse need rapid appraisal and management if the best possible result is to be achieved.

This chapter deals with major pediatric trauma. It addresses the response of a child to trauma, which is different from that of an adult, and seeks to indicate what special equipment and medications should be provided in all EDs for the initial care of injured children of varying ages and sizes. The focus will be on the most severely injured, that is, those patients with multiple trauma in whom clearly defined procedures must be undertaken in their proper sequences in order to ensure the best possible outcome. An overview of the initial assessment of injured children precedes discussion of specific entities related to trauma.

INITIAL ASSESSMENT OF THE INJURED CHILD

There is general agreement that the earlier the child can be definitively treated, the better will be the outcome. In children the first *half hour* is thought to be crucial. The first priority of emergency department personnel is to stabilize the patient's general condition. Generally, the admitting nurse first assesses the child and sets the stage for orderly and progressive care.

Obtaining a rapid history from parents, witnesses, or paramedics is crucial. What were the events leading to the accident? Determine the mechanism and time of injury. Was there a period of consciousness or unconsciousness? If there are open wounds, what is the contaminant? Did the child move his or her extremities when first seen? Determine previous history of chronic illness, past injury, medication, and allergies. Ascertain the time the last meal was eaten. Using the mnemonic "Take an AMPLE history" will guide your assessment. Letters in the acronym stand for allergies, medications, past medical history, last meal, and events leading to the accident (Mayer 1985).

Objective assessment of the patient by the admitting nurse can be completed in less than one minute. The primary survey comprises the ABCs of trauma care:

A = airway maintenance with Cervical (C)-spine control
B = breathing
C = circulation with hemorrhage control
D = disability/level of consciousness
E = exposure

All life-threatening injuries must be corrected during the primary survey. Stage I care is in order. Whenever there is a suggestion of facial or head injury, a fracture of the cervical spine must be assumed to be present. Movement or the lack of movement of the arms and legs should be recorded by the admitting nurse. Excessive manipulation of the neck in evaluating and treating airway obstruction in such patients is absolutely contraindicated. If not already immobilized, moderate traction on the head while moving or examining the child will prevent subluxation and further spinal cord damage.

Airway and Breathing

Observe the adequacy of ventilation. Is the child apneic, not making any effort to breathe, or dyspneic, with labored breathing? Does the chest rise and fall in a symmetric manner? This first impression can be gained in 4 or 5 seconds. More subtle signs of inadequate ventilation are noisy breathing, nasal flaring, pallor or cyanosis, or poor expiratory volume, with little air expelled through the nose and mouth. The presence of injuries to the face, mouth, or neck suggests the possibility of asphyxiation due to aspirated blood clots or crushing and swelling of the pharynx or larynx.

Orotracheal intubation is used more frequently by paramedics as the beneficial effects of controlled respiration are increasingly being recognized. However, most trauma services rely on mask ventilation with high oxygen concentrations. It is important to recognize that gastric dilation is universal in crying and struggling children and that this can be markedly aggravated by positive-pressure mask ventilation. The admitting nurse should note a distended abdomen. Gastric dilation can further compromise respirations and lead to emesis and aspiration.

If ventilation must be supported, endotracheal intubation is instituted. Select size for a comfortable fit in the child's nostril or by measuring the tube to match the diameter of the child's little finger. The use of muscle relaxants will greatly facilitate endotracheal intubation. Succinylcholine, a depolarizing agent, is recommended for infants and children up to the age of five, while pancuronium bromide (Pavulon) may be better for older children and young adults. The effects of succinylcholine will pass spontaneously within 3 to 5 minutes, but those of Pavulon must be reversed. Atropine should be used prior to the administration of both drugs. The dosages are as follows:

Drug	Dosage
Atropine	0.1 to 0.3 mg
Succinylcholine	1 to 2 mg/kg
Pancuronium bromide (Pavulon)	0.1 to 0.6 mg/kg
Neostigmine	0.07 mg/kg (for reversal of pancuronium bromide)

In most significant injuries of childhood, there is usually considerable gastric dilation as the result of crying and the apprehensive gulping of air (Fig. 23–2).

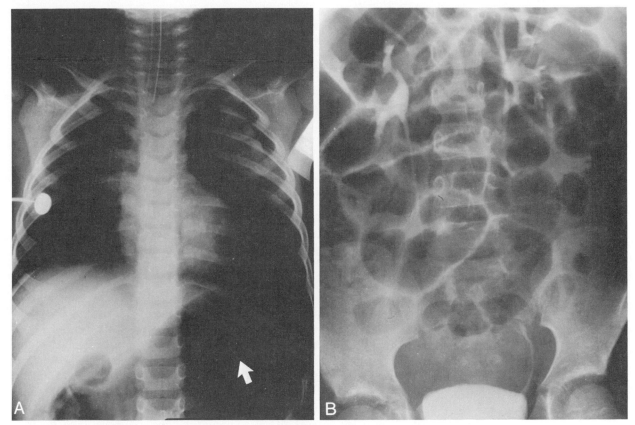

FIGURE 23–2. Gastric dilation (arrow) is always expected.

This diminishes ventilation because it seriously impairs diaphragmatic excursion in children (Mayer 1985, 5). Gastric evacuation allows easier breathing preventing emesis and possible aspiration of vomitus. A double-lumen nasogastric tube is more effective, especially if the child has eaten just prior to the accident. The usual nasogastric (Levin) tube soon becomes clogged with food particles.

Circulation

The state of circulation is determined through palpation of the pulses in the extremities, observation of the neck veins and testing of capillary refill. If the neck veins fill to any degree when the child is lying flat, the blood volume is probably adequate. When the dorsalis pedis pulse of the foot can be felt, there is adequate function of the heart as a pump. A rapid capillary refill after pressure blanching (<2 seconds) will confirm this finding. It should be noted, however, that both capillary refill and the pulses of the extremities may be abnormal if the child is cold.

Quickly expose the patient and observe for obvious injuries. Continued external bleeding is usually evident to even the casual observer, but it may be concealed by

TABLE 23-2
Normal Vital Sign Ranges for Children

Age	Pulse	Respiration	Blood Pressure
0–2 months	120–140	30–50	50–60 systolic
2 months–1 year	110–130	25–40	70–80 "
1–3 years	100–110	20–30	80 "
3–5 years	90–100	20–30	80–90 "
Above 5 years	80–100	15–30	90–100 "

clothing or any bulky dressings that have been applied. The control of bleeding is best achieved by direct pressure on the wound area. Tourniquets are dangerous and should rarely be used. The military antishock trouser (MAST) suit in children is used in massive injuries because increased pressure and tamponade about the pelvis controls bleeding.

Splinting of fractures, if not already done by paramedics, reduces internal bleeding. The goal is immobilization of bone fragments so that the bone ends and the periosteal vessel can seal by clot. A secondary advantage of splinting is that it decreases further injury to surrounding tissues and the larger vessels by sharp bony fragments. It is generally appreciated that 50% or more of the total blood volume may be lost into the tissues following displaced fractures of the pelvis or fracture-dislocations of the upper femur and hip joint (Reichard et al 1980). When blood loss caused by head trauma, hemopneumothorax, or intraabdominal contusion is added to these figures, it is clear that exsanguination is a real possibility whenever a child sustains multiple injuries. Indeed, the most common cause of preventable death in the Maryland Trauma Service experience has been unrecognized blood loss leading to irreversible shock. Support of the circulation therefore is one of the most important measures in resuscitating the trauma patient (McKoy and Bell 1983).

Vital signs including temperature should be monitored closely. Table 23-2 illustrates normal blood pressure, pulse, and respiration appropriate for different ages of children. Although the pulse will rise progressively, blood pressure can be maintained in children until 25% to 50% of the blood volume has been lost. Therefore, blood pressure should not be the sole indicator in determining blood loss. Monitor pulses, skin color and temperature, capillary refill, and urine output in addition.

Electrocardiographic monitoring is essential. Asystole and ventricular fibrillation caused by hypoxia and blood loss can occur in pediatric trauma victims.

The central circulation of injured patients, who are hypovolemic, may be maintained with fluid resuscitation. Electrolyte solutions, plasma, and whole blood or packed red blood cells are the fluids administered. This is discussed later.

The peripheral vasoconstriction experienced by injured children makes intravenous placement difficult. Hot packs to the area selected for venipuncture may increase the diameter of these constricted veins. A few minutes of heat may save a great deal of time as the procedure is attempted. If unable to obtain intravenous access in this way, a cutdown over the saphenous vein at the ankle is the easiest alternative. Placement of an intraosseous catheter for infusion has recently been recommended as another alternative.

Urinary output should be monitored closely. When placing a urinary catheter, use a small size for a child. If there is gross blood on the underclothing or the perineum, a urethral injury should be suspected. In such cases, before a catheter is inserted, a urethrogram must be obtained. Attempts to pass a catheter across a torn urethra may completely disrupt the urethra or result in placing the catheter tip into the periurethral space and not into the bladder.

Disability and Neurologic Status

Note the state of consciousness of the child. Increasing cerebral pressure as the result of head injury is not an immediate threat to life, but it should be treated as soon as possible. The benefits of early treatment facilitate a successful outcome (Wollman et al 1976).

Exposure

The child must be completely undressed during the examination. Care must be exercised to prevent hypothermia. The room (surroundings) should be kept warm if possible, and extra heating lamps should be made available to prevent further hypothermia as the child is being examined.

Once the circulatory and respiratory status have been stabilized, stage II care begins. It must be remembered that the assessment and management of pediatric trauma is a dynamic process. Flexibility is required in order to alternate between stage I and stage II care.

Stage II care involves careful examination of the patient for further injuries. A head-to-toe method can be used, or systems can be assessed according to the urgency with which they should be treated. Of highest priority are the cardiorespiratory and central nervous systems. Injuries to the thorax can further compromise respiratory and circulatory status and therefore are important to assess early. Abdominal bleeding caused by trauma is life-threatening. Assessment of the head and neck, genitourinary system, skin, and the extremities follows (Hazinski 1984).

Severity of Injury

Various attempts have been made to classify injuries according to their severity and probable outcomes in order to compare the rates of success of treatment in different hospitals or with different treatment protocols. Categorization may be according to cause (note e.g., motor vehicle accident to pedestrian or occupant of car; fall from height; beating; and so on). It may also be according to anatomic and physiologic criteria, for example, site of injury, blood pressure, etc. The number of systems injured is another measure of the severity of the accident. Unfortunately, nearly all of the severity scales that have been developed are somewhat complicated and difficult to complete under the emergency conditions associated with injured children (Mayer et al 1980).

The pediatric trauma scoring system outlined in Table 23–3 has currently been advocated as easy to use and accurate (Fig. 23–3). It presents a more simplified

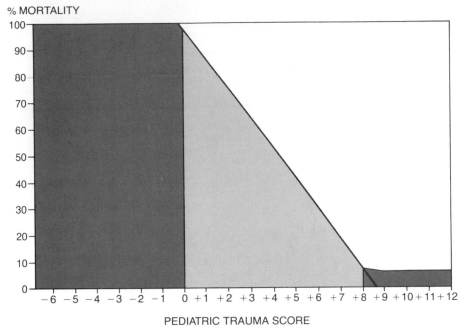

% MORTALITY

FIGURE 23–3. A graphic representation of pediatric trauma scores and associated percentage of mortality. (Modified from Tepas JJ. 1987. Pediatric Trauma Score: A Rapid Assessment and Triage Tool for the Injured Child, 2nd ed. Courtesy of Division of Pediatric Surgery, University of South Alabama, College of Medicine, Mobile, Alabama.)

method than previously developed tools. It can be completed in a few moments through the consideration of six variables: size, airway, mental status, blood pressure, open wounds, and fractures. The pediatric trauma scoring system assesses each of the six components and grades them into one of three categories. The sum of the grades assigned to the six components is the pediatric trauma score (PTS). Statistics have

TABLE 23–3
Pediatric Trauma Score

	Severity Category		
Component	+2	+1	−1
Size	>20 Kg	10–20 Kg	<10 Kg
Airway	Normal	Maintainable	Unmaintainable
CNS	Awake	Obtunded	Comatose
Systolic BP	>90 mmHg	90–50 mmHg	<50 mmHg
Open wounds	None	Minor	Major or penetrating
Skeletal	None	Closed fracture	Open/multiple fractures

Source: Tepas JJ. 1987. Pediatric Trauma Score: A Rapid Assessment and Triage Tool for the Injured Child, 2nd ed. Courtesy of Division of Pediatric Surgery, University of South Alabama, College of Medicine, Mobile, Alabama.
If proper sized BP cuff not available, BP can be assessed by assigning.
+2 = Pulse palpable at wrist
+1 = Pulse palpable at groin
−1 = No pulse palpable

shown that any child with a PTS of eight or less is severely injured and requires the type of care available at major trauma centers (Tepas 1987).

SPECIFIC DISORDERS

Cardiac Irregularities or Arrest

Etiology

Cardiac arrest in the injured child is due to a combination of hypoxia and blood loss (Mayer 1985, 6). Asystole is the dysrhythmia seen most frequently in pediatric trauma. Ventricular fibrillation also occurs, though less commonly than in adults.

Pathophysiology

Hemorrhage leads to hypovolemia. With the decrease in volume of blood ejected by the heart, cardiac output decreases. To compensate for this drop in systemic circulation, the sympathetic nervous system is stimulated, resulting in tachycardia and peripheral vasoconstriction. Occasionally, the systemic arterial vasoconstriction is so profound that a normal blood pressure is maintained in the child despite a very considerable decrease in cardiac output.

    The vasoconstriction also compromises renal perfusion, resulting in a decreased glomerular filtration rate and activation of the renin-angiotensin-aldosterone mechanism. This mechanism causes retention of sodium and water in an attempt to increase the circulating blood volume. In conjunction with this, the vasomotor center increases vascular tone as a means of maintaining blood pressure. Tissue perfusion and oxygenation are therefore compromised, causing the accumulation of lactic acid and resultant metabolic acidosis. If the fluid loss and metabolic acidosis are not corrected, asystole results (Hazinski 1984).

Clinical Manifestations

Early signs of decreasing cardiac output are tachycardia, decreased urinary output, and diaphoresis. The skin is pale as are the mucous membranes and nailbeds. With the onset of shock, extremities are cool and peripheral pulses may be non-palpable. Most children are hypotensive. When an injured child beings to exhibit cardiac extrasystoles or slowing of the heart, cardiac arrest is imminent. A child who has an adequate airway but no pulse should be considered in cardiac arrest. There is no blood flow during either state until cardiac massage is performed.

Treatment and Nursing Care

Decreased Cardiac Output, Related to

- Fluid Volume Deficit Secondary to Hemorrhage

Tissue Perfusion, Altered, Related to

- **Asystole or Ventricular Fibrillation Secondary to Decreased Cardiac Output**

Stage I care for cardiac arrest begins by instituting cardiopulmonary resuscitation (CPR) with 60 to 100 sternal compressions/minute and maintaining adequate ventilation. Intravenous access should be established and volume resuscitation should begin, since a patient with an empty heart will not be resuscitated. The initial medication administered in cardiac arrest is epinephrine. Epinephrine stimulates myocardial contractility and increases cardiac output (Mayer 1985, 7). Sodium bicarbonate may be administered (2 mEq/kg) to correct metabolic acidosis documented on arterial blood gas analysis. Although sodium bicarbonate is no longer recommended as a first-line drug in cardiac arrest, most sources recognize that there is combined respiratory and metabolic acidosis and some form of buffer may be of value. Of course, ventilation via an endotracheal tube is essential in order to rid the lungs of excess CO_2, the by-product of carbonic acid.

Arterial blood gases are obtained and positive-pressure ventilation with 100% humidified oxygen is begun. Cardiac compression assistance should be continued for several minutes after the electrical activity of the heart has resumed, since this evidence of recovery may precede an efficient mechanical thrust by at least that length of time.

In asystole, if medication management fails, transvenous or transthoracic pacemaker insertion may be attempted. Ventricular fibrillation (VF) initially requires the use of the defibrillation at 2 to 5 watt-seconds/kg. If defibrillation is not successful, the dose should be doubled and repeated twice, if necessary. If VF continues, attention should be turned to adequacy of ventilation, oxygenation, correction of acidosis, and hypothermia (Albarran-Sotelo et al 1987).

Evaluation

Expected patient outcomes of medical and nursing measures to correct cardiac arrest include maintenance of adequate tissue perfusion, of normal arterial blood pressure and blood gases for the patient's age, and of normal serum electrolyte concentrations. Nursing measures to achieve this include assessment of temperature of extremities and of quality of peripheral pulses. Capillary refill should be brisk. Vital signs and urinary output are closely monitored and blood gases are assessed for metabolic acidosis, hypoxemia, and hypercapnia (Hazinski 1984).

Shock

Etiology

Pediatric shock differs in its etiology and presentation from shock in adults. Hemorrhagic and septic shock are more commonly seen in children than cardiogenic shock. Because children have a much smaller total blood volume, blood loss from an injury similar to that in an adult can result in a much higher percentage of total blood volume loss in a child. ED nurses must bear this fact in mind when evaluating the pediatric patient for shock.

Pathophysiology

Chapter 5 presents an in-depth discussion of the pathophysiology of shock. Only those points applicable to pediatric patients are discussed here. The general pathophysiology of shock is similar in adults and children. Regardless of the underlying cause, shock is a state of inadequate tissue perfusion resulting in impaired oxygenation at the cellular level (Mayer 1985, 12). In the injured child, shock results from hypovolemia caused by external or internal hemorrhage. Hypoxia may also be a contributing factor. Occasionally, shock in pediatric patients may result from spinal cord injury, pericardial tamponade, or tension pneumothorax. But most of the time, hypovolemia complicated by hypoxia is the critical factor in the development of shock.

Shock is a dynamic process. A child can lose 25% of total blood volume before symptoms are manifested. Compensation through peripheral vasoconstriction occurs. Venous tone also increases. This results in an increase in total peripheral resistance, appearing as a slight increase in *diastolic* blood pressure. Be aware that the systolic blood pressure is not always an accurate measure of impending shock in the pediatric patient. As much as 15% to 25% of total blood volume may be lost, but the patient will still exhibit a "normal" systolic blood pressure. Recognize the early sign of a slight increase in diastolic blood pressure as an indication of impending shock. The pulse rate increases early as a result of beta-adrenergic stimulation of the heart but may then slow very markedly as the shock continues. Prolonged capillary refill caused by vasoconstriction occurs. Both are accurate indicators of shock.

When the patient has lost 25% to 30% of the total blood volume, the compensatory mechanisms fail, and blood pressure decreases. Simultaneously, anaerobic metabolism occurs at the cellular level, and metabolic acidosis results. Remember, this acidosis renders the myocardium less responsive to resuscitative measures. Therefore, the correction of shock should ideally begin before a drop in blood pressure is demonstrated. Anaerobic metabolism can cause failure to the sodium-potassium cellular membrane pump and can result in an increase in intracellular fluid volume with a decrease in the interstitial fluid compartment. This further decreases the total circulating volume (Mayer 1985, 41).

Disseminated intravascular coagulopathy (DIC) is a frequent concomitant of shock in children, and its ill-effects will persist. Head injuries are also made more serious if hypotension is allowed to persist. These common catastrophes of serious childhood injuries are much easier to prevent than they are to treat. Therefore, ED nurses must continually observe for the early signs of hypotension to prevent the progressive development of shock and its complications.

Clinical Manifestations

There are six clinical indicators of hypovolemic shock in the pediatric trauma patient. Vital signs show an increase in pulse rate when approximately 15% of the total blood volume is lost. One must ascertain if this rise is due to anxiety or if other clinical signs indicating shock are present. The rise in diastolic blood pressure is an important early indicator. Respiratory rate also increases. With a 25% loss of total blood volume, hypotension and increased heart rate occur.

Skin temperature and color and capillary refill provide subtle indicators of impending shock. Diaphoresis in response to increased vasomotor tone may be an early sign. As blood loss progresses, the skin becomes cool and mottled, and the capillary refill time increases. With 25% blood loss, extremities may be cyanotic.

Central nervous system responses change with hypoxia. Initially, there may be irritability and anxiety. Frank blood loss presents with confusion, a decreased level of consciousness, or both.

Changes in urinary output also indicate impending shock. When the circulatory blood volume is normal, urine output will be at least 1 ml/kg/hour in children and 2 ml/kg/hour in infants (Hazinski 1984). Urine output drops when more than 25% of the total blood volume is lost.

Laboratory indicators of shock include metabolic acidosis and decreased hematocrit. The hematocrit should not be relied upon as a sole indicator of shock, because 4 to 6 hours is required by the body to restore equilibrium from fluid loss, and the hematocrit may be falsely elevated (Mayer 1985, 14).

Treatment and Nursing Care

The three goals of initial management of hypovolemic shock are (1) restore adequate circulatory volume, (2) maximize oxygen delivery, and (3) detect and control any ongoing blood loss (Mayer 1985, 43–49).

Fluid Volume Deficit, Related to

• **Abnormal Fluid Losses Secondary to Trauma**

Although controversy exists concerning what is the *most* appropriate solution for the initial stabilization of shock, restoration of the circulatory volume is imperative. Adequate intravenous access is established, and a routine type and cross-match specimen is sent. A bolus of 20 ml/kg of Ringer's lactate solution is infused over a 5 to 10 minute time period. The normal child can absorb this much excess fluid without difficulty, while the hypovolemic child will use it to temporarily expand the blood volume. Never use hypotonic solutions such as D5W or 5% D/0.2 saline in injured children. These may lead to hyponatremia and convulsions. It is best to use Ringer's lactate solution without dextrose in this early phase of treatment to avoid hyperglycemia, which may further complicate the care through excessive diuresis and cerebral vasoconstriction (Walker et al 1985).

With exsanguinating hemorrhage, type-specific or O-negative red blood cells plus lactated Ringer's solution will restore circulating volume initially (Hazinski 1984).

Hypovolemic shock requires meticulous monitoring of vital signs to determine the response to the initial bolus of fluid. The initial bolus provides one quarter of the total blood volume to the patient. If no improvement occurs in 5 to 10 minutes, another 20 ml/kg bolus should be administered. Other indicators of improved circulatory volume include an improved sensorium, normal pulse and respirations for age, and brisk capillary refill.

Treatment for ongoing blood loss is accomplished by elevation of the bleeding sites, pressure dressings, and transfusions. The pediatric pneumatic antishock garment (PASG) may be utilized in controlling bleeding from lower extremity or pelvic fractures in the patient who weighs 50 to 150 lbs.

Tissue Perfusion, Altered, Related to

• Hypovolemic Shock

Inadequate tissue perfusion results from inadequate blood flow and oxygen delivery (Mayer 1985, 39). The goal of management is to increase oxygen supply to the tissues and to decrease oxygen demand by the body. Maintenance of an adequate airway and provision of supplemental humidified oxygen are necessary. Blood gases should be monitored and Pao_2 should be maintained at 90 to 100 mmHg (Mayer 1985, 45).

Transfusion with packed red blood cells may be required to increase the oxygen-carrying capacity of the blood. The amount of red blood cells transfused will depend on the amount of blood lost, which can be estimated by careful monitoring for the signs and symptoms of shock.

Once interventions have corrected the immediate threat of shock, stage II care involves continued monitoring of the patient's status and application of additional measures to prevent the complications discussed in the following paragraphs.

Cardiac Output, Decreased, Related to

• Hypovolemic Shock

Some patients may require pharmacologic assistance to restore myocardial contractility following shock. Cardiac output is dependent upon heart rate and stroke volume. Stroke volume depends on the preload (venous inflow) into the heart. Preload is maximized by providing adequate circulatory volume. Dopamine, isoproterenol, or dobutamine may need to be administered after adequate fluid replacement to facilitate left ventricular filling. Assessment for cardiac output and response to treatment is discussed above.

TABLE 23-4
Talwin Dosage
in Children

Age (weight)	Amount
6 months (7 kg)	5 mg
1 year (10 kg)	10 mg
2 years (15 kg)	15 mg
4 years (20 kg)	20 mg
10 years (30 kg)	25 mg

Pain, Related to

- **Injury or Traumatic Event**
- **Fear and Anxiety Secondary to Impending Procedures, Prognosis**

Pain and anxiety (fear) cause an increased demand for oxygen by the cells of the body. Likewise, a temperature elevation or decrease in body temperature raises the consumption of oxygen by 12% for each degree of change (Mayer 1985). Therefore, these must be controlled to decrease the patient's oxygen demands and to prevent oxygenation status from being further compromised. Explanation of examinations and procedures and a calm, gentle approach help alleviate a child's fear and anxiety.

Many physicians fear the use of sedatives and analgesics in injured children, as they may mask developing craniocerebral problems or a deterioration in the child's general condition. However, small amounts of sedative given intravenously will quiet the child and will often improve his or her general condition. Pentazocine lactate (Talwin) is preferred for both sedation and relief of pain in children up to the age of 10 years. Appropriate doses for age and weight are listed in Table 23-4. The child will remain awake but will be drowsy and will experience great relief from discomfort, even though painful sites can still be determined by examination.

After the cardiorespiratory system has been stabilized and treatment of shock has been instituted, stage II care begins with a careful assessment of the patient. Specific body system trauma will be discussed. Only specific treatment and nursing measures and evaluation different from stage I nursing will be discussed.

SPECIFIC SYSTEM INJURIES

Thoracic Trauma

Etiology

Chest trauma in children is not as common as it is in adults. The ribs are more compliant, and the mediastinum is thinner and more mobile. Despite this, chest trauma can cause difficulties if not recognized early. Boys are two to three times more susceptible to chest injury. Most injuries occur in association with abdominal or head trauma (Mayer 1985, 254). Delayed diagnosis and treatment of thoracic trauma contribute significantly to the morbidity and mortality of pediatric patients.

Pathophysiology

Chest injuries are classified as penetrating and blunt (nonpenetrating) injuries. Non-penetrating injuries are the most common type in children. They result from automobile or pedestrian accidents and are associated with multiple trauma. Chest compliance allows internal injuries to occur without external indications. The mediastinum is also more mobile in the child, and organs therefore are more susceptible to dislocation or angulation.

Pneumothorax is the most common injury in pediatric chest trauma and is the focus of this section. The reader is referred to a textbook about trauma for further discussion of injuries. Pneumothorax is classified into four types: open, closed, tension, and hemothorax. Collapse of the lung is caused by loss of negative pressure in the pleural space. Any injury that allows air to accumulate under pressure in the pleural space results in a tension pneumothorax (Fig. 23–4). Hemothorax is an accumulation of blood in the pleural cavity and can result in shock. Hemorrhage into the lung tissues results from pulmonary contusion and bruising.

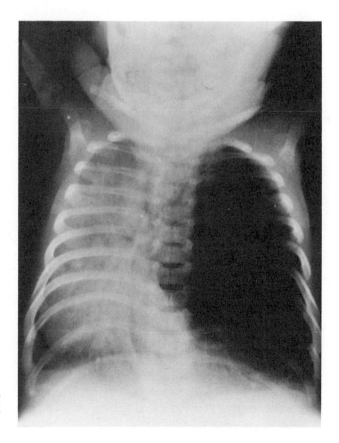

FIGURE 23–4. Tension pneumothorax, with heart pushed to right.

TABLE 23-5
Clinical Manifestations of Pneumothorax in Children

Condition	Observation	Palpation	Percussion	Auscultation
Pneumothorax	Dyspnea Tachypnea	Subcutaneous emphysema Decreased chest wall movement	Dullness	Decreased or absent breath sounds
Hemothorax		Same as pneumothorax		
Tension pneumothorax	Cyanosis Neck vein distention Dyspnea	Tracheal deviation toward side opposite injury Unilateral or decreased chest wall movement	Hyperresonance	Decreased or absent breath sounds

Penetrating injuries are less common and usually result from rib or clavicle fractures. They can also occur as the result of early treatment measures such as use of ventilators, nasogastric tubes, and suction catheters (Mayer 1985, 254).

Clinical Manifestations

Table 23–5 illustrates the clinical manifestations of the three types of pneumothorax. Tension pneumothorax is life-threatening because of the severe cardiorespiratory compromise that occurs with mediastinal shifts or compression of the great vessels. The over-distention of air in the pleural space leads to a shifting of the mediastinum. This compresses the heart and impedes venous return. As a result, cardiac output decreases. This compression and the decreased venous return also compromise the ventilation of the opposite lung.

Treatment and Nursing Care

Tissue Perfusion, Altered, Related to

- **Inadequate Ventilation Secondary to Blunt or Penetrating Chest Trauma**

The goals of treatment are to ensure adequate ventilation and oxygenation and restore circulatory status. The measures discussed under Shock apply to the care of thoracic injuries and are repeated here. Most thoracic injuries in children can be treated without surgery. Maintenance of the blood volume and the insertion of a chest tube for pneumothorax are usually adequate early measures.

Continued bleeding from a thoracotomy tube, progressive widening of the mediastinum, massive air leaks seen on radiography, or an inability to provide adequate Pao_2 (over 70 mmHg) all indicate severe injury. Associated flail chest, pericardial tamponade, rupture of the esophagus or a bronchus, intercostal artery lacerations, or traumatic aortic aneurysms (Fig. 23–5) may be present, and all are indications for aggressive surgical management.

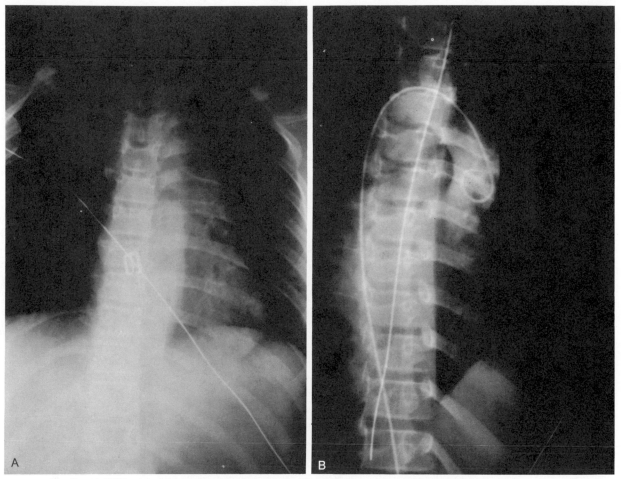

FIGURE 23–5. *A,* Widening of upper mediastinum; *B,* the cause is a ruptured occluded aorta.

Head and Neck Injuries

Etiology

A common type of trauma in children, head injury, is also the leading cause of morbidity and mortality. Seventy-five percent of children who sustain multiple trauma suffer head injury. Several factors predispose the child to this injury. The head of a child constitutes a greater percent of body area and weight than the head of an adult and therefore is more likely to be injured. Common mechanisms of injury in children (motor vehicle accident [MVA], falls, and so forth) also predispose them to head injury. In addition, the cranial bones are thinner, and the brain is less myelinated in children than in adults, making it more vulnerable to injury.

Cervical spine injuries are rare in children under the age of 12. Suspect a fracture of C4–C5 and C5–C6 if the child complains of neck pain, is unconscious, or has sustained head or face trauma. Sixty-seven per cent of children with fractures initially show no radiographic abnormalities (Hazinski 1984).

Pathophysiology

The response to head injury is different in a child than in an adult. Mass lesions are less common in children. Instead, generalized brain swelling is observed in 80% of injured children with head trauma (Mayer 1985, 272). For this reason, children are increasingly susceptible to secondary brain injury as the result of hyperemia. As noted by Walker, Storrs, and Mayer (1985)

> Children often suffer from a unique form of brain injury, previously known as "malignant brain edema." Nearly 50% of children develop this entity, which actually consists, not of brain edema, but of significant cerebral hyperemia in the immediate phase after the head injury.

Operative therapy for head injury in children generally is not of value during the acute phase. Two problems that may require early operation are the *acute subdural hematoma* and *extradural hemorrhage* caused by rupture of the middle meningeal artery or other extrinsic arteries. Children with subdural hematomas usually have a much worse prognosis than do those with extradural hematomas, for they have almost always sustained severe intracerebral damage related to high-speed injuries. On the other hand, fractures of the skull, which may occur at lesser velocities, are more likely to be associated with arterial tears in the extradural space, whereas the brain itself is less commonly affected.

Intracerebral damage that requires operative intervention is rare in childhood. Cerebral hematomas, brain necrosis, and extradural bleeding are not common. As noted above, the main early lesion is cerebral *hyperemia* with consequent swelling of the brain.

Clinical Manifestations

Clinical manifestations of head/neck injury in children are similar to those discussed in detail in Chapters 18 and 19. Early clues are pupillary abnormalities, developing paresis (impairment of movement), and changes in the vital signs.

Treatment and Nursing Care

Sensory-Perceptual Alteration, Related to

- **Change in Mental Status Secondary to Head/Neck Injury**
- **Impaired Mobility Secondary to Head/Neck Injury**

The most important steps in initial management of head injury include airway management, maintenance of adequate ventilation (via hyperventilation), C-spine protection, and maintenance of blood pressure. Table 23–6 summarizes the initial

TABLE 23-6
Initial Treatment of Head Injury

Provision of airway (PA_{O_2} = 80–90 mmHg)
Controlled hyperventilation (PA_{CO_2} = 25–28 mmHg)
Maintain blood pressure (BP ≥ 80 + 2 × age in years)
Elevate head 30–45 degrees
Head and neck in midline position
Minimize stimuli (pain, suctioning, movement, and so on)
Treat seizures
    Dilantin (delayed or persistent seizures) 10 mg/kg
    Diazepam (status epilepticus) 0.1–0.3 mg/kg
Antibiotics (penetrating injuries, open fractures, pneumocephalus)
    Ampicillin 200 mg/kg
    Methicillin 200 mg/kg
Diuretics (for documented deterioration)
    Mannitol (mass lesions) 1 g/kg
    Furosemide (hyperemia) 1–2 mg/kg
Burr holes (rarely necessary)

Source: from Walker ML, Storrs BB, Mayer TA. 1985. In: Mayer TA, ed. Emergency Management of Pediatric Trauma. WB Saunders, 283.

treatment measures. Blood pressure should be maintained at levels appropriate for age (see Table 23–2). Hyperventilation will prevent hypercarbia and its deleterious effects on cerebral vasodilation. Restoration of blood volume promotes effective cerebral capillary blood flow in the face of a potentially increased intracranial pressure.

Pharmacologic treatments, some controversial, include the use of mannitol as an osmotic diuretic, barbiturates, anticonvulsants, and steroids to preserve the cerebral circulation and brain cell function (Table 23–7). Maintenance of moderate hypothermia (between 30 and 32°C) also decreases cerebral edema.

Glasgow Coma Scale evaluations may be done in older children who understand commands (see Chapter 18). Improvement in the overall condition of a child who is admitted with hypotension, a low Po_2, and abnormal electrolytes frequently leads to an improvement in the cerebral function as well. Stage II care also includes the

TABLE 23-7
Head Injury Medications

Mannitol	1 gm/kg IV stat, then 0.25 gm/kg (monitor ICP)
Phenobarbital	20 mg/kg IV stat (up to 30 kg body weight)
Dilantin	10 mg/kg IV stat, then 6 mg/kg/day (children)
	10 mg/kg IV stat, then 100 mg Q8H (adults)
Valium	0.2 mg/kg IV Q1H prn
Pancuronium	0.04–0.10 mg/kg IV stat, then
	0.01–0.02 mg/kg Q30 minutes prn
Dexamethasone*	0.5–1.0 mg/kg IV stat, then
	1.5–2.0 mg/kg Q6H for maintenance

* The use of steroids in head injury is controversial and has largely been discontinued.

meticulous monitoring of respiratory function and systemic perfusion. Brisk capillary refill, strong peripheral pulses, and adequate urine output indicate adequate cardiac output and perfusion.

Evaluation

The expected outcome of nursing measures instituted for head injury is that the child will not demonstrate deterioration in neurologic status. Nursing activities include frequent assessment of level of consciousness (LOC), pupillary response, heart rate and blood pressure, respiratory status and observing for abnormal posturing.

Abdominal Trauma

Etiology

Blunt trauma to the abdomen may initially give rise to few symptoms and is often difficult to diagnose. The causative trauma can be MVA, fall, bicycle or sledding accident, and child abuse. Hemorrhage or visceral perforation results in peritonitis, hypovolemic shock, or both. The goal of assessment is to determine the existence of an acute abdominal injury that requires surgical intervention. Surgery is indicated when (1) the hematocrit persistently declines along with signs of hypovolemia, despite adequate fluid replacement, and (2) severe abdominal tenderness and rigidity exist (Hazinski 1984). Penetrating abdominal trauma is less common in children and frequently requires immediate surgical intervention.

Pathophysiology

Hemoperitoneum from blunt or penetrating trauma does not usually result in signs of peritonitis. Blood is not chemically irritating unless the cells lyse; the released hemoglobin and iron do cause peritoneal irritation. Upper gastrointestinal (GI) perforation results in peritonitis from leakage of hydrochloric acid, digestive enzymes, and bile. Bowel rupture or perforation results in the leakage of fecal material, with the passage of aerobic and anaerobic bacteria into the peritoneum.

Peritoneal irritation results in increased blood flow and capillary permeability in the abdomen. This results in "third spacing" of fluids into extravascular areas. The loss of intravascular fluid contributes to further hypovolemia and decreased cardiac output. The bowel also decreases its motility, and an ileus, with abdominal distention and compromised ventilation, results.

The two most commonly injured intraabdominal organs in blunt trauma are the spleen and the liver, with intestinal rupture a distant third. Whenever there are fractures of the lower left ribs or contusions of the upper abdomen, the spleen is almost always affected.

Perisplenic hematomas are present to a greater or lesser degree, and in most cases, the blood will clot, sealing the opening in the spleen and coating the inferior surface of the diaphragm and the intestines.

The pancreas can be bruised, split around an intact ductal system, or completely transected. It is particularly vulnerable in its midportion as it passes over the vertebral column. A significant injury to the duodenum is often associated with pancreatic injury as well.

A common problem after blunt trauma to the abdomen is the periduodenal hematoma. In this condition, the serosa of the third portion of the duodenum is elevated by a large clot as the result of shearing damage to the subserosal vessels. This results in complete duodenal obstruction, with lack of peristalsis in the affected area.

Clinical Manifestations

Table 23–8 illustrates the signs and symptoms of specific organ involvement in abdominal trauma. In general, the most common symptom is pain. Pain caused by peritonitis increases with any movement. As voluntary and involuntary contractions of muscles occur (guarding), the child lies very still and looks ill. On palpation, the abdomen is tender, and rebound tenderness is present. The bowel sounds are decreased or absent. Nausea and vomiting may be present.

The abdominal pain and tenderness compromise ventilation, and breathing is rapid and shallow. With increased abdominal distention caused by an ileus or third-space volume losses, hypoventilation results, and the child is hypoxic and hypercapnic. Signs of hypovolemia will be present (Hazinski 1984).

TABLE 23–8
Signs and Symptoms of Specific Organ Injury
Caused by Trauma

Organ	Signs and Symptoms
Spleen	Gastric dilation with tympany on percussion and decreased bowel sounds
	Kehr's sign: referred pain in left shoulder
	Ileus
	Decreased hematocrit
Liver and biliary tract	Increased pulse, increased temperature
	Abdominal distention
	Decreased hematocrit
	Severe right shoulder pain with dyspnea
Pancreas and duodenum	Increased temperature
	Abdominal tenderness and rigidity with distention
	Marked leukocytosis
	Epigastric pain
Small bowel and colon	Ileus with abdominal distention
	Tachycardia despite adequate blood replacement
	Presence of free air on film (not often present with small bowel perforation)

Treatment and Nursing Care

Breathing Patterns, Ineffective, Related to

- **Hypoventilation Secondary to Pain, Abdominal Distention, or Both**

Children with actual or suspected intraabdominal injuries require supplemental oxygen to increase Fio_2 and improve oxygenation status. Soft vinyl pediatric masks may be tolerated by children. A face tent may be better tolerated by children than a mask. An oxygen concentration equal to that of the gas source can be delivered if a high flow (10 to 15 L/minute) is provided, although stable concentrations in excess of 40% Fio_2 are not reliable (Albarran-Sotelo 1987, 261).

For the nonhypotensive child, elevating the head of the bed 30 degrees once C-spine integrity is assured may alleviate diaphragmatic pressure from abdominal distention and improve respiratory function.

Fluid Volume Deficit, Related to

- **Internal Hemorrhage**
- **Fluid Shift to Third Space**

Initial management of abdominal trauma begins with measures to correct hypovolemia and shock, as previously discussed. Abdominal girth should be measured and the area clearly demarcated for repeat measurements. A double-lumen nasogastric tube is inserted, and any drainage is evaluated for the presence of blood. Abdominal examination is repeated at least every 15 minutes because of the insidious onset of signs and symptoms associated with intraabdominal injury.

Peritoneal lavage for the diagnosis of any of these conditions in children is rarely performed. Computed tomography (CT) scanning is the procedure of choice in diagnosis, particularly if the child is unconscious from a head injury and has associated abdominal signs. Repeated physical evaluations in conjunction with the CT scan will yield sufficient information in time to plan surgical correction.

Pain, Related to

- **Abdominal Injury**

A child with abdominal injury will experience pain, discomfort, and anxiety. A gentle calm approach should be used to decrease pain and anxiety. While it will be impossible to administer analgesics during the diagnostic phase of care, allowing and encouraging parental support and reassurance will assist the child in tolerating the discomfort. Parents should be allowed to stay with the child as much as possible.

Evaluation

Recognition of the early signs of abdominal trauma is the responsibility of the ED nurse. Expected patient outcomes include absent signs of peritonitis or hemorrhage,

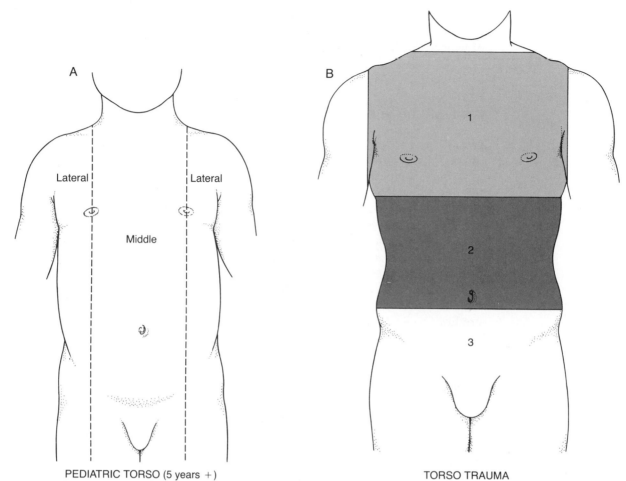

FIGURE 23–6. Pediatric torso trauma can be divided as follows: *A, Middle* (mediastinum and heart) or *lateral* (ribs, lungs, and great vessels). *B,* (1) *Supradiaphragmatic* (heart, lungs, and great vessels), (2) *upper abdominal* (spleen, liver, kidneys, pancreas, and upper small bowel), (3) *lower abdominal* (bladder, urethra, sigmoid colon, and rectum).

normal fluid volume and tissue perfusion, normal respiratory status, and minimal abdominal pain. Continued meticulous assessment is crucial to the success of these outcomes. It helps to divide the torso into segments, looking for both external and internal injuries in the various areas (Fig. 23–6).

Genitourinary Trauma

Etiology

Any significant impact may damage the kidneys or lower urinary tract. Pelvic fractures are frequently associated with both kidney and bladder injuries, for they result from high-impact accidents. Injuries to the kidneys occur more often in children than adults because of the lack of perirenal fat and the thin Gerota's fascia, both of which contribute to a high degree of kidney mobility.

Pathophysiology

Renal injury is commonly caused by blunt trauma. Mechanisms of injury include MVA, sport injuries, and child abuse (Mayer 1985, 341).

Ureteral injuries are rare. The bladder is frequently ruptured because it is often full and located partly in the abdomen in smaller children. With pelvic fractures, bladder or urethral injuries are almost the rule. They must be assumed to be present until specific studies (urethrogram and cystogram) have ruled them out.

Blood at the urethral meatus suggests a urethral injury. Before attempts are made to pass a catheter, a retrograde urethrogram should be obtained. Leakage of urine at the membranous portion of the urethra will often be documented in this way. If such extravasation is seen, attempts to pass a Foley's catheter may be disastrous, completing a tear that originally extended through only a part of the circumference of the urethra.

Clinical Manifestations

Suspect a renal injury whenever there is evidence of trauma to the flank, back, lower chest, or abdomen. Abrasions, contusions, and ecchymosis may be present over the flank or lower abdomen. Pelvic or rib fractures may be present. The signs and symptoms vary depending on the type and extent of genitourinary injury (Table 23–9). Abdominal or flank tenderness is usually present. Hematuria is the hallmark of renal trauma and occurs in 80% to 90% of patients with kidney injuries (Mayer 1985, 343). Remember, the degree of hematuria does not correlate with the extent of injury. Microscopic hematuria may herald a severe injury. The different types of injuries are illustrated in Figure 23–7.

Treatment and Nursing Care

Urinary Elimination, Altered Patterns of, Related to

• **Blunt Trauma**

Urinalysis should be performed to determine the presence of hematuria. Catheter or percutaneous suprapubic decompression should be instituted unless contraindicated. To rule out renal damage, an emergency intravenous pyelogram (IVP) is indicated. The IVP should also be done when there is flank bruising or the mechanism of injury is such that a renal avulsion might have occurred.

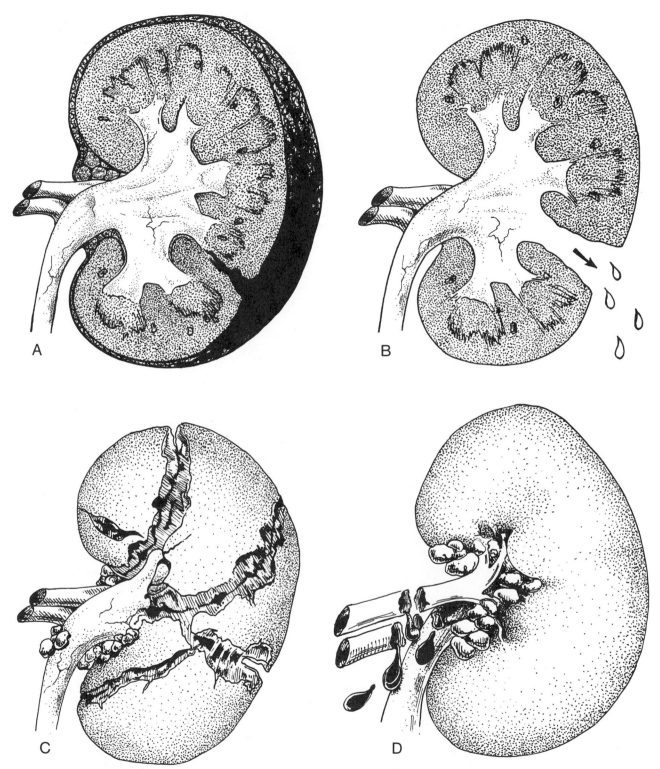

FIGURE 23-7. Kidney injuries. *A,* Contusion with hemorrhage contained by Gerota's fascia; *B,* single fracture into pelvis; *C,* multiple rupture-lacerations; *D,* complete avulsion of hilar vessels.

TABLE 23–9
Physical Signs of
Genitourinary Injury

Renal
   Hematuria
   Flank or abdominal pain
   Flank abrasion, contusion, or ecchymosis
   Flank mass
   Previous renal abnormality
Bladder
   Hematuria
   Abdominal pain
   Inability to void
   Pelvic fracture
   Renal injury
Ureteral
   Deceleration injury with hyperextension
   Flank pain
   Flank mass
   Penetrating injuries
   Hematuria
Urethral
   Blood at urethra
   Inability to void
   Lower abdominal/pelvic pain
   Scrotal hematoma/perineal swelling
   High-riding prostate
   Hematuria

Source: Middleton RG, Matlak ME, Nixon GW, et al. 1985. In: Mayer TA, ed. Emergency Management of Pediatric Trauma, WB Saunders, 343.

Evaluation

Children with suspected renal trauma should be monitored closely. Urinary output should be consistent with fluid intake, and urine should be monitored for hematuria. Vital signs should remain stable with no signs of instability caused by blood loss or shock. If the clinical course worsens, further evaluation may be required.

MUSCULOSKELETAL INJURIES

Musculoskeletal injuries and their treatment are discussed in Chapter 16. All patients should be systematically evaluated for orthopedic injuries. Eighty per cent of missed diagnoses in patients with trauma are orthopedic injuries (Mayer 1985, 31). Although there are few life-threatening orthopedic injuries, there are injuries that seriously threaten the viability of the injured limb. A limb can be lost as the result of a major joint dislocation, amputation, compartment syndrome, and open fracture, with devastating consequences to the child. Therefore, these should be promptly treated. Also, as the result of a missed fracture, a child can develop irreparable nerve damage, deformity, or infection. It is essential to recognize the amount of bleeding

TABLE 23–10
Estimated Local Blood
Loss in Fractures
(Adults)

Bone	Loss (in Liters)
Humerus	1.0–2.0
Elbow	0.5–1.5
Forearm	0.5–1.0
Pelvis	1.5–4.5
Hip	1.5–2.5
Femur	1.0–2.0
Knee	1.0–1.5
Tibia	0.5–1.5
Ankle	0.5–1.5

Source: Walt AJ, ed. 1982.
Early Care of the Injured Patient.
WB Saunders, 284.

into soft tissues that can result from fractures (Table 23–10). This not only compromises the injured limb but complicates the treatment of other injuries. Prompt recognition and treatment of skeletal injuries that threaten the viability of the limb are essential. The degree of angulation that can occur, and its correction, are illustrated in Figure 23–8.

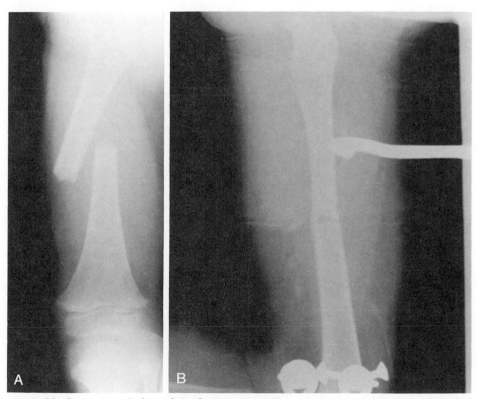

FIGURE 23–8. *A,* Angulation of the femur can totally occlude the arteries and veins of the lower leg. *B,* Correction of angulation by splinting.

Evaluation involves systematic palpation of extremities and radiographic studies of suspected areas. Motor and sensory function is included in the evaluation. Initial treatment consists of splinting. Again, the two exceptions that require immediate attention are evidence of distal neurovascular compromise or when bone fragments from an open fracture cause skin necrosis (Mayer 1985, 31).

PSYCHOLOGIC IMPACT OF TRAUMA TO A CHILD

Few emergency situations create as much anxiety and psychologic trauma as does the injury of a child. The child, the parents, babysitters, nurses, physicians — in fact, all involved in the care — feel the impact of the injury. The injury is usually sudden and unexpected, and the child is not prepared for the injury or the events involved in treating it. The ED is frightening and confusing, and the caregivers are unfamiliar to the child. Strange sights and sounds as well as painful procedures are thrust upon them. Since children's intellectual capabilities are less well developed than those of adults, they may interpret pain inflicted upon them as punishment and are unable to distinguish pain caused by necessary treatment from that of punishment (Mayer 1985).

The parents are traumatized as well. Guilt is the predominant emotion and is often displayed as anger toward the health care providers. Fear and anxiety also complicate their response to the child's injury. The helplessness they feel may be overwhelming.

Treatment and Nursing Care

It is essential that the parents' and the child's level of anxiety be kept to a minimum to ensure the proper delivery of care. With the child, use a calm, gentle, organized approach. Explain what you are doing clearly and simply. Utilize distraction to decrease anxiety — discuss friends, a favorite sport, or a pet. Return to this discussion after a painful treatment or procedure to distract the child from remembering the pain.

Parents should be provided emotional and psychologic support. A calm, simple explanation of the situation frequently will alleviate some anxiety. Be honest about necessary procedures and allow them time to verbalize the fears and frustrations they may be experiencing. Referral to social services or religious affiliates in the hospital may be beneficial.

This kind of attention to the psychologic impact of trauma on both the child and the parents will facilitate the care delivered and a successful outcome.

CONCLUSION

Once the general nature of the child's injuries has been assessed and breathing and circulation have been stabilized, a determination can be made as to whether (1) the child can be observed for a short period of time and sent home, (2) the child can be transferred to the pediatric unit for overnight observation, (3) the nature of the injuries require more definitive studies, or (4) immediate surgery is required because of continued deterioration.

Nursing care in the ED includes careful observation and monitoring of the child for signs of deterioration as well as the provision of skilled technical assistance for rapid diagnostic tests and treatment. An extremely important part of care is reassurance of parents and relatives of injured children, keeping them informed of the progress, and facilitating their processing of guilt feelings. The prognosis is usually good if the child survives the initial injuries and is kept in optimal physiologic condition by prompt and effective treatment in the ED.

REFERENCES

Albarran-Sotelo R, Atkins JM, Bloom RS, 1987. Textbook of Advanced Cardiac Life Support. Dallas, American Heart Association, 268.

Brooks BF, ed. 1985. The Injured Child. Austin, University of Texas Press.

Burke JF. 1964. Wound infection and early inflammation. Monogr Surg Sci 1:301.

Caniano DA, Beaver BL, Boles ET Jr. 1986. Child Abuse. An update on surgical management in 256 cases. Ann Surg 203:219–224.

Carter DC, Polk HC Jr, eds. 1981. Trauma. London, Butterworths.

Churchill ED. 1947. The American surgeon. Surg Gynecol Obstet 84:529–539.

Committee on Trauma, American College of Surgeons. 1988. Advanced Trauma Life Support Course. Chicago, American College of Surgeons, 1–157.

Committee on Trauma, American College of Surgeons. 1982. Early Care of the Injured Patient, 3rd ed. Philadelphia, WB Saunders.

Cooney DR. 1981. Splenic and hepatic trauma in children. Surg Clin North Am 61:1165–1180.

Cowley RA, Dunham CM, eds. 1982. In: Shock Trauma/Critical Care Manual. Initial Assessment and Management. Baltimore, University Park Press.

Crussi FG. 1985. Reflections on child abuse. In: Notes of an Anatomist. New York, Harcourt Brace Jovanovich, 72–90.

De la Torre JC. 1981. Spinal cord injury: review of basic and applied research. Spine 6:315–335.

Douglas GJ, Simpson JS. 1971. The conservative management of splenic trauma. J Pediatr Surg 6:565–570.

Eichelberger ME, Stossel-Pratsch G, eds. 1984. Pediatric Emergencies Manual. Baltimore, University Park Press.

Frankowski RF. 1985. Head injury mortality in urban populations and its relation to the injured child. In: Brooks BF, ed. The Injured Child. Austin, University of Texas Press, 20–29.

Garcia V, Eichelberger M, Ziegler M, et al. 1981. Use of military antishock trouser in a child. J Pediatr Surg 16:544–546.

Haller JA, Shorter N, Miller D, et al. 1983. Organization and function of regional pediatric trauma center: does a system of management improve outcome? J Trauma 23:691–696.

Harris BH, ed. 1985. The 1st National Conference on Pediatric Trauma Proceedings, Boston, September 26 and 27, 1985. Nobb Hill Press.

Hazinski MF. 1984. Nursing Care of the Critically Ill Child. St. Louis, CV Mosby.

Howel CG, Ziegler MD. 1985. Acute management of major trauma and burns. Clin Emerg Med 7:79–106.

Karp MP, Cooney DR, Berger PE, et al. 1981. The role of computed tomography in the evaluation of blunt abdominal trauma in children. J Pediatr Surg 16:316–323.

Karp MP, Cooney DR, Pros GA, et al. 1983. The non-operative management of pediatric hepatic trauma. J Pediatr Surg 18:512–518.

Kitahama A, Elliott LF, Overby JL, et al. 1982. The extrahepatic biliary tract injury. Ann Surg 196:536–540.

Koop CE. 1985. In: Brooks BF, ed. The Injured Child. Austin, University of Texas Press, 97.

Livne PM, Gonzales ET Jr. 1985. Genitourinary trauma in children. Urol Clin North Am 12:53–65.

Matlak ME. Abdominal injuries. In: Meyer TA, ed. Emergency Management of Pediatric Trauma. Philadelphia, WB Saunders, 232–235.

Mayer TA, Matlak ME, Johnson DG, et al. 1980. The modified injury severity scale in pediatric multiple trauma patients. J Pediatr Surg 15:719–726.

Mayer TA, Matlak ME, Nixon GW, et al, eds. 1985. Emergency Management of Pediatric Trauma. Philadelphia, WB Saunders, 1–51.

Mayer TA, Walker ML. 1982. Emergency intracranial pressure monitoring in pediatrics: management of the acute coma of brain insult. Clin Pediatr 21:391–396.

McKoy C, Bell MJ. 1983. Preventable traumatic deaths in children. J Pediatr Surg 18:505–508.

Moore EE, Eiseman B, VanWay CW III, eds. 1984. Critical Decisions in Trauma. St. Louis, CV Mosby.

O'Neill JA Jr, Meacham WF, Griffin JP, 1973. Patterns of injury in the battered child syndrome. J Trauma 13:332–339.

Overgaard J, Tweed WA. 1974. Cerebral circulation after head injury I. Cerebral blood flow and its regulation after closed head injury, with emphasis on clinical correlation. J Neurosurg 41:531–541.

Ramenofsky ML, Luterman A, Curreri PW, et al. 1983. EMS for pediatrics: optimum treatment or unnecessary delay? J Pediatr Surg 18:498–503

Reichard SA, Helikson MA, Shorter H, et al. 1980. Pelvic fractures in children—review of 120 patients, with a new look at general management. J Pediatr Surg 15:727–734.

Reyes HM. 1985. Management of trauma in the pediatric trauma patient. In Vidyasagar D, Sarnaik AP, eds. Neonatal and Pediatric Intensive Care. Littleton, Mass, PSG Publishing Co., 204.

Rivara FP. 1985. Traumatic deaths of children in the United States. Currently available prevention strategies. Pediatrics 75:456–462.

Rosenberg NM, Meyers S, Shackleton N. 1982. Prediction of child abuse in an ambulatory setting. Pediatrics 70:879–882.

Tepas JJ. 1987. Pediatric Trauma Score: A Rapid Assessment and Triage Tool for the Injured Child, 2nd ed. Division of Pediatric Surgery, University of South Alabama, College of Medicine, Mobile, Alabama.

Touloukian RJ. 1983. A protocol for the non-operative treatment of obstructing intra-mural hematoma during childhood. Am J Surg 145:330–334.

Walker ML, Storrs BB, Mayer TA. 1985. Head injuries. In: Mayer TA, ed. Emergency Management of Pediatric Trauma. Philadelphia, WB Saunders, 272–273.

Wesson DE, Filler RM, Ein SB, et al. 1981. Ruptured spleen—When to operate? J Pediatr Surg 16:324–326.

Wollman H, Smith TC, Stephen GW, et al. 1976. Effects of extremes of respiratory and metabolic alkalosis on cerebral blood flow in man. J Appl Physiol 24:50–65.

Young B, Rapp RP, Norton JA, et al. 1981. Early prediction of outcome in head-injured patients. J Neurosurg 54:300–304.

CHAPTER 24

June Kaiser, RN MS
Elaine Scorza, RN MS

Psychiatric Emergencies

Psychiatric emergencies constitute a significant percentage of patient visits to emergency departments (EDs) annually. One primary reason for this has been the deinstitutionalization of the mentally ill, spawned by the introduction of psychotropic drugs in the 1950s, which was not met with adequate community mental health planning. As greater numbers of mentally ill persons were released from state hospitals, more mentally ill persons began living in communities with very few outpatient resources to aid them. Consequently, we are now recognizing the existence of mental illness in a good part of our homeless population today. The only port of entry into the health care system for many of these people is through the ED.

Other factors that contribute to the high rate of use of the ED for psychiatric emergencies include the increase in psychiatric disorders in the general population, the greater acceptability of voluntarily seeking psychiatric help, and the frequency with which acute emotional reactions occur in ED settings in response to acute illness, traumatic injury, or sudden death.

DEFINITION

There is no one exact definition of a psychiatric emergency; however, it is believed that one exists when a person's coping abilities are no longer able to maintain that person at his or her usual level of functioning. A behavioral or mental status change, or both, results. This change is frequently sudden, although at times it may be much more insidious in onset. In either case, the person is experiencing significant mental anguish, which, if not responded to, may result in life-threatening, suicidal, violent, or psychologically damaging behavior. Psychiatric emergencies may be defined by patients themselves, family members or significant others, or agents of society (Parker 1984). Although some health professionals distinguish psychiatric emergencies from psychiatric crises (Talley and King 1984), crises tending to be more situational and less characterological in nature than emergencies, they both overwhelm the functional coping abilities of the person and the terms will be used interchangeably throughout this chapter.

In addition to those psychiatric emergencies that are characterized primarily by identifiable mental status or behavioral changes, crisis situations that require acute medical management as the result of an underlying psychiatric problem (e.g., suicide attempts), or as the result of pharmacologic intervention for a psychiatric problem (e.g., dystonic reactions, lithium toxicity) are also frequent occurrences in EDs. In these instances, and in instances in which psychiatric symptoms may be the primary manifestation of a physiologic disorder (metabolic disturbances, brain tumors), medical and life-saving interventions (stage I care) take priority over psychiatric evaluation and treatment.

When we recognize that the causes of psychiatric symptoms or emergencies may be as varied as the treatments for each of them, and when we recognize that psychiatric problems may manifest themselves primarily with physical symptoms (e.g., anxiety attacks, somatic complaints), the importance of ED nurses possessing excellent assessment skills becomes evident.

For all of the reasons stated previously it is imperative for ED nurses to have the ability to accurately assess, recognize, describe, document, and evaluate psychiatric symptoms. Additionally, they should be able to differentiate functional from organic disorders,* identify major psychiatric illnesses, and be able to initiate a therapeutic treatment plan. This chapter will assist ED nurses in achieving these goals.

ASSESSMENT

Assessment of the person who comes to the ED in psychiatric crisis consists of three parts: the history, physical examination, and mental status examination.

History

The history is usually initiated by the triage nurse, who must quickly determine the urgency of the crisis based on the reason for which the patient is seeking care and his

---

* It is recognized that genetic, biologic, and biochemical aberrations play a significant role in the causes of major psychiatric illnesses. It is therefore increasingly difficult to discuss psychiatric disorders as having a purely organic or functional basis. For operational purposes, however, organic disorders will be considered as those disorders that have a grossly identifiable (and potentially reversible) physiologic cause (e.g., endocrine and metabolic imbalances, neurologic disorders, drug induced disorders, and so forth). Functional disorders will be considered those disorders without a grossly identifiable physiologic cause.

or her capacity to wait. Life-threatening conditions or severe mental anguish must be identified at this time. The onset, nature, and duration of symptoms must be ascertained. Appropriate questions to ask at triage include the following: "What brought you to the emergency room?", "Are you hearing voices or seeing things?", or "Have you thought of harming yourself or anyone else?" When possible, a medication history, including current medications, recent changes in medications, and compliance with medication regimens, and any allergies the patient may have should also be obtained. Objective data collection by the triage nurse should include vital signs and signs of pallor, flushing, diaphoresis, agitation, or dystonic movements.

It is important that the triage nurse recognize that he or she may be the patient's first contact with the health care system. An attitude of acceptance, empathy, and respect along with a genuine desire to help should be conveyed to the patient at this time. It is this first contact with the triage nurse that may significantly influence the patient's acceptance of emergency care and his or her receptivity to future treatment. The triage nurse must also recognize that the majority of people experiencing psychiatric crises who come to the ED do want help. Often they are aware that they have lost control and are frightened. They may be experiencing extreme mental pain, and at no time should their care take second place to a less urgent medical problem of another patient.

Once inside the treatment area, unstable medical conditions or life-threatening emergencies must be dealt with appropriately and expediently. Further details of the history of present illness (HPI) must be ascertained. In the case of a drug overdose, every attempt to determine the type, amount, and time of ingestion (or injection) should be made. The patient's clothing may need to be searched for empty pill containers, and family or friends may need to search the patient's car or living quarters for clues to determine the substance(s) with which the patient overdosed. Precipitating events that may have preceded or contributed to the patient's current crisis should be explored. Recent life stressors or changes in medications are frequently found to trigger psychiatric crises, whether it be a first occurrence or an acute exacerbation of a chronic illness.

Changes in the patient's level of functioning socially, mentally, occupationally, and physically should be determined, as should any history or pattern of substance abuse. Somatic complaints and recent changes in appetite, weight, sleep, digestive function, and sexual interest also should be ascertained. Past experiences and responses to crises and the interpersonal support available to the patient should be sought out. Often, successful coping mechanisms found beneficial to the patient in past crises may again be helpful.

Having obtained data regarding the patient's chief complaint and HPI—life-threatening emergencies having been ruled out or no longer being a danger—attention should be directed toward significant past and present medical, psychiatric, and family histories. Information regarding the patient's medical history may alert the emergency nurse to possible organic causes that may be responsible for or contributing to the patient's presenting symptoms. Endocrine dysfunctions, electrolyte abnormalities, and head trauma are some medical conditions that may manifest themselves primarily as changes in mental status (see Table 24–1).

Medical and psychiatric histories should include diagnosed disorders, patient's age at their onset, and responsiveness to treatment. All hospitalizations, including the reason for each, the length of stay(s), treatments, responses to treatments, and fol-

TABLE 24–1
Organic Illnesses or Conditions
that Can Produce Psychiatric
Symptoms

Alcohol intoxication
Alcohol withdrawal
Alzheimer's disease
Brain tumors or bleeding
Drug ingestions or poisonings
    Hallucinogens (PCP, LSD)
    Amphetamines or cocaine
    Lead poisoning
    Steroid toxicity
    Atropine psychosis
Endocrine abnormalities
    Hyperthyroidism
    Hypothyroidism
    Hyperparathyroidism
    Hypoparathyroidism
    Hypoglycemia
    Cushing's disease
    Hypopituitarism
    Postpartum states
    Addison's disease or adrenal insufficiency
Head trauma
Hepatic insufficiency or failure
Hypoxia
Infections
    Meningitis
    Brain abscess
    Tertiary syphilis
    Encephalitis
Metabolic abnormalities
    Hypokalemia
    Hyponatremia
    Acid-base imbalances
Nutritional deficiencies
Renal failure or uremia
Seizure disorders

---

low-up, should be recorded. Psychiatric family history should include the psychiatric diagnosis (or a description of the disorder) and the relation of the involved family member to the patient. The occurrence of all major psychiatric disorders in the patient and his or her family should be asked about (e.g., anxiety, hysteria, personality and depressive disorders, bipolar illness, thought disorders, and schizophrenia).

Following a thorough history and prior to the actual physical examination, the ED nurse should obtain a brief review of systems (ROS) on the patient. Special attention should be focused on the head and neck and on endocrine, musculoskeletal, and neurologic systems. In this way, no important clues that may be indicative of an organic problem will be overlooked.

While obtaining the patient's psychiatric history, it is important that the nurse promote an atmosphere of trust that is conducive to patient self-disclosure. A private area where noise and interruptions are minimal should be utilized for the interview. If the patient is uncooperative, unreliable, or unable to give an accurate history, a collateral history from friends, relatives, and or rescue workers who may have brought the patient to the ED may be quite helpful. If the patient is currently under treatment, the physician or counselor should be called. Old records, when available, should be obtained.

Physical Examination

A physical examination should be done on all patients in psychiatric crisis to detect any underlying organic problems that may be causative or contributory to the patient's presenting problem. Psychiatric patients do become physically ill, and physical illness can exacerbate or contribute to psychiatric symptoms. Laboratory and radiographic studies along with electrocardiograms should be ordered as the patient's condition dictates. These tests may be ordered for diagnostic reasons to confirm or rule out organic causes responsible for the presenting symptoms (e.g., electrolyte imbalances), or they may be ordered to rule out physiologic problems either resulting from psychiatric causes (e.g., drug toxicities) or physical illness separate from psychiatric illness.

The third part of the assessment of a patient in psychiatric crisis is the mental status examination (MSE). This is similar to the physical examination in that both are based on objective findings. Whereas the physical examination has as its primary focus the identification of organ system pathology, the purpose of the MSE is to assess the cognitive and psychologic status of a patient. Caution is advised, however, that the administration and interpretation of the examination be done in accordance with the patient's social, educational, and cultural background. Although much of the MSE may be integrated into the history and physical examination, some components of it may require more direct and purposeful questioning. The MSE is therefore described separately and in its entirety.

Mental Status Examination

Behavior and general appearance, speech patterns, affect and mood, mental content and thought processes, judgment and insight, perception, and cognitive ability are the major components of the MSE. The skills required to perform the examination are those of structured and purposeful interviewing, direct observation, and careful listening. Definitions of commonly used psychiatric terms that are helpful in describing patient findings or status obtained during the psychiatric assessment are listed in Table 24–2.

Behavior and General Appearance

Appropriateness of the patient's behavior and general appearance has probably already been noted during the history and physical examination. Observe and describe the patient's size, shape, and relation of appearance to his or her stated age. Note the patient's dress, grooming, and hygiene. Is he or she disheveled or dressed inappropriately for the circumstances or season? Is there evidence of acute decompensation? Special attention should be given to the patient's posture, gait, and motor activity. Is

TABLE 24-2
Definitions of Commonly Used Psychiatric Terms

Blocking	Interruption of a train of speech as a result of the individual losing his/her train of thought
Clanging	Pattern of speech in which sounds rather than meaning govern word choice
Circumstantial speech	Speech which gives unnecessary detail delaying communication of the central idea
Delusion	A false fixed belief based on incorrect inference about external reality that cannot be changed by reason or logic; delusions may be grandiose, somatic, persecutory, or nihilistic
Derealization*	A feeling of detachment from one's environment
Depersonalization	Feeling as if one is outside one's body or as if part of it does not belong
Flight of ideas	A nearly continuous flow of accelerated speech with abrupt changes from topic to topic usually with only a thread of connection between ideas
Ideas of reference	A belief that occurrences, objects, or persons in the subject's immediate environment have a particular meaning for him or her
Illusion	Misperception of an external stimulus which is real
Hallucination	A sensory perception in the absence of external stimulation of the relevant sensory organ; hallucinations may be auditory, visual, olfactory, gustatory, or somatic
Loosening of association	Speech reflective of thinking in which ideas shift from one subject to another without any connection between them
Neologism	New word, distortion of word, or a standard word to which the subject has given new meaning
Obsession	A recurrent, persistent, senseless idea, thought, image, or impulse
Poverty of speech	Restriction in amount of speech, so that spontaneous speech and replies to questions are brief and unelaborated
Pressure of speech	Speech that is increased in amount, accelerated, and difficult to interrupt
Rumination*	Adapted from the Latin word meaning "to chew the cud"; a frequent return of thinking to a particular idea
Tangential speech*	A style of speech containing irrelevant or oblique responses to questions asked (e.g., when asked about his or her sleep, the patient tells about the cat's twitching while it sleeps)
Thought broadcasting	Belief that one's thoughts are being broadcast outside one's head, allowing others to hear them
Thought insertion	Belief that thoughts that are not one's own can be inserted into one's mind
Word Salad*	A characteristic of schizophrenia, a mixture of words that lack meaningful connections

Source: Based on definitions from American Psychiatric Association, 1987. Diagnostic and Statistical Manual of Mental Disorders, 391–405.
  * Based on definitions from Waldinger RJ, 1986. Fundamentals of Psychiatry. Washington, DC, American Psychiatric Press, 64–67.

it stiff and tense, or is it relaxed? Is psychomotor retardation present, or does the patient exhibit excessive fidgeting or agitation? Is there tremulous activity or involuntary movements? Note the patient's attitude and facial expressions. Do they match? Do they seem suspicious, friendly, hostile, or cooperative?

Speech

Note the volume, rate, clarity, and quality of speech. Is it loud or soft, slow or fast, clear or muffled? Is there poverty of speech or pressured speech? Does the patient's speech reflect flight of ideas, loosening of associations, blocking, circumstantiality, or tangentiality? Does he or she use rhyming, clanging, word salad, or neologisms?

Mood and Affect

Note whether or not the patient describes his or her mood state similarly to how you perceive it. Is it depressed, elated, angry, or hostile? Is it stable, labile, appropriate?

Does the patient express a sense of hopelessness, worthlessness, despair, anger, or rage that might be indicative of suicidal or violent intent? Does the patient's affect match his or her mood? Is it stable, labile, appropriate? Does it display a full range of emotions or is it blunted and flat?

Thought Processes or Mental Content

Note the rationality, coherency, and organization of the patient's thought processes. Do his or her thoughts display ruminations or obsessional or delusional thinking? Does the patient feel compelled to carry out certain acts? Are his or her delusions recent and circumscribed, or are they widespread and systematized? Are they grandiose, persecutory, or somatic in nature? Does the patient have ideas of reference, thought insertion, or thought broadcasting? Does he or she exhibit flight of ideas, looseness of association, blocking of ideas, tangentiality, or circumstantiality?

Perception

Is the patient experiencing illusions or hallucinations? If so, are the hallucinations auditory, visual, gustatory, olfactory, or tactile? When do they occur and how often do they occur? Does the patient plan on acting on them? Does the patient express feelings of derealization or depersonalization?

Judgment and Insight

Be aware of the patient's ability to form opinions and make social judgments. Ask what he or she would do if his or her car were stalled on a train track and a train was coming. What would the patient do if he or she smelled fire in a high-rise building? Determine if the patient understands why he or she is where he or she is. What does the patient feel should be done about his or her present condition or situation?

Cognitive Ability

Much of the person's cognitive ability will have emerged during the history and physical examination. If a deficit is evident, more formal testing may be performed. If no deficit is suggested, the need to perform these tests in the ED setting is greatly lessened.

Attention span and concentration, basic fund of knowledge, ability to reason abstractly, orientation, and memory are the major components of a mental status examination that best reflect a person's cognitive abilities.

Attention and Concentration • In order to assess a patient's attention and concentration span, ask him or her to repeat a series of unsequenced digits after you. Usually a person can remember and repeat six to eight digits forward and four backward. You may also have the patient count backward from 100 subtracting seven each time. Most individuals are able to perform this within 2 minutes with fewer than four mistakes.

Basic Knowledge • Basic knowledge may be assessed by asking the patient to define a variety of vocabulary words, which range in complexity from simple to difficult. Questions such as the following may also be asked: "How many objects are there in a dozen?" or "How many inches are there in a foot?" Often a person's premorbid level of functioning can be estimated in this way.

Abstract Reasoning • When attempting to determine the abstract reasoning ability of a patient, state several proverbs and ask him or her to explain them. The patient's level of concreteness or abstractness in his or her explanations should be assessed. Examples of proverbs are "People in glass houses shouldn't throw stones," and "A rolling stone gathers no moss."

Orientation • Ask the patient to tell you his or her name, where he or she is, and the date. If the exact date is not known, you may ask the patient if he or she knows the day of the week, month, year, or season. Patients with functional causes of psychosis are more likely to be bizarrely disoriented than those with organic etiologies (e.g., a schizophrenic may believe he or she is Jesus Christ whereas a patient with organic brain syndrome may just not know who he or she is).

Memory • Both recent and remote memory reflect a patient's cognition. Ask the patient to name three objects (not immediately visible or related to each other), and ask him or her to then list them for you again 10 minutes later. Remote memory may be evident by the ability of the patient to give you a past medical or psychiatric history of himself or herself. The person may be asked to identify past presidents and historical events to test remote memory. Persons with psychiatric symptoms from organic causes are more likely to exhibit memory deficits (especially with recent memory) than those with psychiatric symptoms from functional causes.

Much time has been spent on the assessment of patients in psychiatric crisis. Its importance cannot be overemphasized, for it is only by way of accurate and astute assessment that the most appropriate and therapeutic interventions for any given patient can be provided.

Often, given the nature of the ED setting (and the brief duration of patient stays), decisions regarding psychiatric intervention and treatment must be made on the basis of symptoms rather than on a definitive diagnosis. It is not expected (or recommended) that ED nurses (or physicians) label ED patients with definitive diagnoses that imply chronic mental illness. Many times the accurate diagnosis of a psychiatric disorder requires ongoing evaluation and cannot be made on the basis of a one-time contact. For this reason, the remainder of this chapter discusses the most prevalent emotional and behavioral manifestations of psychiatric crises or disorders and their emergency management. First, however, standards that are applicable to the treatment of all psychiatric patients in any setting, along with some precedent legal cases on which our current standards of care of psychiatric patients are based, are discussed. The chapter ends with a description of iatrogenic emergencies resulting from the use of psychotropic drug therapy.

STANDARDS OF CARE FOR PATIENTS WITH PSYCHIATRIC DISORDERS

The provision of safe and effective care for persons experiencing psychiatric crises must be primary goals for ED personnel. The modalities available for providing such care, however, are not always so clear-cut. As society's views toward psychiatric crises or illnesses evolve, so too do our laws. Balancing the rights of patients with their families' and society's rights is not an easy task and often poses a host of moral and ethical dilemmas. Hence, the emergency treatment (or lack of) of persons experiencing psychiatric crises poses a tremendous challenge to ED personnel. In an effort to guide treatment decisions for these people, the ED nurse should be familiar with ethical standards of care taught in schools of nursing, operational policies and procedures suggested by the setting in which he or she works, and also state and local mental health codes.

This section is not intended to identify the particular details of each state's mental health code, but to focus on behaviors that support the standards aimed at the delivery of safe and effective emergency psychiatric nursing care.

The Standards of Psychiatric and Mental Health Nursing Practice first published in 1973 by the American Nurses' Association, set forth guidelines (utilizing the nursing process as their structure) that are intended for the practice of psychiatric and mental health nursing regardless of setting. As the ED is a common setting for treatment of psychiatric patients, these standards are applicable to the ED nurse.

For your convenience, the standards themselves (as revised in 1982) are listed without rationale or detail in Table 24–3. The reader is referred to the official publication for full details.

It is suggested in the aforementioned publication that the Standards of Psychiatric and Mental Health Nursing Practice be used along with ANA publications entitled Standards of Nursing Practice; Statement on Psychiatric and Mental Health Nursing Practice; Nursing: A Social Policy Statement; and Code for Nurses with Interpretive Statements.

The standards outlined in Table 24–3 and the preceding discussion are not intended to serve as a legal guide to practice but are intended to be a matrix for activities carried out by the ED nurse when participating in the care of psychiatric patients in the ED setting.

Although the ED nurse may not have the occasion to write detailed care plans and provide personally for all of the standards outlined in Table 24–3, he or she should be aware of them and also of the major legal issues related to the delivery of care of psychiatric patients. These issues include (but are not limited to): (1) the right to treatment, (2) the expectation that involuntary treatment will effect an improvement in condition, and (3) public safety and the rights of others.

Several recent court decisions have related to the right of patients to treatment (Wilson and Kneisl 1983). For example, cases such as *Rawse vs. Cameron* and *Mason vs. Bridgewater* illustrate the right to treatment while hospitalized. Cases such as *Wyatt vs. Stickney* and *Wyatt vs. Anderhalt* point out that patients held involuntarily have a constitutional right to specialized treatment that offers an opportunity for improvement or a cure (Wilson and Kneisl 1983). The case of *Donaldson vs. O'Connor* has ruled that it is a constitutional right not to be treated if the patient can be safe

TABLE 24-3
ANA Standards of Psychiatric and Mental Health Nursing Practice

---

Professional Practice Standards
   I. *Theory:* The nurse applies appropriate theory that is scientifically sound as a basis for decisions regarding nursing practice.
  II. *Data Collection:* The nurse continuously collects data that are comprehensive, accurate, and systematic.
 III. *Diagnosis:* The nurse utilizes nursing diagnoses or standard classifications of mental disorders to express conclusions supported by recorded assessment data and current scientific premises.
  IV. *Planning:* The nurse develops a nursing case plan with specific goals and interventions delineating nursing actions unique to each client's needs.
   V. *Intervention:* The nurse intervenes as guided by the nursing care plan to implement nursing actions that promote, maintain, or restore physical and mental health, prevent illness, and effect rehabilitation.
      A. *Intervention: Psychotherapeutic Interventions* — The nurse uses pychotherapeutic interventions to assist clients in regaining or improving their previous coping abilities and to prevent further disability.
      B. *Intervention: Health Teaching* — The nurse assists clients, families, and groups to achieve satisfying and productive patterns of living through health teaching.
      C. *Intervention: Activities of Daily Living* — The nurse uses the activities of daily living in a goal-directed way to foster adequate self-care and physical and mental well-being of clients.
      D. *Intervention: Somatic Therapies* — The nurse uses knowledge of somatic therapies and applies related clinical skills in working with clients.
      E. *Intervention: Therapeutic Environment* — The nurse provides, structures, and maintains a therapeutic environment in collaboration with the client and other health care providers.
      F.* *Intervention: Psychotherapy* — The nurse utilizes advanced clinical expertise in individualized group and family psychotherapy, child psychotherapy, and other treatment modalities to function as a psychotherapist and recognizes professional accountability for nursing practice.
  VI. *Evaluation:* The nurse evaluates client responses to nursing actions in order to revise the data base, nursing diagnoses, and nursing care plan.
      In addition to providing direct nursing care (in accordance with the professional practice standards listed above) to patients experiencing psychiatric crises, the ED staff must also be accountable for the following professional performance standards.
Professional Performance Standards
 VII. *Peer Review:* The nurse participates in peer review and other means of evaluation to ensure quality of nursing care provided for clients.
VIII. *Continuing Education:* The nurse assumes responsibility for continuing education and professional development and contributes to the professional growth of others.
  IX. *Interdisciplinary Collaboration:* The nurse collaborates with other health care providers in assessing, planning, implementing, and evaluating programs and other mental health activities.
   X.* *Utilization of Community Health Systems:* The nurse participates with other members of the community in assessing, planning, implementing, and evaluating mental health services and community systems that include the promotion of the broad continuum of primary, secondary, and tertiary prevention of mental illness.
  XI. *Research:* The nurse contributes to nursing and the mental health field through innovations in theory and practice and participation in research.

   Source: From American Nurses' Association. 1982. Standards of Psychiatric and Mental Health Nursing Practice. Kansas City, American Nurses' Association, 3–19.
      * Standards that apply particularly to the specialist.

without it. Other landmark cases have set precedents for issues such as right of refusal of psychiatric medications, nonemergency seclusion, and administration of medication. Public safety must be considered, as must patient confidentiality in rendering treatment.

As mentioned previously, it is up to the nurse to identify the details of the mental health code in the locale in which he or she works. Here we review the general types of admission to hospitals: informal voluntary, voluntary, and involuntary. The nurse, however, must bear in mind that each state's laws may differ.

Informal voluntary admission is the least restrictive type of admission and is similar to a medical admission. A verbal request is used for admission and discharge.

Voluntary admission is more restrictive and requires the patient or patient's guardian to choose in writing to be admitted. All but two states have a grace period for recession of consent, which can last from 48 hours to 15 days. Each practice setting should be checked on the particulars related to this type of admission.

Involuntary admission is the most restrictive type of admission, and within this category, there are several types of involuntary confinement. These include emergency, observational, and indeterminate. Times and conditions of each may vary; however, the basic reason for such admissions is to provide care for those who are a danger to themselves or to others, and to determine whether the patients are competent or not (Wilson and Kneisl 1983). Formal papers of commitment, which contain clear reasons for confinement as well as other requirements dictated by law, must be filed. The nurse should contact the facility and local government for laws and policies regarding documentation of such commitment.

In summary, patients have the right to treatment while hospitalized in the least restrictive and most humane environment. They or their guardians have the right to refuse treatment so long as they are in no danger of harming themselves or others. If the patient is dangerous to self or others, protection of the patient and others becomes the priority. If the patient is committed, issues of competency, treatment (with expected outcomes effected in the least restricted way), and finally, consideration of the risks versus benefits of treatment must be documented accurately.

COMMON EMOTIONAL OR BEHAVIORAL MANIFESTATIONS OF PSYCHIATRIC CRISES OR DISORDERS

Emotional Responses to Stressful Events

Sudden illness, traumatic injury, and untimely death are frequent occurrences in EDs that evoke a wide range of emotional responses in both victims of these occurrences and their significant others. Among these are anger, hostility, guilt, and fear. The display of these emotions, however, does not necessarily constitute a crisis (crisis being characterized by escalating levels of tension and anxiety with resulting cognitive, emotional, and behavioral disorganization); rather they are often "normal" responses to stressful events. According to Aguilera and Messick (1986), what is significant in determining whether a person's response to a stressful event will evolve into a crisis is the interplay between the following three balancing factors: (1) the person's perception of the event, (2) his or her available support systems, and (3) his or her functional coping mechanisms (Table 24–4). ED nurses are in a position to have a therapeutic impact on these balancing factors when a person is experiencing a stressful life event, thereby diminishing the likelihood that a dysfunctional crisis will develop. One specific approach to accomplishing this goal is that of crisis intervention. Therefore, prior to discussing the assessment and management of grossly overt psychopathology, attention is directed toward the assessment and management of persons experiencing stressful life events and how concepts of crisis intervention may be used by the ED nurse to aid such people.

TABLE 24–4
The Effect of Balancing Factors on a Stressful Event

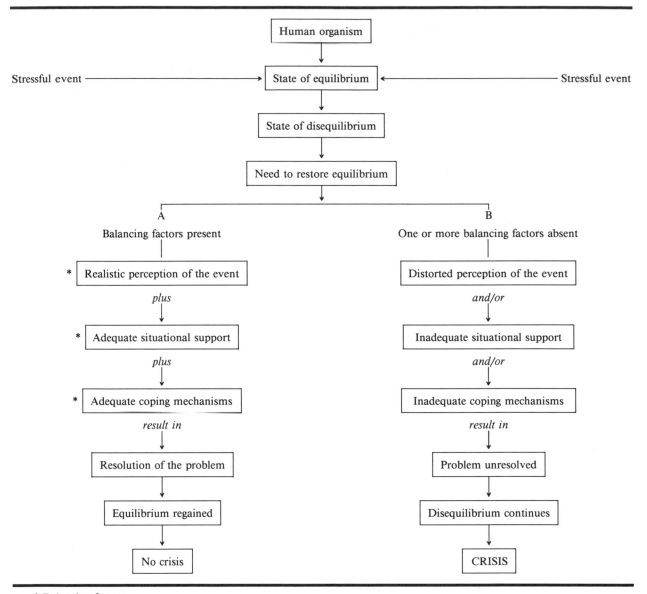

* Balancing factors.
Source: Adapted by permission from: Aguilera D, Messick J, Crisis Intervention: Theory and Methodology, St. Louis, 1986, The C.V. Mosby Co.

A primary feature of crisis intervention is that it focuses on prevention and resolution of an impending or immediate crisis, as opposed to the restructuring of a person's basic personality via long-term psychotherapy. The approach used in crisis intervention is much like that of the nursing process: assessing, planning, intervening, and evaluating.

During the assessment stage of crisis intervention, data must be collected in an attempt to determine the cause of a patient's present feeling state, in addition to information on the balancing factors that influence either the development or the resolution of crisis. Goal-directed interviewing and careful listening are imperative in assisting the person to identify the link between his or her feeling state and the stressful event causing it. Often this link is overtly evident, (e.g., hysteria or confusion following the sudden death of a spouse), but other times it is not.

Appropriate questions to ask include "What brought you to the emergency room?", "When did you start to feel this way?" and "Has anything changed in your life recently?" These may assist the ED nurse in helping the patient identify the link between current symptoms and their causes. Identifying this link in and of itself is often helpful in alleviating some of the patient's anxiety and fear. Listening and acknowledging the thoughts and feelings of the patient, as well as reassuring him or her that he or she is not alone, also are helpful.

Exploration of the person's past experiences and coping mechanisms and identification of his or her available support systems also are important. Appropriate questions include "Has anything like this ever happened to you in the past?" or "How do you usually handle stress?" Often people are not even aware of how they have coped in the past and what has helped them. Bringing these things into their consciousness helps them realize that they have coped with stress in the past and could do it again.

It is also necessary to determine what the person's support systems are. Is there anyone to whom the person is close? Does the person live with someone else? In whom can he or she confide? Cultural variables that may influence the reliance a person places on his or her support systems also must be considered.

Once the aforementioned information is obtained, the ED nurse can appropriately plan therapeutic intervention. It is unrealistic, however, to think that crisis can be thwarted in the ED by the ED nurse for every patient experiencing a stressful life event. Therefore, planning therapeutic intervention for these persons must be realistic and incorporate assessment data obtained relating to the aforementioned balancing factors. Often the most therapeutic interventions that the ED nurse can implement are those of assisting the person in identifying his or her coping abilities and support systems and offering community and follow-up referrals for social services that may benefit the patient and his or her significant others. Some therapeutic principles that should guide the ED nurse during interactions with patients or their significant others experiencing stressful life events include the following:

1. Give permission to patients and their significant others to experience, recognize, and express emotion (this assists them in developing an awareness of their feelings and supports the beginnings of the normal grief process).

2. Observe and acknowledge feelings accompanying stressful life events.

3. Describe clearly each person's strengths and capabilities. Support helpful aspects of each which the persons possess.

In addition to the aforementioned therapeutic principles, which may be applied to any person experiencing a stressful life event, it is imperative that the ED nurse be able to interact with the surviving significant others following a loved one's death. Some suggestions follow.

1. Following a death, if significant others are not present in the ED, they should be contacted immediately. They should be told that the patient was seriously ill or

injured and was brought into the ED in critical condition. They should be asked to come to the ED as soon as possible. Every effort should be made so that notification of a death is not given over the telephone.

2. If significant others are present in the ED (or upon their arrival), they should be brought into a quiet room and told of the patient's death by the physician. The nurse should be present during this time so that he or she may offer additional support or clarification if needed. (A factual account of the events and interventions preceding the patient's death should be given.)

3. Reactions of shock, disbelief, denial, hysteria, crying out, or confusion may be manifested by surviving significant others. These reactions by significant others should be allowed and even encouraged in order to express these emotions and thoughts. The quiet presence of a nurse is often helpful. Sedation should be avoided if possible, as oversedation may delay the normal grieving process.

4. Significant others should be allowed to see the deceased person after blood, emesis, or any other material is cleaned away. If any gross disfigurement is present, however, they should be prepared beforehand by the nurse prior to viewing the body. Viewing the body often assists survivors to acknowledge the death and progress through the grieving process.

5. Survivors should be discouraged from going home alone, especially if severely distraught. A friend or relative should be encouraged to stay with the grieving person, as suicide among survivors of sudden death and trauma is a very real concern. A clergy person or social worker may be called to assist and support the surviving significant other(s) while necessary arrangements are being made.

The evaluation of how well a person has coped with a stressful life event often cannot be assessed in the ED. Ideally, however, successful coping results in the person's achieving an even higher level of functioning, coping ability, and personality integration than prior to the event. At the very minimum, however, it is hoped that the person will return to at least his or her previous level of functioning and coping ability and that appropriate and therapeutic emergency nursing interventions contributed to that outcome. Often follow-up calls in the succeeding days, weeks, and months to these persons will allow the nurse to make this determination.

Anxiety

Anxiety is an emotional sense of impending doom, a mental sense of known or unknown terror, or fear of losing one's mind. Anxiety may range in severity from mild to panic and is manifested by a multitude of physiologic and psychologic behaviors that reflect the severity of the anxiety. Anxiety is a universal problem. Everyone has experienced it to some degree; however, it becomes pathologic when it becomes so severe that it interferes with a person's ability to function and make decisions.

Etiology

Anxiety may be situational, a symptom of other illnesses or conditions (medical or psychiatric), or a disorder in itself. Situational anxiety in ED patients and their significant others is not uncommon and may be precipitated or provoked by sudden, unexpected medical or traumatic events, the unfamiliarity of the hospital environment and treatment protocols, the discomforts of illness and injury, or the uncertainty of recovery. Illnesses in which anxiety may be a prominent feature include angina pectoris, hypoglycemia, chronic obstructive pulmonary disease (COPD), hyperthyroidism, and tachydysrhythmias. Anxiety may also be evident with excessive caffeine intake, substance abuse (e.g., cocaine, amphetamines), and substance abuse withdrawal (e.g., alcohol, barbiturates). Specific psychiatric conditions in which anxiety can be a component are phobias, hyperventilation syndrome, generalized anxiety disorder, alcohol amnestic disorder, fugue states, the schizophrenias, conversion disorder, posttraumatic stress disorder, and drug intoxication. Anxiety as a disorder itself is usually chronic, and research suggests there may be a genetic basis for its origin (Waldinger 1986, 186).

Pathophysiology

Anxiety can be classified according to its level of severity: mild, moderate, severe, or panic (Wilson and Kneisl, 1983). Each level has a marked effect on how a person is able to interact with, interpret, and process information relating to his or her environment and his or her self.

In mild anxiety, a person's sense of alertness and observation are increased. The perceptual field is actually enlarged and he or she is motivated toward optimal functioning. A mild degree of anxiety is at times beneficial. As anxiety progresses to moderate degree, however, the perceptual field narrows. The person can concentrate on only one task or event and filters out all other insignificant stimuli. Cognitive abilities decrease. If anxiety progresses to the level of severe, the person's perceptions are markedly skewed. He or she may be able to concentrate on only a specific detail of a task or event, or he or she may even focus on a multitude of insignificant details. Panic is the ultimate manifestation of anxiety, which evolves into complete disorganization and loss of control. The patient at this stage is terrified and often is in need of external controls to avoid harm.

Clinical Manifestations

Anxiety in any given person may be experienced and manifested in a multitude of ways reflective of the level of anxiety experienced. Common subjective complaints that patients may exhibit include feelings of jumpiness, nervousness, apprehension, and even the fear of "going crazy." The sensations of butterflies in one's stomach, of "jelly" legs, of numbness of the extremities, and of one's hair standing on edge are also common complaints. Objective findings often reveal a person who is perspiring with cool and clammy skin and who is tachycardic and tachypneic. In severe anxiety and panic states delusions and hallucinations may also be evident. Because patients who are acutely anxious are also often quite agitated, they should be brought to the treatment area as soon as possible. The nurse may then determine the circumstances surrounding the onset of anxiety and conduct a thorough physical examination to rule out an organic cause. In attempting to rule out organic causes of anxiety, it is helpful for the ED nurse to realize that tachycardia in persons experiencing panic usually does not exceed 140 beats/minute, whereas in paroxysmal supraventricular tachycardias (SVT) it often does (Urbaitis 1983). Additionally, SVT is more likely to respond to vagal stimulation than tachycardia with anxiety as its origin.

Treatment and Nursing Care

Assessment of the meaning of anxiety to the person experiencing it is critical to its proper management, which according to Walker (1983) is best accomplished via the following activities: (1) establishment of an atmosphere conducive to free discussion of the patient's problems, (2) active listening by the ED nurse with acknowledgment of the patient's physical and emotional complaints, (3) an understanding of the events associated with the anxiety, and (4) identification of the ways in which the patient has successfully and unsuccessfully dealt with similar experiences in the past. Additionally, it is imperative that the nature of the anxiety be identified, especially when keeping in mind that anxiety may be a manifestation of a serious organic disease or that it may escalate, contributing to significant psychiatric decompensation for the patient.

Anxiety, Related to

- **Situational Stress, Underlying Medical or Psychiatric Disorder, or Anxiety Disorder**

Effective intervention strategies for patients experiencing anxiety support the following goals: (1) identify the nature of the anxiety so that the appropriate actions are taken to resolve it, and (2) arrange follow-up care. Whatever the cause, the following guidelines are effective in dealing with the anxious patient:

1. Allow the patient to ventilate his or her concerns.
2. Identify the nature of the anxiety.
3. Provide a safe environment for the patient on arrival to the ED and throughout his or her ED stay.
4. Reduce external sources of stimulation, and if a panic attack occurs, on consultation with the physician, rebreathing into a paper bag may be necessary to reduce further escalation.
5. Use problem-solving approaches to avoid medication dependency and identify practical solutions to problems.
6. Administer antianxiety agents as ordered, and monitor their response.
7. Medical treatments as ordered are given for organic causes of anxiety.
8. Assist in coordinating necessary support services for aftercare (e.g., social services, family assistance, outpatient follow-up).

The blanket use of antianxiety agents is usually avoided because they can mask an organic cause or cause the patient to put off dealing with the underlying conflict. Patients may be more likely to follow up with outpatient treatment when support succeeds in reducing anxiety, drugs are de-emphasized, and follow-up is arranged.

In summary, regardless of the cause, the patient experiencing anxiety requires constant monitoring, reflective listening, problem solving, possible medication, medical intervention for organic causes, and follow-up to reduce the possibility of continued dysfunction.

Depression

Depression is a universal problem, which will affect most people at one time or another in the course of their lives. It is classified as an affective disorder that is most commonly characterized by a saddened mood, loss of interest in activities that previously provided pleasure, and alterations in sleep, appetite, and digestive or eliminatory patterns. The cause, manifestations, intensities, and duration of depression may vary in any given person, or even within the same person at different times. As a result, the prevalence of depression is difficult to determine.

Etiology and Pathophysiology

It is beyond the scope of this book to discuss all of the theories, concepts, and potential causes of depression. However, stated most simply, depression may be classified as resulting from either endogenous or exogenous causes. Endogenous causes suggest that there is a physiologic basis for depression, thereby supporting biochemical and genetic theories of depression. Exogenous causes arise from events without a physiologic basis and suggest a more psychoanalytic approach to depression, although medications may be used in these cases as well. Examples include grief reactions and responses to illness.

Regardless of cause, it is critical for ED nurses to recognize the intense pain and suffering that depressed persons experience and that the potential link which depression has with suicide is very real.

Clinical Manifestations

Depressed persons may come to the ED exhibiting a wide range of symptoms, depending on the nature and severity of their depression. Subjective symptoms may include feelings of sadness; a lack of interest and motivation in work, recreational, or family activities; a sense of helplessness, hopelessness, and worthlessness; and a diminished sense of pleasure when performing activities that previously were enjoyable. Alterations in sleeping, eating, or eliminatory patterns are usually present, and often a decrease in libido occurs. Feelings of self-reproach, deprecation, and low self-esteem are usually evident. Objective observations often reveal a quiet, withdrawn individual with a blunted or flat affect and saddened mood. Poor posture, slow gait, and generalized psychomotor retardation or agitation may also be evident. Disturbances in thought content and processes (e.g., delusions, ruminations, or hallucinations) and distorted perceptions of themselves and their environment may also be present.

TABLE 24-5
Factors Associated with Increased Lethality or Severity of a Suicide Plan or Attempt

Details of suicide plan or attempt carefully thought out over time
Believes or believed plan or attempt could or would be successful
Precautions considered or taken to avoid interruption
Precautions considered or taken to avoid discovery
Final arrangements planned or completed (e.g., purchasing life insurance, writing suicide note, saying
    goodbye to significant others)
Means of carrying out suicide plan available
Plan or method leaves little or no opportunity for survival or reversal
Wish to die is strong or wish to live is minimal or absent
In addition to the foregoing, other indications of ongoing suicide risk in persons who have already
    attempted suicide include
    Suicide attempt did not accomplish what it was intended to (e.g., death, reaction from significant others)
    Patient expresses regret at being discovered or recovered

The nurse must not forget that, in addition to the aforementioned symptoms, depression is often manifested as physical ailments and somatizations. Low back pain, fatigue, and headaches are commonly reported in depressed patients. Additionally, nurses must recognize that depressed patients do get physically sick and that physical illness may exacerbate underlying depression.

Once depression is identified in a patient, assessment of that person's suicide risk is imperative—especially when it is realized that the lifetime incidence of suicide among depressed persons is 15 per cent (Guze and Robins 1970).* Assessment of suicide risk, however, is no easy task. Measurement scales that focus on seriousness of intent (Pierce 1981; Weisman and Worden 1972), ideation (Beck et al 1979), and even degree of hopelessness (Beck et al 1974)—which is an important variable linking depression to suicide (Beck et al 1975)—have been developed in an attempt to identify persons at greatest risk for suicide. Key factors indicative of increased lethality (severity) of suicide behavior are listed in Table 24-5. Those items correlated most positively with hopelessness are listed in Table 24-6.

TABLE 24-6
Attitudes Positively Correlated with Hopelessness

I might as well give up because I can't make things better for myself
I can't imagine what my life would be like in 10 years
My future seems dark to me
I just don't get the breaks, and there's no reason to believe I will in the future
All I can see ahead of me is unpleasantness rather than pleasantness
I don't expect to get what I really want
Things just don't work out the way I want them to
I never get what I want, so it is foolish to want anything
It's very unlikely that I will get any real satisfaction in the future
The future seems vague and uncertain to me
There's no use in really trying to get something I want because I probably won't get it

Source: From Beck AT, Weissman A, Lester D, et al. 1974. J Consult Clin Psychol 42:862.

---

* Although depression has clearly been implicated as a significant precursor in completed suicide attempts, it is by no means the predominant feature present in all suicide attempts (Rund and Hutzler 1983). Therefore, suicide risk assessment should not be limited only to those persons with depression.

TABLE 24–7
High-Risk Factors Associated with Suicidal Behavior

Demographic Factors

Adolescence or older than 45 years
Male
White
Separated, divorced, or widowed
Living alone
Unemployed

Antecedent Life Circumstances

Previous suicide attempts
   Recent attempt(s) with serious intent
   Previous attempt(s) with resultant physical or mental sequelae
   Previous attempt(s) that did not effect desired response(s)
Family history of suicide or suicide attempts
Inadequate or unavailable support systems
Major life changes
   Major losses (e.g., spouse, job, money)
   Major illnesses (of self or significant others)

Psychiatric Conditions

Depressive illnesses
Alcoholism
Schizophrenia

Source: Adapted with permission of Macmillan Publishing Company from Psychiatric Emergencies: Nursing Assessment and Intervention (p. 91) by S. Talley, M.C. King. Copyright 1984 by Macmillan Publishing Company.

Demographic and social characteristics as well as antecedent life circumstances (Sletten and Barton, 1979; Tuckman and Youngman, 1968) and psychiatric conditions (Barraclough et al 1974; Dorpat and Ripley, 1960; Kraft and Babigian, 1976) most commonly correlated with suicidal behavior have also been identified and are listed in Table 24–7.

Although the factors outlined in Tables 24–5 to 24–7 have generally been accepted as characteristic of persons exhibiting high suicide risk, unfortunately many of them are nonspecific and are also widely represented in the general population (e.g., white men living alone). As such, the ED nurse who is aware of high-risk characteristics but who also recognizes that the absence of them does not necessarily guarantee low risk is in the best position to recognize suicide potential, fostering the likelihood of therapeutic intervention and suicide prevention.

Treatment and Nursing Care

The therapeutic interventions used in the treatment of depressed patients in the ED must strive to achieve the following goals:

1. Medical stabilization if a suicide attempt was made.
2. Identification of persons at continued or future risk of suicide.
3. Maintenance of a safe environment for suicidal people.

4. Identification of the need for hospitalization.

5. Reduction, diffusion, or elimination of the immediate mental anguish and suffering that depressed persons experience.

Potential for Injury, Related to

- **Consequences of Suicide Attempt**
- **Suicide Risk**

If the person has attempted suicide and a life-threatening condition is either in danger of occurring or present, stage I care must be instituted. A brief, yet thorough history and physical examination must be undertaken with treatment directed at the presenting injury(ies). Intravenous access must immediately be established. Airway, breathing, and circulatory status must be supported and scrupulously monitored. Intubation equipment should be readily available. Depending on the nature of the suicide attempt, interventions to repair, reverse, or neutralize the effects of the attempt must be instituted. If wrists were slashed and blood loss is significant, the wounds must be sutured and extracellular fluid volume replaced. Gunshot wounds may require surgery and the patient should be prepared for it. In the case of a drug overdose, syrup of ipecac may need to be given if the patient is still alert, followed by gastric lavage. (See Chap. 26.) Simple explanations and clear instructions relating to what is being done and what needs to be done should be communicated to both the patient and significant others.

Awareness of the risk factors and variables outlined in Tables 24–5 to 24–7 should aid the ED nurse in identifying those persons who are at continued or future risk of suicide. Direct questioning, uncomfortable as it may be, is the best way to ascertain such information. Appropriate questions to ask include "Do you feel things will never get better?", "Have you ever thought of ending your life?", or "Do you wish you were dead?" If a positive response is elicited, the nurse should then ask "Have you thought of how you would end your life?" or "Have you made any plans to end your life?" Those who have attempted suicide and who express regret at being found, whose method was very likely to have caused death in the absence of immediate medical intervention, and who have a poor attitude toward help are probably at high risk for repeated attempts. Such persons need to be protected from harm and, if they are not willing to be hospitalized voluntarily, will require commitment. Other persons who may not be deemed high suicide risks but who have become dysfunctional as a result of depression, and who have inadequate support systems and coping mechanisms, also are candidates for hospitalization.

The following therapeutic guidelines may be utilized by the ED nurse in an effort to diminish a depressed or suicidal person's anguish:

1. Reassure the patient that depression is reversible.

2. Assist the person in identifying and exploring choices he or she may have as well as available support systems, which may not be overtly obvious to him or her.

3. Convey an attitude of compassion, empathy, and understanding.

4. Do not attempt to talk a patient out of his or her depression. (Recognize that people are no more able to "snap out" of depression than they are able to "snap out" of a diabetic coma.)

5. If a person has attempted suicide, point out his or her ambiguity about death (e.g., the suicide attempt demonstrated a wish to die whereas the person's survival demonstrates a wish to live).

Occasionally, depressed persons who do not display high-risk suicidal behaviors, who have available support systems, and who declare a willingness to seek help may be discharged home. For these persons appropriate follow-up must be arranged.

The initiation of antidepressant drug therapy for depressed persons on discharge from the ED is usually not recommended for several reasons. First and foremost, therapeutic responses to antidepressants are not immediate. Their desired effects are usually not achieved for several weeks to months following their initiation, during which time the patient's progress should be closely monitored. Second, antidepressant overdoses may be lethal. Therefore, if they are prescribed from the ED, only a limited number of pills should be dispensed. Appropriate follow-up for continuation of therapy must then be arranged.

Because in rare instances antidepressant therapy is initiated in the ED, and because often persons on antidepressant therapy may come to the ED with problems directly related to their usage, some discussion of antidepressants is in order.

Antidepressants

Antidepressants, when properly used, can literally be life-saving for some patients with severe depressions. In many cases, vegetative symptoms, including severe insomnia, anorexia, depressed mood, and low energy can be relieved to allow a depressed patient to become functional again if these symptoms have interfered with the activities of daily life. Improper use of medications can result in a poor response at best, and in serious side effects or death at worst, if overdoses are taken.

There are several classes of antidepressants, each with a different chemical structure and mode of action. As research continues others may be added. The basic function of antidepressants is to diminish symptoms of depression by increasing the availability of certain brain neurotransmitters (e.g., norepinephrine and serotonin) whose absence is implicated in causation of depressive symptoms. The antidepressant agents used today can bring dramatic relief within weeks but are not entirely without side effects. These are discussed in more detail later. According to Gold and Hamlin (1986), of particular current interest is the evolving information that dysfunction of catecholaminergic neurons may be responsible for both depression and a host of other psychiatric disorders.

One major class of antidepressants is the tricyclics (TCA), so named for their chemical structure. Although their exact mechanism of action is not known, it is believed that they exert their effect by interfering with the reuptake of norepinephrine, subsequently potentiating catecholamine action. Of this class, drugs currently in use are imipramine (Tofranil), amitriptyline (Elavil), desipramine (Norpramin, Pertofrane), nortriptyline (Aventyl), doxepin (Sinequan), and protriptyline (Vivactil). Tetracyclic antidepressants, too, are so named because of their chemical structure. Maprotiline (Ludiomil) is an example. Other medications that are thought to exert some antidepressant effects are carbamazepine (Tegretol), alprazolam (Xanax), and lithium carbonate (Lithane, Lithonate, Eskalith). Although these do not have primary use as antidepressants, their effect may be of utility in the search for viable treatment alternatives in resistant patients.

Kaplan and Sadock (1985) state that 70 per cent of depressed patients respond to TCAs. Gold and Hamlin (1986) note that 35 to 50 per cent of patients with endogenous depression treated with TCAs fail to respond. Several factors may be responsible for this, including variability in established diagnosis, degree of response, and other possible ameliorating factors. In any case, TCAs, to be optimally effective, must be prescribed with consistency of dose, attention to blood levels, and enough time to evaluate the effects. In establishing efficacy, it is suggested that the drug of choice be prescribed at a dose within therapeutic range and the blood level of that drug be maintained within its therapeutic range for 21 consecutive days to determine whether the patient's symptoms are responsive or not to the drug. After that time, another drug in the same class may be tried. On the average, plasma half-life of the TCAs is between 16 and 24 hours, but it can be longer, even up to 5 days after the last dose.

Another major class of antidepressants is the monoamine oxidase inhibitors (MAOIs). TCAs and MAOIs are not usually prescribed together, and some combinations of them may produce potentially serious side effects. Some clinicians may combine certain of these drugs to produce desired effects; however, this would require exquisite supervision. MAOIs were first developed in the 1950s, with iproniazid being the first. Currently, the most commonly used MAOIs are phenelzine (Nardil) and tranylcypromine (Parnate). MAOIs exert their effects by inhibiting monoamine oxidase (MAO), an enzyme required for the breakdown of norepinephrine. As a result, levels of norepinephrine increase, diminishing depressive symptoms. MAO is also responsible for the breakdown of other amines: serotonin, dopamine, and tyramine. With the inhibition of MAO, levels of the aforementioned amines rise. Sympathomimetic activity increases, and hypertension may ensue. Subsequent ingestion of foods, beverages, or medications that contain tyramine, dopamine, or epinephrine may further potentiate the effects of MAOIs, resulting in hypertensive crisis. Therefore, patients on MAOIs must be cautioned to avoid foods, beverages, and drugs which contain these substances (Table 24–8).

As noted previously, antidepressants, although often highly effective, are not without side effects. Side effects common to the TCAs are associated with their action in inhibiting reuptake of norepinephrine and their atropine-like effects. These include dry mouth, blurred vision, palpitations, postural hypotension, tachycardia, dizziness, nausea, vomiting, faintness, constipation, aggravation of narrow angle glaucoma, and edema. Rarer side effects of paralytic ileus, urinary retention, and agranulocytosis have been documented. TCAs also may have a quinidine-like effect and act on electrical conduction of the heart. Side effects associated with the MAOIs are precipitation of latent mania, restlessness, anxiety, agitation, confusion, irritability, and possible paranoia (Kaplan and Sadock 1985).

Psychosis

Psychotic patients experience impaired reality testing. They are unable to distinguish between what is real and what is not. Their thought content and processes are disordered and often characterized by hallucinations, delusions, ideas of reference, thought broadcasting, and thought insertion.

TABLE 24-8
Foods, Beverages, and Drugs to be Avoided While Taking MAOIs*

Foods

Broad beans (lima, kidney, and Italian green beans)
Raisins
Bananas
Avocados
Aged cheese (cheddar)
Yeast preparations (bread allowed)
Licorice
Sour cream
Chocolate
Pickled herring
Yogurt
Foods and seasonings that contain monosodium glutamate (soy sauce, meat tenderizers)
Peanuts
Peanut butter
Pizza
Beef liver
Smoked salmon

Beverages

Whiskey
Cider
Beer
Wine
Caffeinated beverages
    Soda
    Coffee
    Tea

Medications

Amphetamines (e.g., diet pills)
Narcotic analgesics
Barbiturates and sedatives
Tranquilizers
Diuretics
L-Dopa
Cold remedies (e.g., antihistamines, decongestants, cough medicine)
Tricyclic antidepressants
Methyldopa

   * The foods, beverages, and drugs listed should be avoided while taking MAOIs and for at least 2 weeks after discontinuing their use.
   Source: Adapted by permission of Elsevier Science Publishing Co., Inc. from Hart C, Turner MS, Orfitelli MK, et al. 1981. Introduction to Psychotropic Drugs, 71. Copyright 1981 by Medical Examination Publishing Company, Inc.

Etiology

Currently there are many theories relating to the cause of major mental illnesses in which psychosis is a prominent feature. Most are either psychoanalytic, biochemical, biologic, or genetic in nature. However, discussion of these theories is not relevant here as the emergency management of psychotic persons does not require detailed understanding of causation. What is imperative for the ED nurse is that he or she be able to differentiate psychosis that results from a potentially reversible organic cause from psychosis that is more functional in nature (e.g., schizophrenia). Additionally, the ED nurse should be able to initiate therapeutic interventions for psychotic persons regardless of cause.

Clinical Manifestations

Recognizing persons with florid psychosis in the ED usually is not difficult. Overt manifestations are present in speech and behavior. The chief complaints and HPIs of such persons are usually disorganized, chaotic, and difficult to understand. This is because their attempts to communicate rationally are hampered by psychotic thinking and abnormal speech patterns. It is not uncommon for psychotic people be brought to the ED by significant others.

Evidence of hallucinations may be apparent in the behavior. Persons experiencing hallucinations of any type may appear preoccupied and are unable to follow or concentrate on the conversation at hand. They may appear to be intently listening or to be cautious in the absence of environmental stimuli that warrant intense listening or caution. Additionally, psychotic patients may talk to themselves.

In contrast, other psychotic persons may have much more subtle symptoms. Identification of such patients may be possible only after detailed interviewing and direct questioning.

Asking patients if they ever hear voices when no one else is present or if they ever see strange things is appropriate. If their answers are affirmative, the nurse should ask further questions as to what the voices say or what they see that seems strange.

Treatment and Nursing Care

Treatment for persons with psychoses first and foremost must be based on whether or not an organic cause has been identified. If so, treatment must be aimed at correction of this cause. Generally speaking, organic causes of psychoses are more likely to have an abrupt onset with an abnormal mental status examination and less bizarre delusions than functional causes of psychoses (Rund and Hutzler 1983). Although management principles for all psychotic persons are similar (diminishing the fear and potential harm to self or others in response to alterations in a person's thought content and perception), pharmacologic intervention may differ depending on the origin of symptoms. For example, psychotropic drug therapy may not be used at all or may be cautiously used in a patient experiencing transient psychosis resulting from the use of amphetamines or hallucinogenic drugs.

Fear, Related to

- **Alteration in Thought Content Secondary to Delusions, Ideas of Reference, Thought Broadcasting, or Thought Insertion**
- **Alteration in Perception Secondary to Hallucinations or Illusions**

Fear in a person with alterations or distortions in his or her thought content or perceptions is highly dependent on the nature of these alterations or distortions.

Delusions may be grandiose, sexual, religious, paranoid, or somatic in nature. Although all are characterized by false, fixed beliefs that are misinterpretations and distortions of reality, those that are paranoid or somatic in nature are usually most frightening. People with delusions may believe that the FBI is out to get them or that they are surely dying of a dreaded disease. Beliefs that external events have special significance to them, that other people are able to read their thoughts, or that others are able to control their thoughts are likewise frightening to these people.

The presence of hallucinations (auditory, visual, tactile, gustatory, or olfactory) or illusions also contributes to fear in psychotic persons. They may be hearing accusatory voices and threats directed at them or they may be seeing snakes crawling all over them. It is understandable how frightening these distorted thoughts and perceptions must be to the patient.

Therapeutic principles that must guide the ED nurse in caring for persons experiencing fear related to distortions in thought content and perception include the following:

1. Attempt to establish a trusting relationship with the patient. Reassure him or her that you want to help and that he or she is in a safe place now and will not be harmed.

2. Attempt to determine if there was a precipitating event that triggered the psychotic episode. If so, evaluate it thoroughly.

3. If an organic, reversible cause is identified, reassure the patient that his or her feelings and thoughts are temporary.

4. Minimize external stimulation. Psychotic persons may be having trouble processing thoughts and often are hearing voices. By decreasing external stimulation, you may help decrease sensory stimulation to which the patient may be responding.

5. Do not attempt to reason, challenge, or argue the patient out of his or her delusions or hallucinations. Often these patients need to believe their delusions in an attempt to decrease their anxiety and maintain control.

6. Do not imply that you believe the person's hallucinations or delusional system in an attempt to win his or her trust. Statements implying that you do not hear what the patient is hearing but you are interested in knowing what it is he or she is hearing are recommended.

7. Do not underestimate the significance of a person's psychotic thoughts. Remember they are very real to the patient and he or she cannot just "put them aside."

8. Unless restraint is required, physical contact with psychotic persons or sudden movements should be avoided as they may induce or validate the patient's fears.

Potential for Injury, Related to

- **Distorted Thought Content**
- **Distorted Perceptions**

The potential of psychotic people to inflict injury on themselves or others in response to their distorted thoughts or perceptions is a very real concern. It is appropriate to ask these persons directly what they plan to do about the voices they hear or things they see in an attempt to determine the likelihood that the persons will act on their distorted thoughts and perceptions. If it is deemed that the patient is potentially harmful to self or to others, and if the person is uncooperative, he or she may require physical restraint or rapid tranquilization with antipsychotic medication.

Physical restraint, when employed, should be done quickly in an organized and efficient manner. Four attendants should be assigned, to hold and restrain each of the patient's four extremities simultaneously. Additionally, one person (preferably the ED nurse) must take charge during the procedure to signal its initiation. Leather restraints should be used, and they should be fastened to the bed frames as opposed to the siderails. During the procedure the charge nurse should explain to the patient that he or she is being restrained to help him or her and for safety reasons, as opposed to punishment. Once all restraints are fastened and the patient is secure the charge nurse signals release to all the attendants assisting. Extremity pulses are then checked to ensure circulation remains intact. Men should be restrained with their legs apart for comfort and women with legs together. In every instance the patient's privacy should be respected (especially if clothing is restricted). The nurse is referred to the locality in which he or she practices for particulars related to policy and procedure there.

When rapid tranquilization of a patient is required, haloperidol (Haldol) is used most commonly. This is because Haldol is highly potent (thereby requiring a lower dose) and has strong antipsychotic properties, few cardiovascular side effects, and a rapid onset of action. It is usually administered at doses of 2.5-10 mg intramuscularly every 30 to 60 minutes until its desired effects are reached. Nursing responsibilities during such time include explanation of the rationale for therapy to the patient and to his or her significant others and close patient monitoring and documentation of the patient's responses to therapy (desired and adverse). Adverse effects that are most notable include hypotension, sedation, and acute dystonic reactions. These adverse effects are described in more detail later in this chapter with a full discussion of antipsychotic medication.

Mania

Mania is characterized by an abnormally increased expansiveness in a person's feeling, thinking, and doing. Reality testing and judgment are grossly impaired. As a result, if mania is not controlled, the patient is at risk of harming self or others.

Etiology

Manic behavior is most commonly the result of manic-depressive illness. Organic causes for its existence, however, must also be ruled out. Common considerations include endocrine abnormalities (e.g., hyperthyroidism), hypertensive disorders, amphetamine toxicity, and steroid psychosis.

Clinical Manifestations

Mania may be manifested by a wide array of behaviors. When mild, patients may appear humorous and gregarious. When severe, florid psychosis and grandiosity are present, often requiring restraint and rapid tranquilization. Typically, however, manic patients have elevated and expansive moods. Feelings of euphoria and elation may vacillate with feelings of irritability and hostility. The patient is usually very impulsive and can be loud, aggressive, and grandiose in his or her thinking. Speech is often pressured and characteristically reflects flight of ideas and grandiose delusions. These grandiose delusions put the patient at high-risk behavior (e.g., believing he or she can fly). Often, manic persons are insulting toward others, with expressions of sexual desires and frequent use of obscenities. They are distracted easily and place a great deal of significance on small details of their external environment.

During the history, it is not uncommon to find changes in dosage or compliance from persons who have been or are managed on lithium therapy.

Treatment and Nursing Care

Although, at times, it may be easy to find manic patients amusing, it is important that the ED nurse not get drawn into the patient's behavior. Giving attention to manic behavior may only serve to escalate it. Nursing care of these persons must center on protecting them (and others) from injury while measures to control mania are instituted.

Potential for Injury, Related to

- **Delusions of Grandeur**
- **Lack of Sleep**

Persons who are manic often are at high risk for injuring themselves or others as the result of their grandiose delusions and consequent impaired judgment and reckless behavior. They may believe they can fly and want to jump off a building, or they may overspend money, emptying their bank accounts. As a result, the suicidal or homicidal risk of these persons must be assessed. If it is strong, restraints may be required, as these patients are usually high elopement risks also. First, however, firm verbal limit setting should be attempted with continuous surveillance of the patient while he or she is in the ED. At all times, clear and simple explanations and directions should be provided to the patient and lengthy conversations avoided. Additionally, external stimuli should be minimized. Tranquilization with antipsychotic medication (most commonly Haldol) for persons who are severely manic may also be instituted to decrease agitation in response to external overstimulation. Hospitalization is most always required. Lithium levels should be obtained on all patients who have been or are on lithium carbonate therapy.

Although therapy with lithium carbonate is not usually initiated in the ED, its role in the management of mania or bipolar disorder (as defined by the Diagnostic and Statistical Manual, third edition) (American Psychiatric Association 1987), is significant. Lithium carbonate is a metallic salt, identified for use in controlling mood swings in the early 1970s. It is thought to have the ability to stabilize mood, thus reducing the possibility of elation and severe depression. Because lithium affects several body systems and since its therapeutic levels are close to its toxic levels, blood concentrations of the salt need to be obtained after the first week of therapy and at 2-

to 4-week intervals until stabilized, or more frequently at the discretion of the attending psychiatrist. Tegretol is used by some physicians for extremely resistant patients who fail to respond to lithium control. However, at this writing, this drug is still experimental and not widely approved for this use.

IATROGENIC EMERGENCIES RESULTING FROM PSYCHOTROPIC DRUG THERAPY

Although psychotropic drugs have revolutionized the treatment of major mental disorders, they are not without adverse effects and may, at times, produce emergencies in their own right. Consequently, it is imperative that ED nurses understand not only the indications and rationale for the administration of psychotropic drugs, but also how to manage the adverse reactions that can occur as a direct result of their use. Often, it is these adverse reactions that are the sole reason for which individuals seek emergency services. Adverse reactions that can be most deleterious to patients if undetected and left untreated will be discussed in this section.

Hypertensive Crisis

Hypertensive crisis (or Parnate-cheese reaction) as the result of MAOI use is truly a life-threatening occurrence.

Etiology

MAOIs exert their effects by inhibiting MAO, an enzyme responsible for the deamination of a variety of monoamines, primarily norepinephrine, dopamine, serotonin, epinephrine, and tyramine. When MAO is inhibited, levels of the aforementioned monoamines increase. Sympathomimetic activity is increased, and hypertension may ensue. Subsequent ingestion of foods, beverages, or medications that contain tyramine, dopamine, or epinephrine may further potentiate the effects of MAOIs, resulting in hypertensive crisis.

Clinical Manifestations

Hypertensive crisis is often characterized by the sudden onset of a severe headache, dizziness, nausea, and vomiting. Chest and neck pain, palpitations, and malignant hyperthermia (which is the usual cause of death in patients experiencing hypertensive crisis) may also be present. Systolic and diastolic blood pressures can range in the hundreds; however, individual responses to increased vascular pressure may vary. History most likely will reveal the ingestion of foods, beverages, or medications known to precipitate hypertensive crisis.

Treatment and Nursing Care

Hypertensive crisis can be fatal. Immediately upon diagnosis, stage I care is required. Interventions are aimed primarily at reducing the patient's blood pressure and temperature.

Tissue Perfusion, Altered, Related to

- **Elevated Blood Pressure Secondary to Hypertensive Crisis**

    Reducing blood pressure in a patient experiencing hypertensive crisis may be accomplished by the use of phentolamine mesylate (Regitine), 1 mg/min intravenously to a total of 5 mg. Regitine is an adrenergic blocking agent, which has a direct vasodilator effect. Other drugs that may also be employed include sodium nitroprusside (Nipride), chlorpromazine (Thorazine), and diazoxide (Hyperstat). Other supportive measures include urinary acidification and forced diuresis. Hypertensive crisis should resolve in 1 to 3 hours following initiation of treatment.

Thermoregulation, Ineffective, Related to

- **Hypertensive Crisis**

    Constant temperature monitoring while employing measures to reduce the hyperthermia associated with hypertensive crisis is imperative. Measures to reduce hyperthermia may include the use of cooling blankets, ice packs, and sponging. Some authors suggest the use of ice water enemas for severe hyperthermia (Walker 1983).

Extrapyramidal Reactions

Extrapyramidal reactions that are the result of antipsychotic medication use may be of several types. Most common are the dystonias, akathisia, akinesia, parkinsonism, and tardive dyskinesia. Only the dystonias, akathisia, and akinesia are discussed here as they are the extrapyramidal reactions most likely to require emergency services. First, however, a brief overview of antipsychotic medication is in order as knowledge of how antipsychotic drugs exert their effects will facilitate an understanding of their associated hazards.

Antipsychotic Medication

Antipsychotic drugs are those medications that are used to treat symptoms of psychosis. There are currently five major classes of antipsychotic drugs: phenothiazines, butyrophenones, thioxanthines, dihydroindolones, and dibenzoxazepines. The majority of antipsychotic compounds are phenothiazines, of which there are three subclasses: aliphatics, piperazines, and piperidines (Table 24–9). Although each class of antipsychotic drugs differs somewhat chemically, none has been found to be

TABLE 24-9
Antipsychotic Drugs and Their Potencies and Associated Side Effects*

Generic (Trade Name)	Approximate Oral Dose Equivalencies (milligrams)	Anticholinergic Effects	Extrapyramidal† Effects	Sedative Properties
Phenothiazines				
Aliphatics				
Chlorpromazine (Thorazine)	100	++/+++	++	+++
Piperidines				
Thioridazine (Mellaril)	100	++/+++	+	+++
Mesoridazine (Serentil)	50	++	+	+++
Piperazines				
Trifluoperazine (Stelazine)	5	+	+++	++
Perphenazine (Trilafon)	10	+	+++	+/++
Fluphenazine (Prolixin)	4	+	+++	+/++
Thioxanthines				
Thiothixine (Navane)	5	+	++/+++	+
Dihydroindolones				
Molindone (Moban)	10	++	++/+++	++
Dibenzoxazepines				
Loxapine (Loxitane)	10	+/++	++/+++	++
Butyrophenones				
Haloperidol (Haldol)	4	+	+++	+

* Relative potency in producing side effects: +, low; ++, medium; +++, high.
† Excludes tardive dyskinesia, which can be produced to the same degree by all antipsychotic agents.
Source: Reproduced by permission from: Beck CK, Rawlins RP, Williams RS, Mental-Psychiatric Nursing—A Holistic Life-Cycle Approach, St. Louis, 1988, The C.V. Mosby Co.

superior to another in abating psychotic symptoms. Persons with similar symptoms often show varied responses when given the same drug(s). Within each class, however, compounds do vary in potency and associated side effects. Generally speaking, the higher the potency of a drug,* the greater its associated extrapyramidal reactions and sedative properties, and the lower its anticholinergic effects (Table 24-9).

Antipsychotics are most commonly used in the ED setting to effect rapid tranquilization for psychotic individuals. Other indications for their use include acute and chronic schizophrenia, organic mental disorders, and the control of mania prior to and sometimes during lithium carbonate therapy.

Although the exact mechanism of action of antipsychotic drugs is unknown, they are believed to exert both their therapeutic and adverse effects via their antidopaminergic, anti-H_1-histaminic, anti-alpha-adrenergic, and anticholinergic properties (Schwarcz 1982).

Antidopaminergic effects of antipsychotic drugs are exerted by blocking the effects of dopamine (a chemical neurotransmitter) at postsynaptic neurons throughout the brain. It is believed that by blocking the action of dopamine (particularly in

---

* High potency does not imply greater therapeutic efficacy. Rather it implies that therapeutic effects can be achieved at lower doses.

the mesolimbic terminals of the CNS) psychotic thinking is abated. Dopamine blockade in the nigrostriatal terminals, however (Walker 1983), is believed to be responsible for the aforementioned extrapyramidal reactions.

Dystonic Reactions

Dystonic reactions may develop within 1 hour to 5 days after initiation of antipsychotic drug therapy. The clinical features of dystonic reactions depend on the muscle groups involved. Essentially, dystonic reactions are prolonged, tonic contractions of muscle groups. When muscles of the tongue, jaw, and neck are involved, this is called torticollis. Torticollis combined contractions of the extraocular muscles whereby the eyes are rolled upward with the head turned to one side is called oculogyric crisis. Opisthotonos, or hyperextension of head and neck, is yet another type of dystonia. Spasms of the lips, tongue, face, and throat may also occur. Although these muscle contractions are extremely frightening to both the patient and others nearby, they can usually be reversed easily. The administration of 25 to 50 mg of diphenhydramine hydrochloride (Benadryl) intramuscularly or 2 mg of benztropine mesylate (Cogentin) intramuscularly or intravenously quickly reverses the contractions. During this time it is important that the nurse stay with the patient and reassure him or her until symptoms abate, as dystonic reactions are quite alarming to the individual experiencing them.

Akathisia

Akathisia is another type of extrapyramidal reaction resulting from antipsychotic drug therapy, which usually appears 5 to 50 days from the start of treatment. It is the subjective feeling of restlessness that a patient has, accompanied by an inability to sit still. Often patients experiencing this will pace back and forth, rock, and shift their weight back and forth. Although not typically an emergency, this inability to sit still can be annoying to patients and their significant others. Additionally, akathisia can be mistaken for agitation associated with the patient's primary disorder. Antiparkinsonian agents (e.g., Cogentin) effect significant relief from akathisia; however, altering antipsychotic drug therapy or discontinuing it temporarily may need to be considered.

Akinesia

Akinesia is another extrapyramidal reaction and is characterized by signs and symptoms of decreased motor activity. The patient experiences fatigue and muscle weakness. Akinesia, too, can be easily controlled with an antiparkinsonian agent.

Although antiparkinsonian drugs are the treatment of choice for most of the extrapyramidal side effects resulting from antipsychotic drug therapy, they too must be used with caution. Antiparkinsonian agents have anticholinergic properties, and their use in combination with antipsychotics or antidepressants (which also have varying degrees of anticholinergic effects) can cause anticholinergic or atropine crisis, which is discussed later in this chapter.

The antihistaminic effects of antipsychotic drugs are responsible for their sedative effects, whereas the anti-alpha-adrenergic effects are responsible for orthostatic hypotension. The adrenergic blocking properties of antipsychotic drugs must be recognized in the face of cardiovascular collapse or arrest. Patients taking antipsychotic medication should not be given epinephrine under such circumstances because its alpha-receptor stimulatory effects would have little effect on already blocked alpha-receptors while its beta-receptor stimulatory effects would paradoxically worsen orthostasis. As such, alpha-adrenergic stimulators such as norepinephrine (Levophed) should be used. The anticholinergic effects which persons taking antipsychotic drugs experience most commonly include thirst, urinary hesitancy or retention, constipation, and blurred vision.

Anticholinergic Toxicity or Crisis (Atropine Psychosis)

As stated previously, antipsychotic drugs, tricyclic antidepressants, and antiparkinsonian agents all contain varying degrees of anticholinergic properties. As such, persons taking any one or combination of these drugs is at risk for developing anticholinergic crisis as a result of their cumulative antivagal effects.

Clinical Manifestations

Unfortunately, the clinical manifestations of atropine psychosis closely resemble those of a deteriorating psychiatric condition. Central nervous system signs of mental confusion, restlessness, and hallucinations may be evident. The patient's skin is hot and dry, and he or she often is febrile. Mydriasis and tachycardia also are usually present.

Treatment and Nursing Care

Initiating treatment for atropine psychosis should help the clinician differentiate anticholinergic toxicity from that of a worsening psychiatric condition. Physostigmine, 1 to 2 mg by slow intravenous push, should reverse symptoms of atropine psychosis (whereas increasing the dose of psychotropic medication would worsen it). Physostigmine acts to increase parasympathetic stimulation by inhibiting the action of cholinesterase, thereby prolonging the effects of acetylcholine. Physostigmine may be repeated in 15 to 30 minutes.

Neuroleptic Malignant Syndrome

Neuroleptic malignant syndrome (NMS) is a potentially fatal result of treatment with antipsychotic medications. It is estimated that up to 1 per cent of patients taking neuroleptic agents show signs of NMS, and of these, 20 to 30 per cent die (Keltner and McIntyre 1985). NMS may occur anywhere from hours to months following initiation of neuroleptic therapy. The exact cause of NMS is unknown; however, it is believed to result from the dopamine blockade at dopamine receptor sites in response to neuroleptic therapy.

Clinical Manifestations

Like anticholinergic crisis, NMS may manifest itself much like that of a worsening psychiatric condition—specifically, much like that of catatonia. Alterations in the patient's mental status along with emotional withdrawal, autonomic instability (tachycardia, tachypnea, diaphoresis, and so forth), muscle rigidity, and hyperpyrexia are characteristic.

Treatment and Nursing Care

Stage I care is required for patients with NMS. Cessation of all neuroleptic drug therapy must constitute the initial treatment.

Mobility, Impaired (Physical), Related to

- **Increased Muscular Rigidity Secondary to NMS**

     Increased muscular rigidity secondary to NMS has been treated with various classes of drugs. Anticholinergics (e.g., benztropine mesylate), minor tranquilizers (e.g., diazepam), and skeletal muscle relaxants (e.g., dantrolene sodium) are some. Benztropine mesylate (Cogentin), although effective in alleviating some muscle rigidity (and other extrapyramidal symptoms associated with NMS), may serve to increase the patient's tachycardia and as such should be used with caution. Diazepam (Valium) has been found to be transiently beneficial in chlorpromazine-induced NMS, and dantrolene aids in the relief of muscle contractions, thereby decreasing subsequent hyperthermia (Parker 1987).

Thermoregulation, Ineffective, Related to

- **Hyperthermia Secondary to NMS**

     Hyperthermia secondary to NMS, as stated previously, may be lessened by decreasing muscular rigidity, which—in addition to dopaminergic hypoactivity in the hypothalamus—contributes to hyperthermia. Dantrolene (Dantrium) given orally (50 to 300 mg/day) or intravenously (0.8 to 10 mg/kg/day) for 2 to 3 days may be used for this purpose. Dantrolene and bromocriptine mesylate (Parlodel) have been used concurrently without complications (Parker 1987). Bromocriptine mesylate is a dopamine agonist with hypothermic activity.

In addition to the aforementioned drug therapy, nursing care of patients with NMS is supportive, with need for close monitoring being crucial. Cooling blankets, sponging, and antipyretics may also be used for fever reduction. Frequent position changes with range of motion exercises to minimize skin breakdown and muscle rigidity should be employed. Neuroleptic malignant syndrome usually resolves in 5 to 10 days. Patients unresponsive to treatments discussed previously may require electroconvulsive therapy (ECT).

AFTERCARE FROM THE EMERGENCY DEPARTMENT

Comprehensive, coordinated, and continuous care for persons arriving in EDs for emergency psychiatric intervention is extremely important. If the patient is to be hospitalized, the ED nurse should provide the receiving service with information relating to the patient's HPI, past medical and psychiatric history, current medical and psychiatric findings, treatment(s) rendered, response(s) to treatment, significant others, and available support systems. Patients who require transfer to a state-run facility require the foregoing information as well as monitoring until they leave the premises and possibly even enroute. Informed consent is especially important in this instance and must be done skillfully to ensure safety and preserve the patient's rights.

If the patient is to be discharged home, the home environment must be assessed to see if it still contains the precipitants of the emergency visit. If so, the ED nurse should assist the patient in problem solving to eliminate them. Enlisting the services of home health nurses, social services, or significant others may be beneficial. Appropriate referrals in accordance with medical and nursing treatment plans should be offered. Many municipalities provide listings of services for the mentally ill in addition to social agencies. Local chapters of the National Alliance for the Mentally Ill (NAMI)* and the Manic Depressive and Depressive Association (MDDA)† may also be helpful in offering support, education, and referrals for psychiatric patients and their significant others. These listings should be kept updated periodically for most accurate reference. If the patient is referred for follow-up to a clinic, provide the patient with clearly written instructions about where to go, whom to see, what to do if something goes wrong, and so forth. In record keeping, clearly identify the data gathered about the patient, treatment rendered, and referrals made so that the information is easily accessible when needed.

CONCLUSION

Patients who come to EDs with psychiatric emergencies deserve the best of the art and science of nursing in assessment, planning, implementation, and evaluation of care.

---

* National Alliance for the Mentally Ill, 1-703-524-7600.
† Manic Depressive and Depressive Association, 1-312-993-0066.

These patients pose particular challenges to nurses as a result of their often aberrant behavior, which may occur as the result of organic, functional, or iatrogenically induced disorders. In conclusion, the timely and humane treatment that the psychiatric patient receives in the ED may literally be the bridge to life or the road to death.

REFERENCES

Aguilera D, Messick J. 1986. Crisis Intervention: Theory and Methodology, 5th ed. St. Louis, CV Mosby Co.

American Nurses' Association. 1982. Standards of Psychiatric and Mental Health Nursing Practice. Kansas City, MO, American Nurses' Association.

American Psychiatric Association. 1987. Diagnostic and Statistical Manual of Mental Disorders, 3rd ed. (revised). Washington, DC, American Psychiatric Association.

Barraclough B, Bunch J, Nelson B. 1974. A hundred cases of suicide: Clinical aspects. Br J Psychiatry 125:355–373.

Beck AT, Kovacs M, Weissman A. 1975. Hopelessness and suicidal behavior. JAMA 234:1146–1149.

Beck AT, Kovacs M, Weissman A. 1979. Assessment of suicidal intention: The scale of suicide ideation. J Consult Clin Psychol 47:343–352.

Beck AT, Weissman A, Lester D, et al. 1974. The measurement of pessimism, the Hopelessness Scale. J Consult Clin Psychol 42:861–865.

Beck CK, Rawlins RP, Williams RS. 1988. Mental Health–Psychiatric Nursing: A Holistic Lifecycle Approach, 2nd ed. St. Louis, CV Mosby Co.

Dorpat TL, Ripley HS. 1960. A study of suicide in the Seattle area. Comprehensive Psychiatry 1:349–359.

Gold MS, Hamlin CL. 1986. The Biological Foundations of Clinical Psychiatry. New York, Elsevier Science Publishing Co.

Guze SB, Robins E. 1970. Suicide and primary affective disorders. Br J Psychiatry 117:437–448.

Hart C, Turner MS, Orfitelli MK, et al. 1981. Introduction to Psychotropic Drugs. Rochester, NY, Medical Examination Co.

Kaplan HI, Sadock BJ. 1985. Modern Synopsis of Comprehensive Textbook of Psychiatry IV, 4th ed. Baltimore, Williams & Wilkins.

Keltner NL, McIntyre CW. 1985. Neuroleptic malignant syndrome. J Neurosurg Nurs 17:363–366.

Kraft DP, Babigian HM. 1976. Suicide by persons with and without psychiatric contacts. Arch Gen Psychiatry 33:209–215.

Parker JG. 1984. Emergency Nursing. New York, John Wiley & Sons.

Parker WA. 1987. Neuroleptic malignant syndrome. Crit Care Nurse 7:40–48.

Pierce DW. 1981. The predictive validation of a suicidal intent scale: a five-year follow-up. Br J Psychiatry 139:391–396.

Rund DA, Hutzler JC. 1983. Emergency Psychiatry. St. Louis, CV Mosby Co.

Schwarcz G. 1982. A rationale ordering of the actions of antipsychotic drugs. J Family Pract 14:263–267.

Sletten IW, Barton JL. 1979. Suicidal patients in the emergency room: A guide for evaluation and disposition. Hosp Commun Psychiatr 30:407–411.

Talley S, King MC. 1984. Psychiatric Emergencies: Nursing Assessment and Intervention. New York, Macmillan.

Tuckman J, Youngman WF. 1968. A scale for assessing suicide risk of attempted suicides. J Clin Psychol 24:17–19.

Urbaitis JC. 1983. Psychiatric Emergencies. Norwalk, CT, Appleton-Century-Crofts.

Walker JI. 1983. Psychiatric Emergencies: Intervention and Resolution. Philadelphia, JB Lippincott.

Waldinger RJ. 1986. Fundamentals of Psychiatry. Washington, DC, American Psychiatric Press.

Weisman AD, Worden JW. 1972. Risk-rescue rating in suicide assessment. Arch Gen Psychiatr 26:553–560.

Wilson HS, Kneisl CR. 1983. Psychiatric Nursing, 2nd ed. Menlo Park, Calif., Addison-Wesley.

Daniel Sheridan, RN MS

Family Violence

For centuries family violence was a well-kept secret within the home. Health care providers have come to recognize, first with child abuse, then with battered women (spouse abuse), and now with elder abuse, the life-long health issues found in abusive families.

Family violence affects millions of people each year in this country. Its survivors are mostly women and children; however, family violence can occur against men or spread to extended family members.

The cost of this form of violence in human suffering and pain is almost immeasurable. There are scant data on the financial cost of family violence. Preliminary data from one urban hospital emergency department (ED) in Chicago estimates its cost of family violence to be $1 million per year (Sheridan 1988). This figure reflects the cost of emergency treatment and hospitalization of family violence survivors at this hospital.

Trauma from family violence can be emotional or physical. Injuries to its victims may range from mild to life-threatening situations resulting from multisystem injuries, homicide, or suicide attempts. The ED is an ideal health setting to identify family violence and institute nursing interventions that may break a vicious cycle of violence.

This chapter explores the following family violence topic areas: child abuse and neglect, battered women, and elder abuse.

611

CHILD ABUSE AND NEGLECT

All 50 states require nurses to report suspected cases of child abuse and neglect to an appropriate child protective agency. As a result, ED nurses (as mandated reporters) must report suspected abuse or neglect or face possible disciplinary action from the state. It is therefore essential that ED nurses have a thorough understanding of state and local statutes concerning child abuse and neglect. Although every state has child protective legislation, there is wide variance in legal definitions of child abuse and neglect, notification procedures, documentation requirements, and penalties for failing to report. Besides state reporting requirements, there may be regional and local laws that require the nurse to notify other agencies, such as the police or local boards of health.

Defining Child Abuse

As already mentioned, legal definitions of child abuse may vary from state to state. The following working definition of child abuse should, however, assist the ED nurse in recognizing and defining child abuse in the clinical setting (this definition is used throughout this chapter):

> **child abuse:** the willful infliction of bodily harm onto a child under the age of 18 by a parent, a person acting as a parent, a family member, or a legal guardian.

Consistent with most state statutes, the foregoing definition excludes willful injury to a child by a noncaregiver assailant, such as a stranger or a neighbor. However, states are increasingly classifying as child abuse injuries inflicted onto a child by an institutional caregiver, such as a day care worker, a school teacher, or a hospital worker.

Defining Child Neglect

Like child abuse, the definition of child neglect also varies considerably from state to state. Because child neglect is defined more broadly, the following working definition of child neglect should assist the ED nurse in recognizing and defining child neglect in the clinical setting (this definition is used throughout this chapter):

> Actions taken, or not taken, by a parent, a person acting as a parent, a family member, or a legal guardian that place a child under the age of 18 in actual or potential risk of harm, or that result in harm through negligent treatment such as failure to provide adequate food, shelter, clothing, medical care and treatment, and emotional support.

As with child abuse, institutional caregivers may be charged with neglect if their actions or lack of actions result in harm or place a child at risk of harm.

Reporting Child Abuse or Neglect

Because the legal definitions of child abuse and neglect can be interpreted subjectively, and because child neglect is defined even more broadly than child abuse, intraprofessional conflict over the need to report or not report suspected abuse or neglect often occurs.

In such instances, the ED nurse must realize that states do not require absolute certainty of abuse or neglect for reporting purposes. Child protective agencies should be notified of all instances in which there is reasonable cause to believe that abuse or neglect has or is occurring. All states provide nurses with immunity from civil or criminal liability as long as he or she reports his or her suspicions in good faith.

Historical Overview

Child abuse and neglect is not a new phenomenon. Humphreys (1984), in an extensive review of literature on the origins of child abuse, demonstrated how for thousands of years children were killed as sacrifices to deities. Other children were put to death if they were born with birth defects or were thought to be possessed by a devil. Historically, in patriarchal cultures first-born female children were at greater risk of abuse or death. Even today, the greater importance of male children is reflected when many expectant couples readily state that they want their first-born to be male. This attitude is based in part on old property laws that did not allow property to be passed from father to daughter and in part on the view that women were second-class citizens. Women and the children they bore and reared were considered chattels or the property of the man. He could, and often did, do whatever he wanted to his family without any sanctions.

During the first half of the twentieth century the United States made great strides in changing its view of children and passing protective legislation for them. However, it was not until 1962 that the term *battered child syndrome* was introduced (Kempe et al 1962). Kempe and a few of his contemporaries were successful crusaders for improved treatment and identification of child abuse victims, so much so that within a handful of years all 50 states had passed comprehensive mandatory child abuse and neglect reporting laws. Most of these laws are now routinely updated and amended to increase the protection of children.

Etiology

Numerous frameworks or theories have been explored to attempt to explain the causes of child abuse. The most notable nursing framework on the causes of abuse is Millor's (1981). This multifactorial perspective explains on a continuum how families can be abusive to nonabusive or neglectful to non-neglectful and looks at the behavioral outcomes of the interactions among stress, culture, child, parent, and family. Millor incorporates principles from the following theories: stress, symbolic interaction, and temperament theory of personality.

Generally, this complex yet comprehensive framework states the likelihood of abuse or neglect increases when several specific conditions are present. Among these

TABLE 25–1
Common Indicators of Child Abuse

Physical Indicators
Alterations in Skin Integrity
  Abrasions to palms, elbows, or knees from being pushed down
  Burns resulting from
  • Cigarettes and cigars
  • Curling irons, clothes irons
  • Chemicals
  • Friction (being dragged on the ground)
  • Immersion in hot liquid or "dunking" injury pattern
  • Splashes
  External genitalia lacerations or abrasions
  Vaginal bleeding, discharge, or infections
  Penile bleeding, discharge, or infections
  Rectal bleeding, discharge, or infections
  Patterned bruises such as from a whip, belt, or other implement
  Bruises in various stages of healing
Alterations in Musculoskeletal System
  Multiple fractures
  Fractures in various stages of healing
  Spiral or midshaft fractures of long bones
  Skull fractures
Neurologic impairment
  Acute onset of paresis
  Post concussion symptoms
  Intracranial hemorrhage
  Visual impairment resulting from retinal detachment
Nonphysical Indicators
  Conflicting histories obtained from parent(s) or adult(s) and child
    regarding the nature of the child's injuries.
  Children who are not allowed by the parent(s) or adult(s) to verba-
    lize a history despite the fact that they are developmentally and
    chronologically old enough to.
  A history given by the parent(s) or adult(s) that does not fit the
    nature of the presenting injuries.
  Children who display fearful body language (e.g., guarding when a
    sudden movement is made).
  A delay in bringing a child into an ED for treatment of any injury or
    illness that indicates abuse or neglect.

---

are parents who feel inadequate in their roles, parents who have unrealistic expectations of their children, parents who endured abuse or neglect in their childhoods, and children whose attitudes and behaviors differ from their parents' expectations.

Clinical Manifestations

ED nurses must always be alert for signs of child abuse or neglect. Identifying these victims, however, is not always an easy task.

Child abuse and neglect occurs in all cultures, races, religions, and socioeconomic backgrounds. At times, there are overt physical indications of abuse or neglect. At other times, however, the nurse must be able to recognize more insidious physical and nonphysical indicators of abuse or neglect. Tables 25 – 1 and 25 – 2 identify many common indicators of child abuse and neglect. Whether obvious or subtle signs of

TABLE 25-2
Common Indicators of Child Neglect

Physical Indicators
  Poor hygiene
  Clothing that does not protect a child from the weather
  Chronic signs of malnutrition and dehydration
  Poor oral hygiene or untreated dental problems
  Failure to receive immunizations
  Child abandonment
  Delays in seeking prompt medical care for an acute injury or illness
  Failure to give child a prescribed medication, which results in the
      child's developing more severe symptoms
  Failure to thrive in infants
Emotional and Behavioral Indicators
  Delay or absence of age-appropriate behaviors, especially in infants
      and young children
  Lethargy in the absence of illness
  Social withdrawal or depression
  Relentless attention-seeking behavior
  Minimal response to painful medical interventions
  Suicide ideation or attempts

abuse or neglect are present, once the suspicion of either is raised, a thorough history is needed. The nurse must seek details of how and when the injury or illness happened or began, and whether or not the child has been seen in the ED (or one or more other health care settings) for similar injuries or complaints. In the case of trauma, ascertaining whether or not witnesses were present and talking with them may be extremely helpful. (Nurses should realize that discipline by a parent that results in abrasions, ecchymosis, or prolonged erythema is reportable as child abuse.) In the case of neglect, the ED nurse should ascertain if the neglectful behaviors of the adult(s) or parent(s) were the result of inadequate resources, information, or education; erroneous information received by another health professional; or an understandable misunderstanding of complicated medical regimens. Often the ED nurse is guided in assessing neglect by determining if the harm or risk of harm could have been prevented by another reasonably competent adult.

A major assessment technique that is frequently overlooked by ED personnel is that of interviewing the child directly. If the child is old enough to talk, ask him or her directly if someone has caused the observed injuries. How the ED nurse asks this, however, is extremely important. Ideally, the nurse should spend some time with the child to build an initial trust relationship. Techniques such as making a balloon out of an examination glove or enlisting the "help" of the child in setting up the examination room take little time yet may be vital in building a beginning trust relationship. If possible, it is best to interview the child alone. The words chosen by the nurse must be age appropriate, culturally understandable, nonthreatening, and nonblaming of either the child or the parent(s). Children must be repeatedly assured that it is alright to share "secrets" with the nurse. The following dialogues have been used by ED nurses to elicit a history of abuse from a child:

"Sometimes grown-ups do things with kids and then say that it's a secret. Has this happened to you?"

If the child responds positively, the nurse may then ask:

> *"Secrets can be pretty important and pretty scary. You're safe with me. Can you tell me more about the secret?"*

or

> *"Sometimes kids are hurt by a grown-up. If that happened to you, it's safe to tell me. Has someone hurt you?"*

The nurse must remember that children have short attention spans. It is unrealistic for the nurse to expect a young child to tolerate a prolonged interview. The interview may best be conducted during frequent but short sessions. The use of play therapy via dolls may also be useful in the identification of child abuse.

Never make false promises to a child no matter how good the intent. For example, do not say to a child, "If you tell me who hurt you, I'll see that no one will hurt you again." This is a promise that cannot be enforced.

Treatment and Nursing Care

Injury, Related to

- ### *Physical or Psychoemotional Trauma Secondary to Child Abuse or Neglect*

Treatment of child abuse or neglect victims depends on the nature and severity of the abuse or neglect and is dictated by the patient's presenting condition. All life-threatening conditions will need immediate attention and will require stage I care. Intubation and artificial ventilation may be required in unconscious victims of head trauma. Intravenous fluids, blood, or blood products may need to be administered to children who are massively bleeding (internally or externally) or who have suffered extensive burns. As such, intravenous access must be established as soon as possible. Fast-acting intravenous medications may be required in instances of neglect if a parent failed to administer prescribed medications to a diabetic or asthmatic child who now comes to the ED in diabetic ketoacidosis (DKA) or acute respiratory distress. Survivors of child abuse or neglect who require stage I care and treatment will almost always be admitted to the hospital, often to a pediatric intensive care unit.

Thousands of children die each year in this country from child abuse or neglect, and many survivors of such trauma are brought to EDs in need of stage II care. As with stage I care, stage II care will be dictated by the patient's presenting condition. Although nursing care and treatment of the child's physical needs remain paramount, the emotional needs of the child and the parent(s) must also be addressed.

Children who have been abused or neglected are often in great fear of the health team's interventions and of possible future abuse or neglect because the "secret" is now known by people outside the family. The child needs to be informed in an age appropriate way of all tests, procedures, and interventions. Computed tomographic (CT) scanning, radiographs, blood specimens (e.g., complete blood count, platelet count, coagulation times, typing and cross-matching) and urine specimens may be obtained as deemed appropriate. The parent(s) should be told of a need to notify child protective agencies and the police. Communication between the ED nurse, the patient, and the child's family must be direct and nonjudgmental. This can be a difficult task. The presence in the ED of a possibly abusive parent(s) can evoke feelings of anger and hostility in the nurse. For nursing interventions to be effective with the child and the parent(s), these feelings must be controlled. Counseling referrals for an allegedly abusive parent(s) should be available in all ED settings.

The appropriate child protective agency should be notified of suspected abuse and neglect cases by the ED physician or nurse as soon as possible. The responsibility of calling the child abuse hotline should not be diverted to someone unfamiliar with the child or postponed until the patient is transferred to the in-patient unit. In general, whoever has the most information or direct knowledge about possible child abuse and neglect should be the person to notify the child protective agency. Protocols that dictate that only the physician or social worker can call the hotline are illegal in most states and fail to acknowledge that nurses are mandated reporters. In addition to notification of the appropriate child protective agencies, most EDs have a policy regarding who should be notified internally of such situations (e.g., hospital administration).

In all cases of suspected child abuse or neglect, the ED nurse must provide thorough, unbiased documentation in the medical record. Only data that were heard and seen by the ED staff should be documented. There is no place in the medical record for inferences and judgments.

It is appropriate to write verbatim or as closely as possible any allegations of abuse or neglect, noting who made them, who was present at the time, and so forth. Photographic documentation of suspected abuse or neglect has been extremely helpful in subsequent court actions. It is recommended that two sets of photographs be taken, one set for inclusion in the medical record and a second set for evidence. Child abuse is a crime and standard evidence-collection procedures should be utilized. If a camera is not available, body maps should be used to diagrammatically document the nature and extent of the observed trauma. Documentation that a report was made to the appropriate child protection agencies and that appropriate notification was given to internal hospital personnel should also be included in the medical record.

No child should be discharged from the ED if this places him or her at risk of further harm. Most states allow a physician, a child protective services worker, or a police officer to take temporary protective custody. Hospital admission of a medically stable survivor of suspected child abuse or neglect is an option, especially during off hours. A brief hospital admission provides a safe environment and allows for better coordination of follow-up services for the abused or neglected child.

Evaluation

Emergency department nurses, although they are often first to suspect child abuse or neglect, frequently never know the outcome of their suspicions and interventions. The development of hospital-based, multidisciplinary child protective teams who follow up with abused and neglected children and external child protection agencies may be effective in providing feedback to ED staff nurses. Additionally, this team can be responsible for periodically reviewing and updating protocols for reporting and treating abused or neglected children.

BATTERED WOMEN

The role of the ED nurse in providing prompt, comprehensive care to battered women cannot be overemphasized. The ED nurse is often the first person outside the home to recognize that a woman is being victimized by her husband or boyfriend.

Battered women come to EDs with physical and emotional injuries. To treat just their physical injuries without addressing their emotional needs will do little to break a cycle of violence that may one day result in the victim's death.

Defining Battered Women

The following working definition of a battered woman should assist the ED nurse in identifying and defining battered women in the clinical setting (this definition is used throughout this chapter).

> A battered woman is a woman aged 16 or older who is physically, emotionally, or psychologically abused by a husband or significant other.

Historical Overview and Etiology

Patriarchal cultures have dominated societies for thousands of years, and women have endured in the privacy of their homes untold acts of violence. Historically, a woman has been considered chattel, or the property of first her father and then of her husband, to be used or abused as her "owner" saw fit. A woman's historical role in the family was limited to helping her husband, bearing children (preferably male), cooking, and caring for the household.

As more women have expanded their roles outside the home, the social isolation that often keeps women figuratively and sometimes literally prisoners in their own homes has become less significant. Women have found support from other women. The women's movement that began in the 1960s further challenged many traditional patriarchal views, and new roles for women have and are still emerging. In groups first composed of other women, then in society at large, women began to tell about the severe beatings and verbal abuse they endured from their husbands or boyfriends. The secret is out, but society has been slow to accept the truth. Although the causes of family violence are beginning to be researched, many experts believe that at the root of violence against women is power and control. Men have it, women do not (Dobash and Dobash 1979; Martin 1981; Walker 1979). This perspective is based on an acknowledgment that our society is rooted in a patriarchal system in which women and children have little ability to effectively control many significant aspects of their lives. That control is held by men, who often use violence or the threat of violence to maintain it.

During the late 1960s and early 1970s battered women began to seek help from health professionals in increasing numbers. Early health articles often blamed the victim and viewed the battered woman as the one in need of psychiatric help. The rationale was that if a woman stayed in an obviously painful and abusive relationship she must be receiving some sort of masochistic pleasure (Hilberman 1980). This view still has some advocates, but it is now known that battered women stay in abusive relationships for many understandable reasons (Campbell and Humphreys 1984).

The woman may stay because she fears further, more serious beatings or even a deliberate attempt to kill her if she tries to leave. She stays because she fears for the safety of her children. Often isolated from family and friends, she stays because of lack of a family support network. A battered woman may endure years of violence owing to a religious belief that a marriage is for life, through good times and bad. In addition, many battered women would like to leave abusive relationships but remain in them because there are simply not enough community services to meet their health and safety needs.

Clinical Manifestations

There is no race, religion, or socioeconomic background exempt from this form of violence. Battered women may be very poor or very wealthy. They may be unemployed, single mothers on welfare, or married to corporate executives.

Battered women often go unrecognized by ED professionals. In a classic study, approximately 25 per cent of the women who presented to one ED with injuries were battered woman; however, the ED staff identified as battered only a fraction of these women (Stark et al 1979). Although some women will openly state that they are victims of family violence, many women are reluctant to admit to a history of violence on the part of their husbands and boyfriends. This reluctance often is based on a realistic fear of further violence from the abuser and also on shame, humiliation, and a shattered self-image. Recognizing the need for improvement in the identification and treatment of battered women by health professionals, the U.S. Surgeon General stated in 1985 that interpersonal violence has become one of the major public health issues of our time (Cron 1986).

ED nurses must be familiar with general indicators of abuse so that battered women are appropriately identified (Table 25–3). Additionally, they should be familiar with injuries most commonly associated with this type of abuse (Table 25–4). Generally speaking, injuries to battered women tend to be proximal in nature as opposed to accidental injuries, which are more likely to occur to distal body parts.

TABLE 25–3
Common Indications in Battered Women

Women who minimize the frequency or seriousness of their injuries
Injuries that are not likely to have been caused by the accident reported
Women who come for treatment one or more days following the sustained injuries
Radiographic evidence of fractures in different stages of healing
Repeated ED visits with injuries becoming more severe as frequency of visits increases
Overprotective mates who do not allow the women to be alone with the health care professional
Child abuse in patient's or partner's background

TABLE 25–4
Injuries Commonly Seen in Battered Women

Physical Indicators
Alterations in Skin Integrity
  Burns resulting from
  • Splashes
  • Friction (being dragged on the ground)
  • Chemicals
  • Cigarettes or cigars
  Knife wounds
  Scalp, facial lacerations
  Oral mucosa lacerations
Alterations in Musculoskeletal System
  Facial or nose contusions or fractures
  Skull fractures
  Patterned bruises
  Torso injuries
  • Breast contusions
  • Fractured ribs
  • Abdominal contusions (especially during pregnancy)
  • Back or spine injuries
Neurologic Impairment
  Altered consciousness from strangulation attempts
  Intracranial hemorrhage
  Post concussion symptoms
  Visual impairment resultant from corneal abrasion or retinal de-
    tachment
Other
  Miscarriages

Battered women often come to the ED with nontraumatic or somatic complaints, especially if they believe that they are about to receive another beating. Psychologically, they are likely to display a low self-esteem, a sense of helplessness and hopelessness, and an overwhelming sense of apprehension and worry. Sleep disturbances, depression, and suicidal ideation are not uncommon.

If the suspicion of abuse is raised, the most effective way to determine if a woman is a victim of family violence is to separate her from any family or friends that have accompanied her to the ED and ask her directly in a supportive manner if abuse is present in the home. Some statements (such as "Are you a battered woman?" or "So your husband beat you; You're a battered woman") are labeling and may well result in defensiveness and hostility toward the ED nurse. The following sample questions have been used extensively in EDs and other settings and have been shown to be very effective in eliciting a history of abuse.

"It seems that the injuries you have could have been caused by someone hurting or abusing you. Did someone hurt you?"

"Sometimes when people come to the ED with physical symptoms like yours, we find that there may be trouble at home. We are concerned that someone is hurting or abusing you. Is this happening to you?"

"Sometimes when people feel the way you feel it is because they may have been hurt or abused at home. Is this happening to you?" (Sheridan et al 1985.)

Although experience has shown that a battered woman who comes to the ED in obvious physical and emotional distress is more likely to mobilize extra support from the staff, not all battered women are in crisis. Many women in chronically abusive relationships view their injuries as "just another beating; no big deal." These women may have difficulty believing that there is an alternative to abusive relationships because of a lack of self-esteem and overwhelming feelings of helplessness and hopelessness. Although the chronically abused woman may be less likely to believe that she has choices, the ED nurse must still explain to the woman that she does have choices and if and when she is ready to seek alternatives to the abusive relationship there are people who will support her decisions.

Treatment and Nursing Care

Injury, Related to

- *Physical or Psychoemotional Trauma Secondary to Abuse*

Battered women may come to EDs with severe trauma requiring stage I care. Specific stage I care will be dictated by the nature and severity of the trauma. Most battered women who require stage I care will be admitted to the hospital. However, the majority of battered women who come to the ED for treatment will not be admitted to the hospital and are in need of stage II care.

Of utmost importance is the patient's immediate and ongoing safety. The battered woman who is not going to be admitted to the hospital has basically two choices. She can return to the abusive relationship, or she can seek alternative living arrangements. The ED nurse needs to explore with the woman the risks and benefits of either decision. For example, if the woman opts to leave her abuser, does leaving place her children at risk or place her at risk of being accused of abandoning her children? Does leaving increase her chances for future beatings, or of being killed by her abuser in the near future?

The nurse needs to ask the woman if abuse has occurred in the past. For example, has the woman previously used shelters or left her abuser to stay with family or friends? If the woman needs to make arrangements to leave the abusive relationship, have her call her family, friends, or a battered women's shelter. Most shelters insist on talking directly with the battered woman so that the shelter staff can assess if the woman is appropriate for and really wants to utilize the shelter.

If the local battered women's shelter is fully occupied (as they often are) the nurse should explore with the woman the option of utilizing a shelter for the homeless. Although these types of shelters are less than ideal to meet the complex needs of battered women, they can provide a safe environment for several days until the woman can explore other options or until space becomes available at a battered women's shelter.

Before the nurse encourages the battered woman to stay with family or friends, the nurse needs to assess with the woman the risk of homicide from her abuser.

Campbell (1986) has developed a danger assessment tool to assist nurses in all health settings to explore with the battered woman her likelihood of being killed by

TABLE 25-5
Key Factors Identified with Increased Homicidal Risk

The presence of a gun in the home
An abuser who has threatened to kill the woman or a woman who
   believes her abuser is capable of killing her
An abuser who is violent to nonfamily members
An abuser who is overly jealous
An abuser who also has an alcohol or drug abuse problem

---

her abuser. Key factors for increased homicidal risk identified by this tool are listed in Table 25-5.

The ED nurse should never attempt to minimize the potential for homicide. Women who are murdered in this country are most often killed at home by men intimately known to them, not by a stranger on the street.

If the battered woman states that she wants to or must return to the abusive relationship, the nurse must respect the woman's choice. This can be difficult for the nurse, especially if the alleged abuser is in the ED waiting room. An alleged abuser should never be "confronted" by the ED staff without the woman's consent. Such confrontation may place her at risk of future abuse. However, if she insists that the ED staff talk to the alleged abuser about his violent behavior, the discussion should center on his responsibility for choosing violence. He should be informed that there are nonviolent ways to resolve conflict and he should be given abuser counseling referrals.

It may be helpful for the nurse to remember that, as already noted, the battered woman may stay in an abusive relationship for many understandable reasons. The woman may have to seek help and support numerous times before she develops the courage and understands her options well enough to leave her abuser. The battered woman may need to return to her abuser for a period of time to save money, to prepare her children for the separation, to gather necessary documents such as health records and birth certificates, or sometimes to wait until there is room at the local shelter.

No matter what the reason, the battered woman who returns to an abusive relationship will benefit from teaching on survival tactics by the nurse. For example, the patient may be coached on how to obtain prompt police response if her abuser begins to beat her. Many police departments place low priority on emergency calls that involve domestic violence. The police may respond more quickly if the woman states, "There's some man in my home and he is beating me" instead of saying, "my husband (or boyfriend) is beating me."

Battered women should be given battered women telephone hotline and community referral numbers. Many communities operate 24-hour crisis hotlines that may assist the women during crisis. Some battered women will state that they can predict that a beating is about to occur. The nurse should encourage these women to leave home, call the police, or call the community agency before the beating occurs.

The nurse needs to inform battered women in a supportive manner that no woman deserves to be beaten. They need to hear that battery is a crime in all states; that they are victims of crime and not the cause of it.

Until recently, no one has asked the abuser, "Why did you hit her?" Health professionals are just now insisting that the abusive man take responsibility for his violent behavior. In keeping with stage II care, the ED nurse should begin to work with battered women to help them understand that they are not responsible for the abuser's violent behavior. Although this understanding may take weeks of support (usually via battered women's support groups or individual counseling), the ED nurse is in an ideal situation to help these victims rebuild their self-esteem. Many community agencies are beginning to develop services for abusive men in an effort to break their cycles of violent behavior. Battered women should be given these referrals and also informed that increasing numbers of criminal justice court systems are mandating that abusive men receive counseling.

The nurse must be aware of any legal requirements to notify the police if a battered woman comes for treatment. Most states require hospital personnel to notify the police if a person comes for treatment of injuries received during a criminal act. Hospital legal departments can provide the nurse with specific legal requirements.

Historically, the police have been trained to view family violence as a domestic problem, best resolved by social interventions. Although the attitudes of many police departments are changing to recognize the serious criminal aspect of wife battering, the individual officer who responds to the ED may still view family violence solely as a domestic problem. As with all victims of sexual assault, the battered woman should never be interviewed alone by the police. The nurse (or battered woman's advocate) should be present during the entire police interview and advocate for the victim as needed (Sheridan 1987a). Except for a few communities that have adopted mandatory arrest policies for alleged abusers, it is the woman's choice if she wants to file criminal charges.

Thorough and accurate documentation by ED nurses is vital. The medical record is a legal document, and what the ED nurse writes or does not write may play a crucial role in future criminal or civil court proceedings. The hospital's legal counsel can address specific concerns of the individual ED nurse; however, in general, most states protect hospital and medical personnel from criminal and civil liability if the charting of a patient's history of abuse is presented in the words of the patient and without malice on the part of the writer.

The SOAP (Subjective, Objective, Assessment, Plan) charting format is an effective method of documenting a battered woman's history and the ED nurse's plan of care. The use of photographs or body maps to document the nature of the woman's injuries is strongly recommended.

Evaluation

Nursing interventions with battered women survivors may greatly reduce the likelihood of future abuse or death. Evaluating these interventions, however, may be difficult. Battered women may not utilize community referrals for weeks after an ED visit.

Establishing a networking relationship with community-based battered women's agencies can be invaluable in assessing if battered women seen in EDs have utilized shelter or support services. This networking can also generate additional ED referrals from women and children who come to the community program with untreated injuries. Family violence programs based in ED settings can also be extremely effective in obtaining consistent follow-up and in providing ongoing counseling for battered women survivors (Sheridan 1987b).

ELDER ABUSE

Family violence is being increasingly viewed as a life-cycle health issue that may begin when the patient is an infant, continue into early adulthood, and culminate as abuse of the elderly. Elder abuse is just now becoming a national issue with nurse practitioners as a major force in the identification and treatment of this large group of family violence survivors (Beck and Phillips 1984; Fulmer and Wetle 1986; Hirst and Miller 1986). Reporting elder abuse to authorities is mandatory in many states; however, some states have only voluntary reporting statutes or no reporting statutes. There may be reluctance by health professionals to involve outside reporting agencies (such as the police, departments of aging, health departments). When outside agencies are contacted, there is often a reluctance to provide any concrete services to elder abuse survivors, especially if the patient is unable or unwilling to tell authorities the nature of the abuse.

Defining Elder Abuse

The following working definition of elder abuse should assist ED nurses in identifying elder abuse in the clinical setting (this definition is used throughout this chapter).

> Elder abuse is the willful infliction of bodily harm onto a person aged 60 or older by a spouse, a child, a family member, a legal guardian, or a primary caregiver.

This definition would cover physically abusive acts such as slapping, hitting, punching, sexual abuse, weapon injuries, burns, and other physical injuries. Elderly persons, however, are also often the targets of material abuse (e.g., theft of assets, such as money or property). This is especially true when elderly persons are confused or give unsupervised consent to another person to handle their financial affairs. This is a concern to ED nurses because if such abuse is identified law enforcement authorities should be notified.

The following working definition of material abuse should assist the ED nurse in recognizing it in the clinical setting (this definition is used throughout this chapter).

> Purposeful actions taken, or not taken, by a spouse, a child, a family member, a legal guardian, or a primary caregiver that financially benefit this person while financially harming the elderly person without the elderly person's giving informed consent.

Excluded from this definition are financial gifts by a competent elderly person that may be financially unwise but are made after informed consent and have not been coerced by another. Also excluded from this definition is material abuse by salespersons or contractors that take money from the elderly person for services that either are not needed or are grossly overpriced.

Defining Elder Neglect

Definitions of elder neglect are even broader than definitions of child neglect. When assessing for the presence of neglect, it is important to try to determine if the neglect is purposeful or unintentional.

The following working definition of elder neglect should assist the ED nurse in identifying victims of it in the clinical setting (this definition is used through this chapter).

> Passive or active withholding of medicine, food, clothes, treatments, basic hygiene, and emotional support by a spouse, a child, a family member, a legal guardian, or a primary caregiver.

Excluded from this definition is neglect that results from a true knowledge deficit on the part of the caregiver, or neglect by another aged person whose best efforts to care for the patient are less than adequate. This type of neglect can be viewed as unintentional and without malice. Nursing and social support services are urgently needed for such persons.

Etiology

Although abuse of the elderly is not a new health problem, little has been published on its origins within our society. There is a growing recognition that family violence is exactly that — violence within a family that affects all members, young and old. Stark (1986) states that the majority of elder abuse survivors are battered women now over age 60 who are still being abused by their husbands. He believes the next largest group of elder abuse patients are women being abused by their daughters. This is empirically logical for two reasons. First, women live longer than men, and therefore the frequency of abuse among them is greater. Second, societal norms still place the primary responsibility of caring for aged parents on the daughter, even if she is less able to provide the necessary care than are her brothers. Sons who accept the responsibility of caring for aged parents often transfer the responsibility to their wives; thus daughters-in-law often are at risk of abusing or neglecting the elderly. Older men who are being abused may have been abusive in years past. The child abuse survivor may now be the perpetrator of elder abuse, completing a cycle of family violence.

Although issues of power and control may be common in many instances of elder abuse, so are issues of stress and frustration. With the implementation of prospective payment systems, elderly patients have markedly shorter hospitalizations. Older patients are now routinely sent home requiring extensive and often highly technical care. Much of this care is performed by the family with visiting nurse teaching and assistance. Although prospective payment systems have created an increased demand for home health care, studies to determine if shorter hospitalizations and earlier discharges have helped to place the elderly at greater risk for abuse or neglect still need to be conducted.

Clinical Manifestations

Elder abuse and neglect occurs in all races, religions, and socioeconomic classes. Like other types of abuse, however, elder abuse or neglect often goes undetected. Common myths that contribute to this underdetection of elder abuse include the following:

- No one would purposefully abuse an elderly person.
- Older people fall all the time and are constantly bruising or breaking something.
- Older people are confused and you cannot believe what they say.
- Older people are paranoid about their money. They always think someone in the family is out to steal their money.
- Skin breakdown in the bedridden older patient is inevitable. They all get decubiti.
- Older people forget to eat and drink, and they constantly mix up their medications. No wonder they become dehydrated or malnourished and have subtherapeutic or toxic drug levels.

Recognizing misconceptions about elderly patients is essential for accurate identification of abuse or neglect. The most common indicators of physical abuse of the elderly are quite similar to those of battered women, as listed in Table 25–4. Additionally, however, elder abuse should be suspected in all cases of hip fracture. Although hip and proximal femoral fractures are common after accidental falls, identical injuries can occur if the patient has been pushed or tripped. The presence of multiple untreated or poorly treated decubiti is an important physical indicator of elder neglect. As with child neglect, indicators of elder neglect are quite numerous and vary from mild to severe. Each case must be assessed separately.

For the elderly patient who is alert and oriented, assessment of abuse or neglect should occur in a similar manner to that of the assessment of battered women. Assessing elder abuse and neglect of the disoriented or unconscious elderly patient is much more difficult. Suspicions of elder abuse should be raised if physical indicators of such abuse are present. In many instances it may be appropriate to ask any accompanying family members about possible abuse. Slight modifications of the nonjudgmental sample questions for assessing battered women have been effective in eliciting a history of elder abuse from family members. For example, the ED nurse could ask the family the following questions:

> *"It appears that the injuries your mother has could have been caused by someone. Do you think someone may have caused them?"*

> *"It must be really difficult and frustrating at times to care for your father. He needs so much care. How do you deal with your frustration?"*

Treatment and Nursing Care

Injury, Related to

- ***Physical or Psychoemotional Trauma Secondary to Elder Abuse or Neglect***

Elder abuse or neglect survivors may come to EDs with severe trauma or neglect requiring stage I care. As with the battered women, stage I care must be specific to the patient's presenting condition. These persons usually require hospitalization. During this time, social services must be consulted and involved in discharge planning for the patient. Most elder abuse survivors, however, are in need of stage II care and will not require hospitalization.

Interventions with the alert, oriented, and competent elder abuse or neglect survivors are very similar to those for battered women. The nurse's primary responsibility is to provide these people with choices. Elder abuse is a crime in all states, and increasingly states are passing specialized elder abuse and neglect statutes that provide additional protection to this vulnerable and growing segment of our population.

The section on Treatment and Nursing Care for battered women in this chapter is appropriate for most elder abuse survivors as well. Most battered women shelters will accept the elderly into shelters as long as they are capable of independent living and do not have disabilities that require specialized equipment. Few shelters are accessible for wheelchairs, and if a shelter has a lot of stairs, the elderly person who uses a walker, crutches, or cane may not be accepted into the shelter for liability reasons.

Creative discharge planning for elder abuse or neglect victims is essential. This author has negotiated with local shelters to accept elderly women with home health needs by scheduling visits by home nurses and health aides. Most shelters are not staffed sufficiently to address health needs of clients professionally. The burgeoning home health care industry would find a receptive audience if networked with family violence shelter directors.

The elderly person who does not need or want shelter, or who is not eligible for acceptance into existing shelters, needs alternative safety interventions. Extensive outreach to other family members, friends, community, or church groups is needed. Among these populations the nurse can often find persons who will assist in helping abuse or neglect survivors. Involvement of police and state departments on aging are also helpful in breaking the cycle of violence.

Abuse of the elderly that is rooted in stress and frustration on the part of the abuser may well subside when respite is provided. Working with family, community, and church services to have someone come into the home one day per week, for example, can give an overburdened exhausted caregiver a much-needed break.

Elder abuse or neglect survivors may be considered legally competent but in reality may be disoriented, suffer from severe dementia, or have marked alterations in their level of consciousness. The ED nurse needs to be able to advocate with the ED physician or the primary physician to consider instituting formal legal guardianship proceedings in such instances. If the patient is incapable of understanding his or her choices on how to stop abuse, the state needs to give that decision-making authority to another. Guardianship is best given to a concerned family member or close friend who will be concerned for the patient's welfare. If, however, the patient's only family member is suspected of the abuse, the court can appoint a private, state, or court guardian.

Being familiar with guardianship options has not been a routine part of ED nursing; however, as the acknowledgment and assessment of elder abuse increases, this type of training will be a great asset to elder abuse patients.

Some individuals may have profound disabilities that prevent them from protecting themselves or leaving an abusive home. However, if these individuals are mentally competent, they have the right to choose whether or not to return to such a home. If the abused person chooses to return to the abusive situation, the nurse should respect that choice and ensure that the patient has emergency referral numbers and other information, as previously discussed under Battered Women.

As in other cases of abuse, documentation in the medical record and the use of photographs is vital. Also as in other cases, the alleged perpetrator of elder abuse or neglect may be present in the ED. Interactions with *all* family members and significant others must be conducted professionally in a nonjudgmental manner. Nursing interventions that are accusatory or inflammatory may not only place the patient at risk of future harm but also may precipitate aggression or violence against the ED staff. Referrals for counseling and social support services for significant family members should be available in the ED.

Evaluation

Nursing interventions with elder abuse or neglect survivors can be as challenging as with battered women. For many elderly people, family violence has been a lifelong problem, and they may not believe that a violence-free home is ever possible. Elderly persons who are being abused or neglected by a son or daughter may endure the abuse in an effort to protect the "child." Elderly persons may state that having an abusive caregiver is better than being alone, with no caregiver. Victims of elder abuse or neglect may feel even more trapped in an abusive relationship than battered women do.

The ED nurse needs to have available all referral numbers for battered women plus referral numbers specific to elder abuse. Additionally, numbers for community services for the elderly should also be available.

CONCLUSION

Effective nursing intervention with family violence survivors is an ED nursing challenge that will continue to require creative nursing responses. Child abuse has been addressed for over 20 years by the health professionals, and the number of reported cases is still increasing. The plight of battered women has prompted concern from nurses around the country. The Nursing Network on Violence Against Women (NNVAW)* is organizing nurses throughout the country to improve nursing care of battered women, young and old. Elder abuse survivors are just now being recognized, and nursing interventions for them are on the forefront.

Nurses who choose to work in EDs thrive on challenge. Caring for survivors of family violence is one such challenge.

---

* For additional information on NNVAW, write Daniel J. Sheridan, Family Violence Program, Rush-Presbyterian-St.Luke's Medical Center, 1753 W. Congress Parkway, Chicago, IL 60612.

REFERENCES

Beck CM, Phillips LR. 1984. The unseen abuse: Why financial maltreatment of the elderly goes unrecognized. J Gerontol Nurs 24(10):28–34.

Campbell J, Humphreys J, eds. 1984. Nursing Care of Victims of Family Violence. Reston, VA, Reston Publishing Co.

Campbell JC. 1986. Nursing assessment for risk of homicide with battered women. Adv Nurs Sci 8(4):36–51.

Cron T. 1986. The Surgeon General's workshop on violence and public health: Review of the recommendations. Public Health Rep 101(1):8–14.

Dobash RE, Dobash R. 1979. Violence Against Wives: A Case Against the Patriarchy. New York, Free Press.

Fulmer T, Wetle T. 1986. Elder abuse screening and intervention. Nurse Pract 11(5):33–38.

Hilberman E. 1980. Overview: The "wife-beater's wife" reconsidered. Am J Psychiatry 137:1336–1347.

Hirst SP, Miller J. 1986. The abused elderly. J Psychosoc Nurs Ment Health Serv 24(10):28–34.

Humphreys J. 1984. Child abuse. In Campbell J, Humphreys J, eds. Nursing Care of Victims of Family Violence. Reston, VA, Reston Publishing Co., 119–144.

Kempe CH, Silverman FN, Steele BF, et al. 1962. The battered child syndrome. AMA 181:17–24.

Martin D. 1981. Battered Wives. San Francisco, Volcano Press.

Millor GK. 1981. A theoretical framework for nursing research in child abuse and neglect. Nurs Res 30:78–83, March/April.

Sheridan DJ, Belknap L, Engel B, et al. 1985. Guidelines for the Treatment of Battered Women Victims in Emergency Room Settings. Chicago, Chicago Hospital Council.

Sheridan DJ. 1987a. Advocacy with battered women: The role of the emergency room nurse. Response 10(4):14–16.

Sheridan DJ. 1987b. Creating a hospital-based family violence program. Paper presented at Violence: From Fear to Action. Indianapolis, IN, Indiana State Board of Health.

Sheridan DJ. 1988. Family violence survivors: ED cost analysis. Unpublished data.

Stark E, Flitcraft A, Frazier W. 1979. Medicine and patriarchal violence: The social construction of a "private" event. Int J Health Serv 9:461–493.

Stark E. 1986. Personal communication.

Walker L. 1979. The Battered Woman. New York, Harper & Row.

David N. Zull, MD FACEP

Poisoning and Drug Overdose

The list of agents that are potentially toxic to humans is virtually endless. In fact, most drugs, household and industrial products, and environmental agents are toxic when taken in large enough quantities. Table 26–1 is a list of nontoxic products; however, any of the compounds listed can be harmful in large quantities. From 5000 to 6000 deaths occur annually from toxic ingestions. Although children less than 5 years old account for 75 per cent of all cases of poisoning, they constitute only 2 per cent of the deaths, with 95 per cent of deaths occurring in adults and adolescents (Epstein and Eilers 1983).

ASSESSMENT OF THE POISONED VICTIM

Obtaining a history from a patient suspected of poison ingestion frequently is very difficult. Often the patient is lethargic and confused and thereby unable to recount events accurately. The suicidal patient may give false information to avoid embarrassment. Patients intoxicated with recreational drugs may fear retribution from the law or wish to avoid family embarrassment and therefore also give inaccurate information.

Because of this inherent unreliability of the history in ingestion cases, the nurse or physician must seek verification and further details from friends or family. In addition to the obvious questions regarding the identification of the drug or toxic

TABLE 26–1
Agents with Low Toxicity on Ingestion

Adhesives	Glues and pastes
Antacids	Laxatives
Ballpoint pen ink	Lipstick
Bathtub floating toys	Matches (potassium chloride)
Battery (dry cell)	Paint (indoor and latex)
Bleach (<5% sodium hypochlorite)	Pencil (graphite)
Bubble-bath soaps	Felt-tip markers
Candles (beeswax or paraffin)	Putty (<3 oz)
Caps (toy pistol) (potassium chlorate)	Rubber cement
Chalk (calcium carbonate)	Shampoos (liquid)
Clay (modeling or Play Doh)	Shaving cream (soap, perfume, menthol)
Cigarettes or cigars (nicotine)*	Silly Putty (silica, 1% boric acid)
Cosmetics (most, except perfumes)	Soap
Contraceptive pills	Sweetening agents (saccharin, cyclamate)
Corticosteroids	Teething ring
Crayons (marked AP or CP)	Thermometer (mercury)*
Dehumidifying packets (silica)	Toothpaste
Detergents (most, except electric dishwasher)	Vitamins without iron
Deodorants	Writing ink
Fish-bowl additives	

* Low toxicity except in large amounts.
Source: Adapted from Mofenson HC, Greensher J. 1970. Pediatr Clin North Am 17:583.

compound, there is a series of critical questions that should be asked in all poisoning cases (Table 26–2).

In-depth questioning with regard to the patient's psychiatric history may be awkward and inappropriate on initial contact with the patient; this information is better obtained from family, friends, and private physician. When beginning to interview the patient, do not be thwarted by the patient's hostility and lack of communication. Also, be aware that any feelings of disapproval and disgust may show through and confound any attempts to achieve rapport with this patient. Being supportive of the patient's plight on this first contact is important, yet an objective and professional attitude should prevail. It may be more productive to open the history with questions such as, "How are you feeling?" or "What happened?", rather than ask "Why did you do it?" Further information on assessment of the suicidal patient is found in Chapter 24.

TABLE 26–2
Critical Questions in the Interview of the Overdose Patient or Observers

1. What was ingested? Was anyone present at the time to verify the history? Are there empty or partially filled pill bottles at home?
2. How much was taken? If pill bottles are available, the nurse should calculate the number of missing tablets from the initial amount prescribed, taking into account the date on the prescription.
3. What was the time of the ingestion? The nurse must take into account the time at which the person was last seen and when symptoms of intoxication began if the timing is not clear.
4. What is the route of poisoning? (Oral, intravenous or subcutaneous, snorted, smoked, inhaled, and so forth)
5. Does the patient have a history of depression, schizophrenia, drug abuse, or alcoholism?
6. What is the patient's past medical history, and history for prescription drugs, allergies, and so forth?

Physical Assessment

The initial priorities in stage 1 assessment of the poisoned patient are airway, breathing, and circulation. Is the airway patent? Does the tongue fall back and obstruct the airway? Is the patient able to protect the airway from secretions and gastric reflux? The gag reflex is an easy way to help answer the last question. Is the patient moving air well? What are the blood pressure, pulse, and peripheral skin color and perfusion?

At this point in evaluation, tracheal intubation and establishment of venous access may be necessary. A trauma survey should also be part of the immediate assessment. Intoxicated patients often fall or are involved in accidents; therefore, if there is any suspicion of trauma by history or physical examination, the cervical spine should be immobilized. If intubation is needed, the nasotracheal route is a safer option until a lateral cervical spine radiograph is obtained, because extension of the neck for oral intubation may aggravate neck injury.

The next priority in evaluation is the patient's neurologic function. Emergency department (ED) nurses should be responsible for brief, ongoing assessments of patient behavior, level of consciousness, pupillary size and reactivity, and sensory and motor function. Neurologic assessment is discussed in greater detail in Chapter 17. Documentation is important so that the patient's improvement or deterioration can be followed over time.

Etiology

Poisonings can be categorized into three groups: accidental, intentional, and iatrogenic. Accidental ingestion includes playful exploration in young children, inadvertent ingestion from mislabeling or not following directions, and environmental exposures. Intentional ingestion includes recreational drug abuse and suicide attempts. Iatrogenic poisoning usually results from unanticipated drug interactions or misdosing in patients with renal or hepatic insufficiency.

In dealing with any patient with overdose or poisoning, awareness of the risk factors for suicidal potential may give the nurse insight into the patient's motivations and help identify patients at risk of repeat attempts. Often there has been some precipitating personal crisis regarding loved ones, finances, health, or other factors. Patients should be asked if they have contemplated suicide in the past, and if so, had they made any concrete plan. The presence of a suicide plan is an ominous sign. A personal or family history of suicide attempts is also a major risk factor. The initial interview should also look for symptoms or history of depression, psychosis, drug abuse, and alcoholism. The schizophrenic or manic-depressive patient should not be assumed to be too disorganized to put together a suicide plan. More importantly, the drug- or alcohol-intoxicated patient who makes a suicide attempt should not be dismissed from mind because he or she is "stoned"; rather the intoxication should be viewed as a factor that releases inhibitions to underlying suicidal intent (Warner 1983).

Clinical Manifestations

The nurse should be aware of the various clinical presentations in which drug overdose should be highly suspect, even if there is no history of poisoning (Table 26–3).

TABLE 26–3
Circumstances Highly Suspect for Poisoning
or Drug Overdose

Coma or any alteration in consciousness
Cardiac dysrhythmias or angina in a young person
Acute pulmonary edema in a young person
New-onset seizure disorder
Unexplained metabolic acidosis
Gastrointestinal symptoms in a young child

Such suspicious situations include the following: the patient with any alteration in mental status, ranging from coma to acute psychosis; cardiac dysrhythmias and pulmonary edema in the young patient; the new-onset seizure disorder; the patient with unexplained metabolic acidosis; and gastrointestinal symptoms of nausea, vomiting, diarrhea, and abdominal pain (Haddad 1983b).

Coma or any depression in level of consciousness should lead to a search for possible sedative or hypnotic, narcotic, or antipsychotic drug use. Acute psychosis or any bizarre behavior may be caused by hallucinogens such as phencyclidine (PCP) or lysergic acid (LSD), stimulants such as cocaine or amphetamines, or any of the sedatives.

Cardiac dysrhythmias, including sudden death, in the young patient or one with no cardiac risk factors, should arouse suspicion of drug intoxication. The tricyclic antidepressant drugs are the most notorious and lethal agents to consider. In addition, other drugs prescribed to psychiatric patients, such as phenothiazines and lithium, are potentially cardiotoxic. Sympathomimetic drugs such as cocaine, amphetamines, and over-the-counter diet pills are also common causes of acute dysrhythmias, and in some cases have resulted in myocardial infarction (Pasternack et al 1985; Weiss 1986). The nurse should also bear in mind that many prescription cardiac and asthma medications (e.g., digoxin, theophylline) may result in rhythm abnormalities (Benowitz and Goldschlager 1983).

Pulmonary edema, especially in the young person, should also make the nurse suspect drug toxicity. Any intravenous drug abuse can cause acute noncardiogenic pulmonary edema, either by an idiosyncratic capillary leakage or by particulate embolization. Heroin is the intravenous drug that most commonly causes acute respiratory insufficiency, but any drug taken intravenously can have a similar effect. Methaqualone (Quaalude) and ethchlorvynol (Placidyl) also can cause pulmonary edema by oral overdose. Even aspirin intoxication can result in pulmonary edema, although this generally occurs in the elderly patient with renal insufficiency (Taviera da Silva 1983).

Seizures in a person with no prior history of seizure disorder should raise the suspicion of drug abuse. Alcohol withdrawal, not intoxication, is the most common drug-related cause of new seizures. Drugs of abuse, such as cocaine and PCP; suicide drug overdose, especially the ingestion of tricyclic antidepressants; iatrogenic poisoning, particularly with theophylline compounds; and environmental exposure to carbon monoxide are other intoxications that may result in seizure activity.

Unexplained metabolic acidosis in a patient who appears to be intoxicated with alcohol should alert the nurse to the possibility of toxic alcohol substitutes such as methanol (wood alcohol), ethylene glycol (antifreeze), and paraldehyde. Aspirin is the most common therapeutic drug to cause metabolic acidosis in the overdose setting (Emmett and Narins 1977).

Sometimes nausea, vomiting, diarrhea, and abdominal pain may be clues to a toxic ingestion, particularly for poisonings in young children. Withdrawal syndromes associated with alcohol, sedative, or narcotic abuse may all be manifested in this manner.

In addition to the already mentioned clinical presentations (coma, psychosis, seizures, cardiac dysrhythmias, pulmonary edema, metabolic acidosis, and gastroenteritis), certain other patients might be suspected to be suffering from drug abuse or overdose. These would include victims of trauma, drowning, and housefires, as well as the alcoholic or psychiatric patient and the criminal.

Psychosocial Considerations

To effectively interview the patient whose ingestion may have been suicidal, the interviewer should have some understanding of the psychology of suicide. Ambivalence is characteristic of suicidal thinking. Although the prospect of self-annihilation is terrifying, killing one's self may be attractive for several reasons. Suicide may be a means of withdrawing from a situation or assuming final control; it may also be a form of self-punishment or an attempt to extract love from another or inflict guilt. Indeed, the patient's suicidal thoughts usually revolve around at least one other person. With feelings of helplessness, the patient's thought processes become very childlike and egocentric. The medical team, on the other hand, may react with feelings of anger and disgust. It is important to be supportive and be aware of the patient's comfort. Do not be thwarted by the patient's hostility or lack of communication. As mentioned in stage I assessment, the nurse should not confront the patient about motive but, instead, focus on the sequence of events and the patient's physical and emotional symptoms (Fought and Throwe 1984).

Physical Examination

Once the initial priorities of airway, breathing, and circulation are attended to and brief neurologic and trauma surveys are completed, the focus can shift to the remainder of the physical examination. Many clues to the cause of the poisoning may be obtained from a careful examination. With regard to the vital signs, the following associations can be helpful. Bradycardia may suggest poisoning with beta-blockers, digitalis, organophosphate insecticides, or cyanide. Severe tachycardia and hypertension are often found in cocaine, amphetamine, and phencyclidine intoxications. Fever may be an indication of overdose from salicylates, anticholinergics, and stimulants (Arena 1979; Dreisbach 1980; Epstein and Eilers 1983; Schwartz 1986).

The skin should be surveyed for evidence of trauma, as noted earlier, as well as needle tracks and pitted scars from "skin popping" (subcutaneous injections). Needle tracks and skin pops may be blackened if the intravenous drug abuser uses a match to sterilize the needle, thereby depositing carbon on the needle, which tattoos the skin. Large cutaneous blisters are seen in barbiturate overdoses and sometimes are noted with other sedative intoxications and after carbon monoxide exposure. Cyanosis in the presence of normal respiratory status may indicate that the patient had an elevated level of methemoglobin in the blood, which can result from nitrates, nitrites, sulfa drugs, and clothes dyes. In chronic intoxications, thallium may cause alopecia, and arsenic results in hyperkeratosis of the skin. Finally, some patients advertise their preferred drug of abuse in the form of skin tattoos.

Assessment of the eyes in the overdose patient can be very revealing. Pinpoint pupils suggest intoxication from narcotics, chloral hydrate, phenothiazines, and organophosphate insecticides. Dilated pupils tend to be less specific but are very prominent in intoxications from alcohol, amphetamines, cocaine, belladonna derivatives, tricyclic antidepressants, and glutethimide (Doriden). Pupils that are fixed and dilated generally indicate a structural brain lesion; however, glutethimide is notorious for producing these pupillary changes and thereby mimicking brain death.

Eye movement may also be a clue as to the cause of an apparent intoxication. In coma, "doll's eye" movements are usually preserved in overdose, but not in a structural brain lesion. Nystagmus on lateral gaze is a common finding in alcohol and various sedative intoxications from inhibition of cerebellar and vestibular function. Phenytoin (Dilantin), even at therapeutic levels, often causes nystagmus. PCP abuse demonstrates the most dramatic ocular motility abnormalities, with spontaneous horizontal and vertical nystagmus.

Examination of the mouth may reveal burns to the lips and mucosa from acid or alkali ingestion. Paraquat, a herbicide, produces a white film or pseudomembrane on the posterior pharynx. Note the patient's breath during this examination also. Hydrocarbons, such as gasoline, kerosene, toluene, and carbon tetrachloride, have characteristic odors. Prescription drugs and drugs of abuse generally produce no odor on the intoxicated patient, except for ethchlorvynol (Placidyl) and paraldehyde, both of which produce a pungent, volatile scent. Poisons such as cyanide and arsenic are notorious for their odors (bitter almond and garlic, respectively).

Examination of the lungs may reveal diffuse rales indicative of pulmonary edema, as discussed earlier. Local crackles and wheezes suggest pneumonia secondary to aspiration, which is a common complication of severe intoxications. Wheezing can occur in nonasthmatics from poisonings of organophosphate insecticides and from inhalation of toxic fumes, such as chlorine gas. In the asthmatic patient, wheezing can be aggravated by the aforementioned factors, but the most common drugs to exacerbate bronchospasm are the beta-adrenergic blockers. Tachypnea in a patient with a normal pulmonary examination may be secondary to compensatory hyperventilation for drug-induced metabolic acidosis, as seen in poisonings from aspirin, methanol, and ethylene glycol.

Examination of the heart in the overdose patient should focus primarily on the rate and rhythm, as noted previously in the discussion of the patient's vital signs.

On examining the abdomen, attention should focus on the presence or absence of bowel sounds. Their absence points toward opiates or anticholinergic drugs, which slow bowel motility. The finding of Hemoccult-positive stool on rectal examination is common in overdoses from iron and the nonsteroidal anti-inflammatory agents.

Although physical assessment may provide many clues as to the cause of the poisoning, the examination frequently is normal, or the findings are too nonspecific. As a result, the medical team must rely on a careful repeat history from the patient as well as from family and friends. Data from laboratory tests, electrocardiogram

(EKG), and radiographs may also provide very useful information at this point (Arena 1979; Dreisbach 1980; Epstein and Eilers 1983; Schwartz 1986).

Laboratory Evaluation

Most severe poisonings and overdoses will require a complete blood count and determination of serum electrolytes, BUN, glucose, ethanol, and arterial blood gases. These data may reveal drug-related changes in acid-base balance, electrolyte shifts, hypo- or hyperglycemia, CO_2 retention from respiratory depression, or hypoxia from aspiration or pulmonary edema. Of course, the alcohol level should be documented in any patient suspected of poisoning because it is such a common associated factor.

Any patient with suspected toxic ingestion should be placed on a cardiac monitor to carefully follow the heart rhythm and rate. The nurse should also note the QRS and Q-T intervals, because prolongation of these intervals points toward overdosage with tricyclic antidepressants, phenothiazines, and quinidine. If there is any suspicion of cardiac toxicity, a 12-lead EKG should also be obtained.

A chest radiograph is recommended if there is any respiratory distress or abnormal pulmonary findings, to look for evidence of pulmonary edema or aspiration pneumonia.

An abdominal radiograph may show a drug-induced ileus, but its main utility in overdose is to look for radiopaque pills. The acronym CHIPE (chloral hydrate, heavy metals, iron, phenothiazines, and enteric-coated tablets) is a useful mnemonic for recalling which medications will be visible on radiographs.

Urine and gastric contents should be sent for toxicologic screening. Although the results may reveal unexpected ingestions, the clinician should not await these data before initiating therapy. This patient should be treated immediately, on the basis of the history and physical assessment. Only in a few specific instances are quantitative blood levels helpful in determining treatment and assessing prognosis. These would include overdoses of salicylates, acetaminophen, ethanol, iron, methanol, lithium, and tricyclic antidepressants.

Treatment and Nursing Care

When a patient with known or suspected poisoning or overdose arrives in the ED, initial attention is focused on the basics of airway, breathing, and circulation. If ventilations are slow and shallow or the patient is unable to guard the airway, immediate intubation is indicated. Cervical spine precautions may be necessary if there is associated trauma. Elective intubation may be needed in the lethargic patient who will require gastric emptying, even if the gag reflex is intact.

The patient should be placed on a monitor and an intravenous line established. A bolus of normal saline solution may be needed to correct hypotension, but caution is needed if the poison is one that may cause pulmonary edema, such as heroin and various sedatives or hypnotics. Frequent auscultation of the lungs should be done and a baseline chest radiograph obtained. If any signs of pulmonary edema develop, intubation is indicated and fluids should be restricted. If hypotension persists, dopamine or norepinephrine infusion may be necessary (Benowitz et al 1979).

Thought Processes, Altered, Related to

• *Hypoglycemia and Substance Abuse*

For a patient in coma, or with any alteration in mental status, hypoglycemia must be considered as a possible cause. Blood should be obtained for glucose determination, then 50 ml of 50% dextrose (one ampule of D50) should be given by intravenous push. This should be followed by thiamine, 50 or 100 mg intramuscularly, as a large glucose bolus may precipitate acute thiamine deficiency in an alcoholic or other malnourished patient (Sullivan et al 1979).

Any patient with a depressed level of consciousness should receive a test dose of naloxone (Narcan), which is a specific antagonist to the narcotics. The usual recommended dose is 2 mg by intravenous push. If narcotic addiction is suspected, a 0.4-mg intravenous push of naloxone is a more prudent starting point. With this smaller dose, it should be possible to titrate between arousal and gross withdrawal symptoms. Even if narcotic withdrawal is precipitated, it persists for only a few minutes, and the associated vomiting provides efficient gastric emptying. Naloxone dosage higher than 2 mg may be needed for certain narcotic congeners such as propoxyphene (Darvon), pentazocine (Talwin), butorphanol (Stadol), nalbuphine (Nubaine), and diphenoxylate (Lomotil) (Allen 1983).

Decreased Cardiac Output, Related to

• *Electrical Dysfunction Secondary to Ingestion of Cardiotoxic Agent*

Careful cardiac monitoring should be emphasized at this stage for any severe overdose, but particularly when the compound ingested is cardiotoxic. Poisonings that are most notorious for inducing cardiac dysrhythmias include tricyclic antidepressants, phenothiazines, lithium, cocaine, and all cardiac and asthma medications. A defibrillator and lidocaine for bolus injection should be kept close at hand in these instances.

Potential for Injury, Related to

• *Absorption of Poisoning Agent*

Finally, it is important to stop further exposure to a toxic agent and minimize ongoing absorption, if the poisoning has occurred via inhalation, through ocular and other mucous membrane exposure, or transcutaneously. For inhalation exposure, the victim should have been removed from the toxic environment immediately and 100 per cent oxygen administered if carbon monoxide exposure is suspected. Ocular exposure to drugs or chemicals mandates immediate, copious irrigation with saline solution or water for 10 to 15 minutes. Alkali exposure to the eye often requires 30 minutes of irrigation. For cutaneous absorption of poisons, all clothes should be removed immediately to minimize further exposure of toxin absorbed in the clothing, and the skin should be copiously washed and irrigated (Arena 1978; Haddad 1983b; Nicholson 1983).

At completion of the stage I assessment phase, the patient may have been intubated to protect the airway from aspiration or in order to assist respirations. A large-bore intravenous line is in place and a saline bolus should have been given if there was initial hypotension. The patient is on a cardiac monitor, and emergency equipment should be easily accessible to the patient's room. Also, at this point, any skin or mucous membranes exposed to poisons should have been thoroughly washed and irrigated, and clothing removed if tainted. The nurse can now move on to stage II care, which addresses gastric dilution, gastric emptying, charcoal administration, catharsis, diuresis, and dialysis.

Potential for Injury, Related to

• *Tissue Destruction Secondary to Ingestion of Caustic Agents*

The majority of poisonings encountered in the emergency department are by oral ingestion. In some cases, dilution of the toxin by milk or water may be the first line of therapy. This is particularly true of compounds whose primary toxicity is by mucous membrane irritation, with little systemic absorption, such as strong alkalis and acids. Lye and other caustic alkalis are the prototype poisonings treated by immediate ingestion of large quantities of milk or water. Generally, no other therapy is necessary; in fact, gastric emptying is contraindicated because of the risk of worsening esophageal burns by retransit of the caustic material back up through the esophagus (Howell 1986).

Dilution therapy alone is also indicated for hydrocarbons, such as gasoline, with gastric emptying best avoided because of the risk of aspiration or prolonged inhalation of fumes, leading to pulmonary injury. Indeed, dilution therapy may be the only intervention needed for a variety of poisonings considered to be nontoxic in small quantities (Table 26–1). The only precaution in dilution therapy is not to push fluids if the patient is becoming nauseated or bloated, especially if emesis is contraindicated, as when corrosives and hydrocarbons were ingested.

Potential for Injury, Related to

• *Absorption of Toxic Amounts of the Ingested Substance*

For the preponderance of serious poisonings, gastric emptying is the mainstay of treatment. Dilution alone in drug ingestions may increase dissolution of capsules or tablets and promote rapid transit, thereby increasing absorption. Contraindications to gastric emptying include ingestion of corrosive compounds and petroleum distillates, as noted earlier. A relative contraindication is alteration in state of consciousness with loss of gag response. In this situation, endotracheal intubation should be performed before gastric decompression is attempted (Tandberg and Troutman 1985).

The sooner that gastric emptying is achieved, the higher the yield; preferably emptying should be done within 2 hours of ingestion. However, gastric emptying up to 6 hours after ingestion may show significant returns in specific circumstances. Drugs that inhibit peristalsis, such as opiates and anticholinergic drugs, or drugs that form concretions in the stomach, such as salicylates and meprobamate, are very slow to transit out of the stomach. Therefore, attempts to empty gastric contents up to 6 hours after ingestion of these drugs may show good yields. Any severely intoxicated patient or one with an alleged massive ingestion should have gastric emptying regardless of the timing, because an accurate history of time of ingestion is often not available, and further delays in treating the critically ill patient should be avoided.

Giving syrup of ipecac or gastric lavage is the preferred method for gastric emptying. A history of spontaneous emesis by the patient prior to arrival to the hospital should not lead to a false sense of security on the part of health care providers. This post-ingestion vomiting is ineffective in removing sufficient quantities of the toxic material from the stomach (Easom and Lovejoy 1979). Also, self-induced emesis by gagging produces inefficient vomiting and should not be recommended to patients over the phone, nor should it be performed in the ED. Apomorphine by subcutaneous injection is not a recommended form of treatment for ingestion despite its effective and rapid stimulation of emesis. It has highly sedative properties and tends to cause protracted vomiting. In addition, apomorphine requires on-the-spot preparation of solution for injection from a tablet form.

Administration of syrup of ipecac is the preferred method for gastric emptying in the home, the prehospital setting, and the ED if the patient is alert and has an intact gag reflex. The active constituents of ipecac are the alkaloids emetine and cephaeline. Small amounts are absorbed into the circulation and stimulate the brain's chemoreceptor trigger zone, the vomiting center. Onset of action is in 10 to 30 minutes, with a duration of effect from 15 to 30 minutes. However, the patient often is not able to tolerate any oral intake for 1 to 2 hours.

The dose of ipecac is 15 ml for children less than 12 years of age and 30 ml for adolescents and adults. Ipecac should be avoided for infants less than 6 months, and a dose of 10 ml is recommended for children 6 months to 2 years of age. If emesis does not occur within 20 minutes, the dose should be repeated. After administration of syrup of ipecac, the patient is given water to drink, 10 to 12 ounces for an adult and proportionately less for a child. Repeated movement and stimulation of the patient may hasten the effect of ipecac. This fact is best taken advantage of in small children, who can be bounced on their mother's knee. If no emesis occurs after a second dose of ipecac, gastric lavage should be instituted, not only to empty the stomach of the original ingestion, but also to eliminate the ipecac, which has potential cardiac toxicity (Manno and Manno 1977).

A frequently raised question is which method achieves the most efficient gastric evacuation, ipecac or gastric lavage? Studies have shown a clear cut advantage of ipecac over gastric lavage with a 16 French nasogastric tube (Arnold et al 1959). These results seem relevant for children, but in adults, in whom a tube of much larger bore, such as a 36 French Ewald tube, could be used, the difference may be negated or reversed.

In what instances is gastric lavage recommended over ipecac? In the unresponsive, comatose patient, in which the airway must be protected by an endotracheal tube, nasogastric lavage is the only method feasible. In the obtunded patient who fights off intubation but allows a nasogastric tube, lavage is risky without meticulous attention to the airway (Tandberg and Troutman 1985).

In the awake patient, gastric lavage may be indicated over syrup of ipecac in certain circumstances. The delay in onset of ipecac and its prolonged emetic effect may be dangerous in an overdose in which there is a rapid decline in the mental status of the patient. In addition, a patient may find it difficult to tolerate charcoal by the oral route after ipecac administration, even if over an hour has elapsed before the charcoal is tried. As a result, nasogastric lavage may be the preferred approach in the severely poisoned patient, by which rapid gastric emptying and efficient charcoal administration may be achieved without the usual regurgitation (Haddad 1983b).

If the substance ingested is an antiemetic, such as prochlorperazine (Compazine), trimethobenzamide (Tigan), or promethazine (Phenergan), use of syrup of ipecac may not be effective (Thoman and Verhulst 1966). Although there is controversy regarding this, nasogastric lavage may be advised for antiemetic overdose. The awake, unruly patient may refuse syrup of ipecac or charcoal, in which case he or she may need to be restrained and a nasogastric tube passed. Finally, if food or milk has been ingested about the same time as the toxic compound, this may cause a significant delay in action or obviate the effect of syrup of ipecac. Gastric lavage, although often recommended in this circumstance, may be fraught with great difficulty because even large-bore tubes may get clogged with food particles.

For best results in lavage, the largest tube that can be tolerated should be used, such that intact pills can be aspirated easily. A tube smaller than a 24 French is generally useless for aspiration unless the toxin is a liquid, or unless the tube is to be used for charcoal administration alone. In an adult, a tube of up to 36 French size can be passed through the nose, and tubes up to a 50 French size can be put through the mouth. Before gastric lavage is begun, as much of the gastric contents as possible should be aspirated. The patient should then be placed in the left lateral decubitus position to minimize passive gastric emptying into the duodenum and also to decrease risk of aspiration (McDougal and McLean 1981).

Lavage can be done with water or saline solution, and the lavage aliquots should be 150 to 200 ml. Smaller amounts will barely fill the lumen of the tube. Lavage should be continued until the aspirate is clear. Then the patient should be repositioned and external abdominal massage performed. If there are adherent concretions of drug, repeat lavage at this point will be of high yield. Warming of lavage fluid may also increase the yield, but generally this is not practical. For certain specific poisonings, neutralizing agents could be used both in the lavage fluids and as a substitute for charcoal. These neutralizers include sodium bicarbonate and desferoxamine for iron poisoning, starch for iodine ingestion, and potassium permanganate for strychnine, nicotine, and quinine poisonings.

Potential for Injury, Related to

- ### *Internal Effects of Toxins Secondary to Ongoing Absorption from the Intestinal Tract*

In most poisonings and overdoses, charcoal administration should follow gastric evacuation. In fact, some data suggest that charcoal administration alone, without previous gastric emptying, may be more efficacious and efficient if a long interval has elapsed since ingestion (Kulig et al 1985; Park et al 1986). Charcoal works by adsorbing the drug to its surface. The complex then passes through the gut and is eliminated unchanged in the stool. Certain compounds are not well adsorbed by charcoal, such as iron, electrolytes (potassium, magnesium), strong acids and alkalis, alcohols, cyanide, solvents, and hydrocarbons. There may be potential harm in giving charcoal in corrosive and hydrocarbon poisonings because of the risk of reflux and aspiration. In addition, if there is a specific antidote that should be given by mouth, such as *N*-acetylcysteine (Mucomyst) for acetaminophen overdose, charcoal administration should be avoided (Greensher et al 1979).

Activated charcoal is given as a slurry by mouth after syrup of ipecac–induced vomiting has subsided, or by nasogastric tube after the lavage fluid clears. If in powder form, charcoal should be prepared by slowly adding water and mixing thoroughly to avoid lumps. A premixed slurry, if available, is much faster and cleaner.

Most authors recommend 50 to 100 g of activated charcoal for serious adult poisonings, and an absolute minimum dose of 30 g. For children, 1 g/kg body weight is the recommended dosage. Theoretically, the addition of flavorings to charcoal or mixing it with magnesium citrate should be avoided because of diminution of the binding capacity of the charcoal. However, in a practical sense, these measures are acceptable if they improve patient acceptance, thereby expediting therapy.

Household sources of charcoal, such as burnt toast or barbecue coals, should not be recommended in the prehospital setting because their adsorptive capacity is very low. Activated charcoal in a fine slurry has a high margin of safety. Even if aspirated, it is relatively nontoxic to the lungs, unless there are large charcoal plugs or admixture of gastric contents (Pollack et al 1981).

In severe intoxications, it may be useful to repeat charcoal administration in a dose of 15 to 20 g at 3- to 4-hour intervals. Certain drugs, after absorption from the gut, are secreted back into the bowel lumen via bile or gastrointestinal secretions. Repeated doses of charcoal can bind additional drug that enters the gut by this enterohepatic and enteroenteral recirculation. The tricyclic antidepressants and the sedative glutethimide are common examples of drugs that undergo this enteral recirculation and thereby benefit from repeated doses of charcoal. In addition, even if there is no drug in the bowel lumen, charcoal seems to leach drug from the circulation into the bowel lumen, thereby hastening drug elimination. This "gastrointestinal dialysis" has been shown to significantly decrease blood levels of theophylline and phenobarbital, even after these drugs were given intravenously (Berg et al 1982; Berlinger et al 1983).

Catharsis

Following charcoal administration, it is traditional to hasten elimination with a cathartic. However, there are little clinical data to support the efficacy of this practice. Table 26–4 lists a number of cathartics that are available. Generally, magnesium citrate is the most commonly used cathartic because it is so readily available.

There are certain contraindications to cathartic use. A cathartic should not be used if a corrosive agent has been ingested, to minimize the risk of reflux into the esophagus. In addition, cathartics should be avoided when bowel sounds are absent,

TABLE 26–4
Cathartics

Magnesium citrate	Adults:	200 ml
	Children:	5 ml/kg
Magnesium sulfate	Adults:	250 ml of 10% solution
	Children:	2.5 ml/kg of 10% solution
Sorbitol	Adults:	100–150 ml of 70% solution
	Children:	1 ml/kg of 70% solution
Fleet's Phosphasoda	Adults:	30–60 ml
	Children:	10–15 ml

when ileus or bowel obstruction is present, or in poisonings that cause vomiting, diarrhea, or gastrointestinal bleeding. Also, laxatives should not be used in children less than 6 months of age or in elderly or medically debilitated adults, because the fluid losses by catharsis may cause serious dehydration in these patients.

Although magnesium citrate is the preferred cathartic, it should not be used if there is pre-existing renal disease or a nephrotoxic ingestion, because hypermagnesemia may develop. Sorbitol is the best substitute in this situation. Fleet's phosphasoda should be avoided in infants and renal patients because of the tendency to accumulate phosphate. Sodium sulfate (Glauber's solution) should be avoided in patients with heart failure. Finally, castor oil should never be used because of its tendency to cause a prolonged cathartic effect with colicky abdominal pain (Riegel and Becker 1981).

Antidotes

Considering the vast number of potential poisons that exist, few poisons have specific antidotes. Table 26–5 is a listing of various poisonings and their antidotes. The mechanisms of action of these various antidotes differ for each agent. Direct binding of antidote to poison, drug receptor site competition or receptor modification, alteration in poison metabolism, and directly counteracting physiologic effects are the principal means by which antidotes work (Epstein and Eilers 1983; Litovitz 1984).

Diuresis

Because most drugs undergo metabolism by the liver and many others are strongly protein or tissue bound, it is not surprising that diuresis has a very limited role in poisoning management. In addition, certain poisons are associated with noncardiac pulmonary edema, such that saline loading would be detrimental.

If a poison is excreted primarily by the renal route and a potentially life-threatening situation exists, fluid diuresis should be considered. Saline loading will increase glomerular filtration of the toxin, and if there is not significant renal tubular reabsorption, increased excretion in the urine will be accomplished. The goal is to achieve and maintain a urine output of 3 to 6 ml/kg/hour (Barkin et al 1984). To achieve such a diuresis, an initial bolus of 20 ml/kg of saline over the first hour, with the addition of a diuretic such as furosemide (Lasix) or mannitol, may be needed.

TABLE 26–5
Acute Antidote Therapy

Poison	Antidote	Dosage
Acetaminophen	N-Acetylcysteine	140 mg/kg orally
Anticholinergics		
Antihistamines		
Atropine		
Antispasmodics	Physostigmine	1–2 mg slow IV push (adult)
Phenothiazines		0.1–0.5 mg slow IV push (child)
Tricyclic antidepressants		
Carbon monoxide	Oxygen	100% by non-rebreather mask
Cyanide	Amyl nitrite, then	Inhale crushed pearl every 2 minutes
	sodium nitrite, then	0.33 ml/kg of 3% solution to maximum of 10 ml IV push over 2 minutes
	sodium thiosulfate	1.65 ml/kg 25% solution to maximum of 50 ml over 10 min
Ethylene glycol	Ethyl alcohol	1 ml/kg of 10% solution in D5W over 30 min as loading dose
Methanol		
Digoxin	Fab fragments	
	(digoxin antibodies)	3–5 vials IV push acutely
Heavy metals		
Arsenic		
Mercury	Dimercaprol (BAL)	5 mg/kg IM
Gold		
Iron	Desferoxamine	90 mg/kg IM, up to 1 g maximum
		10 mg/kg hr IV infusion if coma or shock
Lead	EDTA	5 ml ampule of 20% solution in 250 ml D5W over 5 hrs
Calcium channel blockers	Calcium chloride	3–5 ml of 10% solution over 10 min
Beta blockers	Glucagon	1–2 mg IV push over 5 min
Organophosphate insecticides	Atropine	1–2 mg IV push
	Pralidoxime	25–50 mg/kg IV up to 1 g
Narcotics	Naloxone (Narcan)	0.01 mg/kg IV push (children)
		0.4 to 2 mg IV push (adults)
Coumadin	Vitamin K	5 to 25 mg subcutaneously
	Fresh frozen plasma	2 to 4 units IV

EDTA, ethylenediamene tetraacetic acid.

If the toxin is a weak acid, alkalinization of the urine will enhance excretion. Alkaline diuresis is accomplished by placing two 50-mEq ampules of sodium bicarbonate in 1 L of 5% dextrose in water (D5W) with 10 to 20 mEq of KCl. The infusion is started at 10 ml/kg/hour. The infusion is adjusted to maintain a urine pH of 8.0 or greater. If the toxin is a weak base, acid diuresis may hasten excretion. Urine acidification is accomplished with ammonium chloride, 75 mg/kg to a maximum of 1.5 g given by nasogastric tube or intravenously at 6-hour intervals to maintain a urine pH less than 5.5.

Drug elimination by diuresis, specifically alkaline diuresis, has proved most efficacious for salicylate and phenobarbital overdoses. In all other poisoning situations, diuresis has never shown any clinical benefit, although a definite decrease in blood levels may be demonstrable. For overdoses of the following agents, drug excretion can be enhanced by diuresis, although clinical benefit is questionable: alkaline diuresis: lithium, isoniazid; acid diuresis: PCP, amphetamines, strychnine; saline diuresis: meprobamate, ethanol, methanol, ethylene glycol (Maher 1977).

Dialysis

Although rarely indicated for drug overdose, hemodialysis should be considered immediately if the poisoning is associated with a severe metabolic acidosis, such as after ingestion of ethylene glycol, methanol, and massive amounts of salicylates. Charcoal hemoperfusion may be considered in life-threatening poisonings from theophylline, paraquat, and various sedative or hypnotic overdoses (excluding the benzodiazepines). In addition to the aforementioned situations, hemodialysis or hemoperfusion must be considered in any severe intoxication in which there is progressive deterioration marked by respiratory arrest, hypotension, pulmonary edema, or impairment of renal or hepatic function (Maher 1977).

Health Maintenance, Altered, Related to

- *Perception or Cognitive Impairment as Manifested by Substance Abuse*

The psychiatry service should be involved in the patient's care from the very beginning of his or her hospital stay. If the overdose proves to be very minor and the patient does not require medical admission, the psychiatrist should take over further care. No overdose should be considered too trivial or presumed accidental. Psychiatric admission is mandatory for virtually all medically cleared patients, unless there is no question that this was an accidental or recreational poisoning. The only patient who can safely go home is the young child who can be monitored closely at home by the parents. However, even the latter situation should raise the question of parental neglect.

Evaluation

The overall evaluation of the effectiveness of stage II care (gastric emptying, charcoal administration, catharsis, and so forth) follows both the patient's physiologic status and his or her psychologic status. Stable vital signs and an improvement in the patient's level of consciousness imply that the therapy is effective.

SPECIFIC POISONINGS

Alcohol

Ethanol ingestion is by far the most common intoxication in the emergency setting, either alone or in combination with other drugs. The clinical features of alcohol intoxication are familiar to us all. With increasing severity, there is marked mental and sensory impairment, incoordination, ataxia, slurred speech, and nystagmus.

Ultimately, respiratory failure and coma lead to death (McMicken 1983; Urso et al 1981).

Marked individual variability occurs in correlating ethanol levels to clinical presentation. The legal definition of intoxication in most communities is a blood alcohol level of 100 mg/dl. For the unconditioned adult, an alcohol level greater than 400 mg/dl may be lethal, whereas a chronic drinker may be ambulatory and only moderately intoxicated at that same level (Hammond et al 1973; Tintinalli 1985).

Alcohol levels will drop at a fairly constant rate of 20 to 40 mg/dl per hour, depending on the degree of hepatic conditioning. If a large amount of alcohol remains in the stomach on presentation, the level may initially rise or remain constant for some time before finally dropping. Gastric emptying may eliminate this problem and hence shorten the patient's stay, but charcoal poorly binds alcohol and saline diuresis has limited efficacy. Indeed, gastric emptying followed by charcoal usually is not recommended unless other drugs have been ingested with the alcohol. As a result, there is little that can be done to hasten elimination and the patient must be patiently observed until he or she becomes sober.

The usual protocol in the obtunded patient should be followed with naloxone (Narcan) and D50. With or without administration of dextrose, thiamine (50 to 100 mg intramuscularly) should be given to prevent the Wernicke-Korsakoff syndrome. Magnesium sulfate, 2 g intramuscularly, is recommended in alcoholics to correct magnesium deficiency and thereby minimize the risk of seizures in the withdrawal state. Because alcoholics often fall down and get into fights, the ED personnel should be wary of the possibility of cervical spine and head injury whenever an intoxicated patient is evaluated.

Alcohol withdrawal is a common emergency. The withdrawal syndrome will vary with the duration and intensity of drinking, but it can follow even an isolated binge. There is no absolute alcohol level associated with withdrawal symptoms, but rather a relative change from a steady state level. In fact, the initial symptoms of tremor, irritability, and insomnia, which begin 6 to 12 hours after the last drink, may be associated with an alcohol level of anywhere from zero to 200 mg%. Dehydration may occur in the first 24 hours from vomiting, diarrhea, and diaphoresis.

Alcohol withdrawal seizures, or "rum fits," are usually seen in the first 36 hours of abstinence and are typically tonic-clonic. Ordinarily there is only a single seizure, but sometimes two or three occur in close succession. Status epilepticus is generally not a part of this syndrome.

Also occurring in the first 36 hours is alcoholic hallucinosis, which is usually visual and tactile rather than auditory in nature. The patient's senses become extremely heightened to all sights and sounds and he or she is easily frightened. The patient does recognize that the insects and strange people he or she sees and feels are not real, yet nevertheless these are very threatening.

The full-blown syndrome of delirium tremens ("DTs") develops 48 to 96 hours after the last drink. Fever is the hallmark of delirium tremens, usually accompanied by hypertension, tachycardia, diaphoresis, hallucinosis, tremors, and paranoia. Generally, the initial withdrawal symptoms of tremulousness, seizures, and hallucinosis precede full-blown delirium tremens, but this is not always the case (Victor and Adams 1983).

A patient in alcohol withdrawal is generally dehydrated and may be orthostatic, requiring intravenous volume replacement. Hypokalemia and hypomagnesemia are common, and replacement therapy should be initiated; potassium is supplemented in intravenous fluids, and 2 g of magnesium sulfate is given intramuscularly, as noted for acute intoxication (Geiderman et al 1979).

Hypoglycemia is common in the alcoholic person both with acute intoxication and during withdrawal. If dextrose is given to an alcoholic, an acute thiamine deficiency state, called the Wernicke-Korsakoff syndrome, may be precipitated. This syndrome consists of ocular muscle palsies, nystagmus, ataxic gait, and progressive mental impairment. Therefore, thiamine is given routinely for both intoxication and withdrawal states (Follender 1977).

Alcoholics in the intoxicated or withdrawal state may also manifest acidosis. Usually this results from ketoacidosis, which can occur in the nondiabetic drinker who develops protracted vomiting and has poor caloric intake over a 1- to 2-day period. Generally, the acidosis is mild and will be corrected with saline and glucose infusion. If the patient's urine is negative for ketones, the acidosis may be secondary to poisoning from ethylene glycol or methanol, which are alcohols sometimes consumed inadvertently by the desperate alcoholic. Isopropyl alcohol (rubbing alcohol) will result in ketones in the urine but will not cause metabolic acidosis (Fulop and Hoberman 1975).

In addition to correction of dehydration and electrolyte abnormalities, the patient may also require sedative therapy. Minimal tremulousness in a patient with a normal mental status may not require any tranquilizer therapy. However, the patient who is agitated, who is hallucinating, who is having seizures or who has evidence of autonomic hyperactivity (such as fever and tachycardia) should be calmed rapidly. Any tranquilizer may be effective, but diazepam (Valium) is the preferred agent, given intravenously in 2- to 5-mg boluses every 10 to 15 minutes as needed for calming effect. The dose required to quiet the delirium tremens patient is quite variable. Chlordiazepoxide (Librium) is another commonly used sedative for the treatment of alcohol withdrawal. The dose is 25 to 50 mg every 4 to 6 hours, administered intramuscularly or by mouth (Sellers and Kalant 1976; Thompson 1978).

The patient should be monitored closely for respiratory depression and hypotension during drug administration. In addition, physical restraints are usually necessary. Drugs such as haloperidol (Haldol) or chlorpromazine (Thorazine) generally are avoided because they increase the risk of seizures. Paraldehyde, in doses of 5 to 15 ml, has a limited role in alcohol withdrawal because of difficulty in titrating dose to effect, restriction of route of administration to oral and rectal only, and the very noxious odor, which is repulsive to the patient and staff alike. The hallucinosis and agitation of alcohol withdrawal can be confused with acute psychosis; therefore, a careful alcohol history is important in all psychiatric patients.

If seizures occur, intravenous diazepam (Valium) is the treatment of choice. If seizures recur, phenytoin (Dilantin) loading and maintenance therapy for 3 days may be useful (Sampliner and Iber 1974). Patients with full-blown delirium tremens should have a careful evaluation for infection, because sepsis is the most common cause of death in this population.

Sedatives and Sleeping Pills

The barbiturates, the benzodiazepines, and the nonbarbiturate sedatives such as glutethimide, methaqualone, ethchlorvynol, meprobamate, and chloral hydrate all produce their major toxicity by sedation and respiratory depression. In severe overdose, respiratory arrest and shock may occur. Benzodiazepines are the least likely to cause respiratory depression unless combined with other sedatives. Glutethimide and ethchlorvynol can cause very prolonged coma, as well as hypotension and pulmonary edema. Glutethimide (Doriden) is unique in that it causes dilated, poorly reactive pupils and may cause unexpected laryngeal spasm and wide swings in level of consciousness. Chloral hydrate overdose, on the other hand, is associated with cardiac dysrhythmias.

Protection of the airway and ventilatory support, as well as volume resuscitation for hypotension, are the mainstays of treatment in sedative overdoses. Gastric evacuation followed by administration of charcoal and a cathartic should be routine. Hastening excretion with alkaline diuresis is effective only for phenobarbital; otherwise treatment is supportive in an intensive care unit (ICU) until the patient awakens (Flomenbaum et al 1986; Lankin and Baltarowich 1983).

Narcotics

Opiate overdose causes the typical triad of coma, respiratory depression, and constricted pupils. Sudden onset of pulmonary edema can lead to death and is most commonly associated with intravenous heroin abuse. Seizures also may occur. It should be kept in mind that such drugs as propoxyphene (Darvon) and diphenoxylate (Lomotil) are also opiates. Routine poisoning management should be performed. Naloxone (Narcan) should cause prompt arousal; however, its duration of effect is only a few minutes. The dosage of Narcan is 0.4 to 2.0 mg as an initial test dose, with subsequent repeat boluses or an intravenous infusion.

Patients with narcotic withdrawal syndrome may have vomiting, diarrhea, diaphoresis, gooseflesh, and twitching. Fluid replacement and methadone therapy, 10 to 15 mg orally, should be administered. Other than dehydration, opiate withdrawal is not life threatening; therefore, replacement narcotics should not be given unless clear-cut objective signs are present (Allen 1983).

Tricyclic Antidepressants

Tricyclic antidepressant overdoses can be highly lethal and should be treated very aggressively. Confusion and coma are seen initially, but it is the cardiotoxicity that results in death. QRS interval duration greater than 10 ms is correlated with a high risk of cardiac arrhythmias, particularly ventricular tachycardia, ventricular fibrillation, and heart block. Status epilepticus, another serious complication of tricyclic antidepressant overdoses, is heralded by QRS prolongation and carries a bad prognosis. Hypotension and pulmonary edema also may ensue (Boehnert and Lovejoy 1985; Callaham 1979; Hollister 1978; Marshall and Forker 1982; Salzman, 1985).

The patient should immediately be placed on a monitor and an intravenous line placed. Routine gastric lavage, charcoal, and cathartics should follow, with appropriate airway precautions. Alkalinization of the serum with sodium bicarbonate, which diminishes circulating drug by enhancing serum protein binding, is the mainstay of treatment. Two 50-mEq ampules of sodium bicarbonate in 1 L of D5W should be started as an infusion to maintain a blood pH of 7.5. Alkalinization can also be accomplished by hyperventilation if the patient is intubated. If cardiac dysrhythmias persist, specifically tachyarrhythmias, physostigmine (1 to 2 mg intravenously over several minutes) may be helpful, but severe bradyarrhythmias are a danger. Phenytoin loading is another option in treatment of dysrhythmias and in seizure prophylaxis (Hagerman and Hanashiro 1981; Mayron and Ruiz 1986). ICU monitoring is necessary for most overdoses with tricyclic antidepressants, unless there is no sedation or EKG abnormalities after 4 hours of observation in the ED (Callaham and Kassel 1985).

Aspirin and Acetaminophen

Aspirin and acetaminophen are in so many over-the-counter and prescription medications that it is not surprising that they are common causes of intentional overdose in the adolescent and adult and of accidental poisoning in the child.

Salicylates have multiple metabolic effects that contribute to their toxicity. They are gastric irritants leading to vomiting and gastric bleeding. They cause a metabolic block at oxidative phosphorylation, leading to acidosis. Salicylates have a toxic effect on the central nervous system, leading to initial confusion and irritability, followed by lethargy, stupor, and convulsions. Stimulation of the brain stem respiratory center accounts for the characteristic deep, panting respirations of these patients. Finally, salicylates interfere with glucose metabolism, resulting in either hypo- or hyperglycemia (Temple 1981).

The earliest symptoms of salicylate toxicity are vomiting, tinnitus, and decreased hearing. Moderate intoxication is first manifested by hyperventilation with possible mild lethargy or irritability. More severe intoxication is characterized by increasing hyperpnea, dehydration, fever, delirium, stupor, and coma. Arterial blood gases show a mixed metabolic acidosis and respiratory alkalosis, with the former being predominant in young children, and the latter seen more frequently in adults. Pulmonary edema may develop in older patients with renal insufficiency (Anderson et al 1976; Walters et al 1983).

Therapy in salicylate overdose includes standard gastric evacuation, followed by charcoal and cathartics. At the same time, fluid deficits should be corrected by 5% dextrose in lactated Ringer's solution. Significant toxicity and need for medical observation can be anticipated by use of the Done nomogram (Fig. 26–1), on which the salicylate level 6 hours or more after ingestion is plotted (Done 1960). Alkaline diuresis may be useful in moderate intoxications, but more severe poisonings may require dialysis (Done 1978; Temple 1981).

Acetaminophen's toxicity is characterized by a delayed hepatic necrosis, resulting from the accumulation of toxic metabolic products that result when the normal metabolic pathways are overwhelmed. The clinical course of acetaminophen overdose typically progresses through three phases. The first phase occurs within hours of ingestion and is characterized by repeated vomiting and malaise. The second phase, which encompasses the next 48 hours, may be a period in which the patient is completely asymptomatic or has mild persistent gastrointestinal symptoms. The third phase occurs after 3 to 5 days and is marked by signs of acute hepatic necrosis, including jaundice, right upper quadrant pain, and encephalopathy.

In the acute management of acetaminophen overdose, correction of dehydra-

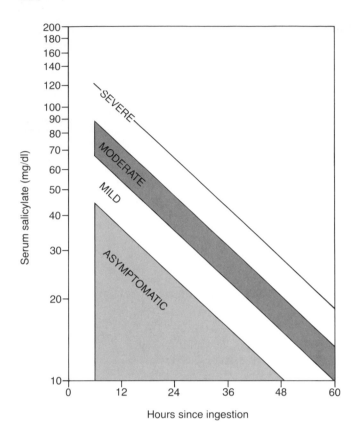

Serum salicylate (mg/dl)

SEVERE

MODERATE

MILD

ASYMPTOMATIC

Hours since ingestion

FIGURE 26-1. Done nomogram for salicylate poisoning. Note that this nomogram is not accurate for chronic ingestions. (Modified by permission from Pediatrics, Vol 26, page 800, Copyright 1960.)

tion and gastric emptying should be accomplished. In contrast to routine poisoning management, charcoal administration should be withheld if the patient is being considered for antidote therapy, as the charcoal would bind both the antidote and the offending drug. N-Acetylcysteine (Mucomyst), the specific antidote for acetaminophen overdose, increases the hepatic production of glutathione, which metabolizes the hepatotoxic intermediate, thereby protecting the liver. An acetaminophen level, determined 4 hours or more after ingestion, correlates well with the risk of hepatotoxicity when plotted on the graph (Fig. 26-2) (Rumack and Mathew 1975). If the level falls within the toxic range, 140 mg/kg of Mucomyst by mouth is given initially, and subsequent doses of 70 mg/kg are repeated at 4-hour intervals for 72 hours. To be effective, the antidotal therapy must begin within 18 hours of ingestion (Linden and Rumack 1984; Rumack et al 1981).

Cocaine and Phencyclidine

Cocaine use has gained enormous popularity over the past decade in the United States. Intranasal administration or "snorting" is the principal route of abuse; how-

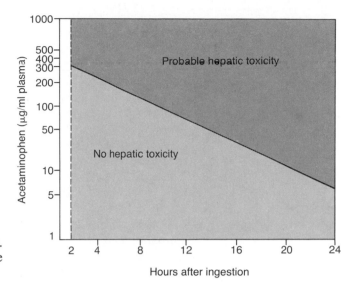

FIGURE 26-2. Plasma acetaminophen levels over time. (Modified by permission from Pediatrics, Vol 55, page 871, Copyright 1975.)

ever, the drug can also be smoked or injected. "Free-based" cocaine, known as "crack," is a more purified form that is usually smoked, giving a similar acute "rush" as intravenous use. The dose of cocaine by nasal insufflation is typically spoken of in gram quantities. One gram of cocaine can be arranged into 30 to 40 lines (1/8 inch by 1 inch) and then inhaled through a straw at 15- to 30-minute intervals. The typical abuser has three to four lines in succession, but the addict may be on a "run" of repeated insufflations over one to two days.

Cocaine produces central and autonomic nervous system stimulation by blocking neurotransmitter uptake, thereby causing a build-up of catecholamines. The central nervous system effects start with excitement and euphoria and, with increased intoxication, progress to apprehension, anxiety, delirium, and ultimately seizures. Profound intoxication has a biphasic response of initial stimulation followed by CNS depression, characterized by coma and paralysis (Haddad 1983a; Kleber and Gawin 1984).

Physical assessment of the patient intoxicated with cocaine usually reveals tachycardia, hypertension, pallor, dilated pupils, and hyperreflexia. The EKG may reveal ventricular dysrhythmias, and in some instances myocardial infarction has been reported (Pasternack et al 1985; Weiss 1986).

Treatment of cocaine intoxication is primarily supportive. The patient is placed on a monitor and observed for dysrhythmias. An intravenous line is placed to correct dehydration as well as to provide a port to administer drugs. Seizures are treated with intravenous diazepam and ventricular ectopy with lidocaine. If hypertension is extreme, use of nitroprusside may be necessary. Agitation usually responds to observation in a quiet environment, but delirium or psychosis may require Thorazine or Haldol. There is no effective method to prevent absorption of cocaine, and acid diuresis does not affect outcome (Gay 1982).

Phencyclidine (PCP), which was initially introduced as a veterinary anesthetic, has become a common street drug. PCP is usually smoked, but it can be snorted, injected, or taken by mouth. Frequently it is an adulterant of other street drugs, and as a result, the abuser often is not aware that he or she is using PCP. PCP often causes a state of disorientation, inability to concentrate, and altered judgment. In fact, patients under its effects generally are acutely psychotic, exhibiting extreme agitation, violence, hallucinations, and delusions, alternating with a catatonic state. In severe poisoning, death can result from coma, seizures, and hypertensive crisis.

The classic physical findings in PCP intoxication are spontaneous horizontal and vertical nystagmus and severe hypertension. A urine toxicologic screen will identify PCP, but there are no other characteristic laboratory findings (McMarron et al 1981; Rumack 1980).

There is no effective method to stop absorption of PCP from the nasal or respiratory route. Indeed, the drug is so potent in such small quantities that gastric elimination and charcoal are of little benefit, even if the charcoal is taken by the oral route. Treatment is primarily supportive, placing the patient in a quiet, dimly lit room, and avoiding any physical or verbal stimuli. Restraints often are necessary, but this will certainly further agitate the patient. Acid diuresis can increase the excretion of PCP; however, this therapy does not detoxify the patient any faster. Cardiac monitoring and seizure precautions should be routine (Aronow and Done 1978; Rappolt et al 1979).

CONCLUSION

Poisoning is a common clinical problem in the ED setting. An intoxication may be an intentional overdose, a recreational drug abuse, or an accidental environmental, or iatrogenic poisoning. Several clinical presentations should heighten suspicion for poisoning, including cardiac dysrhythmias, pulmonary edema, coma, bizarre behavior, seizures, gastroenteritis, and unexplained metabolic acidosis. History taking in poisonings and overdose is notoriously unreliable. The physical assessment may give valuable clues, but they are rarely specific.

Poisoning management focuses initially on the basics (airway, breathing, and circulation). If the patient is lethargic and has a poor gag response, protection of the airway with an endotracheal tube is recommended before gastric emptying is attempted. Depression in sensorium should be treated with Narcan and D50 on a routine basis. Gastric emptying should be accomplished, either by use of a nasogastric tube or by administration of syrup of ipecac. This is followed by administration of a charcoal slurry, and lastly a cathartic-like magnesium citrate. Diuresis and dialysis have a very limited role in overdose management. Specific antidote therapy in selected situations may be life-saving.

Most poisonings will not be life threatening, and some may not require any therapy at all other than pushing fluids. However, all potential intoxications should be approached in an aggressive, thorough manner, because morbidity and mortality in this setting are easily preventable.

REFERENCES

Allen T. 1983. Narcotics. In Rosen P, Baker FJ, Braen GR, et al, eds. Emergency Medicine, Concepts and Clinical Practice. St. Louis, CV Mosby Co., 1535–1548.

Anderson RJ, Potts DE, Gabow PA, et al. 1976. Unrecognized adult salicylate intoxication. Ann Intern Med 85:745.

Arena JM. 1979. Poisoning: Toxicology— Symptoms—Treatments, 4th ed. Springfield, IL, Charles C Thomas.

Arena JM. 1978. The treatment of poisonings. Clin Symp 30:3.

Arnold FJ, Hodges JB, Baria RA, et al. 1959. Evaluation of the efficacy of lavage and induced emesis. Pediatrics 23:286.

Aronow R, Done AK. 1978. Phencyclidine overdose: An emerging concept of management. J Am Coll Emerg Phys 7:56.

Barkin RM, Kulig KW, Rumack BH. Poisoning and overdose. In Barkin RM, Rosen P, eds. Emergency Pediatrics. St. Louis, CV Mosby Co., 266–305.

Benowitz NL, Goldschlager N. 1983. Cardiac disturbances in the toxicologic patient. In Haddad LM, Winchester JF, eds. Clinical Management of Poisoning and Drug Overdose. Philadelphia, WB Saunders Co., 65–99.

Benowitz NL, Rosenberg J, Becker CE. 1979. Cardiopulmonary catastrophes in drug-overdosed patients. Med Clin North Am 63:267–296.

Berg MJ, Berlinger WG, Goldberg MJ, et al. 1982. Acceleration of the body clearance of phenobarbital by oral activated charcoal. N Engl J Med 307:642.

Berlinger WG, Spector R, Goldberg MJ, et al. 1983. Enhancement of theophylline clearance by oral activated charcoal. Clin Pharm Ther 33:351.

Boehnert MT, Lovejoy FH. 1985. Value of the QRS duration versus the serum drug level in predicting seizures and ventricular arrhythmias after an acute overdose of tricyclic antidepressants. N Engl J Med 313:512.

Callaham M. 1979. Collective review of tricyclic antidepressant overdose. J Am Coll Emerg Phys 8:413.

Callaham M, Kassel D. 1985. Epidemiology of fatal tricyclic antidepressant ingestion: Implications for management. Ann Emerg Med 14:1.

Done AK. 1960. Salicylate intoxication: Significance of measurements of salicylates in blood in cases of acute ingestion. Pediatrics 26:805.

Done AK. 1978. Aspirin overdose; incidence, diagnosis, and management. Pediatrics 62(Suppl): 890–897.

Dreisbach RH. 1980. Prevention, Diagnosis and Treatment: Handbook of Poisoning. Los Altos, CA, Lange Medical Publications.

Easom JM, Lovejoy FH. 1979. Efficacy and safety of gastrointestinal decontamination in the treatment of oral poisoning. Pediatr Clin North Am 26:827.

Emmett M, Narins RG. 1977. Clinical use of the anion gap. Medicine 56:38.

Epstein FB, Eilers MA. 1983. Poisoning. In Rosen P, Baker FJ, Braen GR, et al, eds. Emergency Medicine: Concepts and Clinical Practice. St. Louis, CV Mosby Co., 237–244.

Flomenbaum N, Goldfrank L, Roberts JR. 1986. Selected clinical toxicologic presentations: Evaluation and management. In Schwartz GR, Safar P, Stone JH. Principles and Practice of Emergency Medicine, 2nd ed. Philadelphia, WB Saunders Co., 1688–1699.

Follender AB. 1977. Neurologic problems prevalent in alcoholics. Postgrad Med 61:166.

Fought SG, Throwe AN. 1984. Psychosocial nursing care of the emergency patient. New York, John Wiley and Sons, 131–146.

Fulop M, Hoberman HD. 1975. Alcoholic ketosis. Diabetes 24:785.

Gay GR. 1982. Clinical management of acute and chronic cocaine poisoning. Ann Emerg Med 11:562.

Geiderman JM, Goodman SL, Cohen DB. 1979. Magnesium: The forgotten electrolyte. J Am Coll Emerg Phys 8:204.

Greenblatt DJ, Allen MD, Noel BJ, et al. 1977. Acute overdosage with benzodiazepine derivatives. Clin Pharmacol Ther 21:497.

Greensher J, Mofenson HC, Picchioni AL, et al. 1979. Activated charcoal updated. J Am Coll Emerg Phys 8:261.

Goodman JM, Bischel MD, Wagers PW, et al. 1976. Barbiturate intoxication: Morbidity and mortality. West J Med 124:179.

Haddad LM. 1983a. Cocaine. In Haddad LM, Winchester JF, eds. Clinical Management of Poisoning and Drug Overdose. Philadelphia, WB Saunders Co., 443–447.

Haddad LM. 1983b. General approach to the emergency management of poisoning. In Haddad LM, Winchester JF, eds. Clinical Management of Poisoning and Drug Overdose. Philadelphia, WB Saunders Co., 4–17.

Hagerman GA, Hanashiro PK. 1981. Reversal of tricyclic antidepressant-induced cardiac conduction abnormalities by phenytoin. Ann Emerg Med 10:82.

Hammond KB, Rumack BH, Roderson DO. 1973. Blood ethanol: a report of an unusually high level in a living patient. JAMA 226:63.

Hollister LE. 1978. Tricyclic antidepressants. N Engl J Med 299:1106, 1168.

Howell JM. 1986. Alkaline ingestions. Ann Emerg Med 15:820–825.

Kleber HD, Gawin FH. 1984. The spectrum of cocaine abuse and its treatment. J Clin Psychiatry 45:18.

Kulig K, Bar-Or D, Cantrill SV, et al. 1985. Management of acutely poisoned patients without gastric emptying. Ann Emerg Med 14:562–567.

Lankin DL, Baltarowich LL. 1983. Sedative hypnotics. In Rosen P, Baker FJ, Braen GR, et al, eds. Emergency Medicine: Concepts and Clinical Practice. St. Louis, CV Mosby Co., 1516.

Linden CH, Rumack BH. 1984. Acetaminophen overdose. Emerg Med Clin North Am 2:103–119.

Litovitz TL. 1984. The anecdotal antidotes. Emerg Med Clin North Am 2:145.

Maher JF. 1977. Principles of dialysis of drugs. Am J Med 62:475.

Manno BR, Manno JE. 1977. Toxicology of ipecac: A review. Clin Toxicol 10:221.

Marshall JB, Forker AD. 1982. Cardiovascular effects of tricyclic antidepressant drugs. Am Heart J 103:401.

Mayron R, Ruiz E. 1986. Phenytoin: Does it reverse tricyclic antidepressant-induced cardiac conduction abnormalities? Ann Emerg Med 15:876–880.

McDougal CB, McLean MA. 1981. Modifications in the technique of gastric lavage. Ann Emerg Med 10:514.

McMarron MM, Schulze BW, Thompson GA, et al. 1981. Acute phencyclidine intoxication: Incidence of clinical findings in 1000 cases. Ann Emerg Med 10:237.

McMicken DB. 1983. Alcohol related disease. In Rosen P, Baker FJ, Braen GR, et al, eds. Emergency Medicine, Concepts and Clinical Practice. St. Louis, CV Mosby Co., 1486.

Nicholson DP. 1983. The immediate management of overdose. Med Clin North Am 67:1279–1293.

Park GD, Spector R, et al. 1986. Expanded role of charcoal therapy in the poisoned and overdosed patient. Arch Intern Med 146:969–973.

Pasternack PF, Colvin SB, Baumann FG. 1985. Cocaine induced angina pectoris and acute myocardial infarction in patients younger than 40 years. Am J Cardiol 55:847.

Pearlson GD. 1981. Psychiatric and medical syndromes associated with phencyclidine abuse. Johns Hopkins Med J 148:25.

Pollack MM, Dunbar BS, Holbrook PR, et al. 1981. Aspiration of activated charcoal and gastric contents. Ann Emerg Med 10:528.

Rappolt RT, Gay GR, Farris RD. 1979. Emergency management of acute phencyclidine intoxication. J Am Coll Emerg Phys 8:68.

Riegel JM, Becker CE. 1981. Use of cathartics in toxic ingestions. Ann Emerg Med 10:254.

Rumack B. 1980. Phencyclidine overdose: An overview. Ann Emerg Med 9:595.

Rumack B, Mathew H. 1975. Acetaminophen poisoning and toxicity. Pediatrics 55:871.

Rumack BH, Peterson RG, Kock GG, et al. 1981. Acetaminophen overdose: 662 cases with evaluation of oral acetylcysteine treatment. Arch Intern Med 141:380.

Salzman C. 1985. Editorial: Clinical use of antidepressant blood levels and the electrocardiogram. N Engl J Med 313:512.

Sampliner R, Iber FL. 1974. Diphenylhydantoin control of alcohol withdrawal seizures: Results of a controlled study. JAMA 230:1430.

Schwartz GR. 1986. Emergency management of the toxicologic patient. In Schwartz GR, Safar P, Stone JH, eds. Principles and Practice of Emergency Medicine, 2nd ed. Philadelphia, WB Saunders Co., 1671.

Sellers EM, Kalant H. 1976. Alcohol intoxication and withdrawal. N Engl J Med 294:757.

Sullivan JB Jr, Rumack BH, Peterson RG. 1979. Management of the poisoned patient in the emergency department. In Bayer MJ, Rumack BH, eds. Poisonings and Overdose. Rockville, MD, Aspen Systems Corporation, 1–12.

Tandberg D, Troutman WG. 1985. Gastric lavage in the poisoned patient. In Roberts JR, Hedges JR, eds. Clinical Procedures in Emergency Medicine. Philadelphia, WB Saunders Co., 762–770.

Taviera da Silva AM. 1983. Principles of respiratory therapy. In Haddad LM, Winchester JF, eds. Clinical Management of Poisoning and Drug Overdose. Philadelphia, WB Saunders Co., 198–220.

Temple AR. 1981. Acute and chronic effects of aspirin toxicity and their treatment. Arch Intern Med 141:364.

Thoman ME, Verhulst HL. 1966. Ipecac syrup in antiemetic ingestion. JAMA 196:433.

Thompson WL. 1978. Management of alcohol withdrawal syndromes. Arch Intern Med 138:278.

Tintinalli JE. 1985. Alcohols. In Tintinalli JE, Rothstein RJ, Krome RL, eds. Emergency Medicine, A Comprehensive Study Guide. New York, McGraw-Hill Book Co., 309–315.

Urso T, Gavaler JS, Van Thiel DH. 1981. Blood ethanol levels in sober alcohol users seen in an emergency room. Life Sci 28:1053.

Victor M, Adams RD. 1983. Alcohol. In Petersdorf RG, Adams RD, Braunwald E, eds. Harrison's Principles of Internal Medicine. New York, McGraw-Hill Book Co., 1285–1295.

Walters JS, Woodring JH, Stelling CB. 1983. Salicylate induced pulmonary edema. Radiology 146:289.

Warner RB. 1983. Psychiatric intervention with the suicidal patient. In Haddad LM, Winchester JF, eds. Clinical Management of Poisoning and Drug Overdose. Philadelphia, WB Saunders Co., 268–274.

Weiss RJ. 1986. Recurrent myocardial infarction caused by cocaine abuse. Am Heart J 111:793.

David N. Zull, MD FACEP

Anaphylaxis

An acute allergic reaction is an easily preventable cause of death, but immediate recognition and treatment are critical. Severity may range from nuisance symptoms, such as a rash or lip swelling, to sudden death secondary to upper airway obstruction or shock. However, even the patient who presents with hives alone, if left untreated, may go on to develop hypotension, bronchospasm, or laryngeal edema. Therefore, all acute allergic reactions should be treated with similar urgency (Fisher 1987, Sheffer 1985, Terr 1985, Lockey 1974).

The terms *anaphylaxis* and *anaphylactoid reaction* are used to denote a generalized allergic reaction following exposure to a foreign substance. Clinical characteristics include urticaria, angioedema, bronchospasm, hypotension, laryngeal edema, and abdominal colic. In the first half of this century, the most common cause of lethal anaphylaxis was horse serum. In the past 35 years, penicillin and penicillin derivatives have led the list (O'Leary 1986). The second and third most common causes of death from anaphylaxis currently include bee stings (Patterson 1982) and iodinated contrast media (Greenberger 1984), respectively, followed closely by foods (Amlot 1987, Golbert 1969, Novey 1983) and nonsteroidal antiinflammatory drugs (Stevenson 1984, Sandler 1985).

PATHOPHYSIOLOGY

The allergic constellation of symptoms occur from a massive release of chemical mediators from mast cells and basophils throughout the body. For anaphylaxis to

655

occur there must be previous sensitization to a foreign substance in which antibody-producing B lymphocytes of the host make immunoglobulin E (IgE) in reaction to the substance. Whether a host will make specific IgE that causes allergy depends upon genetic predisposition, antigen potency, dose, and timing of exposure. Once IgE is made, it binds to mast cells and basophils throughout the body. On re-exposure of the host, the antigen will bind to the IgE on mast cells and basophils, and this interaction induces release of chemical mediators from these cells. If immunoglobulin G (IgG) is made in preference to IgE, as is the hope in allergy injection therapy, the circulating IgG will bind the antigen before it can get to IgE on mast cells. The term *anaphylactoid reaction* is often used to denote a clinical syndrome identical to anaphylaxis but distinguished by the fact that no role of IgE can be identified in causing mast cells to release their mediators (Ishizaka 1983, Weiszer 1985).

Mast cells have preformed granules containing histamine, platelet-activating factor, and kallikrein, which are released in allergic reactions. In addition, arachidonic acid metabolism is stimulated in the mast cell at the same time that granules are released, producing prostaglandins and leukotrienes (slow-reacting substance of anaphylaxis, SRS-A). Histamine, prostaglandins, and kallikrein lead to vasodilation and capillary leaking resulting in hypotension; angioedema of the skin, upper airway, and

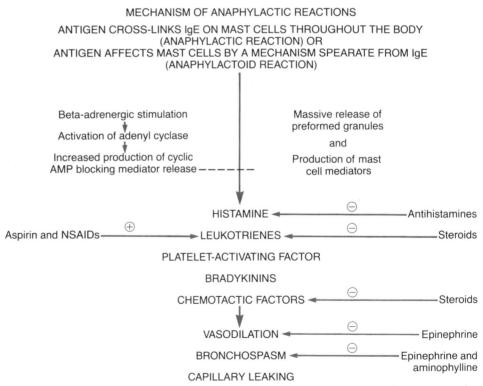

FIGURE 27–1. Mechanism of anaphylactic reactions. Anaphylaxis results from the massive release of chemical mediators from mast cells. Beta-adrenergics block this mediator release. Other drugs may have a therapeutic or an aggravating effect, depending upon direct end-organ effects or interaction with specific chemical mediators.

gastrointestinal tract; and urticaria. The leukotrienes are extremely potent broncho-constrictors. Cyclic AMP (cAMP) in mast cells inhibit degranulation and mediator synthesis. The beta-adrenergic receptor stimulates the enzyme adenyl cyclase, which promotes the synthesis of cAMP in the mast cell. Thereby, a potent adrenergic stimulus such as epinephrine will increase cellular cAMP and thus stop further mediator release from mast cells. Epinephrine therefore is the mainstay of anaphylaxis therapy, because it stops the ongoing reaction. Antihistamines compete directly with histamine at tissue histamine receptor sites, and steroids block arachidonic acid metabolism, making these agents useful additions to therapy (Ishizaka, 1983; Lucke, 1983; Weiszer, 1985) (Fig. 27–1).

EPIDEMIOLOGY AND PREDISPOSING FACTORS

It is estimated that 15% to 20% of the population will develop urticaria during their lifetime and that 2% of hospitalized patients will develop allergic skin reactions (Monroe 1977). Urticaria is a localized form of anaphylaxis and occurs by the same pathophysiologic mechanisms; its incidence, however, is some 20-fold greater than anaphylaxis. The reaction rate to penicillin, for example, is less than 1%, most of these being urticaria alone. Of 100,000 patients treated with penicillin, it is estimated that 25 will have severe anaphylaxis, and one patient will die (O'Leary 1986). In the United States, between 100 and 200 deaths per year are reported from penicillin anaphylaxis. For comparison, the allergic reaction rate to bee stings is about 0.4%, with 50 to 80 anaphylactic deaths per year (Patterson 1982). Iodinated contrast media administration, particularly in intravenous pyelography (IVPs), results in anaphylactoid reactions in 1% to 2% of patients, with 1 to 10 of 100,000 cases resulting in death. There are some 40 to 50 deaths per year reported from contrast media in the United States (Greenberger 1984).

Are there patient characteristics that identify a patient at risk? Male to female ratios appear equal. Reactions tend to be more common and more severe as patients age from adolescence to adulthood, presumably from repeated exposures. However, this increasing incidence with age tends to reverse in the elderly, secondary to decline in the immune system (Weiszer 1985). A startling example of these age relationships in anaphylaxis occurs with regard to bee sting allergy. Ninety percent of bee stings are seen in patients less than 20 years of age; however, 93% of the deaths from such envenomations occur in patients over 20 years old (Patterson 1982). There also appears to be a higher risk in patients with a personal or family history of atopy, such as asthma or allergic rhinitis. The correlation to atopy is not seen however, for such potent allergens as penicillin and hymenoptera (bee) venom (O'Leary 1986). Exercise may be an important aggravating factor and in some cases a cause in itself (Sheffer 1984, Kidd 1983).

Dosing and the route of antigen exposure may also be important in the development and severity of anaphylaxis. Frequent administration of a substance or drug with interruptions in exposure increase the risk of sensitization. The more direct the route to the systemic circulation the greater the likelihood and the severity of reac-

TABLE 27-1
Etiologic Agents in Anaphylaxis

Proteins
  Insect venoms
  Foods
  Allergy extracts
  Foreign serum and whole blood
  Insulin
  Streptokinase
  Vaccines
  Seminal fluid

Haptens
  Penicillin and cephalosporins
  Other antibiotics
  Local anesthetics

Prostaglandin Inhibition
  Aspirin (not sodium salicylate or salsolate [Disalcid])
  Nonsteroidal antiinflammatory drugs (e.g., ibuprofen, tolmetin,
    etc.)

Physical factors
  Exercise-induced anaphylaxis
  Food or NSAID anaphylaxis unmasked by exercise
  Cold-induced urticaria and anaphylaxis

Complement Activation/Mast Cell Degranulators
  IVP dye and other radiocontrast materials
  Polysaccharides
  Thiamine, vitamin K, morphine

Idiopathic Anaphylaxis

tion; therefore, routes of exposure in descending order of severity would be intravenous, intramuscular, subcutaneous, intradermal, oral, other mucous membrane surfaces, and skin.

Onset of symptoms is usually less than 30 minutes and often is immediate. However, antigens by the oral route may have a 2-hour delay before onset of reaction. In general, the more immediate the reaction, the more life-threatening it may be. Duration of symptoms may last only a few minutes even without therapy, but on the average they persist 3 to 4 hours. Rarely, symptoms will last for more than 24 hours (Weiszer 1985, Sheffer 1985). In a small percentage of patients, a secondary exacerbation of symptoms will occur within 24 hours despite earlier complete resolution of symptoms. It is in the prevention of the late exacerbation that steroids appear to be most useful (Stark 1986).

ETIOLOGIES

There is a virtually endless list of agents that can cause anaphylaxis or anaphylactoid reactions (Table 27-1). Anaphylaxis is an IgE-mediated reaction to a complete protein antigen or a hapten. A hapten is a low-molecular weight organic compound that must bind to a tissue protein to be immunogenic; examples include penicillin and other antibiotics. Complete protein antigens include hymenoptera venom (Patterson and Valentine 1982), blood products (Leikola et al 1973), foods (Amlot et al 1987), chymopapaine (Hall and McCulloch 1983), insulin (Lieberman et al 1971), allergy shots, and seminal fluid (Friedman et al 1984). In anaphylactoid reactions, no IgE mechanism can be demonstrated; these include iodinated radiocontrast agents (Greenberger 1984), aspirin and nonsteroidal antiinflammatory agents (Stevenson 1984), vitamins, local anesthetics (DeShazo and Nelson 1979), and physical factors such as exercise (Sheffer and Austen 1984).

CLINICAL MANIFESTATIONS

At the very onset of an anaphylactic reaction, certain premonitory symptoms are common. Patients often complain of pruritus of the palms and soles, tingling about the mouth and tongue, or a feeling of generalized warmth. Tightness in the chest or a lump in the throat are also common complaints. Occasionally, patients will note a feeling of impending doom or dizziness or may have acute loss of consciousness from hypotension (Table 27–2).

Over 90% of patients have some combination of urticaria and angioedema. Urticaria is edema and vasodilation of the upper dermis. It appears as raised erythematous wheals covering most of the body surface in evanescent patches. It is intensely pruritic. Angioedema is edema of the deep dermis and appears as a puffy, nonpitting, swollen area of skin. It is not inflamed, and there is no pruritus. Patients complain of the swelling and a tingling or numb sensation. Angioedema tends to be

TABLE 27–2
Symptoms and Signs of Anaphylaxis

Reaction	Symptom	Sign
Urticaria	Itching	Raised wheals, diffusely distributed and evanescent
Angioedema	Nonpruritic tingling	Swelling of lips, eyes, hands no heat or erythema
Laryngeal edema	Hoarseness dysphagia lump in throat airway obstruction sudden death	Inspiratory stridor intercostal and clavicular retractions, cyanosis
Bronchospasm	Cough, dyspnea chest tightness	Wheezing, high respiratory rate retractions
Hypotension	Dizziness syncope confusion	Hypotension (mild to severe) tachycardia oliguria
Rhinitis	Nasal congestion itching and fluid	Mucosal edema
Conjunctivitis	Tearing itching	Lid edema and injection
Gastroenteritis	Cramping diarrhea vomiting	Normal examination

most prominent about the face and lips, followed by the hands and arms. Angioedema of the lips should alert the examiner to the high likelihood of associated angioedema of the oropharynx (Fisher 1987, Sheffer 1985, Terr 1985).

The respiratory tract is the next most common site of involvement in anaphylaxis, which consists here of bronchospasm and laryngeal edema. Bronchospasm is common but tends to be quite mild unless the patient has a pre-existing history of asthma. Laryngeal edema is much less common, but it is the principal cause of death from anaphylaxis. Upper airway obstruction from laryngeal edema can be sudden and dramatic and may present as sudden death or "café coronary." Angioedema of the lips, uvula, tongue, and oropharynx are less likely to obstruct the airway completely but must be treated aggressively because of the likelihood of concomitant edema of the larynx. The uvula, in particular, is a helpful marker in the physical assessment, warning of imminent upper airway obstruction. Angioedema of the uvula has a gelatinous appearance, similar in appearance to a peeled white grape. Rhinitis and conjunctivitis are other common manifestations of mucous membrane involvement but are not life-threatening (Weiszer 1985, Patterson and Valentine 1982, Fisher 1987). Pulmonary edema is not part of anaphylaxis but has rarely been reported as a terminal event (Carlson 1981).

Refractory hypotension is a leading cause of death from anaphylaxis, second only to laryngeal edema. A 20- to 30-mmHg drop in blood pressure is typical, but there is much variability in degree and rate of development. When sudden in onset, syncope or sudden death may occur. Because the mechanism is vasodilation and capillary leaking, the hypotension in anaphylaxis is responsive to volume loading (Silverman et al 1984; Smith et al 1980).

Abdominal cramping is common in anaphylaxis but is usually overshadowed by other symptoms of the syndrome. Angioedema of the gut lining causes this colic as well as nausea and vomiting, and, rarely, hematochezia.

Although there have been case reports of myocardial infarction and ventricular tachycardia and fibrillation in anaphylaxis, these are not considered part of the anaphylaxis syndrome. Nonspecific changes in S-T segments are also common on EKG. All these cardiac abnormalities are thought to be secondary to hypotension, hypoxia, and overzealous epinephrine therapy (Levine 1976, Booth and Patterson 1970).

Last, there have been case reports of stroke associated with anaphylaxis. Cerebrovascular accident is a rare complication of severe Hymenoptera envenomation but is otherwise not part of anaphylaxis from other causes.

ASSESSMENT

The most common presentation for a patient with an acute allergic emergency will be a rash. If the rash is diffuse it is likely to be urticaria. The severity of the reaction is proportional to the acuteness of the onset; hence an eruption occurring over a few minutes is much more urgent than one that developed over several hours or days. Since the major threat to life is upper airway obstruction, one should ask if the patient feels a lump in the throat, hoarseness, difficulty swallowing, or inability to breathe in air. These symptoms are all indicative of laryngeal edema. One should also ask if the tongue, lips, or uvula feel swollen or tingle, since these symptoms are also harbingers of airway obstruction. Wheezing, tightness in the chest, and dyspnea are complaints more indicative of bronchospasm than of laryngeal edema and should also be a routine part of the history (Weiszer 1985, Fisher 1987).

One should question whether the patient has lost consciousness at any time or feels dizzy, events suggestive of hypotension. Confusion also indicates shock in this clinical situation.

Other symptoms which should be asked about are eyelid swelling, nasal congestion, abdominal cramps, nausea, vomiting, diarrhea, or swelling of the hands and feet. These latter symptoms are common in anaphylaxis but in themselves pose no immediate threat to life.

If the patient is stable and there are no symptoms of laryngeal edema or hypotension, one may proceed with the remainder of the history and physical. Is the patient on any medication, particularly antibiotics, antiinflammatory drugs, or over-the-counter medications. When was their last meal, and what did they eat? Where were they, and what were they doing at the onset of symptoms (e.g., exercise, bathing, sex, and so forth)? Was there any topical exposure such as a bee sting, chemicals, or soap? Does the patient have any past history of asthma, hay fever, urticaria, or similar allergic reactions? Any family history of allergy?

Vital signs often reveal hypotension, tachycardia, and tachypnea. The temperature should be normal. Fever is not seen in anaphylaxis and if present should suggest a delayed drug reaction such as serum sickness. The patient usually appears apprehensive and should be reassured that the symptoms will respond promptly to therapy. Examine the mouth, lips, uvula, and tongue for evidence of angioedema. Look for supraclavicular retractions and listen with the stethoscope over the upper sternum for inspiratory stridor, indicative of laryngeal edema. Also note if the patient's voice sounds hoarse or raspy. Listen to the lungs for air movement and wheezing. And of course, survey the skin for urticarial lesions, erythema, angioedema, and possible inoculation sites.

TREATMENT AND NURSING CARE

Breathing Patterns, Ineffective, Related to Airway Compromise

The immediate threat to life in anaphylaxis is airway compromise, hypotension, or both. When either of these symptoms are present stage 1 care is in order. If there are symptoms of laryngeal edema even without physical findings, the treatment must be administered immediately. Epinephrine is the keystone of all allergic therapy. Beta-adrenergic effects stop the ongoing release of mediators from mast cells and basophils, and dilates bronchial smooth muscle. Epinephrine's alpha-adrenergic effects shrink edematous tissues and cause the blood pressure to rise by vasoconstriction. By these means, epinephrine stops the ongoing anaphylactic reaction, opens the airway, and improves the blood pressure. Epinephrine is given subcutaneously in a 1 : 1000 dilution, 0.3 ml for an adult, and 0.01 ml/kg to a maximum of 0.3 ml for a child. Concomitantly, the patient should be placed on oxygen, an intravenous line with normal saline or lactated Ringer's solution should be established, and the patient should be placed on a cardiac monitor. If airway obstruction persists, the epinephrine may be repeated at 5- to 10-minute intervals. If air movement is poor or absent, cricothyroidotomy may be necessary, since edema usually obliterates visualization of the vocal cords, thereby making endotracheal intubation extremely difficult. If laryngeal edema is refractory to subcutaneous epinephrine or if complete obstruction is imminent, as evidenced by extreme stridor and little air movement, cautious administration of intravenous epinephrine is suggested. The intravenous dose of epinephrine is 1 ml in a 1 : 10,000 dilution, further diluted in 10 ml of normal saline, given by IV push over 5 to 10 minutes. Aerosolized epinephrine has variable efficacy and should not be relied upon.

Decreased Cardiac Output (Potential), Related to

• *Dysrhythmias Secondary to Drug Therapy*

Careful monitoring should be done during this therapy, since there is a high risk of ventricular dysrhythmias. Elderly patients (older than 60 years of age) or those with heart disease pose a difficult therapeutic problem because of fear of precipitating chest pain or cardiac dysrhythmias with the use of epinephrine. In general, however, epinephrine should not be withheld in this type of patient if life-threatening laryngeal edema or hypotension is present (Barach and Nowack 1984, Weiszer 1985).

If the patient is hypotensive, one should proceed with epinephrine therapy as outlined above, but in addition, a fluid bolus of saline or lactated Ringer's solution should be given (the patient should be placed in a modified Trendelenburg position). Most adults will require at least 1 or 2 liters in the first hour. If the patient is in profound shock, epinephrine may need to be administered intravenously from the very beginning of therapy. In addition, the military antishock trouser (MAST) suit may be a useful adjunct to massive fluid boluses and intravenous epinephrine. If reversal of hypotension and airway edema cannot be maintained by subcutaneous epinephrine, one should consider an epinephrine drip of 1 mg in 250 ml of D5W at 1 to 4 μg/minute infusion. An infusion pump must be used to assure accurate administration and avoid untoward reactions (Perkin and Anas 1985, Oertel and Loehr 1984, Bickell and Dice 1984). A dopamine drip may also be used in refractory shock secondary to anaphylaxis.

The majority of patients with anaphylaxis will not require such intensive therapy. In general, two or three doses of epinephrine subcutaneously at 15- to 20-minute intervals, based on resolution of symptoms, and a liter of fluid administered intravenously will be adequate for milder cases. Even if skin involvement is the only manifestation of an acute allergic reaction, it is reasonable to administer epinephrine to stop progression of the reaction. Bronchospasm in anaphylaxis is treated in the same manner as asthma, including an aminophylline loading dose of 5.6 mg/kg over 30 minutes if there is no response to epinephrine (Lucke and Thomas 1983, Fisher 1987, Weiszer 1985).

Useful adjuncts in the therapy of anaphylaxis are antihistamines, specifically diphenhydramine (Benadryl), 25 to 50 mg, orally, intravascularly (IM), or IV, depending on the severity of symptoms. Benadryl is primarily useful for control of the rash and its associated pruritus but has little effect on angiocdcma, bronchospasm, or hypotension.

Steroids are another important adjunct to anaphylaxis therapy. Although they have no immediate benefit in the acute reaction, steriods are felt to prevent reexacerbation of symptoms, which may occur several hours later. The recommended dose is hydrocortisone (Solu-Cortef), 250 to 500 mg or methylprednisolone (Solu-Medrol), 50 to 125 mg IV push. This dose may be repeated every 4 hours in patients whose symptoms persist despite standard therapy (Sheffer 1985, Fisher 1987).

For patients over 60 years of age or those with a cardiac history, if there is life-threatening laryngeal edema or hypotension unresponsive to fluid boluses, epinephrine should not be withheld. Test doses of 0.1 to 0.15 ml subcutaneously can be used with continuous monitoring. If no chest pain or dysrhythmias develop, one should follow with the usual adult doses of 0.3 ml subcutaneously. Intravenous epinephrine should not be used in patients over 50 years of age or those with heart disease, unless death appears imminent without this therapy. If anaphylaxis is present without signs of airway compromise or hypotension unresponsive to volume loading, these patients should be treated with Benadryl, steroids, and IV fluids alone (Barach and Nowack 1984).

Last, but certainly not least, it is critical to stop further exposure to antigen: place a tourniquet above an injection site, flick off the stinger of a honey bee, wash off any offending chemicals, stop the intravenous line.

Evaluation

Throughout therapy, the vital signs should be assessed frequently, the airway should be checked for angioedema of the uvula or oropharynx, and the patient should be questioned for symptoms of laryngeal edema or bronchospasm and examined for signs of stridor, retractions, or wheezing. These checks should be at 1- or 2-minute intervals at first, and the intervals should be lengthened as the patient stabilizes (Table 27–3).

The nurse should continue periodic monitoring as previously outlined until final disposition is made. If there was complete and rapid resolution of all symptoms with initial therapy, the patient could be observed in the emergency department without further treatment. If there is no recurrence of symptoms in the next 3 hours, the patient may safely go home but should continue on a two- to three-day course of prednisone 40 mg once daily and Benadryl 25 mg every 4 hours as needed for any itching or rash. If the symptoms were urticaria alone, without progression, the patient could be discharged on Benadryl prn, with or without prednisone for three days.

Discharge Instructions

Of course, discharge instructions should caution the patient about avoidance of any suspected inciting cause such as medications, foods, chemicals, or even exercise. If

TABLE 27–3
Treatment of Anaphylaxis

Remove antigen; delay absorption
Maintain an adequate airway

Epinephrine
  0.3 ml 1 : 1000 dilution subcutaneously (0.01 ml/kg in a child)
    Repeat at 10 to 20 minute intervals
    May give IM if severe episode
  If patient in shock or has incipient airway obstruction
    1 : 100,000 dilution intravenously, 1–2 ml/min to a total of 10 ml (0.1 mg)
    if persistent shock, may start a drip:
      1 mg in 250 ml D5W, 1–4 μg/min
  If patient older than 50 or heart disease and life-threatening symptoms exist:
    Test dose of 0.1–0.15 ml subcutaneously or IM
    Close cardiac monitoring is mandatory
    If shock resistant to other measures or airway closure imminent consider drip (above)

Volume Expansion with Saline or Lactated Ringer's Solution
  For shock:
    Adult, 1 L over 15 min then reassess
    Child, 20 ml/kg bolus

Methylprednisolone
  50–125 mg IV push, may repeat every 4 hours if symptoms persistent (hydrocortisone
    250–500 mg is alternative)
  If discharging home, prednisone 40 mg/day for 2 to 3 days

Diphenhydramine
  25–50 mg IV push, then every 2 to 4 hours as needed
    If being discharged, 25 mg q6h prn for 3 days

If Resistant Hypotension
  MAST suit
  Dopamine infusion

---

the etiology is unknown or avoidance not possible (e.g., foods in restaurants), the option of portable epinephrine ([Epi]Pen, Ana-Kit) could be discussed and usage could be demonstrated to the patient. Instructions should be given to return to the ED immediately if there are any symptoms suggesting laryngeal edema, bronchospasm, or hypotension, or if the cutaneous eruption worsens despite home therapy with Benadryl and steroids. All patients should be encouraged to follow up with an allergist, particularly if no obvious cause of the incident has been determined in the ED.

If the initial symptoms of anaphylaxis were life-threatening or if response to therapy was not prompt, in most cases, the patient will be admitted to the hospital. If reassessment reveals worsening, the patient should be treated as outlined in stage I care.

CONCLUSION

Anaphylaxis is an easily preventable cause of death if recognition and treatment are immediate. All patients presenting to the ED with signs of an acute allergic reaction should be treated with similar urgency. The most common causes of acute allergic reactions are penicillin, bee stings, and iodinated contrast media. Urticaria, angioedema, or both occur in most cases, and the respiratory tract is the next most common site of involvement, which consists of bronchospasm and laryngeal edema. This chapter has detailed the assessment, management, evaluation, and appropriate discharge teaching for the patient who has suffered an allergic reaction.

REFERENCES

Amlot PL, Kemeny DM, Zachary C, et al. 1987. Oral allergy syndrome (OAS): symptoms of IgE-mediated hypersensitivity to foods. Clin Allergy 17:33–42.

Barach EM, Nowack RM. 1984. Epinephrine for treatment of anaphylactic shock. JAMA 25:2118–2122.

Bickell WH, Dice WH. 1984. Military anti-shock trousers in a patient with adrenergic-resistant anaphylaxis. Ann Emerg Med 13:189–190.

Booth BH, Patterson R. 1970. Electrocardiographic changes during human anaphylaxis. JAMA 211:627–631.

Carlson RW, Schaeffer RC, Puri VK, et al. 1981. Hypovolemia and permeability pulmonary edema associated with anaphylaxis. Crit Care Med 9:883–885.

DeShazo RD, Nelson HS. 1979. An approach to the patient with a history of local anesthetic hypersensitivity: experience with ninety patients. J Allergy Clin Immunol 63:387–394.

Fisher M. Anaphylaxis. 1987. Dis Mon 33:433–479.

Friedman SA, Bernstein IL, Enrione M, et al. 1984. Successful long-term immunotherapy for human seminal plasma anaphylaxis. JAMA 251:2684–2688.

Golbert TM, Patterson R, Pruzansky JJ. 1969. Systemic allergic reactions to ingested antigens. J Allergy 44:96–107.

Greenberger PA. 1984. Contrast media reactions. J Allergy Clin Immunol 74:600–605.

Hall BB, McCulloch JA. 1983. Anaphylactic reactions following intradiscal injection of chymopapain under local anesthesia. J Bone Joint Surg (AM) 65:1215–1219.

Ishizaka K, Ishizaka T. 1983. Immunology of IgE-mediated hypersensitivity. In: Middleton E, Reed CE, Ellis EJ, eds. Allergy: Principles and Practice, 2nd ed. St. Louis, CV Mosby.

Kidd JM, Cohen SH, Sosman AJ, et al. 1983. Food-dependent exercise-induced anaphylaxis. J Allergy Clin Immunol 71:407–411.

Leikola J, Koistinen J, Lehtinen M, et al. 1973. IgA-induced anaphylactic transfusion reactions: a report of four cases. Blood 42:111–119.

Levine HD. 1976. Acute myocardial infarction following wasp sting. Am Heart J 91:365–374.

Lieberman P, Patterson R, Metz R, et al. 1971. Allergic reactions to insulin. JAMA 215:1106–1112.

Lockey RF, Bukantz SC. 1974. Allergic emergencies. Med Clin North Am 58:147–156.

Lucke WC, Thomas TH. 1983. Anaphylaxis: pathophysiology, clinical presentations, and treatment. J Emerg Med 1:83–95.

Monroe EW, Jones HE. 1977. Urticaria. Arch Dermatol 113:80–90.

Novey HS, Fairshter RD, Salness K, et al. 1983. Postprandial exercise-induced anaphylaxis. J Allergy Clin Immunol 71:498–504.

Oertel T, Loehr MM. 1984. Bee-sting anaphylaxis: the use of the military antishock trousers. Ann Emerg Med 13:459–461.

O'Leary MR, Smith MS. 1986. Penicillin anaphylaxis. Am J Emerg Med 4:241–247.

Patterson R, Valentine M. 1982. Anaphylaxis and related allergic emergencies including reactions due to insect stings. JAMA 248:2632–2636.

Perkin RM, Anas NG. 1985. Mechanisms and management of anaphylactic shock not responding to traditional therapy. Ann Allergy 54:202–208.

Sandler RH. 1985. Anaphylactic reactions to zomepirac. Ann Emerg Med 14:171–174.

Sheffer AL. 1985. Anaphylaxis. J Allergy Clin Immunol 75:227–233.

Sheffer AL, Austen KF. 1984. Exercise-induced anaphylaxis. J Allergy Clin Immunol 73:699–703.

Silverman HJ, Van Hook C, Haponik EF. 1984. Hemodynamic changes in human anaphylaxis. Am J Med 77:341–344.

Smith PL, Kagey-Sobotka A, Bleecker ER, et al. 1980. Physiologic manifestations of human anaphylaxis. J Clin Invest 66:1072–1080.

Stark BJ, Sullivan TJ. 1986. Biphasic and protracted anaphylaxis. J Allergy Clin Immunol 78:76–82.

Stevenson DD. 1984. Diagnosis, prevention, and treatment of adverse reactions to aspirin and nonsteroidal anti-inflammatory drugs. J Allergy Clin Immunol 74:617–622.

Terr AI. 1985. Anaphylaxis. Clin Rev Allergy 3:3–23.

Weiszer I. 1985. Allergic emergencies, In: Patterson R, ed. Allergic Diseases: Diagnosis and Management, 3rd ed. Philadelphia, JB Lippincott, 418–439.

Benita Reed, RN BSN MPh

Infectious Diseases

A multivehicle accident has just occurred. Your emergency department (ED) receives four of the eight injured persons.

Patient number 1, a 34-year-old man, was driving one of the cars. He is lethargic and responding slowly. His speech is garbled. You note a gash on his left leg that is bleeding profusely. He also has labored breathing with asymmetric chest expansion. He looks pale. You have been told that his male passenger was killed in the accident.

Patient number 2, a passenger in the second car, is a pregnant 23-year-old woman, with profuse vaginal bleeding. She is assessed to be about seven months pregnant. She is in tears, holding her abdomen, and constantly repeating, "My baby! My baby!" Her husband, who was driving the car, and another man and woman in the car were taken to a different hospital and you are uncertain of their condition.

Patient number 3, a 56-year-old man, was the driver of the third car. You note a bone protruding from his right leg. He is also holding his chest and complaining of a crushing pain. He is diaphoretic, complains of nausea, and has a cough. You note he is expectorating blood-tinged sputum. He then has a cardiac arrest, requires intubation, and becomes unresponsive.

Patient number 4, a 54-year-old female, is the wife of Patient number 3. She presents with multiple contusions on her torso and extremities. After trying to obtain information from her, you find she is disoriented to time and place. She will respond to her first name.

Do any of these patients present an infection control risk? Will you or any of the other personnel or patients be at risk to develop infections at a later date because of exposure to one or all of these patients? Can you make quick assessments in order to determine if there is an infection risk? Do you know what controls to implement? Do you have a monitoring system to evaluate your infection control methods for effectiveness? At the end of this chapter we will return to these patients and discuss ways to prevent infection transmission.

This chapter reviews and discusses (1) whether your ED is at high risk for admitting infectious patients, (2) what constitutes an exposure and your potential for infection, and (3) specific infectious diseases.

IS YOUR ED AT HIGH RISK FOR ADMITTING INFECTIOUS PATIENTS?

The number and type of infectious patients an ED will admit depends on a variety of factors: (1) seasonal incidence of infection, (2) infections common in the community, (3) size of hospital and services available, (4) category and location of hospital, (5) specific infections in specialized hospitals, (6) the level of emergency services offered, and (7) the type of population served (Fig. 28–1).

Seasonal Incidence of Infection

Some infectious diseases are more prevalent during specific seasons. ED personnel should be aware of the seasonal infectious diseases occurring in their potential patient population. Some examples include (1) the common cold, the incidence of which increases in the fall, winter, and spring; (2) influenza, occurring most frequently

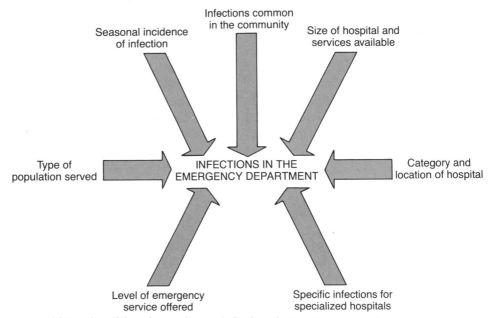

FIGURE 28-1. Conditions impacting on infections in the Emergency Department.

during winter and early spring; and (3) mosquito-borne viral encephalitis, of which incidence is highest in summer and early fall. Emergency department personnel should contact their infectious disease department or the local health department on a seasonal schedule to identify increased incidences of infectious diseases.

Infections Common in the Community

The type of infectious diseases that patients are most likely to present with depends primarily on the type of infections most prominent in the community. Some of the infectious diseases that the ED personnel should be aware of are acquired immune deficiency syndrome (AIDS), hepatitis, gonorrhea, syphilis, chlamydia, tuberculosis, and herpes.

The ED log book could contain a column for infectious diseases as one means to monitor what infections are prominent. Emergency personnel could call other EDs in the area to find out what infectious disease patients they are seeing. Other resources are the hospital's infectious disease department and the local public health department.

Size of Hospital and Services Available

Large hospitals that offer more intense medical, surgical, and specialty services probably see more patients with infectious diseases than a small hospital with limited services. Conditions that can change the type and number of infectious diseases a hospital ED would admit are (1) seasonal infections and (2) infections common in the community.

Category and Location of Hospital

For sake of comparison, this chapter categorizes hospitals as county, federal, university, or private. Although all of these hospitals care for patients with diagnosed infectious and noninfectious diseases, it must be recognized that in addition to a noninfectious disease, a patient may also have a concurrent active infection such as hepatitis B. Whether a hospital is urban or rural has a bearing only on the number of patients admitted with infectious diseases. The likelihood of seeing patients with infectious diseases is greater in urban hospitals serving populous areas than in rural hospitals.

Specialized Hospitals

Hospitals that serve specific patient populations (e.g., women's, rehabilitation, oncology, and orthopedic hospitals) see less varied infectious diseases in their EDs, compared with the general hospitals. Although infections are primarily limited to those associated with their specific patient population, a false sense of security may expose personnel to chronic infections such as hepatitis B. Therefore, it is advisable to remember that any person can be a carrier of a chronic infection.

Level of Emergency Services

The emergency services an ED provides are classified into four levels, according to the Joint Commission on Accreditation of Hospitals (JCAH). A Level 1 ED offers comprehensive 24-hour care for medical, surgical, orthopedic, obstetric and gynecologic, and pediatric emergencies, with anesthesia availability on site.

A Level 2 emergency room offers 24-hour care with a physician on duty and has specialty consultation (of the aforementioned specialties) available within 30 minutes of the site.

A Level 3 emergency room offers 24-hour care with a physician on call (within 30 minutes of the site).

A Level 4 emergency room can offer reasonable care to the patient until transfer to the nearest facility capable of providing adequate care is possible. Emergency personnel should be aware of the level of emergency services offered by their ED. Emergency departments of all levels see patients with infectious diseases; however, the potential for frequency of exposure is the greatest in Level 1 EDs and decreases as the levels decrease.

Type of Population Served

Emergency personnel should be aware of the population they serve and the groups of patients that are noted to be at risk for specific types of infections. Examples include malnourished alcoholics, who frequently have tuberculosis and pediculosis, and IV drug abusers, who are at high risk for hepatitis B and non-A, non-B; AIDS; gonorrhea; syphilis; and chlamydia.

Identification of patients in an ED who have an infectious disease is difficult. However, if a few helpful hints are at hand, infectious diseases can often be identified, and the spread of infections to others can be prevented. Know your ED, the community in which it is located, and the infectious diseases common to the community.

EXPOSURE AND POTENTIAL FOR INFECTION

Exposure to a communicable disease does not necessarily result in an infection. Exposures may be specific or nonspecific, and each may occur via air, blood, body fluids, and/or direct contact with the organism(s) (Table 28–1).

TABLE 28–1
Type of Exposure and Relative Risk of Infection

Type	Exposure	Outcome (Nonprotected)	Outcome (Protected)
Specific	Inhaling organisms Entrance of organisms by Needle stick Open skin sites Direct contact with organisms	High risk for infection	No risk for infection
Nonspecific	Exposure by air, blood, body fluids, or direct contact without entrance of organisms into host because of Lack of organisms Lack of entrance site	Minimal or no risk of infection	No risk for infection

Specific exposures occur when a person is exposed to a disease spread by (1) the airborne route and actually inhales the microorganisms, (2) blood and other body fluids and suffers a needle-stick injury or has blood or other body fluids splashed on an open wound, (3) direct contact, such as suctioning a patient without gloves with an open wound of the finger. (Herpes whitlow can be spread in this manner, which is the reason a two-glove technique is recommended for suctioning.)

Nonspecific exposures occur when a person is exposed to a disease spread by the airborne route but there are no organisms in the air, because the infected person has not coughed or sneezed, or a person is exposed to a disease spread by contact with blood or other body fluid but his or her skin is intact.

Exposures are protected when an individual is exposed to a disease spread by any route or by direct contact, but the person is immune.

Exposure and infectivity involves microbial conditions: the number, virulence, and viability of microorganisms; entrance for microorganisms; and host factors (Fig. 28–2).

Number of Microorganisms

Are there enough microorganisms present to cause infection? The specific disease determines the number of microorganisms needed to cause infection. Some diseases may require a number of contacts before infection occurs.

Virulence of Microorganisms

Are the microorganisms capable of causing an infection? Microorganisms lose their virulence during the last few days of illness or in the presence of antimicrobials, and sometimes they are just a less pathogenic strain.

Viability of Microorganisms

Are the microorganisms still alive when transmitted? Most microorganisms need a special environment to live — nutrients, compatible temperature, and moisture. If the time lapse between leaving the host and entering the next host is prolonged, the microorganisms may no longer be viable and are unable to produce infection.

Entrance for Microorganisms

If there are enough virulent and viable microorganisms, do they have an appropriate entrance? Airborne infections must be transferred through the airborne route. Infection spread by blood must be transferred to the prospective host's blood. In those infections spread by direct contact, the microorganisms must have an appropriate entrance. If all the conditions are not present and favorable, infection will not occur. In summary, three conditions must be present for infection to occur: (1) microorganisms capable of producing infections, (2) a means for the organism to exit the infected source and enter the new host, and (3) a host that is capable of acquiring an infection.

Host Factors and Infection

Host factors are also important in infection transmission. Consider the number of times you have been exposed to an infectious disease but did not succumb to it. Have

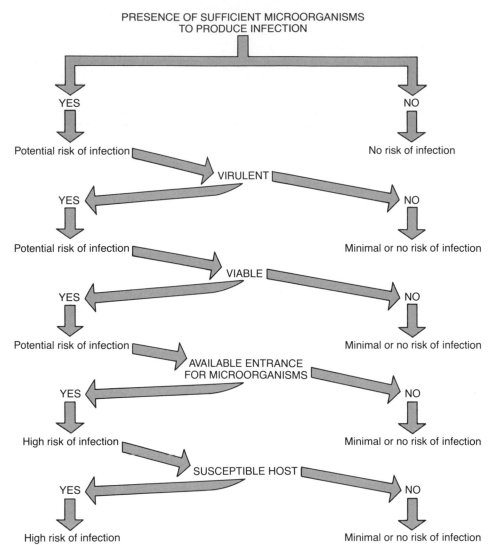

FIGURE 28-2. Microbial conditions and relative risks of infection.

you seen a co-worker become ill when you did not? Why is one person susceptible to an infection, whereas another is not?

Bodies have natural defense mechanisms and an immunologic defense system. Some natural defense mechanisms include integrity of skin and mucosa, complex protective mechanisms of the respiratory tract, and the gastrointestinal tract defenses: normal motility, immunoglobulins in the gut, and gastric acid (Castle 1980, 63). The immunologic defense system includes complex interactions of various factors: lymphocytes; phagocytic cells; the vascular system; antibody, complement, and other components (Alexander and Good 1977, 7).

Immunity from some infectious diseases is achieved by vaccination. It is to the

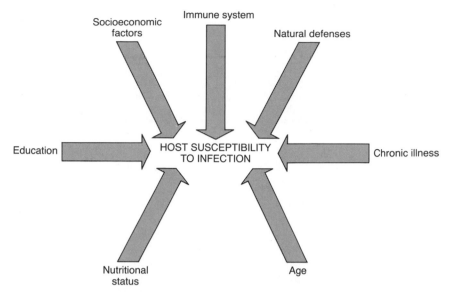

FIGURE 28-3. Factors influencing host susceptibility to infection.

advantage of emergency personnel to receive available vaccinations (e.g., rubella, hepatitis B, and influenza).

Some disease states make a person more prone to infection: cancer, diabetes, and chronic illnesses (e.g., cardiac, pulmonary, and renal), among others. Susceptibility to infection is also influenced by age (the very young and very old), nutritional status, crowded living conditions, social and economic factors, and knowledge deficits related to elements of maintaining good health (Fig. 28-3).

SPECIFIC INFECTIOUS DISEASES

Acquired Immunodeficiency Syndrome (AIDS)

AIDS, a syndrome of puzzling occurrences, unusual malignancies, opportunistic infections, and immune system abnormalities that mysteriously developed in previously healthy individuals, was first reported in 1981, but cases had occurred in the USA as early as 1978. The United States has reported the largest number of cases; however, many other countries have also reported cases among the varying high-risk groups. Populations at high risk for AIDS have been identified, but as the disease continues to spread, not all cases will continue to occur in only those groups (Table 28-2).

By December 1988, 82,764 cases of AIDS had been reported in the United States (Centers for Disease Control, 38 [14] 1989). The fatality rate for patients diagnosed with AIDS prior to 1984 exceeds 75% (Cole and Lundberg 1986, 22-23).

TABLE 28–2
Populations at High Risk for AIDS

Sexually active homosexual and bisexual men
IV drug abusers (past or present)
Persons with hemophilia and other coagulation disorders
Heterosexual contacts of someone with AIDS or at risk for AIDS
Persons who have had transfusions with blood or blood products between 1978–1985
Infants born to infected mothers

At the time of this writing, it is believed that the prevalence of human immuno-deficiency virus (HIV) infection in the United States is highest in those groups that account for the vast majority of AIDS cases (Centers for Disease Control, 36 (49) 1987): homosexual and bisexual men, intravenous (IV) drug abusers, persons with coagulation disorders, heterosexual partners of persons with HIV infection or at risk of HIV infection, and infants born to infected mothers. Demographic data suggest the prevalence of HIV infection to be greatest on the East and West Coasts and in urban as opposed to rural areas. Additionally, HIV infection has been more common in young and early middle-aged adults than in the elderly population and has been significantly more prevalent in men than in women (Centers for Disease Control, 36 (49) 1987).

Etiology

Currently reported AIDS cases are the result of HIV infection. In order for the infection to occur, a person must have an adequate exposure to HIV, and the virus must enter the bloodstream. To date, the recognized modes of entry are sexual intercourse, injection with infected intravenous needles, and maternal-fetal transmission.

Semen, blood, and vaginal secretions have been found to contain varying concentrations of the AIDS virus, which may gain entry into the bloodstream during intercourse through even small mucosal tears. Although HIV has been isolated in tears and saliva, it is unlikely that transmission of the virus occurs via these secretions, as the concentration of HIV in them is relatively low.

Following adequate exposure and entry of HIV into the bloodstream, a person will show serologic evidence of antibody formation against HIV (seroconversion) in about 6 to 12 weeks. Once seroconversion occurs, the individual is considered to be HIV-infected. Seroconversion however, does not tell whether an individual will ultimately get AIDS. It merely indicates that exposure to HIV was adequate to cause infection. However, a person with HIV infection has the capacity to transmit the virus to others whether or not he or she is symptomatic. Such a person is a carrier.

Pathophysiology

HIV belongs to a class of RNA viruses termed retroviruses. Furthermore, HIV is a type of retrovirus that specifically invades T helper (T_H) cells (a subset of T lymphocytes that augments the immune response). Infection is then evidenced by the presence of viral reverse transcriptase activity within the lymphocyte.* (Reverse transcriptase is an enzyme present in HIV that allows the virus to reproduce itself using the genetic material (DNA) of the T_H cell.) Eventually, the T_H cell is destroyed, replication of the AIDS virus continues, and more T_H cells are invaded and destroyed. The normal 2 : 1 ratio of T_H cells to T suppressor (T_S) cells (which suppress the immune response) becomes decreased. Immunosuppression, with resultant opportunistic infections and malignancies, ultimately occurs.

This is the most serious scenario for HIV infection. The pathophysiologic sequelae and spectrum of clinical symptomatology that follow HIV infection however are actually quite varied; they are discussed in more detail in the following section.

Clinical Manifestations

Once HIV infection occurs, its actual sequelae and clinical symptoms vary. Individuals presenting to the ED with HIV infection may not exhibit any signs and symptoms of illness, or they may exhibit a range of symptoms from nonspecific, generalized, and constitutional complaints to severe symptoms reflecting immunologic defects and cancers. Additionally, HIV-infected individuals may present to EDs with complaints completely unrelated to the HIV infection. For these reasons, it is difficult to describe the "typical" ED presentation. At best, ED nurses should be aware of symptomatology commonly associated with HIV infection (Table 28 – 3). Additionally, ED nurses should be familiar with the CDC definition of AIDS and the diagnostic criteria required for its diagnosis (Centers for Disease Control, 36 (1S) 1987; Centers for Disease Control, 36 (15) 1987).

Individuals with HIV infection may have behavioral pattern changes caused by the uncertainty of their final disease outcome. They may or may not have informed their significant others of their illness. They may or may not have sought information regarding AIDS and its transmission.

Treatment and Nursing Care

Neither a cure nor an effective vaccine has been developed for AIDS at this time. Numerous drugs and treatments have been and are being studied; however, treatment of HIV infection remains basically symptomatic and supportive. Combinations of antibiotic, antiviral, chemotherapy, and radiation therapy are most commonly used for treating the opportunistic infections and malignancies associated with HIV infection.

---

* Reverse transcriptase enables RNA to synthesize DNA from an RNA template—a reversal of the classic dogma that the process of transferring genetic information is one-way, from DNA to RNA. The DNA then acts as a template to produce RNA.

TABLE 28-3
Symptoms and Signs Commonly Present in Individuals with
Symptomatic HIV Infection*

Symptoms

Malaise, generalized weakness
Fever, night sweats
Weight loss
Recurrent viral infections
Diarrhea

Signs

Chronically ill, malnourished appearing individual
Neuro-psychiatric manifestations
   Confusion
   Agitation
   Memory loss
   Inappropriate behavior
Varying degrees of respiratory distress
Lymphadenopathy
Voluminous diarrhea
Purplish lesions on skin and mucous membranes
Mucocutaneous vesicular lesions

Laboratory Findings

Positive HIV antibody test (ELISA and/or Western blot technique)
Positive cultures for any of the opportunistic infections associated with HIV infection
Biopsies conclusive of malignancies and/or opportunistic infections associated with HIV infection
Enlarged ventricles on C-T scan
Abnormal chest x-ray
Abnormal ratio of helper to suppressor T lymphocytes

    * Symptoms presented in this table may also be reflective of conditions other than HIV infection. As such, HIV infection and AIDS should only be diagnosed based upon laboratory evidence of such in accordance with specific guidelines established by the CDC for defining a case of AIDS. Conversely, the absence of symptomatology presented in this table does not rule out HIV infection.

Tissue Perfusion, Altered (Potential), Related to

- **Overwhelming Infection**
- **Severe Dehydration**

    Individuals with HIV infection may have alterations in systemic tissue perfusion for a multitude of reasons. Advanced opportunistic infections place these individuals at high risk for septic shock, which may potentially lead to total organ failure. Cryptosporidial infection often causes voluminous diarrhea, which in addition to a decrease in appetite and oral intake results in severe dehydration with associated electrolyte imbalances. In these instances, it is often necessary to implement stage I care. Intravenous access for the administration of fluids and medications will be required. Emergency resuscitation equipment should be close at hand. (Mouth-to-mouth resuscitation is not recommended; therefore a disposable pocket mask, airway, and ambu bag should be available.) Consultation with the patient's physician, significant others, and the patient when possible should be sought to determine the extent to which life-support procedures are desired.

Infection, Potential (Patient), Related to

- **Immunocompromised State Secondary to HIV Infection**

Treating existing infection while preventing and minimizing the chance of a patient acquiring new infections as a result of the immunocompromised state is the primary therapeutic goal for patients with HIV infection. Antibiotic and antiviral treatment is determined by the specific infection(s) that the individual presents with. Pentamidine isethionate (pentamidine) and azidothymidine (AZT) have been found to show some effectiveness in the treatment of persons with *Pneumocystis carinii*. Because the recommended treatment modalities for individuals with HIV-associated opportunistic infections are changing so rapidly, the readers are referred to recent journal articles for more detailed information on this topic.

In an effort to minimize the chances of individuals with HIV infection acquiring iatrogenically induced or nosocomial infections or both, invasive procedures should be kept to a minimum. This can be done by coordinating blood drawing to avoid unnecessary sticks, minimizing the number of lines and tubes for the patient, and protecting the patient from exposure to external pathogens (e.g., not allowing visitors or staff with colds). Additionally, taking rectal temperatures should be avoided, as the rectum is colonized with numerous microorganisms that can gain access to the blood stream through trauma to the rectum.

Initial blood tests in the ED may include CBC with differential and platelet count, electrolytes, hepatitis B status, VDRL sedimentation rate, liver function tests, and cultures if the patient is febrile. An HIV antibody test can be done only if the patient consents. Stool examination for ova and parasites and other pathogenic microorganisms should be done if possible. If the patient is febrile, a lumbar puncture could diagnose CNS involvement. A chest radiograph can determine pulmonary involvement and arterial blood gas (ABG) analysis may be obtained to determine the individual's oxygenation status.

Infection Transmission, Potential for (Health Care Workers),* Related to

- **Care and Treatment of Individuals with HIV Infection**

Transmission of HIV infection from patients to health care workers, although extremely rare, is possible (McCray 1986). Because HIV-infected patients are not always aware of their HIV status and they may be asymptomatic, precautions to avoid direct contact with blood and body fluids from *all* patients (whether known to be HIV infected or not) are now recommended by the CDC. The use of gloves, gown, mask, and goggles all may be needed (Table 28–4).

---

* Non-NANDA–approved nursing diagnosis.

TABLE 28–4

Recommended Precautions to Prevent Transmission of HIV Infection

---

Protective covering appropriate to the nature of the potential exposure to blood and body fluids should be utilized
  Gloves should be worn when drawing blood, starting IVs, and handling items soiled with blood or other body fluids
  Gowns should be worn when clothing may be soiled with blood or other body fluids
  Masks and/or goggles should be worn when the possibility of aerosolization of blood or body fluids is likely (e.g., endoscopic procedures, obstetric deliveries, and so forth)

Hands and other skin surfaces should be washed immediately if contaminated with blood or other body fluids

Consider all contaminated sharp instruments as potentially infective
  Puncture-resistant containers should be located as close as possible to where sharp instruments are used and all sharp instruments should be placed in them

All specimens should be identified and transported according to hospital policy

Linen and equipment soiled with blood and other body fluids should be handled and processed according to hospital policy

Special housekeeping is not required after an HIV-infected patient leaves a bed upon discharge from the ED. If blood or other body fluid spills occurred on contact surfaces they can be cleaned with 1 : 10 dilution of 5.25% sodium hypochlorite (household bleach) or routine hospital disinfectant

Disposable emergency resuscitation equipment should be nearby to avoid mouth-to-mouth resuscitation

---

Source: Adapted from Centers for Disease Control. 1987. Recommendations for Prevention of HIV Transmission in Health Care Settings. MMWR, 36(2S):3S-18S.

It is recognized that the spectrum of clinical manifestations of HIV infection (and other communicable diseases) may range from subclinical to overt. Therefore, precautions against contact with blood and body fluids should be used with *all* patients at *all* times in *all* settings. In this way, the transmission of HIV infection (and other infectious diseases) will be minimized.

The risk of contracting HIV infection is no greater for pregnant than for nonpregnant nurses. However, HIV infection contracted during pregnancy does place the infant at increased risk of infection via perinatal transmission.

Coping, Ineffective (Potential), Related to

- **Self-Image Changes**
- **Rejection from Significant Others**
- **Uncertainty of Diagnosis, Prognosis, and Treatment Modalities**
- **Sense of Helplessness**
- **Inability to Accept Death and Dying**

Once the certainty of HIV infection is known, a myriad of psychosocial, emotional, and financial problems inevitably emerge. Individuals experience a significantly changed lifestyle as a result of the social stigma that HIV infection carries. Oftentimes they lose their jobs, insurance benefits, and support of significant others. Denial, anger, anxiety, and depression are common coping mechanisms for these individuals in response to such changes.

A multidisciplinary approach to help these individuals cope with their illness and responses to their illness by significant others is needed. Input from the chaplain, psychologist, psychiatrist, social workers, physicians, nurses, the patient, and significant others should be used as necessary.

The patient needs to know all of the caretakers are honest and interested in his or her well being; additionally, the patient needs the opportunity to express feelings and to develop the best strategies to deal with these problems, using the support systems available. In an environment where it is possible to express feelings openly without fear of rejection, the patient may be able to find peace, comfort, and acceptance of his or her illness.

Comfort, Altered, Related to

- **Fever**
- **Pain**
- **Nausea and Vomiting**
- **Diarrhea**
- **Drug Reactions**

Patients with AIDS often relate varied complaints and experience significant discomfort. Nursing care must be supportive and should be aimed at alleviating the patient's specific complaints.

A patient with a fever should have oral or axillary temperatures repeated often to evaluate the effectiveness of the treatments rendered. Antipyretics can be administered as ordered. Cooling blankets and ice packs can also be used as necessary.

A patient with pain should be medicated as ordered and should subsequently be evaluated to determine the effectiveness of the medication, including the duration of relief. Patients who have been IV drug abusers usually require larger doses of analgesics and frequent administration. Inadequate pain relief may be caused by (1) the patient's lack of response to the pain medication, (2) inadequate dose, (3) a need for more frequent administration, (4) degree of illness, or (5) the need for a second medication (i.e., a tranquilizer or sedative).

Nausea and vomiting can usually be controlled with antiemetics and by keeping the patient NPO. Although not generally pertinent to the emergency phase of care, once the initial episode of nausea and vomiting is resolved, the patient should slowly be started again on oral intake. A patient can tell the caregiver which foods are well tolerated.

Diarrhea is sometimes difficult to control, despite the administration of medications and keeping the patient NPO. Nursing interventions should include linen changes as often as needed to keep the patient dry and to prevent skin breakdown.

Because of the various drugs utilized for the treatment of the patient's opportunistic infections and malignancies, drug reactions are not uncommon. These patients are frequently started on toxic or experimental drugs or both. Close observation for any reaction is very important. If a drug reaction is suspected, the drug should be stopped and the physician should be notified. When the potential for a drug reaction is present, it is advisable to keep diphenhydramine hydrochloride (Benadryl) and epinephrine (Adrenalin) close at hand.

Breathing Pattern, Ineffective (Potential), Related to

- **Pulmonary Involvement**

Patients with pulmonary involvement may exhibit a variety of respiratory symptoms. Shortness of breath, tachypnea, increasing dyspnea on exertion, and a dry, nonproductive cough are not uncommon. These patients should frequently be assessed for acute respiratory distress, cyanosis, and airway patency. Although masks are not commonly utilized in caring for patients with HIV infection, if tuberculosis is present or suspected, or if the patient has a productive cough, masks should be worn by the caregiver and by the patient, if traveling through the hospital.

Before any invasive interventions are initiated, the patient's condition should be fully explained to him or her, significant others involved in decision making, or both. The patient's desires regarding resuscitation should be clear to all caregivers.

Knowledge Deficit (Patient and/or Significant Others), Related to

- **Disease Process**
- **Disease Transmission**

Knowledge deficits related to the disease process of AIDS (or HIV infection) and disease transmission are not uncommon in both patients with HIV infection and their significant others. Emergency nurses should be knowledgeable enough to answer questions regarding the patient's condition. It is also important that they be able to explain to the patient and significant others the meaning of a positive HIV antibody test. Patients and their significant others should be referred to AIDS support groups in their community. It is important for ED personnel to be able to explain the mode of transmission of the AIDS virus to the patient and significant others and to describe methods of minimizing the transmission of the AIDS virus. Numerous teaching pamphlets available through AIDS support groups and public health departments can be given to the patient and significant others. Everyone has a responsibility to help prevent the spread of the AIDS virus.

Summary

The clinical spectrum of manifestations of HIV infection range from no signs and symptoms to full-blown AIDS. Additionally, individuals with HIV infection may present to EDs for complaints unrelated to HIV infection. Therefore, it is prudent for ED nurses to develop practices for the safe handling of all blood and body fluids from all patients. ED nurses should also be able to provide information regarding HIV infection, to prevent the transmission of HIV infection, and to institute specific treatments for individuals with complaints and problems related to HIV infection. Patients that present with complaints associated with HIV infection usually need hospital admission. The treatment and teaching initiated in the ED will be a basis for continued treatment and teaching while the patient is hospitalized.

Hepatitis

There are several distinct infections grouped as viral hepatitis. The etiologies, pathophysiology, and clinical manifestations of hepatitis A, hepatitis B, and delta hepatitis are considered here.

Hepatitis A

Hepatitis A is not a new disease; it dates from the time of Hippocrates. Usually described as an icteric illness, hepatitis A has occurred in endemic and epidemic forms with worldwide distribution. There is usually a high prevalence of the disease in areas of the world where there are poor environmental conditions.

Etiology

Hepatitis A is caused by type A hepatitis virus (HAV). An enterovirus, it is chemically, physically, and morphologically distinct. Once exposure occurs, symptoms appear after an incubation period of 15 to 45 days, the average being about 28 days.

Hepatitis A is primarily transmitted through person-to-person spread via the fecal-oral route, especially where unsanitary or overcrowded conditions are present. Contaminated water or foods such as cold cuts, milk, raw vegetables and fruits, and shellfish are common sources of the spread of HAV.

Pathophysiology

A person must ingest the hepatitis A virus for infection to occur. Once a person is infected, the virus can be isolated from fecal cultures. Symptoms become apparent one to two weeks after peak levels of the virus are found in the stool. Some of these symptoms remit with the onset of jaundice or liver impairment. At this time, the serologic test for HAV antibodies becomes positive.

The infected person is most likely to transmit the virus during the last half of the incubation phase and until a few days after the onset of jaundice. Usually, a person is no longer infectious after the first week of jaundice.

Symptoms in individuals with hepatitis A are directly related to liver involvement. Because the liver has the unique ability to regenerate cells while others are being destroyed, the liver cells are usually back to normal in two to three months, and the infected patient is symptom-free. Occasionally, the liver is unable to regenerate the cells as rapidly as they are destroyed, and the infected person then dies. (Wehrle and Top 1981, 302).

Clinical Manifestations

A detailed history is important in the diagnosis of hepatitis A. Whether or not the patient has been in contact with anyone else who has or had hepatitis and whether or not they have eaten shellfish recently should be asked, for patients often are unaware of the process and mode of transmission of their disease. Onset of symptomatology of hepatitis A usually develops quickly within a 24- to 72-hour period. The first symptoms noticed by an infected person may be abdominal discomfort, anorexia, nausea, lack of energy, and a low-grade fever. Three days after the onset of these symptoms, the icteric phase begins: yellow skin and sclera become apparent. Urine is a dark amber, and the stool, clay-colored or pale.

Physical examination reveals an ill-appearing person who complains of fatigue and anorexia. The patient may have a low-grade fever and some abdominal pain (epigastrium or right upper quandrant) or frank jaundice, brownish-colored urine, and scleral icterus. The liver may be palpable at one to two fingers below the right costal margin and is usually tender. Diarrhea may or may not be present.

Laboratory data reveal a positive anti-HAV and an increase in serum total immunoglobulin M (IgM), which is replaced by immunoglobulin G (IgG) during the convalescence period. The ratio of serum alanine aminotransferase (ALT) to aspartate transaminase (AST) is elevated. Serum bilirubin is usually elevated above 4 mg/dl. The prothrombin time is usually increased.

Treatment and Nursing Care

There is no specific treatment for hepatitis A. Stage I care should be initiated only in cases of fulminant hepatitis if coagulation disorders occur. In these instances, vascular access will be needed for administration of necessary blood components, fluids, and emergency medications. The patient's airway, breathing, and circulation must be maintained, so emergency resuscitation equipment must be available.

Most treatment for hepatitis A is supportive and is aimed at maintaining comfort and an adequate nutritional balance. Additionally, education for the patient and significant others regarding the disease process and mode of transmission should be initiated. The administration of standard immunoglobulin (which provides passive immunity) could alter the course of hepatitis A if given immediately after exposure, during the incubation period.

Comfort, Altered, Related to

- *Abdominal pain*
- *Low-grade fever*

Pain medication should be given only as ordered by a physician. It is important not to mask symptoms until all other diagnoses have been ruled out. Helping to position the patient, occasional back rubs, and keeping the bed linen straight will provide some comfort.

Nutrition, Altered, Related to

- *Anorexia*
- *Fatigue*

Although not a treatment priority in the ED, good nutrition is imperative for an uncomplicated recovery. If the patient cannot tolerate oral intake, parenteral nutrition should be initiated. In house, the patient's intake, output, and daily weight should be monitored and skin should frequently be assessed.

Knowledge Deficit (Potential), Related to

- *Disease process*
- *Disease transmission*

Oftentimes, patients with hepatitis A (and their significant others) do not know how they acquired the disease, details of its course, and how it is transmitted. ED nurses should provide instruction to these individuals in these areas. The patient should be reassured that the clinical course of hepatitis A is usually self-limited, with full recovery after a period of two to four weeks. Chronic liver sequelae occur extremely rarely if at all. The importance of good handwashing after using the bathroom, before preparing food, and before eating should be stressed. Patients should be told that they will have lifetime immunity to hepatitis A and that they will not be chronic carriers.

Infection Transmission, Potential for (Health Care Workers),* Related to

- *Care and treatment of patients with hepatitis A*

Since transmission of hepatitis A is usually by the fecal-oral route, isolation precautions in accordance with hospital policy should be initiated. Wearing gloves when handling excretions, wearing gowns if there will be contact with feces, and good handwashing should be adequate. Precautions for handling blood and body fluids as cited in Table 28–4 are also applicable and should be instituted for patients with hepatitis A.

Hepatitis B

Hepatitis B virus was first found in the serum of an Australian aborigine and was called the Australian antigen. This disease is also called serum hepatitis and long-incubation hepatitis.

Hepatitis B is endemic throughout the world. Because of a high antigen carrier state (10% to 15%), there is an increased occurrence of infection in infants and young children in Asia. Worldwide there is a chronic carrier rate of 5% to 10%. The United States has a low carrier rate of 0.3% because of the available medical services. Concurrent HIV infection in individuals with hepatitis B is also possible.

Etiology

Hepatitis B is caused by the hepatitis B virus (HBV). There are three hepatitis B antigens: HBcAg, an antigenic system found in the internal component of the HBV; HBsAg, previously described, which is detected in the serum of infected individuals; and HBeAg, which is associated with relatively high infectivity. These three antigens have specific humoral antibodies directed against them: HBcAb (anti-HBc) is the window phase between the time a person tests HBsAg positive and the time when the person becomes HBsAb positive, which could be a period of infectivity; HBsAb (anti-HBs) shows immunity to the HBV; and HBeAb (anti-HBe) correlates with a relative (but not absolute) lack of infectivity.

Transmission occurs by percutaneous (IV, IM, subcutaneous (SQ), or intradermal) or mucosal exposure to infective blood or body fluids, as may occur in needle-stick accidents or sexual exposure.

Contaminated needles, syringes, and other IV equipment are common modes of transmission, especially among drug addicts. The infection can also be spread through contamination of wounds or lacerations or by exposure of mucous membranes to infective blood. Perinatal transmission is common in the endemic areas of Southeast Asia and the Far East. Accidental percutaneous inoculations by razors or toothbrushes used in common have occasionally been implicated as vehicles of transmission.

The incubation period is usually 45 to 180 days, with an average of 60 to 90 days.

---

* Non–NANDA-approved nursing diagnosis.

Pathophysiology

The primary reservoir for hepatitis B virus is humans. Infection is initiated by direct access of HBV into the bloodstream. Viral transmission to the liver is presumably rapid.

The appearance of HBsAg may precede the onset of clinical disease by as much as four weeks, and the individual is considered infectious during this time. Usually, HBsAg appears 4 to 6 weeks after infection and can persist for 10 to 12 weeks. Soon after the appearance of HBsAg in the serum, HBcAb also appears and persists throughout convalescence and possibly for many years thereafter. The appearance of HBsAb can coincide with the disappearance of HBsAg but more commonly is delayed. The antibody persists and is associated with long-term immunity. The development of a subclinical chronic carrier state and chronic hepatitis, however, is possible.

Clinical Manifestations

Again, a thorough history to determine whether or not an individual is at high risk for hepatitis B should be sought. Hepatitis B usually has a more gradual onset than hepatitis A. The clinical manifestations of hepatitis B are usually difficult to distinguish from hepatitis A. The clinical course of hepatitis B is also similar to hepatitis A.

In some cases (5% to 25%), physical examination can reveal a patient with arthritis, angioedema, and skin problems, including urticaria and maculopapular eruptions. Hepatomegaly is not uncommon. Nausea and vomiting are often severe, and jaundice appears during the icteric phase.

Hepatitis B is diagnosed by a positive HBsAg in the acute phase of illness. If HBsAg has already disappeared, a diagnosis is rendered by finding a high titer of HBcAb in the serum. Other laboratory data often reveal elevated serum liver enzymes, alkaline phosphatase, and indirect serum bilirubin, in addition to an elevated WBC.

Treatment and Nursing Care

Since symptoms of hepatitis B are similar to those of hepatitis A, the treatment is the same (see Treatment and Nursing Care under Hepatitis A). The only significant difference is in the mode of transmission. Isolation precautions in accordance with hospital policy should be initiated. Precautions for handling blood and body fluids as listed in Table 28–4 are also applicable and should be instituted for patients with hepatitis B.

If individuals are exposed to hepatitis B, passive immunoprophylaxis with hepatitis B immunoglobulin (HBIG) is possible. HBIG therapy should be given within seven days of exposure. Vaccination will not prevent infection once exposure has occurred; however, it is recommended for individuals in high risk groups.

Delta Hepatitis

Delta hepatitis, known also as hepatitis D (HDV), has been reported worldwide. This disease is prevalent in the same risk groups as hepatitis B. HBsAG carriers are at high risk for infection with the delta virus, especially if they have repeated exposure to hepatitis B through drug abuse or homosexual practices.

Etiology

The virus causing delta hepatitis is sometimes considered defective because it can only cause infection in the presence of active hepatitis B infection. The virus is described as 35 to 37 nm and as having a HBsAG coating and an inner protein called delta antigen. As many as 50% of the fulminant hepatitis B cases have been associated with coinfection with the delta virus.

Delta hepatitis is probably transmitted in much the same modes as is the hepatitis B virus: blood and blood products, dirty needles and syringes, sharp instruments, sexual contact, perinatal exposure, and organ transplantion.

In all phases of active delta hepatitis, blood may be infectious. The individual is probably most infectious before onset of symptoms, when the delta antigen can be found in the blood.

Pathophysiology

The onset of delta hepatitis resembles hepatitis B, with signs and symptoms occurring suddenly. The infection may be self-limiting or chronic hepatitis may develop. Illness can be severe. It is important to remember that delta hepatitis is always associated with a coexistent hepatitis B virus infection. The delta agent and hepatitis B virus can infect at the same time, or delta hepatitis can occur with a HBV carrier state.

Clinical Manifestations

These patients may or may not be aware of the disease process or its mode of transmission. A complete history that suggests present or prior hepatitis B infection is of utmost importance.

The patient presents with signs and symptoms of hepatitis B. Physical examination can reveal an extremely ill individual.

Diagnostic tests show the viral antigen in the liver, or serum or IgM antibody to the viral antigen can be detected (Benenson 1985, 177).

Treatment and Nursing Care

The same preventive measures that apply to hepatitis B infection also are true for delta agent infection. There is no specific treatment. It is important to remember that neither HBIG, IG, nor HBV vaccine is useful in protecting HBV carriers against the delta agent (Benenson 1985, 178).

Nursing care should be supportive, with special attention to nutrition (see Hepatitis A). During all phases of care, precautions should be taken to prevent exposure to the patient's blood and body fluids.

Summary

ED nurses must continuously be cognizant of the fact that individuals who present to EDs are not always aware that their symptomatology reflects a communicable disease. Additionally, individuals with communicable diseases often present to EDs for complaints of some other illness or trauma. The alert ED nurse who develops astute assessment skills and who uses precautions for the handling of all blood and body fluids from all patients greatly minimizes the transmission of infectious diseases.

Gonorrhea

Gonorrhea is a sexually transmitted disease that is common worldwide. It affects both males and females and is especially prevalent in the young adult population where sexual activity is greatest.

Etiology

The causative agent of gonorrhea is *Neisseria gonorrhoeae.* Transmission occurs by contact with exudates from mucous membranes of infected persons, almost always as a result of sexual activity. However, perinatal transmission (ophthalmia neonatorum) is also possible. The incubation time is usually two to five days. There is no lasting immunity to gonorrhea; therefore subsequent reinfection is possible.

Pathophysiology

Gonorrhea is an infection that most commonly invades the genitourinary tract; however, infection of these other anatomic sites is possible: urethra, endocervix, anal canal, pharynx, and conjunctiva. Infection may remain local or may spread into adjacent organs. Complications that may occur in females from primary site spread are bartholinitis, pelvic inflammatory disease (PID), and perihepatitis. Complications in males include prostatitis, epididymitis, and paraurethral abscess. More serious illnesses occurring as a result of septicemia secondary to dissemination of infection are arthritis, dermatitis, endocarditis, meningitis, and hepatitis.

Clinical Manifestations

Patients with gonococcal infection may present with varying symptomatology, depending on the site of infection and whether or not local spread or dissemination has occurred. Men often seek treatment for gonorrhea early in the course of illness because they are usually symptomatic at an earlier stage of illness than are women. Women often are asymptomatic, and complications of untreated gonorrhea often constitute the reason they seek medical help.

Symptoms in men with gonorrhea of the genitourinary tract classically reflect urethritis: dysuria and a purulent urethral discharge with onset about two to five days following exposure. Women may also experience some dysuria and a vaginal discharge; however, these symptoms are often disregarded by women until infection has spread to the upper genital tract (i.e., uterus and fallopian tubes) and pelvic inflammatory disease (PID) is present. When this occurs, symptoms are usually severe and often constitute the patient's reason for seeking health care. Continuous bilateral abdominal pain beginning several days following the onset of menses is usually characteristic. Fever along with leukocytosis is usually present.

On physical examination, women with PID may appear quite ill and at times are tearful. They usually present walking doubled over with a widened stance to their gait. Pelvic examination reveals adnexal tenderness with significant pain on cervical motion. Leukorrhea is usually present. Definitive diagnosis in both men and women is confirmed by a positive culture for *Neisseria gonorrhoeae*.

Treatment and Nursing Care

Because at least two days are required to obtain gonorrhea culture results and follow-up of ED patients often is poor, treatment for gonorrhea in the ED setting is often initiated on the basis of history and clinical findings. Antibiotics are the mainstay of treatment for individuals with gonorrhea; however, specific treatment protocols may vary, depending on the site of infection, clinical presentation of the patient, and whether or not the patient has any allergies to antibiotics. Currently, cephalosporins (e.g., ceftriaxone 250 mg IM), followed by tetracycline, 500 mg PO qid, or doxycycline, 100 mg PO bid, for seven days, have replaced penicillin therapy for the treatment of genitourinary gonorrhea, as many strains of gonorrhea have become penicillin-resistant. (Tetracycline and doxycycline therapy is also effective in the treatment of concurrent chlamydia infections, an important consideration when one recognizes the incidence of asymptomatic and concurrent chlamydia infection.) Hospitalization and IV antibiotics may be indicated for those patients who present with severe clinical symptoms or in whom disseminated gonorrhea is suspected. Cephalosporins should not be used in patients with penicillin allergies. Because treatment protocol recommendations change so rapidly, the reader is referred to current literature on the subject.

In addition to antibiotic treatment, nursing care of patients with gonorrhea should include promoting comfort measures and education for them and their significant others regarding the disease process, mode of transmission, and importance of compliance with treatment. Overall, stage II care should be adequate, as persons with gonorrhea usually do not present in life-threatening states.

Pain, Related to

- **Local or Disseminated Gonococcal Infection**

Persons with gonococcal infections can experience severe pain, especially when the primary site of infection has spread to other sites, as in pelvic inflammatory disease or epididymitis. They should be medicated for pain according to physician orders. Symptoms should not be masked if there is any question as to diagnosis. Acetaminophen or mild analgesics may be prescribed. Reassurance should be given to the patient that the pain will subside as the infection clears.

Knowledge Deficit (Potential), Related to

- **Disease Process**
- **Disease Transmission**
- **Treatment Modalities**

Education by ED nurses for patients and their significant others related to the disease gonorrhea, its mode of transmission, and treatment protocols is imperative to minimize the chances of incomplete treatment, reinfection, and continued spread of the disease. Instructing the patient to complete all prescribed medications for their full duration is critical. Patients should also be advised to inform all their sexual contacts of their infection and treatment so that their contacts can also be diagnosed and treated. Patients need to be aware that they should refrain from sex for at least two weeks, at which time a follow-up culture should be obtained to be sure that the infection has cleared. Explaining to the patient that reinfection can occur by having sex with an untreated partner (even if he or she is asymptomatic) is of utmost importance.

Infection Transmission, Potential for (Health Care Workers),* Related to

- **Genitourinary Discharge**

If there is obvious drainage or discharge, precautions should be maintained when handling excretions and secretions. Gloves and good handwashing should usually be sufficient.

Syphilis

Syphilis is a sexually transmitted infection that is acquired most commonly during the sexually active years. Most new cases occur in patients between 15 and 29 years of age. The disease is widespread throughout the world, although there is a correlation of increased incidence with lower socioeconomic status. Syphilis is also more prevalent in urban than in rural areas.

Etiology and Pathophysiology

The causative agent of syphilis is a spirochete *Treponema pallidum*. Transmission occurs almost exclusively by direct contact with infectious exudates from obvious or concealed moist early lesions of skin and mucous membranes. (Congenital syphilis occurs as the result of placental transmission from mother to fetus usually after the 16th week of pregnancy.) Indirect transmission by contaminated articles is possible but unlikely, since the organism survives only a short time outside the body. Infection results from accidental inoculation (i.e., touching a syphilitic lesion) and can be transmitted by blood transfusion if the donor was in the early stage of the disease at the time of blood donation. *Treponema pallidum* can be readily destroyed by heat, disinfection, and drying. The incubation period of syphilis is approximately three weeks. There is no lasting immunity against syphilis; reinfection is possible.

Clinical Manifestations

Clinically, syphilis is classified into four stages: primary, secondary, latent, and late. Symptoms vary accordingly.

---

* Non–NANDA-approved nursing diagnosis.

Primary syphilis is characterized by a painless chancre, which usually occurs on the genitalia or in the mouth. Healing occurs within three to six weeks. Every genital lesion should be suspected of being a chancre until proved otherwise by darkfield examination and serologic testing. Serologic blood tests usually become reactive during the month after the appearance of the chancre. Fever and lymphadenopathy may also be present. Vaginal or urethral discharge need not be present. The time elapsing between primary and secondary syphilis can vary from one to several months.

Secondary syphilis is characterized by cutaneous eruptions, mucous patches, condylomata lata (venereal warts), syphilitic alopecia, generalized adenitis, iritis, periostitis, and neurosyphilis.

During latent syphilis, the patient is without recognizable clinical evidence of infection but demonstrates a reactive serologic test. The latent period may persist from 1 to 40 or more years.

Late syphilis can attack any tissue or organ of the body, and principally involves the cardiovascular and central nervous systems. Complications of late syphilis are rare, as syphilis can successfully be treated in any of its earlier stages.

Treatment and Nursing Care

Regardless of stage of infection, antibiotics are the treatment of choice. Penicillin G benzathine, 2.4 million units IM, is currently the treatment of choice for primary, secondary, and latent syphilis. Late syphilis requires the same dosage of penicillin G benzathine injections to be repeated at one-week intervals for three to four weeks. Tetracycline, 500 mg qid for 15 days, is prescribed for individuals with penicillin allergies. All stages of syphilis are treatable. The reader is referred to current literature on recommended treatment protocols for each stage, as treatment protocols change. Serologic blood testing (i.e., VDRL or rapid plasma reagin [RPR]) to screen for syphilis should be done. False-positive VDRL reactions are likely to occur in an individual who was previously treated for syphilis. In those cases, an FTA (fluorescent treponemal antibody test) may be done. (FTA is a more specific serologic test than VDRL or RPR, thus differentiating false-positive tests from true syphilis.)

Patients who receive IM penicillin in the ED should be observed for at least 20 minutes following administration to be sure that anaphylaxis does not occur.

Stage II care is usually all that is required for individuals with syphilis. In addition to the administration of antibiotics, nursing care must include education for the patient and significant others (see the following section). Nurses must use caution when caring for individuals with syphilis to minimize the possibility of contracting syphilis themselves.

Knowledge Deficit (Potential), Related to

- **Disease Process**
- **Mode of Transmission**
- **Treatment Modalities**

Syphilis can be treated successfully and reinfection prevented only by understanding its mode of transmission and the importance of compliance with treatment.

Therefore, emergency nurses have the responsibility of educating patients in these areas prior to their discharge from the ED. Like other sexually transmitted diseases, all contacts of the patient who have been exposed should be notified to obtain serologic testing and subsequent treatment. Patients must understand the importance of abstaining from sex until the infection has cleared and that reinfection is possible through continuing to have sex with untreated partners. The importance of close follow-up for patients and their contacts must be stressed.

Infection Transmission, Potential for (Health Care Workers),* Related to

- **Contact with Exudate from Syphilitic Lesion**
- **Accidental Parenteral Contact**

Exudates from lesions of patients with primary or secondary syphilis are highly contagious. Caretakers of patients have developed primary lesions on their hands following clinical examination of infectious lesions (Benenson 1985, 377). Therefore, the use of gloves when touching any suspected chancre cannot be overemphasized. Good handwashing is also imperative as fluid from a chancre is filled with spirochetes. Because the blood of patients with secondary and latent syphilis contains organisms, needle-stick injuries should be avoided.

Chlamydia

Chlamydia is a sexually transmitted infection that occurs primarily as urethritis in males and mucopurulent cervicitis in females. Infection may coexist with gonorrhea and may persist after the gonorrhea has been successfully treated.

Etiology

The causative agent is *Chlamydia trachomatis,* immunotypes D to K. Chlamydia is transmitted during sexual contact. It can also be transmitted to infants at the time of delivery, causing conjunctivitis, pneumonia, or both.

The incubation period is five to ten days or longer. The period of communicability is uncertain, but relapses are probably common.

Pathophysiology

Male urethritis as the result of chlamydial infection is often confused with gonorrhea. There can also be asymptomatic infections. Possible sequelae of the urethral infection can include epididymitis and male infertility.

Chlamydia infections in females can also be confused with gonorrhea. Salpingitis with subsequent risk of infertility or ectopic pregnancy can be a complication. Infection during pregnancy can result in conjunctival or pneumonic infection of the newborn.

---

* Non–NANDA-approved nursing diagnosis.

Clinical Manifestation

Males with urethritis secondary to chlamydia often present with a urethral discharge, urethral itching, and burning on urination. Females usually complain of mucopurulent discharge from the vagina and possibly dyspareunia.

Diagnosis is confirmed by microscopic examination of the drainage or by culture growths. However, cultures are expensive and often not available.

Treatment and Nursing Care

The treatment of choice for chlamydia infection is antibiotics. Tetracycline, 500 mg qid for seven days, is most commonly prescribed. Stage II care, focused on education, is in order (see the next section). Additionally, nurses must use care to prevent the spread of infection to themselves.

Knowledge Deficit (Potential), Related to

- **Disease Process**
- **Mode of Transmission**
- **Treatment Modalities**

Emergency nurses should be aware of the disease process, mode of transmission, and treatment of chlamydia. Teaching should be considered one of the most important aspects of care for patients with chlamydia (and other communicable diseases) and their significant others. Stressing the importance of completing all medication prescribed and abstaining from sex with infected partners is critical to minimizing the chance of incomplete treatment or reinfection. Follow-up in seven to ten days is recommended for a repeat culture to determine adequacy of treatment.

Infection Transmission, Potential for (Health Care Workers),* Related to

- **Urethral Drainage**
- **Vaginal Drainage**

Emergency nurses should initiate precautions to prevent direct contact with drainage. Gloves and good handwashing should be adequate.

Herpes Simplex

Herpes simplex is a viral infection that is transmitted by direct contact with the lesion, either person-to-person or from one body part to another on the same person. It infects skin surfaces, mucous membranes, and the eyes; it has even been found in the central nervous system. Health care workers have developed herpes lesions (herpetic

---

* Non–NANDA-approved nursing diagnosis.

whitlow) on the fingers when suctioning or performing oral hygiene in patients with a history of herpes simplex and no active lesions.

The infection is usually subclinical; however, when it is clinically apparent, it can be in either acute or recurrent form (Wehrle and Top 1981). Once infected with herpes simplex virus (HSV), the individual is infected for life. Herpes occurs world-wide.

Etiology and Pathophysiology

Herpes simplex virus (HSV) is categorized as types 1 and 2. HSV-1 infections frequently occur during childhood and usually infect body sites above the waist. HSV-2 usually occurs during adolescence and young adulthood and usually infects body sites below the waist (Evans 1982, 351). Either strain, however, can cause disease at any site. Recurrent HSV infections are common. There is also a high rate of HSV infections in immunocompromised patients. Incubation can be any time from 2 to 12 days.

Herpes simplex virus lesions are usually confined to the outermost layer of skin (epidermis) or superficial mucous membranes. Dissemination of the virus is rare. When it does occur, however, the organs most often affected are the brain, liver, adrenal glands, and lungs.

Clinical Manifestations

Herpes simplex virus infections range from mild to severe. A number of factors influence severity, including age of the host, organs involved, whether the host is immunocompromised, and the recurrent nature of the infection.

Generally, individuals with primary HSV-2 infection complain of burning pain at the site of inoculation along with dysuria and possible urinary retention. A purulent vaginal discharge is not uncommon. Systemic manifestations may include fever, chills, malaise, and headaches. Recurrent episodes usually have less severe symptomatology than primary episodes.

On physical examination, the patient may or may not look ill. Vesicular lesions and inflammation will be noted at the site involved. Inguinal lymphadenopathy may also be present. Examination of scrapings from the margins of the vesicle provide the most rapid means of determining a presumptive diagnosis of HSV infection. Diagnosis is confirmed by viral culture of active lesions.

Treatment and Nursing Care

At the current time there is no cure for HSV. Treatment and nursing care are symptomatic and revolve around educating patients and their significant others about the disease process, its mode of transmission and treatment protocols, along with promotion of patient comfort.

Knowledge Deficit (Potential), Related to

- **Disease Process**
- **Mode of Transmission**
- **Treatment Modalities**

Patients and their significant others often have many questions regarding HSV, what it is, how it is spread, and how it is treated. Emergency nurses must be knowledgeable in these areas so that they can educate patients (and their significant others) before they leave the ED.

As transmission occurs via direct contact with exudative lesions, patients with HSV must understand the importance of refraining from sex during infectious outbreaks.

There are a number of antiviral drugs available. Acyclovir (Zovirax) is most commonly prescribed; however, none of the drugs offers a complete cure. However, acyclovir helps in reducing the pain and minimizing the frequency and severity of HSV outbreaks. Additional comfort measures may include mild analgesics, sitz baths several times a day, and wearing loose fitting undergarments and clothing. Antimicrobials for bacterial superinfection may also be necessary.

Infection Transmission, Potential for (Health Care Workers),* Related to

- **Care and Treatment of Patients with HSV Lesions**

Vescicular lesions contain large quantities of infectious viral particles; therefore, direct contact of draining lesions should be avoided. Gloves should be worn, and good handwashing following patient contact is critical to minimizing the spread of infection.

Pulmonary Tuberculosis

Pulmonary tuberculosis is an infection of the respiratory tract. It occurs worldwide. Mortality and morbidity rates increase with the elderly, lower socioeconomic status, and crowded urban living conditions. In areas of low incidence, most tuberculosis develops from a person's own organisms: a reactivation from latent foci remaining from an initial infection. Although tuberculosis ranks low among communicable diseases in infectiousness per time-unit of exposure, with prolonged exposure, household members, especially, have a 30% chance of becoming infected and a 1% to 2% chance of infection progressing to disease within a year.

Etiology

The organisms causing tuberculosis are species of *Mycobacterium*, commonly *M. tuberculosis* in humans. Characteristic of tuberculosis infection is a reactive tubercu-

---

* Non–NANDA-approved nursing diagnosis.

lin skin test without other abnormal changes seen by physical, laboratory, or radiologic examinations. Characteristics of tuberculosis disease are a reactive tuberculin skin test and abnormal changes that can be seen in physical, laboratory, and radiologic examinations.

Transmission occurs from exposure to bacilli in airborne droplet nuclei from sputum of persons with infectious tuberculosis (those with disease).

Pathophysiology

Infection begins with the accidental inhalation of a single dried-droplet containing a viable *Mycobacterium* that becomes implanted in an alveolus. Mycobacteria slowly replicate for three weeks and eventually are carried into the systemic circulation. At sometime between 3 and 12 weeks following initial infection, an immunologic response is generated by the intact system. As a result of this response, the microscopic foci—containing bacteria, located throughout the body, are successfully encapsulated and contained in 85% to 95% of initially infected individuals. These foci continue to remain quiescent for prolonged periods of time, but they retain their capacity to reactivate and invade normal structures to cause disease. Five to fifteen percent of initially infected persons have difficulty controlling initial foci and exhibit evidence of tuberculosis disease several weeks after exposure (Wherle and Top 1981, 679).

Clinical Manifestations

Patients with pulmonary tuberculosis can present with the following symptoms: cough, blood-tinged sputum, weight loss, difficulty breathing, and night sweats. By history, illness is frequently related to prior exposure.

In prolonged untreated disease, physical examination can reveal an emaciated patient with some respiratory distress.

Diagnosis is confirmed with sputum smears positive for acid-fast bacilli and cultures positive for *M. tuberculosis.* In this case, the tuberculin skin test is positive. Chest radiographs reveal abnormal findings (cavitary lesions are usually consistent with pulmonary tuberculosis).

Treatment and Nursing Care

Hospitalization is usually not required for patients with tuberculosis except for diagnostic reasons or when the individual is severely debilitated. Most patients with tuberculosis are treated on an outpatient basis; thus nursing care must have as a primary focus education for the patient and significant others regarding the disease itself, its mode of transmission, and treatment protocols. Additionally, precautions should be taken in the ED to prevent the spread of the disease as soon as tuberculosis is suspected. Stage II care is usually adequate.

TABLE 28-5
Populations Recommended to Receive Antituberculosis Drugs

Persons with known exposure who may be in the process of converting their tuberculin skin test
Persons under 35 years old who have recently converted from a negative to positive tuberculin skin test
Household contacts of persons diagnosed with tuberculosis
Tuberculin reactors over age 35 who are at special risk
    Persons receiving steroids
    Persons receiving immunosuppressive therapy
    Persons with immunologic disorders
Persons with
    Leukemia or lymphoma
    Silicosis
    Insulin-dependent diabetes mellitus
    Gastrectomy

Source: Reproduced by permission from: Brucia J, Phipps WJ, Daly BJ. In: Phipps WJ, Long BC, Woods NF. Medical and Surgical Nursing Concepts and Clinical Practice, 3rd ed, 1323. St. Louis, 1987, The C.V. Mosby Co.

Knowledge Deficit (Potential), Related to

- **Disease Process**
- **Mode of Transmission**
- **Treatment Modalities**

Individuals with tuberculosis (and their significant others) need to know that once they are infected with *M. tuberculosis*, they harbor the organism for life; however, they also need to understand that infection does not mean active disease.

Antituberculosis drugs are the treatment of choice for pulmonary tuberculosis. They are used to treat individuals with active disease and to prevent disease in those persons who are infected but in whom the disease is not active (Table 28-5). More than 96% of initial isolates of mycobacterium tuberculosis from patients native to the United States and without previous history of antituberculosis drug therapy show complete sensitivity to the standard antituberculoisis drugs. However, 14% to 20% of initial isolates from persons in the Asian and Pacific areas and Central America show resistance to these drugs, and drug resistance in these populations must be taken into account. Drug therapy is long-term (several months) and the importance of compliance and close patient follow-up must be stressed.

Because patients are most likely to be treated at home, significant others need to be reassured that transmission does not occur via inanimate objects. Infected individuals with active disease should always cough and sneeze into a handkerchief. Significant others should be instructed to report to their own physician or a health care clinic that they have been exposed to tuberculosis.

Infection Transmission, Potential for (Health Care Workers and Significant Others), Related to*

- **Pulmonary Tuberculosis**

Emergency personnel should be observant and should ask pertinent questions to determine if a patient has any history of exposure to pulmonary tuberculosis. Rapid

---

* Non-NANDA-approved nursing diagnosis.

identification can prevent the spread of infection. If a diagnosis of pulmonary tuberculosis is suspected, isolation precautions should be directed at preventing the accidental inhalation of infectious nuclei. Masks for ED personnel should be worn when entering the patient's room, and if transported to other areas of the hospital, the patient should wear a mask during transport.

Breathing Pattern, Ineffective (Potential), Related to

- **Diminished Lung Capacity Secondary to Tuberculosis**

Stage I care is rarely required for patients with pulmonary tuberculosis. However, extremely ill patients with prolonged untreated illness could have a diminished lung capacity. In these instances, stage I care may be required. The effectiveness of the patient's breathing pattern should be closely monitored. Oxygen should be administered if ordered. In cases of acute distress, intubation may be necessary.

SKIN AND BODY INFESTATIONS AND INFECTIONS

Pediculosis (Lice)

Pediculosis is an infestation of the head, body, or pubic area with adult lice, larvae, or nits (eggs). Infestations occur worldwide; however, outbreaks of head lice are common among school children. Any person can become infested under suitable conditions of exposure.

Etiology

The infesting agents are *Pediculus humanus capitis* for the head, *P. humanus corporis* for the body, and *Phthirus pubis* (crab louse) for the pubic area (Benenson 1985, 247).

The *P. humanus capitis* and *P. humanus corporis* are closely related, interbreedable variants of the same species, despite their different habits. They can usually be seen by the naked eye. Their color is gray-white; they have six legs and are 3 to 4 mm long. Although they are blood sucking insects, they live on the outside of the infested Although they are blood sucking insects, they live on the outside of the infested person's body except when feeding. During a female's life span of 30 days, she produces approximately 140 eggs. The eggs adhere to hair shafts or clothing. After eight to nine days, the young adult (nymph) is hatched; after shedding its outer covering three times over a ten-day period, it becomes an adult.

The *Phthirus pubis* has a smaller, spade-like body and short legs that end in large claws. It is usually invisible to the naked eye because of its skin-like color and small size. In order to survive, it must feed at least every 24 hours on blood. The adult female lives 20 to 30 days and produces approximately 50 eggs. The eggs adhere to a hair shaft, usually in the pubic area, but can also be found in the axillae, eyelashes, and even mustaches.

Transmission occurs by direct contact with an infested person and indirectly by contact with their personal belongings, especially clothing and headgear. Pubic lice are usually transmitted through sexual contact.

Pathophysiology

Lice are hematophagous. As they feed, saliva is introduced into the site of their puncture, causing an erythematous papule within hours. Since the papules itch, scratching them often leads to secondary skin infections.

On microscopic examination, infiltration with lymphocytes and the extravasation of erythrocytes are found. A residual pigmentation of the skin from bleeding and scratching is characteristic of lesions from prolonged infestations, particularly with pubic lice.

Clinical Manifestations

Patients infested with *P. capitis* usually complain of itching of the scalp, neck, and ears. When pyoderma is present at the neck and ears, the possibility of head lice should be included in the assessment. Cervical lymph nodes may be enlarged secondary to skin infections from scratching the papules. Head lice may be seen, but usually only nits are visible about an inch from the scalp.

Patients infested with *P. corporis* usually complain of itching of the trunk and neck. Close inspection of the body may reveal hemorrhagic punctures, wheals, or both from fresh bites. Residual pigmentation and honey crusts from secondary pyoderma are common. Body lice are not usually seen on the skin since they live in the clothing. The body louse is the only one found to have been a carrier of epidemics such as typhus, trench fever, and louse-borne relapsing fever.

Patients infested with *Phthirus pubis* usually complain of itching in the pubic area, groin, lower abdomen, and axilla. Pale, bluish-gray maculae can be seen at the sites of the bites. Secondary pyodermas are not uncommon. A good light and a hand-held magnifying glass are usually needed to see the lice.

The clothing of impoverished persons who have excoriations of the trunk should be inspected routinely for the presence of nits and lice.

Patients may or may not be aware of their infestations and the mode of transmission.

Treatment and Nursing Care

Stage II care is adequate, since the patient will not present in acute distress.

Patients with *P. capitis* should wash their hair with 1% lindane shampoo (Kwell). If used as directed no neurotoxicity will occur with young children. The shampoo is repeated in one week to catch newly hatched lice. Nits moistened a few minutes with vinegar can be removed with a fine-toothed comb. Household contacts should be examined and treated if infested.

Patients with *P. corporis* have to be washed thoroughly with soap and water. If nits are found on the body hairs, 1% lindane lotion (Kwell lotion) can be applied and left in place 8 hours then washed off thoroughly. Lindane should not be used in this way on young children or pregnant women. Clothing and bed linens with which the patient was in contact during the prior month should be washed in very hot water or dry-cleaned. Storage of these for 30 days is also effective. Household contacts should be examined and treated if infested.

Patients with *Phthirus pubis* should have the infested hair shampooed with 1% lindane shampoo (Kwell). Retreatment is usually unnecessary. All sexual contacts should be treated simultaneously; other household contacts are treated only if infested. *Phthirus pubis* infestation of the eyelashes can be treated with yellow oxide of mercury ophthalmic ointment applied to the area twice daily for a few days, after which time lice and nits can usually be squeezed out easily. Since Phthirus infestation is also associated with other sexually transmitted diseases (gonorrhea and trichomonas and to lesser extent scabies, nongonococcal urethritis, condyloma acuminatum, genitourinary candidiasis, and syphilis), patients should be assessed for treatment of these conditions also.

Infestation Transmission (Potential), Related to*

- **Skin Lesions**

‹Caretakers should take precautions whenever a patient presents with any skin disease. The use of gloves and good handwashing are usually adequate. If prolonged close exposure to the patient is anticipated, gowns or aprons should also be used.

Knowledge Deficit (Potential), Related to

- **Infestation Process**
- **Infestation Transmission**

Emergency personnel should recognize the various types of pediculosis infestations and know the means of transmission. It is important that treatment be thorough and infested contacts, clothing, and linens be treated to prevent further infestation.

Evaluation

Initial identification and treatment, teaching, and the establishment of appropriate barriers (gloves, gowns or aprons) are important in preventing the spread of infesta-

---

* Non–NANDA-approved nursing diagnosis.

tions. In the event of hospitalization, the care plan, including the treatment rendered, should accompany the patient.

Adequate treatment can be measured by the absence of spread of infestation.

Scabies (Mites)

Scabies is an infectious disease of the skin found worldwide. Infestations can affect persons from all socioeconomic levels without regard to age, sex, race, or standards of personal hygiene. It is endemic in many developing countries.

Etiology

The infecting agent is the *Sarcoptes scabiei,* a tiny, whitish, eight-legged mite (parasite) shaped like a turtle.

The incubation period is two to six weeks in persons with a first exposure. Persons being reexposed develop symptoms in one to four days (Benenson 1985, 303).

Transmission occurs by direct skin-to-skin contact and to a limited extent from undergarments or soiled bedclothes freshly contaminated by infected persons. The infection is frequently acquired during sexual contact. Norwegian scabies is extremely infectious because of the large number of mites in the exfoliating scales and requires only minimal contact for spreading.

Pathophysiology

Scabies infection is caused by *S. scabiei* penetration of the skin, visible as vesicles or papules or as tiny linear burrows containing the mites and their eggs. Lesions appear around the finger webs, anterior surfaces of the wrists and elbows, anterior axillary folds, belt line, thighs, and external genitalia in men; nipples, abdomen, and lower portion of the buttocks are frequently affected in women.

Diagnosis may be established by recovering the mite from its burrow and identifying it microscopically. Lesions that have not been excoriated by repeated scratching should be used for the scraping or biopsy.

Clinical Manifestations

Patients infested with *S. scabiei* usually complain of intense itching, especially at night. Complications are limited to lesions secondarily infected from scratching. The lesion is a burrow for the mite — a thin, dirty line that is straight, sinuous, or zig zag and 2 to 15 mm long (Wehrle and Top, 1981).

A vesicle or pustule may be present at the point of entry into the skin. Sensitization to the presence of scabies can occur approximately one month after the primary infestation with a follicular, papular eruption distributed over areas where mite burrows are absent.

In immunocompromised individuals, infestation often appears as a generalized dermatitis with extensive scaling. Sometimes extensive vesiculation and crusting occur. The severe itching may be reduced or absent.

Patients may or may not be aware of their infestation and the means of transmission.

Treatment and Nursing Care

Stage II care is adequate as the patient will not present in acute distress.

Treatment for adults and older children consists of lindane (Kwell and others) in a 1% lotion form. It is easy to use, effective, and well accepted by the patient. A single application is usually curative.

Lindane is toxic to the central nervous system. Safe alternative treatments for young children, infants, and pregnant women is 10% crotamiton cream (Eurax) or 5% sulfur precipitate in petrolatum.

The key to success in treatment lies in good timing and adequate communication. All members of the household, including close contacts of family members, should be treated at the same time to prevent reinfestations. Bedding and clothing worn next to the skin should be laundered or dry cleaned. Storage of blankets and outer garments for a week or more is sufficient to clear them of stray mites, since the mite does not survive more than three or four days away from the skin.

Infestation Transmission (Potential),* Related to

- **Skin Lesions**

Caretakers should take precautions whenever a patient presents with any skin disease. The use of gloves and good handwashing are usually adequate. If prolonged close exposure to the patient is anticipated, gowns or aprons should also be used.

Knowledge Deficit (Potential), Related to

- **Infestation Process**
- **Infestation Transmission**

Emergency personnel should recognize infestations with *S. scabiei* and know the means of transmission. Treatment must be thorough, and infested contacts and clothing/linens should be treated to prevent further infestations.

Evaluation

Initial identification and treatment, teaching, and the establishment of appropriate barriers (gloves, gowns or aprons) are important to prevent the transmission of infestations. In the event of hospitalization, the care plan, documenting the treatment rendered, should accompany the patient.

---

* Non–NANDA-approved nursing diagnosis.

Treatment effectiveness can be measured by the absence of spread of the infestation.

CONCLUSION

Let us return to the four patients described at the beginning of the chapter and determine if any or all posed a potential infection control problem.

Patients 1, 2, 3, and 4 all have the potential to transmit infectious diseases via their blood, body fluids, or both. Therefore, appropriate precautions should be instituted when handling all of these patients. Patients 1 and 2 are profusely bleeding and thus are most likely to transmit hepatitis, HIV, or both if they are infected. Patient 3 should be evaluated for tuberculosis as well as for fractured ribs. He has a cough and is expectorating blood-tinged sputum. Wearing a mask would be prudent. Patient 4 may not pose an infection control problem; however, taking a good history as soon as possible is important. She has no drainages, so the likelihood of her exposing anyone to infection is minimal. However, she is the wife of Patient 3 and could be at risk for tuberculosis transmission.

The ED can be a reservoir for infections. Not only should ED personnel treat patients for their obvious symptoms, they should also remember to take a comprehensive history to uncover less obvious causes of potential infection transmission — the "whole" patient must be treated. ED nurses must know about the infectious diseases as well as emergency situations in order to protect themselves and others from unnecessary illness caused by the transmission of infection.

REFERENCES

Alexander WJ, Good R. 1977. Fundamentals of Clinical Immunology. Philadelphia, WB Saunders.

Benenson AS. 1985. Control of Communicable Diseases in Man, 14th ed. Washington, DC, The American Public Health Association.

Castle M. 1980. Hospital Infection Control. New York, John Wiley & Sons.

Centers for Disease Control. 1987. Classification system for human immunodeficiency virus (HIV) infection in children under 13 years of age. MMWR 36(15):225–235.

Centers for Disease Control. 1989. Current update: acquired immunodeficiency syndrome US 1981–1988. MMWR 38(14):229.

Centers for Disease Control. 1987. Revision of the CDC surveillance case definition for acquired immunodeficiency syndrome. MMWR 36(1S):3S–9S.

Centers for Disease Control. 1987. Human immunodeficiency virus infection in the United States. MMWR 36(49):801–804.

Centers for Disease Control. 1987. Recommendations for prevention of HIV transmission in health-care settings. MMWR 36(2S):3S–18S.

Cole HM, Lundberg GD. 1986. AIDS from the Beginning. Chicago, American Medical Association.

Evans AS. 1982. Viral Infections of Humans: Epidemiology and Control. New York, Plenum Press.

McCray E. 1986. Occupational risk of the acquired immunodeficiency syndrome among health care workers. N Engl J Med 314:1127–1132.

Wehrle PF, Top FH. 1981. Communicable and Infectious Diseases, 9th ed. St. Louis, CV Mosby.

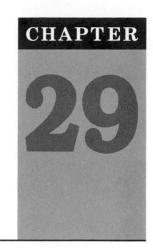

CHAPTER

29

James Mathews, MD

Hypertension and Hypertensive Emergencies

The patient with elevated blood pressure is frequently encountered in the emergency department (ED). Hypertension can be defined as a blood pressure of greater than 140 systolic and greater than 90 diastolic. Approximately 25% to 30% of the United States population has hypertension. The exact incidence of this problem is not known, but screening performed on the general population has shown that at least 20 million people in the United States suffer from some degree of elevated blood pressure (National Center for Health Statistics 1966; Kilcoyne 1973). Often their first encounter with medical care is a visit to the ED (Glass 1978; Kaszuba 1978). Thus it is essential that every patient over the age of 12 years who presents for emergency care have a blood pressure recorded on his or her record. Some authors lower this age limit even further. The emergency nurse has a vital role in assuring that this is accomplished. In addition to identifying hypertension, the emergency nurse needs a working knowledge of the pathophysiology of hypertension; should recognize hypertensive emergencies; and must know the administration, indications, contraindications, and side effects of the antihypertensive medications utilized in emergency care.

ASSESSMENT

Evaluation of an individual with an actual or potential elevation in blood pressure begins with an assessment of the chief complaint. Although an elevated blood pressure may be found incidentally on initial evaluation, "high blood pressure" is rarely a presenting complaint. Moderate hypertension generally causes no specific symptomatology and as such does not incite an ED visit. Consequently, hypertension has come to be known as the "silent killer" in our society today. However, there are several chief complaints that are nonspecific but nonetheless may represent the vague clinical effects of hypertension. Constitutional complaints such as malaise, fatigue, headache, and vertigo may be associated with untreated hypertension. Certain patients may present with multiple complaints including palpitations, rapid heart rate, sweating, anxiety, and epistaxis. In this situation, if markedly elevated blood pressure is also found, a hypertensive emergency must be suspected. Other symptoms associated with acute hypertensive crisis include tremors, headache, and marked apprehension. Patients may also present with complaints related to end-organ damage (e.g., confusion from cerebral ischemia or uremic syndrome from renal failure).

A review of systems should focus on target organs commonly affected by chronic elevations in blood pressure: kidneys, heart, and lungs. An elevated blood pressure discovered on initial examination should alert the triage nurse to inquire about past medical history relevant to hypertensive disease. Has the patient or anyone in his family had renal, cardiac, or pulmonary disease? Are there other risk factors commonly associated with vascular disease: smoking, hypercholesterolemia, or obesity?

Has the patient ever been told he or she has high blood pressure? Ask the patient to describe past and present medications and determine if there have been any changes in prescriptions. Has the patient stopped taking medication without a physician's advice? If so, have the patient describe reasons. Most often, cost of drugs and unpleasant side effects influence such decisions.

Assigning a triage category is dependent upon the patient's clinical presentation. When severe respiratory or cardiovascular compromise or both is overt, the triage nurse should have little difficulty in determining an acuity rating. Any individual with a presenting history compatible with cardiovascular or respiratory insult should be taken immediately to the patient care area, where treatment can begin at once. However, when patients present with symptomatology that is less overt, is somewhat vague, and is not clear-cut as to origin, the triage nurse may assign a less emergent acuity rating to their triage status.

Objective evaluation of the patient's clinical status includes a physical examination and laboratory analysis. Again, special attention may be focused on target organs most likely to be reflective of hypertensive disorders: mainly, the heart, lungs, and kidneys. Assessment of cardiovascular status by determination of vital signs is a priority. Additionally, an electrocardiogram (EKG) and cardiac monitoring may be in order for those individuals with complaints that may reflect an acute cardiac event (chest pain, syncope, shortness of breath, and so forth). Assessment of the patient's respiratory status should include breathing rate and pattern as well as identification of breath sounds on auscultation. Complaints associated with suspected renal pathology will most likely be evaluated through laboratory analysis of blood and urine.

As stated previously, determination of blood pressure is necessary for all patients over the age of 12 presenting for emergency care. Many factors can influence the level of a person's blood pressure, including age, size, degree of anxiety, presence of pain, and other underlying problems. Special cuffs should be readily available for the pediatric population and for the very obese. The blood pressure cuff should be large enough to wrap comfortably around the arm one to one and one half times, attach smoothly at the Velcro surfaces, and remain adjoined when the cuff is inflated. In all situations, the cuff should be deflated slowly to avoid a gap in the cuff pressure and measured pressure on the gauge—a situation that produces an artificially elevated measurement. This is less apt to occur with anaeroid instruments, but these are not as accurate as instruments with a mercury column. Another reason for slow deflation is that a slowly falling needle or column of mercury is much easier to read accurately.

The level of systolic pressure is taken as the first sound is heard during deflation, and in general diastolic pressure best correlates with disappearance of this sound. In certain patients, some sound is heard down to zero, and the diastolic pressure correlates best with the level at which distinct muffling of the sound occurs. As noted earlier, the current upper levels of normal are 140 mmHg systolic and 90 mmHg diastolic. These are arbitrary values for adults but seem to correlate well with the chronic problems of long-standing hypertension (VA study 1970; Kannel 1970, 1967; Multiple Risk Factor Group 1982; The 1984 Report of Joint National Committee 1985). These values are lower for the young, higher for the elderly, and not applicable to the pregnant population, in which blood pressure recordings of greater than 125/70 have been shown to increase fetal risk.

A single, isolated recording of elevated blood pressure does not make a diagnosis of hypertension. Many patients present with moderate elevations secondary to pain or anxiety. If an elevated reading is found, a second recording prior to discharge should be made, and if normal, the initial reading can be disregarded. Elevation suspected to be secondary to stress should not be taken too lightly, however, as it is uncommon for there to be elevation of the diastolic component past 100 to 110 mmHg from stress alone. If a higher level is encountered or if the level is elevated on the second reading, hypertension must be strongly considered, and the patient should be referred for follow-up or should receive further evaluation within the ED.

There are no specific diagnostic laboratory tests for hypertension. However, special tests are discussed with specific etiologies associated with hypertensive disease.

ETIOLOGY

Hypertension does not represent a specific disease; rather, it is a physical finding associated with many underlying processes. In the majority of cases, the specific cause of hypertension is unknown; this is referred to as essential hypertension. Even though a specific cause cannot be found in most cases of hypertension, many risk factors have been identified and include family history, race, increased amounts of sodium in the diet, age, and obesity. The incidence of hypertension increases with age and is more prevalent in the black population. The more factors present in a given individual, the higher the probability of the development of elevated blood pressure (Kilcoyne 1980).

The most common known cause of hypertension is renal disease (Kincaid-Smith 1977; Kincaid-Smith and Whitworth 1987). The direct relationship between most types of renal disease and hypertension is not clear. However, all types of renal disease are associated with an increased incidence of hypertension (Kincaid-Smith 1977).

Excessive catecholamine production, caused by a pheochromocytoma or complications associated with certain drugs, is another cause of hypertension. Monoamine oxidase (MAO) inhibitors may be responsible for profound elevation of blood pressure if tyramine-containing foods are ingested or if certain other therapeutic agents are given to the patient. An identified cause of excessive catecholamines is acute withdrawal of clonidine (Geyskes et al 1979). A careful drug history in all patients is paramount. If the patient is unable to provide a history, all other available sources need to be explored. This is often the purview of the ED nurse and is an important aspect of care.

PATHOPHYSIOLOGY

In relatively recent years, patients with essential hypertension have been divided into two groups based on renin levels (Esler 1975). Renin is formed in renal tissue in response to decreased kidney perfusion. To increase perfusion, the kidney attempts to retain sodium and thus to increase blood volume by secreting renin. Renin leads to the formation of angiotensin, a potent vasoconstrictor. Angiotensin also stimulates the release of aldosterone, a hormone that increases sodium retention (Fig. 29–1).

All of these activities lead to increased blood volume, increased renal perfusion, and subsequent reduction of renin production. If renin levels are obtained, initial drug therapy can be selected more accurately, as those patients with high levels

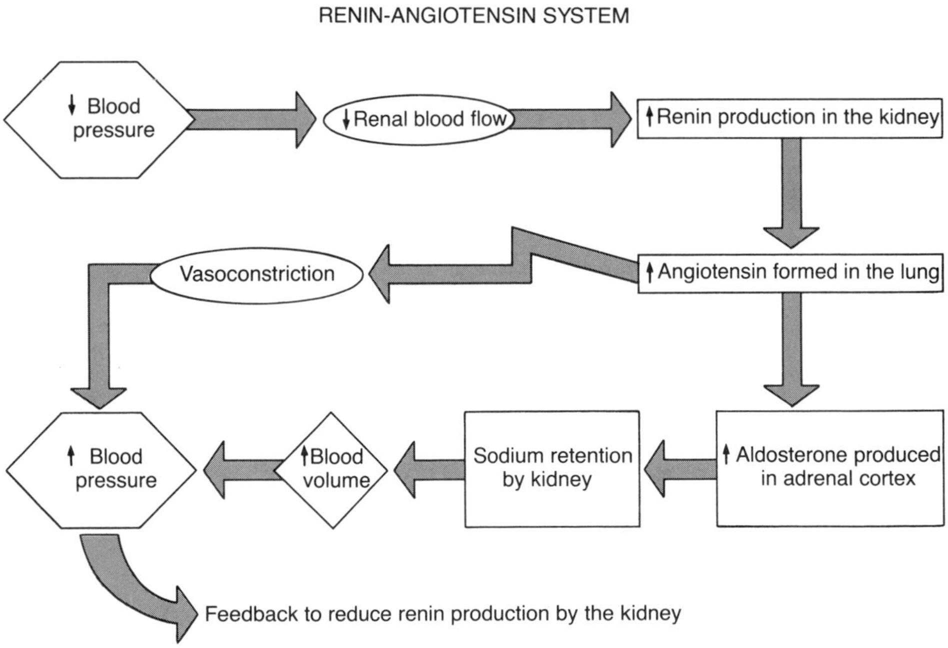

RENIN-ANGIOTENSIN SYSTEM

FIGURE 29–1. Effect of decreased blood pressure on renal blood flow, renin production, vascular tone, and blood volume.

respond better to beta blockade, whereas those with low renin levels do better with diuretics in their initial treatment.

As stated earlier, the direct relationship between most types of renal disease and hypertension is not clear. An exception is the uncommon case of unilateral renal artery stenosis. Renal ischemia leads to a marked overproduction of renin with resultant activation of the angiotensin system. Removal of the affected kidney may lead to complete resolution of the hypertension (Goldblatt et al 1939; Kincaid-Smith 1961; Simon et al 1983). There are other vascular anomalies that may produce similar levels of renin, but unfortunately, these lesions are bilateral, and no simple surgical repair exists.

For many renal diseases, such as chronic pyelonephritis, in which the exact cause of hypertension is not clear, the major thrust of treatment is aimed at the cause of renal disease. Also, it has been well demonstrated that controlling hypertension with medication can retard progression of renal failure.

The presence of excessive catecholamines results in marked, often transitory, elevation of blood pressure. Peripheral vascular resistance is increased as a result of the vasoconstrictor effects of catecholamines. The classic condition associated with excessive catecholamine production is pheochromocytoma, an epinephrine- and norepinephrine-excreting tumor usually occurring in the adrenal medulla. This is a rare disease and accounts for less than 1% of all hypertension. These patients are important to identify, as 90% of them are completely curable with removal of the tumor.

The other causes of excessive production of catecholamines are iatrogenic, caused by potential complications associated with certain drugs. Of primary importance in this group are the monoamine oxidase (MAO) inhibitors. These agents are

TABLE 29–1

Foods and Drugs Contraindicated in Conjunction with MAO Inhibitors*

Foods with Tyramine	Drugs Contraindicated with MAO Inhibitors
Various cheeses (especially aged)	Tricyclic antidepressants
Chicken livers	Reserpine
Yeast	Methyldopa
Citrus fruits	Dopamine
Coffee (large amounts)	Tryptophan
Beer	Guanethidine
Wine	Amphetamines
Pickled herring	Other sympathomimetic amines
Broad beans (contain dopa)	
Chocolate	
Heavy cream	

* Foods that contain tyramine (a catecholamine) are normally deactivated by monoamine oxidase. However, in the presence of MAO inhibitors, the catecholamines in these foods will not be deactivated and potent vasoconstriction will occur, resulting in hypertension.

Certain drugs have been associated with similar results and therefore should not be prescribed if a patient is taking an MAO inhibitor.

used as part of psychotherapy and are a potential problem because of their primary activity, that of reducing the level of monoamine oxidase. This enzyme inactivates circulating catecholamines before they can cause vasoconstriction and elevation of blood pressure. Tyramine is a catecholamine found in many foods. Under normal circumstances, tyramine is rapidly deactivated when ingested and produces no side effects. In the presence of MAO inhibitors, tyramine is not deactivated, and there is a rapid rise of circulating catecholamines with resultant profound elevation of blood pressure. Other agents have also been associated with a similar result when MAO inhibitors are present (Table 29-1).

As mentioned earlier, abrupt withdrawal of clonidine may contribute to excessive catecholamine production. This agent is a potent antihypertensive agent that produces suppression of sympathetic outflow. Abrupt withdrawal may lead to a rebound of sympathetic activity and may result in a severe hypertensive crisis. This usually occurs within 48 hours of stopping the agent.

CLINICAL MANIFESTATIONS

Hypertension is a lifelong disease, and if not controlled, it results in numerous cardiovascular complications (Kannel 1967; Geyskes 1979). The organs at special risk of long-term effects are the brain, the heart, and the kidneys. Patients with long-standing complications related to hypertension often present to the ED when their lives are interrupted by a life-threatening event such as myocardial infarction. Acute elevation of blood pressure is often present but is not, in most situations, the immediate cause of the acute problem. Although these events may be a result of long-standing hypertension, they are not hypertensive emergencies. This definition is limited to hypertensive encephalopathy and malignant hypertension (Koch-Weser 1974).

The primary basis for symptoms in individuals with hypertension is vasoconstriction related to renal disease and subsequent stimulation of the renin-angiotensin system, excessive catecholamine production, or an unknown cause. Tachycardia and a bounding pulse are typical in moderate hypertension. The point of maximum impulse (PMI) on precordial palpation may be displaced laterally and exaggerated as a result of left ventricular enlargement. Retinal changes graded on the basis of arterial narrowing and irregularity or papilledema reflect the vascular effects of hypertension.

Laboratory tests may reflect the effects of hypertension on commonly affected organs. Diagnostic tests should include a urinalysis and serum chemistries. Protein or blood in the urine may represent renal damage as will an elevated blood urea nitrogen (BUN) (> 20 mg/dl), creatinine (> 1.5 mg/dl), and/or potassium (> 5 mEq/L). Disruption of mechanical and electrostatic barriers to protein filtration within the glomerular capillary basement membrane occurs in long-standing hypertension. This leads to large quantities of plasma proteins gaining access to the urine (Anderson 1987). Cholesterol and lipid levels may be elevated in individuals with hyperlipidemia. An EKG and a chest radiograph may show evidence of left ventricular hypertrophy, strain, or both—a common result of long-standing hypertensive disease.

SPECIFIC DISORDERS

As mentioned previously, the two major hypertensive emergencies are hypertensive encephalopathy and malignant hypertension. The clinical manifestations of these two entities are discussed in some detail. To understand hypertensive encephalopathy, the concept of cerebral autoregulation must be introduced. This is the ability of cerebral vessels to vasodilate or vasoconstrict in response to changes in blood pressure to maintain constant blood flow (Reed and Anderson 1986). Blood flow to the brain remains constant as a result of autoregulation when the mean arterial pressure (MAP) is between 60 mmHg and 150 to 200 mmHg. Below a MAP of 60 mmHg there is a maximum dilation of the small arteries, and ischemia rapidly develops. When the MAP rises above 150 to 200 mmHg, the vessels may go into complete spasm or may dilate and become more permeable. The result is intermittent areas of ischemia and brain edema. In patients with long-standing hypertension, the range of autoregulation rises, especially on the lower end, and cerebral ischemia may result at a much higher MAP than 60 mmHg (Strandgaard 1973; Ledingham and Rajagapalan 1979). This explains why vigorous acute reduction of blood pressure in a severely hypertensive patient needs to be avoided. Lowering the blood pressure to a MAP of 90 mmHg may predispose the individual to cerebral ischemia.

Hypertensive Encephalopathy

Hypertensive encephalopathy is an acute event and in most cases is reversible if early treatment is begun (Koch-Weser 1974; Graham 1983). It is defined as neuronal degeneration and cerebral edema related to severe uncontrolled hypertension. Failure of cerebral autoregulation results in hypertensive encephalopathy.

Clinical Manifestations

Patients present with complaints and findings directly related to cerebral ischemia and edema. The most common complaint is of severe, generalized headache associated with vomiting. Increasing mental obtundation may occur, and seizures are often present. Blindness and focal neurologic deficits may occur or may be the primary reason for presenting to the ED. On fundoscopic examination papilledema is often present. There may be numerous findings of long-standing hypertension, including cardiac enlargement and renal failure. If encephalopathy has occurred early in the patient's course, there may be few of these chronic changes, and the rest of the physical examination may be normal. Laboratory evaluation is nonspecific and may be normal. Computed tomographic (CT) scans are generally normal but may be necessary to eliminate the possibility of a cerebral vascular accident. Lumbar puncture is not indicated but if done, reveals clear fluid under increased pressure. Electroencephalograms reveal nonspecific changes.

Hypertensive encephalopathy is a true medical emergency, and if left untreated, the risk of irreversible changes increases; these patients may progress rapidly to coma and death. Reduction of blood pressure by 30% to 40% of pretreatment values is mandatory. Various agents used are discussed under Treatment and Nursing Care.

Malignant Hypertension

Malignant hypertension refers to the clinical triad of uncontrolled hypertension, neuroretinopathy, and renal insufficiency. The majority of cases of hypertension follow a long, slowly progressive course with gradual development of end-organ damage (Dollery 1985). Certain individuals follow a different course, either presenting initially with profound elevations of blood pressure with rapid and progressive end-organ damage or developing such an episode during the course of their disease. This phase is termed malignant hypertension, and represents a medical emergency (Koch-Weser 1974; Clark and Murray 1956).

Clinical Manifestations

These patients appear sick and have a host of complaints and clinical findings, including chest pain, severe headache, dyspnea, blurring of vision, and often acute uremic syndrome. There may be associated hypertensive encephalopathy, but each syndrome may present alone. Malignant hypertension requires urgent therapy, as end-organ damage occurs rapidly and may lead to renal or cardiac failure.

In most cases, the malignant phase is associated with levels of diastolic pressure greater than 130 mmHg, although the syndrome has been reported at levels as low as 100 mmHg. On the other hand, a reading of greater than 130 mmHg does not define malignant hypertension, as most patients with blood pressure readings above this level do not develop either clinical syndrome.

Physical examination reveals evidence of end-organ damage, especially those of heart failure and retinopathy. In general, retinal hemorrhages, cotton-wool patches, and papilledema are present. Urinalysis will reveal hematuria and proteinuria, and the BUN and creatinine levels will be elevated. Other electrolytes may be normal or may reflect a metabolic acidosis secondary to renal failure. In the past, this was a frequent cause of death although the outcome has been altered by the use of dialysis. Electrocardiogram shows evidence of left ventricular strain and hypertrophy, and chest radiographs may show an enlarged heart with signs of congestive heart failure. An unusual aspect in severe cases is the finding on the blood smear of red cell fragments consistent with microangiopathic hemolytic anemia. This reflects the actual pathology of the malignant phase, which involves the small arterioles and is termed fibrinoid necrosis. This pathologic change results when the small arterioles dilate secondary to the rapid increase in blood pressure and can no longer control blood flow to tissues. Rupture leading to leaking of plasma and blood, followed by deposition of fibrin within the arteriolar walls, may occur. Directly visible in the retina, linear hemorrhages represent leaking blood dissecting along nerve fibers. Cotton-wool patches represent swollen, ischemic nerve axions distal to arteriolar obstruction resulting from fibrin deposits. This process, occurring unchecked in all organs, rapidly produces renal failure, cardiac failure, and cerebral damage.

Other Emergencies Associated with Hypertension

There are a number of medical emergencies associated with marked elevation of blood pressure. These include stroke syndromes, pulmonary edema, acute renal failure, and acute congestive heart failure. In the majority of these cases, hypertension is not the cause of the acute problem but is a secondary response by the organism to the stress of the event.

The majority of patients with acute pulmonary edema have marked elevation of blood pressure. Hypertension is usually not the cause of pulmonary edema; rather, it is a result of increased levels of circulating catecholamines.

Many patients who present with acute stroke syndrome have an associated elevation of blood pressure (Cuneo 1977). In by far the majority of patients, the hypertension seen during the acute phase of a cerebral vascular accident is transitory and labile and a short time later may return toward normal or even fall below normal levels.

Treatment and Nursing Care

Stage I care should be initiated when individuals with hypertension present with symptomatology reflecting a life-threatening process secondary to their primary disease—a hypertensive emergency or an acute cardiovascular event. Otherwise, most individuals with hypertension do not require stage I care, and their conditions can be accommodated nicely by stage II interventions.

Tissue Perfusion, Altered (Cerebral), Related to

- **Vasoconstriction Secondary to Excessive Catecholamine Production, Metabolism, or Both; Excessive Renal Renin Production, or Unknown Cause**

The mainstay of treatment for the individual with an alteration in cerebral tissue perfusion is chemotherapeutic. Long-term management of hypertension generally consists of oral pharmacologic therapy with a vasodilator, beta-adrenergic blocking agent, diuretic, or combination of these. Table 29–2 lists common agents and their associated adverse effects.

Individuals suffering acute symptomatology secondary to their hypertensive disease will require more aggressive management in the form of parenteral or oral therapy as listed in Table 29–3.

When a hypertensive emergency exists, nitroprusside is the mainstay of treatment. It is effective in almost all cases, is safe if used appropriately, and response can be easily titrated. The primary effect of nitroprusside is as a powerful vasodilator. This agent exerts its effect on both venous (capacitance) and arterial (resistance) vessels. Nitroprusside is effective in virtually all cases of hypertension. It reduces blood pressure rapidly and after infusion is stopped has a short duration of action. Nitroprusside is metabolized to thiocyanate and excreted by the kidneys. Cyanide is an intermediate metabolite, and in certain situations, it is theoretically possible to develop cyanide toxicity. This is extremely rare but indicates need for caution in

TABLE 29–2
Common Antihypertensive Agents Categorized by Primary Pharmacologic Effects

Category	Agent	Potential Adverse Effects
Diuretic	Thiazide	Potassium depletion
		Elevated BUN
	Furosemide	Electrolyte imbalances
		Hearing loss with high doses
	Spironolactone	↑ Serum potassium
		GI disturbances
		Megaloblastic anemia (rare)
Central sympatholytic	Alpha methyldopa	Postural hypotension
		Impotence
		Hemolytic anemia (uncommon)
		Drug fever
	Clonidine	Sedation
		Rebound hypertension if acutely withdrawn
Peripheral sympatholytic	Propanolol	Congestive heart failure
		CNS effects
		Masks signs of hypoglycemia
		Asthma attack
	Reserpine	Depression, especially in elderly
		GI bleeding
Vasodilator	Minoxidil	Pericardial effusion
	Captopril	Proteinuria
		Agranulocytosis (rare)
		Elevated BUN
		Profound hypotension if CHF present
	Hydralazine	Lupus-like syndrome (up to 10%)
		Peripheral neuropathy
		Flushing
		Headaches and dizziness
		Palpitations
	Labetalol	Paroxysmal hypertension if pheochromocytoma present
		Side effects similar to propanolol, but less common
	Prazosin	Orthostatic hypotension
		Syncope, especially if patient is salt-depleted (may occur after first dose)
		Headache and drowziness

patients with severe renal failure or during prolonged high-dose therapy. A special case is the pregnant woman, in whom the fetus is at a higher risk since thiocyanate appears to concentrate in the uterus and may affect fetal thyroid tissue or produce cyanide toxicity (Nourok et al 1964; Bower and Peterson 1975).

Nitroprusside is given intravenously, and an infusion pump must be used. The effects of this agent require careful and continuous monitoring by measurement of blood pressure at least every 5 minutes and more frequently when the dose is adjusted. Arterial lines should be inserted to assure precise and continuous blood pressure measurement. The usual starting dose is between 0.25 μg and 1.0 μg/kg/minute, and control is usually achieved with 3 μg/kg/minute.

Dosages over 800 μg/min should be avoided, as thiocyanate and cyanide accumulate rapidly. The solution is made by adding a few milliliters of D5W to a 100-mg vial of nitroprusside and then adding this combination to 500 ml of D5W. The agent is broken down by ultraviolet light, and the bottle should be wrapped in aluminum foil or other opaque material. Solutions over 4 hours old should not be used.

TABLE 29–3

Drugs for Hypertensive Emergencies

Drug	Class	Route and Dose	Onset	Duration	Comments
Parenteral					
Nitroprusside (Nipride; others)	Arteriolar and venous vasodilator	IV infusion pump 0.25 μg/kg/min to 8 μg/kg/min	secs	3–5 min	Thiocyanate toxicity may occur with prolonged (>48 hours) or too rapid infusion (>15 μg/kg/min) when thiocyanate concentrations exceed 10 mg/dl (particularly in renal insufficiency). Not used in pregnancy
Diazoxide (Hyperstat)	Arteriolar vasodilator	IV 50–150 mg q 5 min or as infusion of 7.5–30 mg/min	1–5 min	4–24 hr	Should not be used for patients with angina pectoris, myocardial infarction, dissecting aneurysm, or pulmonary edema
Trimethaphan (Arfonad)	Ganglionic blocker	IV infusion pump 0.5–5 mg/min	1–5 min	10 min	Drug of choice for emergency treatment of aortic dissection
Labetalol (Trandate; Normodyne)	Alpha- and beta-adrenergic blocker	IV 2 mg/min or 20 mg initially, then 20–80 mg q 10 min Max cumulative dose 300 mg	5 min or less	3–6 hr	80% to 90% response rate; can be followed by same drug taken orally
Hydralazine (Apresoline)	Arteriolar vasodilator	IV 10–20 mg	10–30 min	2–4 hrs	May precipitate angina, myocardial infarction; not used for aortic dissection; main use is in pregnancy
Propranolol (Inderal; others)	Beta-adrenergic blocker	IV: 1–10 mg load then 3 mg/hr PO 80–640 mg daily	immediate beta-adrenergic blockade	2 hr 12 hr	Useful as adjunct to potent vasodilators to prevent or treat excessive tachycardia; usually will not lower blood pressure acutely
Oral					
Nifedipine* (Procardia; Adalat)	Calcium entry blocker	10–20 mg PO, sublingual or buccal	5–15 min	3–5 hr	Not yet standardized; somewhat variable response
Clonidine (Catapres; others)	Central sympath-olytic	PO 0.2 mg initial then 0.1 mg/hr, up to 0.8 mg total	1/2–2 hrs	6–8 hr	Sedation prominent; rebound hypertension can occur
Captopril (Capoten)	Angiotensin converting enzyme inhibitor	PO 6.5–50 mg	15 min	4–6 hr	Variable, sometimes excessive response

Source: Drugs for hypertensive emergencies. 1987. Med Lett Drugs Ther 29:20.
* Not approved for this indication by the US Food and Drug Administration.

    The therapeutic goal is to reduce blood pressure by 30% to 40% from pretreatment levels. This goal is the same for all hypertensive emergencies and for whatever agent is used. The response to nitroprusside is dose-related, although elderly patients and patients on other antihypertensive agents tend to be more sensitive to nitroprusside and should be started on lower doses. Profound hypotension is the biggest risk of nitroprusside therapy, but it can be avoided by careful use of the agent and close monitoring of the patient. Stopping the agent will cause a return of blood pressure within 1 to 10 minutes. The patient should be placed in the Trendelenburg position, and intravenous saline may be needed to restore blood pressure to adequate levels. Because this agent dilates capacitance vessels, patients should be kept supine, as profound orthostatic changes in blood pressure can occur. Nitroprusside is apt to cause local necrosis if extravasation occurs, and its use requires a good, freely flowing IV line. If used carefully, this agent is safe and effective and remains the drug of choice for severe hypertensive emergencies except those of pregnancy.

Labctalol appears to be a safe alternative to nitroprusside. It is both an alpha- and beta-adrenoreceptor blocker, with the primary antihypertensive effect secondary to alpha blockade of vascular smooth muscle (Cressman et al 1984). Reflex tachycardia, a common occurrence with alpha$_1$ blockade, does not occur because of the beta-blocking effect of this agent.

Labetalol is available for oral use, but for hypertensive emergencies it should be used as an intravenous infusion. The antihypertensive effect is usually seen within 5 to 10 minutes, and maximum effect occurs within one-half hour. Therapy is started with a 20-mg dose infused over 2 minutes, and the blood pressure is checked every 5 minutes. If minimal effect is observed, increments of 20, 40, or 80 mg are given every 10 minutes to a total dose of 300 mg.

When labetalol is used intravenously, the patient must be kept in the supine position, as there is risk of profound orthostatic hypotension. In addition, the beta-blockade effects of labetalol (bronchoconstriction and slowing of myocardial conduction) may potentiate problems in patients with congestive heart failure, asthma, severe bradycardia, or heart block. For this reason, treatment with labetalol should be avoided in these patients.

The major advantage of labetalol over nitroprusside is that its maximum effect is seen early, and if blood pressure has stabilized, these patients may not require intensive care admission; hence, a shorter hospital stay can be anticipated. On the other hand, if an untoward drop in blood pressure occurs, reversal is difficult because of the long duration of action, and treatment for hypotension with fluids and alpha-adrenergic agents may be required.

Diazoxide (Hyperstat) is closely related to the thiazide diurctics and works primarily as a dilator of resistance blood vessels. Since diazoxide is chiefly an arteriolar vasodilator and has no effect on veins, it reduces cardiac afterload, without affecting preload. A dose of 20 to 40 mg IV of furosemide may also be given because of the salt-retaining properties of diazoxide. Extreme care should be taken to avoid IV infiltration, as local extravasation is extremely painful and may produce necrosis of the skin.

Diazoxide therapy is started with a 20-mg dose infused over 2 minutes; blood pressure should be checked every 5 minutes. Increments of either 20, 40, or 80 mg are given every 10 minutes up to a total dose of 300 mg. The therapeutic goal is a 30% to 40% reduction of blood pressure from pretreatment levels.

A regimen deserving comment is the use of the calcium channel blockers, particularly nifedipine, for treatment of hypertensive emergencies (Bertel et al 1983; Erbel et al 1983; Conen et al 1982; Takekoshi et al 1981). Nifedipine is a calcium entry–blocking agent, is administered sublingually or buccally, and causes a drop in blood pressure within 10 to 15 minutes that persists for 4 to 6 hours. Profound hypotension has not been reported, but clinical experience is limited. Nifedipine may come to play a major role in treatment of hypertensive emergencies, particularly in the prehospital setting, where a rapid reduction of peripheral resistance would be advantageous.

Numerous other agents have been advocated for the treatment of hypertensive emergencies. Refer to Table 29–3 for information on additional drugs used as antihypertensive agents.

Breathing Pattern, Ineffective, Related to

- **Pulmonary Congestion Secondary to Acute Myocardial Infarction, Fluid Overload, or Congestive Heart Failure**

Traditional treatment with oxygen, furosemide, morphine, and nitrates usually results in relief of the ineffective breathing pattern secondary to an acute cardiac event. Generally, there also is a rapid fall of blood pressure toward normal. In certain cases, if hypertension persists, nitroprusside or sublingual nifedipine may be used to lower blood pressure.

Tissue Perfusion, Altered (Cerebral), Related to

- **Interruption of Blood Flow Secondary to Vascular Accident or Hypertensive Encephalopathy**

Patients with altered cerebral tissue perfusion will require ongoing mental status evaluations. Mental status changes may be manifested by confusion, memory deficit, distractibility, delusions, inappropriate social behavior, lethargy, or somnolence. The somnolent patient warrants airway protection in the form of oropharyngeal, nasopharyngeal, or endotracheal intubation in conjunction with supplemental oxygen.

The methods for treating hypertension associated with cerebral vascular accident and hypertensive encephalopathy vary. With certain exceptions, hypertension associated with the acute phase of a cerebral vascular accident is not treated, as lowering of the blood pressure may provoke bleeding and lead to extension of the involved area. For the patient with a change in mental status related to hypertensive encephalopathy, nitroprusside is the agent of choice.

Potential for Injury, related to

- **Hypertension Secondary to Toxemia of Pregnancy**

Hydralazine is effective and appears to be safe in reducing the potential for injury related to hypertension secondary to toxemia of pregnancy (Vidt 1986). The drug is given as a 5-mg test dose intravenously, followed by 10-mg boluses every 20 minutes as required. Blood pressure and fetal heart tones need to be monitored closely, and the therapeutic goal is a diastolic pressure of less than 100 mmHg. This end-point is usually achieved with a total dose of 20 mg or less. This agent can also be given as a continuous intravenous infusion. Because of potential risk to the fetus, nitroprusside is relatively contraindicated (Vesey et al 1976; Nourok et al 1964).

TABLE 29–4
High–Salt Content Foods

Type of Food	Examples
Canned foods	Soups, vegetables
Packaged foods	Stove-top stuffing, noodles stroganoff, dried cereal, instant hot cereal, pudding
Cheeses	
Cured foods	Sausage, ham, lunchmeats
Foods in brine	Olives, pickles, sauerkraut
Packaged seasonings	Chili and taco seasonings, spaghetti mixes, spices
Snack foods	Crackers, potato chips, nuts

Knowledge Deficit (Potential), Related to

- **Lack of Health Education**
- **New Onset Hypertension**
- **Anxiety**

Because patients with hypertension, with the exception of those suffering hypertensive emergencies, are frequently discharged from the ED, discharge teaching is an important aspect of total patient care. Education in the ED should stress the importance of follow-up, salt restriction, and information on antihypertensives if the patient is on prescribed medication. Pamphlets or patient information sheets are useful as an adjunct to verbal instructions, and a list of foods with high salt concentration may be useful in patient education (Table 29-4).

However, a wide range of ethnic taste preferences suggests that a few guidelines on limiting salt consumption may prove more effective than a list of specific foods in controlling salt intake. The patient should be instructed to cut down on salt used in cooking, to remove salt shakers from the dinner table, and to use other flavors, such as white wine, garlic, herbs, spices, and lemon juice to season food. In addition, dietary management may consist of caffeine restriction and a reduction in dietary cholesterol, lipids, and saturated fats. Weight reduction or control may be recommended, and an exercise program designed to increase cardiovascular fitness may be suggested. The emergency nurse should be aware of community resources with respect to dietary education, weight control, cardiovascular fitness, and smoking cessation.

EVALUATION

Evaluation of the patient's response to therapy is the key to ongoing assessment of patients with acute alterations in blood pressure. The emergency nurse is responsible for monitoring the effectiveness of pharmacologic regimens through judicious determination of vital signs and tracking of patient complaints. Regulation of pharmacologic infusions according to the physician's orders is dependent upon ongoing evaluation of the patient's response to therapy.

CONCLUSION

Hypertension is an extremely common condition in our society, and numerous agents are used for the long-term treatment of this entity. True hypertensive emergencies are rare, although hypertension is associated with many acute medical conditions seen in the ED. Treatment modalities for these emergencies have been discussed. One of the emergency nurse's most important functions is to ensure that a blood pressure is recorded on all patients presenting for care. Procedures should be developed within the department to make certain that any patient with an elevated blood pressure receives appropriate instructions and follow-up care. This is most critical in those patients with moderate elevation of blood pressure who are discharged. If these patients are brought to early medical attention, many of the catastrophes associated with long-term untreated hypertension can be avoided.

REFERENCES

Anderson RJ, Hart GR, Crumpler CP, et al. 1981. Oral clonidine loading in hypertensive urgencies. JAMA 246:848–850.

Anderson RJ, Schrier RW. 1987. Acute renal failure. In Braunwald E, Isselbacher KG, Petersdorf RG et al, eds. Harrison's Principles of Internal Medicine, Vol 2, 11th ed. New York, McGraw-Hill Book Co, 1143.

Bertel O, Conen D, Radiu EW, et al. 1983. Nifedipine in hypertensive emergencies. Br Med J [Clin Res] 286:19–21.

Blashke T, Melmon K. 1980. Antihypertensive agents and the drug therapy of hypertension. In Gilman AG, Goodman LS, Gilman A, eds. The Pharmacological Basis of Therapeutics, 6th ed. New York, Macmillan.

Bower PG, Peterson JN. 1975. Methemoglobinemia after sodium nitroprusside therapy. N Engl J Med 293:865.

Clark E, Murray EA. 1956. Neurological manifestations of malignant hypertension. Br Med J 2:1319.

Conen D, Pertel O, Dubach UC. 1982. An oral calcium antagonist for treatment of hypertensive emergencies. J Cardiovasc Pharmacol (Suppl 4) 3:8378–8382.

Cressman MD, Vidt DG, Gifford RW, et al. 1984. Intravenous Labetalol in the management of severe hypertension and hypertensive emergencies. Am Heart J 107:980–985.

Cuneo RA, Caronna JJ. 1977. Neurological complications Med Clin North Am 61:569–577.

Dollery CT. 1985. Arterial hypertension. In Wyngarden JB, Smith LH, eds. Cecil Textbook of Medicine, 17th ed. Philadelphia, WB Saunders.

Erbel R, Brand G, Meyer J, et al. 1983. Emergency treatment of hypertensive crisis with sublingual nifedipine. Postgrad Med J (Suppl 3) 59:134–136.

Esler MD, Julius S, Randall OS, et al. 1975. Relation of renin status to neurologenic vascular resistance in borderline hypertension. Am J Cardiol 36:708.

Geyskes GG, Boer P, Dorhout Mees EG. 1979. Clonidine withdrawal: mechanism and frequency of rebound hypertension. Br J Clin Pharmacol 7:55.

Giese J, Aurell M, Munck O. 1972. Peripheral and renal venous plasma renin concentration. Scand J Urol Nephrol (Suppl 15)6:38.

Gilman AG, Goodman LS, Rall TW, et al, eds. 1985. The Pharmacological Basis of Therapeutics, 7th ed. New York, Macmillan.

Glass RI, Mirel R, Hollander G, et al. 1978. Screening for hypertension in the emergency department. JAMA 240:18.

Goldblatt J, Kahn JR, Hanzal RF. 1939. Studies on experimental hypertension. J Exp Med 69:649.

Graham DI. 1983. Ischaemic brain following emergency blood pressure lowering in hypertensive patients. Acta Med Scand (Suppl) 678:61–9.

Kannel W. 1970. Epidemiological assessment of the role of blood pressure in stroke. JAMA, 214:301.

Kannel W, Brand N, Skinner JJ, et al. 1967. The Framingham study. Ann Intern Med 67:48.

Kaszuba AL, Matanoski G, Gibson G. 1978. Evaluation of the emergency department as a site for hypertensive screening. J Am Coll Emerg Phys 7:51.

Kilcoyne MM. 1980. The developing phase of primary hypertension: Part I. Mod Concepts Cardiovasc Dis 49:19.

Kilcoyne MM. 1980. The developing phase of primary hypertension: Part II. Mod Concepts Cardiovasc Dis 49:25.

Kincaid-Smith P. 1977. Parenchymatous diseases of the kidney and hypertension. In Genest J, Koiw E, Kuchel O, eds. Hypertension: Physiopathology and Treatment. New York, McGraw-Hill Book Co.

Kincaid-Smith P, Whitworth JA, eds. 1987. Vascular lesions associated with idiopathic glomerular lesions. In Kincaid-Smith P, Whitworth JA (eds). The Kidney: A Clinicopathological Study, 2nd ed. Oxford, Blackwell Scientific Publishing Co.

Kincaid-Smith P. 1961. Renal ischemia and hypertension: a review of the results of surgery. Med J Aust, 2:130.

Koch-Weser J. 1974. Hypertensive emergencies. N Engl J Med 290:211.

Ledingham JCG, Rajagapalan B. 1979. Cerebral complications in the treatment of accelerated hypertension. QJ Med 48:25–41.

Lowenthal DT, Schwartz CD. 1985. Hypertension update for the 1980s. Prim Care 12:101–115.

McEntee MA, Peddicord K. 1987. Coping with hypertension. Nurs Clin North Am 22:583–592.

Multiple Risk Factor Intervention Trial Research Group. 1982. Multiple Risk Factor Intervention Trial. JAMA 248:1465–1477.

National Center for Health Statistics. 1966. Hypertension and heart disease in adults, U.S.A. 1960–1962. Public Health Service Publication No. 1000, Series 11, No. 13, Washington, DC, USGPO.

Nourok DG, Glassock RJ, Solomon DH, et al. 1964. Hypothyroidism following prolonged sodium nitroprusside therapy. AM J Med Sci 248:129.

Pettinger WA. 1980. Minoxidil and the treatment of severe hypertension. N Engl J Med 303:922–926.

Ram C, Venkata S, Kaplan NM. 1979. Individual of diazoxide dosage in the treatment of severe hypertension. Am J Cardiol 43:627–630.

Reach G, Thibonnier M, Chevillard C, et al. 1980. Effect of labetalol on blood pressure and plasma catecholamine concentrations in patients with pheochromocytoma. Br Med J 280:1300.

Reed WG, Anderson RJ. 1986. Effects of Rapid blood pressure reduction on cerebral blood flow. Am Heart J 111:226–228.

Schlant RC, Tsagaris TS, Robertson RJ. 1962. Studies on the acute cardiovascular effects of intravenous sodium nitroprusside. Am J Cardiol 9:51.

Simon G, Limas CC, Miler RP. 1983. Renovascular hypertension with unilateral atherosclerotic renal artery occlusion: diagnostic use of renal vein renins. Angiology 33:728–737.

Strandgaard S. 1983. Cerebral blood flow in hypertension. Acta Med Scand (Suppl) 678:11–25.

Takekoshi N, Murakami E, Murakami H, et al. 1981. Treatment of severe hypertension and hypertensive emergency with nifedipine, a calcium antagonistic agent. Jpn Circ J 45:852–860.

The 1984 Report of the Joint National Committee on the Detection, Evaluation, and Treatment of High Blood Pressure. 1985. Nurse Pract 10:9–33.

Vesey CG, Cole PV, Simpson PJ 1976. Cyanide and thiocyanide concentrations following sodium nitroprusside infusion in man. Br J Anesthesiol 48:651.

Vidt DG. 1986. Current concepts in treatment of hypertensive emergencies. Am Heart J 111:220–225.

Gary Sollars, MD

Thermoregulatory Emergencies

Thermoregulatory emergencies are a very broad subgroup of the environmental emergency category. They are the most truly "environmental" of the group, for they are the result of interaction between the patient's internal heat-control processes and his or her immediate climatic surroundings. In a simpler day, these were problems of "exposure" and discussed only in relation to military casualties; however, the increased popularity of outdoor pursuits has created an awareness of the disasters awaiting those who head into "uncivilized" environmental extremes, such as barotrauma, high altitude sickness, oxygen-displacement and inhalant toxin exposure, drowning and water deprivation, diseases of microclimate disruption, lightning-strike, and snakebite and other envenomations. Some of these topics are covered elsewhere in this book. This chapter is limited to central and peripheral manifestations of microclimate or thermoregulatory disruption: hyperthermia, hypothermia, frostbite, and other, similar conditions. For those interested in the more esoteric subjects of outdoor medicine, several excellent books cover the field in detail (see References).

Thermoregulatory malfunction can result from a number of subtle, protean diseases or drug ingestions but is most commonly a manifestation of a lack of metabolic reserve in the face of environmental stress. This stress need not be extreme, especially in the neonate or the elderly.

Patients coming to emergency departments (EDs) with these disorders will seldom be able to define the cause of their problem. The thermoregulatory malfunction component of their disease may be missed entirely in the face of more obvious conditions, unless the temperature is taken on all patients coming for treatment. Oral temperatures with a mercury and glass thermometer can serve only as a rough screening device; any temperature found outside the range of 95° to 103.5°F *must* be repeated with an electronic core thermometer and reassessed frequently. (Aphorism 30–1.) Without this critical bit of information, truly life-threatening conditions may be misdiagnosed and mistreated, resulting in significant morbidity or even preventable death.

Aphorism 30–1 If you don't look for it, you'll never find it.

This chapter begins with an overview of the mechanisms of temperature regulation. The peripheral and central effects of temperature disruption are quite diverse. In this chapter disease states are organized by temperature range, and the discussion reviews the clinical presentation, treatment, and nursing interventions for each condition.

THERMOREGULATION

The human body, as a complex chemical factory, has only a narrow range within which the enzymatic reactions are able to proceed reliably. To maintain this narrow range, heat production and dissipation must be precisely balanced in the face of marked environmental variation. This balance is maintained by the hypothalamus, using two basic strategies (Fig. 30–1). Baseline heat production within the body is relatively constant, but it can be markedly increased for short periods, as with exercise. This is, however, a mechanism limited by factors of available energy and conditioning, so that for most people it has only a minor role in thermoregulation. Heat dissipation can be restricted or enhanced by a variety of maneuvers. Convection, radiation, and especially evaporation allow extensive heat loss. Peripheral vasoconstriction provides heat conservation when necessary.

The balance of heat control is mediated by the preoptic anterior hypothalamus, which receives information from central and peripheral thermoreceptors. The central receptors monitor the blood temperature directly at the brain stem. Peripheral skin receptors sense "thermal comfort" of the ambient temperature and stimulate directed, voluntary attempts at temperature control. Thermoreceptor information is received and processed by the hypothalamus, which then activates various physiologic mechanisms to maintain homeostasis. Signals sent to the pituitary modify heat production by stimulating or depressing thyroid and adrenal function. The frontal lobes process information to initiate environmental alteration that will restrict or enhance heat loss. The sympathetic nervous system mediates messages controlling vasoconstriction or dilation, and shivering (a potent heat generator) is controlled via

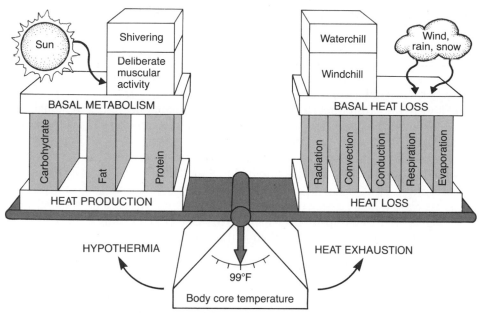

FIGURE 30–1. Factors affecting thermal equilibrium of the body.

the extrapyramidal spinal tracts. These mechanisms work in concert to maintain internal (core) heat at the homeostatic temperature necessary for most efficient function.

Internal chemical reactions produce waste heat. At rest, the constant metabolic processes required for homeostasis generate a predictable amount of heat measurable as the basal metabolic rate (BMR). The amount depends on age, height and weight, sex, and hormonal balance. The largest portion at rest is generated by the liver (26.4%), skeletal muscle (25.6%), and brain (18.3%), which together supply 70% of the total. Although there are detailed BMR tables stratified by age, height, and weight, a simple estimate is to assume that the average young 70-kg person will produce about 70 to 100 kcal/hour. This allows an internal temperature of approximately 101°F at the liver, reflected as the more easily measured rectal temperature of 99.6°F.

Muscular work is the primary source of further internal heat production. Moderate work will generate approximately 300 kcal/hour, and maximal exertion can yield 600 kcal/hour with brief bursts of up to 900 kcal/hour with extreme exertion. Shivering also is a most efficient source of added internal heat generation, producing 500 kcal/hour. Energy supplies to create this heat come from food intake and metabolic stores of glucose, fats, and protein. Metabolic stores provide the driving energy for all internal body processes, but the easily accessible energy supplies can be depleted rapidly in the very young, the very old, or the infirm. Internal body temperature can also be elevated by external sources, such as the sun or an overheated workplace, but these will not figure significantly until the upper limits of the body's dissipation mechanisms have been reached.

The heat dissipation mechanisms of the human body provide the true regulation process for heat control. Without the environmental stresses of cold, wet, or wind, the body surrounds itself with a protective microclimate of laminar heated air at approximately 71°F. When this is abolished by the environment, the body must work to maintain homeostasis. Humans are not cold-adapted organisms and have none of the heat-scavenging mechanisms of true cold-weather mammals such as seals or whales. Heat preservation is limited to higher-level functions to conserve the heat envelope—such as adding clothing, building houses, or moving to Florida.

When these fail, peripheral vasoconstriction must be called upon, which allows blood flow to the extremities to be sacrificed to retain core warmth. Peripheral blood flow is controlled primarily by the sympathetic nervous system, although local vascular reflexes (the "hunting response" of Lewis) serve some protective function. The "standard 70-kg man" at rest in a thermally neutral environment has approximately 200 to 500 ml/minute of total cutaneous blood flow. This can be altered by changes in ambient and internal heat. Total constriction retards flow to 20 to 50 ml/minute; under maximum heat stress, cutaneous blood flow can be as high as 3000 ml/min. The variation is provided primarily by the extremities; in fact, cutaneous blood flow to the head and neck is basically fixed—they are obligate heat losers (Aphorism 30–2).

Aphorism 30–2 Mother was right: If your hands are cold, put on your hat!

Core heat brought to the surface by blood flow can be dispersed via several mechanisms. When ambient temperature is low, radiation (via infrared) and convection (heat exchange between the heat envelope and the environment through wind currents) provide adequate dissipation of excess heat. As the ambient temperature approaches body temperature, or if core temperatures are high, evaporation of sweat allows further cooling. This can be a very efficient heat loss mechanism, as each 1.7 ml of sweat will draw off 1 kcal of body heat on evaporation. Unevaporated sweat absorbed in clothing, or dripping from the body, does not provide effective heat loss. Therefore, as atmospheric humidity increases, evaporative heat loss efficiency decreases.

Conduction, respiration, and excretion are other methods of heat dissipation, but these play an extremely minor role under normal physiologic conditions. The heat lost with breathing, urination, and defecation is only about 10% of the homeostatic dissipation and likewise plays little role in physiologic temperature defenses. However, in extreme thermoregulatory stress states consideration is given to heat conservation and loss through breathing and excretion, because manipulation may affect the patient's total body heat significantly. Conduction is the direct transfer of heat between two contiguous objects of different temperatures. Although it is not part of the usual homeostatic defenses, it has special bearing in cold-water drowning: water is 26 times more efficient than air at extracting heat from a body. Rapid hypothermia may develop in cold water immersion, which may well be the primary *correctable* insult in many apparent drownings.

As is clear, the body has limited defenses against temperature change, but there are no limits to a person's potential for getting into trouble; thus the homeostatic mechanisms are often overwhelmed. When this occurs, the patient can develop any of the several "environmental emergencies," which can range from minor to catastrophic.

COLD WEATHER EMERGENCIES

Both the central and peripheral manifestations of cold stress are results of a patient's attempts to defend core warmth. With that in mind, remember that these problems can and will often appear together and may adversely affect each other: honing in on only one aspect while ignoring the entire patient may frustrate the nurse's attempts at appropriate intervention. Also, it is wise to remember that "hypothermia" is a *relative* state: as humans appear to have evolved in the tropics, and the defended internal temperature is 101°F., central (and at least one kind of peripheral) hypothermia can develop any time the ambient temperature is less than 80°F.

Frostbite

Frostbite can be simply defined as "tissue damage from cold." Usually this requires freezing temperatures, but it can occur even in warmer weather. Under cold stress, the body primarily attempts to maintain core warmth. The peripheral vasoconstrictive response sacrifices blood flow to the extremities. Rapid cooling of the affected area then follows.

Microscopically, there appear to be two different mechanisms of injury. With rapid cooling, formation of interstitial ice crystals and a marked increase in intracellular sodium and chloride ions result in cell membrane disruption and damage to subcellular organelles. This type of injury is seen most often with sudden extreme temperature drop: cold metal exposure, with immersion in gasoline at low ambient temperature or into liquid gases, or with wetness in extreme wind chill or at high altitude. The other, more common form could be called "slow frostbite." This is what is usually seen from cold environmental exposure. Vascular constriction results in a low-flow state, with capillary thrombosis from sludging, tissue ischemia, and subsequent vascular permeability, which produces microscopic and macroscopic tissue edema. However, both entities demonstrate the same macroscopic picture and have a similar course, so for clinical purposes they are indistinguishable.

Clinical Manifestations

The awake patient coming to the ED will usually have made the diagnosis for himself or herself. Presenting symptoms for the victim of frostbite will vary with the person, depending on acclimatization, previous exposures, and severity of the current exposure, but in general the patient will be able to give a history of progressive coldness leading to tingling and then to an anesthetic, "wooden stump" sensation. There will be no pain at all unless some thawing has begun. Information must be obtained concerning length of time of exposure and degree of protection, previous similar injuries, whether any attempts were made to rewarm the area before arrival, chronic medical problems (especially those that may retard healing or pose infection risk), and current tetanus immunity status. The patient should be assessed as well for signs and symptoms of hypothermia, which often will also be present.

Initially the injured area will appear hyperemic, but when the syndrome is fully developed the area will be pale and waxy and feel firm to touch. If a little pressure produces a "crunchy" sensation, like a firm crust overlying softer tissue, a superficial injury is likely. Unfortunately, even light pressure can greatly increase the damage to fragile tissue and should be guarded against. Prognosticating should take a back seat to patient protection: please don't squeeze.

Three other related disease states should be mentioned briefly: frost-nip, chilblains, and trenchfoot (or immersion foot). Frost-nip is an extremely superficial form of cold injury, usually involving the most peripheral extremities or epithelium of exposed skin. Basically an epithelial freezing, it produces tingling or burning skin sensations and a frosty sheen to the involved area. It resolves quickly on removal from cold and has no sequelae.

Chilblains, however, are more akin to "slow frostbite" and are usually seen in cool, damp climates. This is a form of localized vasculitis, producing tender, discrete subcutaneous nodules. Often the condition affects the cheeks, and patients complain of pain and tenderness. Chilblains are also known to occur in infants who have been given popsicles to suck, even in summer weather. The condition is self-limited and without significant complications.

Trenchfoot or immersion foot results from prolonged immersion in water of lower than body temperature. The tissues become edematous and macerated, and a local vasculitis develops. The affected limb will initially appear pale and pulseless, but with drying and elevation it will become hyperemic and very painful. Risk of infection is very high, and the morbidity from this disease is significant. The pathophysiology is very similar to that of frostbite, but this disorder can occur even in tropical climates. Therapy consists of dry rewarming, and tissue protection and conservation remain paramount. As the name implies, this is commonly a disease of warfare conditions and was frequently seen in the Vietnam and Korean conflicts.

TABLE 30–1
Treatment of Frostbite

Always
   Handle tissue gently
   Rewarm with water at 105 to 115°F
   Protect from infection and further injury
   Consider tetanus diphtheria toxin and tetanus
     immune globulin (TIG)
   Check for systemic hypothermia
Never
   Scrub or handle tissue roughly
   Rewarm near a flame or a concentrated heat source
   Discharge patient into cold-stress environment
     immediately after thawing
   Prepare for early amputation

Treatment and Nursing Care

A patient with significant frostbite should be brought into the patient care area immediately and definitive treatment begun (Table 30–1). After basic health evaluation, assessment for occult injuries, and careful monitoring of oral (or if necessary, rectal) temperature, gentle but rapid rewarming of the injured area must begin. A delay in treatment is detrimental to the patient's condition, exposing him or her to risk of greater tissue loss, more pain, and a consequent decrease in rapport with the health care team, and thus less cooperation and understanding during therapy.

Potential for Injury, Related to

- **Tissue Destruction Secondary to Vascular Constriction, Capillary Thrombosis, Tissue Ischemia**

Rewarming is best accomplished with a gently circulating water bath to the injured area. Water should be heated to 105° to 115°F, and placed in a basin large enough that the damaged area will not strike the sides of the container. A small amount of povidone-iodine (Betadine) or chlorhexidine (Hibiclens) may be added to the water, but this is not essential. The water should be agitated frequently and fresh warmed water added often. Be careful *not* to pour the hot water directly onto the skin. If a whirlpool treatment is available, this provides some débridement. The key here is *gentle handling;* this tissue is extremely fragile. Do not scrub the injured area. Warming should continue for 20 to 40 minutes, after which the area should be gently patted dry and subsequently handled with sterile technique. Broken blisters and tissue fragments should be removed at this time, preserving as much tissue as possible. Recent studies (Heggers et al 1987) suggest that hemorrhagic blisters should be left intact, but pale blisters should be débrided. The area should be elevated to reduce swelling. Sterile dressings should be placed in interdigital areas (e.g., between the fingers and toes, or behind the ears) and the area loosely wrapped or left exposed to air.

As the tissue rewarms, it will first appear hyperemic; if this quickly progresses to a purple or burgundy color, the prognosis is grim. The sooner paresthesias and blistering occur, the better the chance of full recovery. Significant edema may begin within 3 hours, although blistering may develop any time between 6 hours and 7 days after the injury. Demarcation of nonviable tissue may take months to be complete; early amputation results in greater tissue loss than may be necessary.

Tissue Perfusion, Altered (Peripheral), Related to

- **Thrombosis**
- **Vascular Spasm**
- **Platelet Aggregation**
- **Leukocyte Adhesion**

Several adjunctive therapies are currently under investigation, and some hold promise in improving tissue salvage. As thrombosis seems to enter into the pathophysiology of frostbite necrosis, some investigators have had success with heparinization or use of low-molecular-weight dextran to reduce microvascular clotting in the underperfused tissue. Although somewhat successful for the local injury, these drugs have systemic effects as well that may be deleterious. Arteriolar spasm has been attacked with sympathectomy, intra-arterial reserpine injections, or systemic use of phenoxybenzamine (Dibenzyline) or prazosin (Minipress). All of these therapies are as yet unproved and controversial.

Recent studies have concentrated on the microphysiology of tissue injury and the role of the arachidonic cascade. This biochemical cascade is responsible for the release of thromboxane and other prostanoids that cause vascular spasm, platelet aggregation, and leukocyte adhesion with resultant tissue ischemia and destruction. Protocols have been devised to remove or inactivate these products, and these seem to result in improved tissue survival. The treatment protocol of Heggers and colleagues (1987) includes débridement of all intact pale (nonbloody) blisters, which contain fluid high in prostaglandins, and application of topical aloe vera cream (a thromboxane inhibitor), as well as oral ibuprofin (Motrin), 12 mg/kg per day. Initial reports appear promising for a significant improvement in frostbite care.

Pain, Related to

• Rewarming Process

The rewarming process is frequently painful, causing paresthesias, burning, or "electric shock" sensations. Release of tissue breakdown and anaerobic metabolic products is the mechanism behind this response. Patients may require parenteral analgesia or even sedation. Often they will experience a marked anxiety or agitation out of proportion to the pain, possibly owing to release of thromboxane and other prostanoids into the circulation. By the time the rewarming is complete, the initial severe pain should have resolved, but significant residual pain may last for weeks to years, and temperature intolerance is usually the rule.

Potential for Injury, Related to

• Tetanus, Re-exposure

Tissue damage may be deep and extensive. Tetanus prophylaxis is required. Because there is potential for large amounts of tissue necrosis, tetanus immune globulin should be suggested as well.

Thawing an injured extremity and immediately returning the patient to an environment in which refreezing is a significant possibility is tantamount to malpractice. Refreeze injuries are much more extensive than primary frostbite and can result in loss of limb. Patients with significant frostbite injuries should be admitted to the hospital for 24 to 48 hours of observation and pain control. During this period, whirlpool débridement and tepid water exercise may improve functional outcome. Elevation to reduce swelling also may be of major benefit: occasionally, edema is so great that escharotomy is necessary to maintain peripheral circulation. Viability of damaged tissue may be assessed beyond the hyperacute stage with digital plethysmography, angiography, or radioisotope scanning, although most surgeons recommend primary tissue demarcation before amputation, as this seems to preserve the greatest amount of viable tissue.

Knowledge Deficit

The patient who presents with frostbite as the presenting feature may unrealistically minimize the seriousness of his or her condition and must be educated concerning further protection. During the acute thawing episode, the patient must be reassured that the pain reactions are normal and appropriate drug control must be made available. Patients must be forewarned of the prolonged sensitivity of the injured limb and its potential for easy injury, and they should be told of the extent to which further cold-weather activities may need to be curtailed. Smoking (which induces vasospasm) and exposure-prone lifestyles should be discouraged. Patients should be encouraged to verbalize their expectations about functional limb recovery and guided to a realistic assessment, with advice about the degree to which a physical therapy regimen may help.

Hypothermia

The term *hypothermia* refers to a condition of decreased body temperature, which results in a continuum of symptoms of progressive severity as the core temperature falls. Controlled hypothermia has been used for centuries as primary treatment or adjunctive therapy for a wide range of conditions, including schizophrenia, breast abscesses, and open-heart surgery (with varying degrees of success). This discussion is limited to accidental hypothermia as the body's thermal homeostatic defenses fail and the core temperature is depressed to 95°F or lower. This condition used to be called *exposure.*

As core body temperature falls, metabolic processes slow and beyond a certain point become significantly deranged. Each organ system is affected, and with each malfunction, the clinical picture worsens. Ultimately, the hypothermic patient may *seem* to be dead: pulseless, apneic, areflexic, and with fixed and dilated pupils. However, slowing of internal chemical processes reduces metabolic demands and slows entropic derangement; thus the patient may recover after rewarming. The lowest reported survivable core temperature in accidental hypothermia was 62°F (Aphorism 30–3). This patient went on to full neurologic recovery, although with complications from concomitant frostbite.

Aphorism 30–3 Nobody's dead till they're warm and dead.

Patients will not complain directly of hypothermia, and the clinical variations in manifestations can be extreme. The syndrome is identified, however, by one of the very basic responsibilities of the triage nurse: taking and recording a temperature *on every patient.* An oral temperature of 95°F or less must be confirmed with a repeated core measurement, usually approximated by a rectal or a tympanic temperature. If low temperature is confirmed, stage I procedures must be begun, with monitoring to include continuous temperature readings by rectal or esophageal thermistor probe.

Etiology

Certain patients are at risk for hypothermia. A mixed bag of conditions occurs, including both primary (cold exposure) and secondary (systemic failure) hypothermia. The "six A's" that predispose to hypothermia are age, activity, adjuvants, accidents, adrenals, *and* CNS (using a little cheating) (Table 30–2).

The common factor among these categories is the basic pathologic mechanism of the disease process: the inability of the patient's internal temperature defenses to protect him or her from an environmental challenge.

The majority of cases reported in large series usually are at the extremes of *age.* The elderly, owing to a combination of factors that include decreased mobility, poor energy reserves, lessened sensory awareness, chronic medical conditions, and poverty, are at significant risk for hypothermia even in relatively mild weather conditions. Furthermore, if they are chronically ill, they may be taking certain medications that may blunt the body's defensive responses. Without careful nursing attention to accurate recorded temperature, such cases are prone to misdiagnosis, as the ataxia, confusion, and withdrawal may be assumed to be evidence of cerebral or metabolic

TABLE 30–2
The Six "A's" or Predisposing
Factors for Hypothermia

Age
  Infants (especially neonates)
  Elderly
Activity
  Campers
  Backpackers, mountaineers
  Swimmers
  Homeless
Adjuvants
  Alcohol
  Barbiturates
  Phenothiazines
  Heroin
Accidents
  Victim exposed to low ambient temperatures
Adrenals
  Adrenal failure or sepsis
  Hypopituitarism
  Hypothyroidism
  Hypoglycemia
"And CNS"
  Cerebral thromboembolism
  Cerebral neoplasm
  Basilar skull fracture
  Parkinsonism
  Spinal cord transection

disturbance. Similarly, neonates and infants often are victims of hypothermia within "low stress" temperature settings: relative immobility, large body surface to weight ratio, minimal metabolic reserve, and small fat stores for insulation all contribute to a high-risk situation for temperature disturbance. Mortality from hypothermia is greatest in neonates and decreases with age; the condition must be especially guarded against with the newborn infant delivered in transit to the hospital without expert assistance (Aphorism 30–4). Infant hypothermia may present, however, with a confusing initial picture: the child may appear pink and healthy but will be cool to the touch and lethargic. The child's skin may seem firm to the touch, although later facial and extremity edema may appear. The presenting complaint may be as vague as "poor feeding"; thus the index of suspicion must be high. In severe or prolonged cases the infant may develop bradycardia, depressed respirations, oliguria, and hypotension. The hypothermic infant's death is usually due to respiratory conditions, although spontaneous ventricular fibrillation is recognized to occur, even several hours after complete rewarming.

Aphorism 30–4 Yellow cab = blue baby.

A small but significant group of patients can develop profound hypothermia due to *activity*. These patients are usually young, healthy persons who have managed to get into circumstances that overwhelm their bodily reserves. Commonest among these situations is immersion hypothermia, which must always be given major consideration in any attempted resuscitation from a drowning. As a heat absorber, water is 26 times more efficient than air; this fact, coupled with highly effective conduction losses and cutaneous vasodilation from the work expended in struggling, can produce rapid, deep hypothermia, which can be the primary physiologic derangement in such settings. More indolent, but often as severe, is the temperature derangement brought about by exposure to unexpected freezing temperatures, cold winds, or wetness, especially when accompanied by physical exhaustion, inadequate clothing, inexperience, or lack of training. Without the protection of sure, heated shelter, the outdoors adventurer has less room for error. Mother Nature does not forgive accidents, alcohol, unpreparedness, or lack of judgment; these factors are usually significant components in victims in this group. But no matter how physically conditioned and prepared a person is, bodily reserves can always be overcome (Aphorism 30–5).

Aphorism 30–5 Backpackers' Rule of 3s
The human body can survive:
    3 weeks without food
    3 days without water
    3 hours without shelter
    3 minutes without air
    3 seconds of panic

When the environmental stresses become significant, homeostatic responses must be activated quickly, fully, and accurately. If these mechanisms are blunted by drugs *(adjuvants),* a situation that otherwise would be merely taxing can easily become overwhelming. Many metabolically active substances can affect this system, including a wide range of common medications; drugs with depressant properties are especially likely to create a hypothermia victim.

The primary offender is alcohol: in addition to its ubiquitousness and its tendency to confuse and immobilize its users, this substance has some specific pharmacologic properties that increase the risk of hypothermia. As a peripheral vasodilator, it increases the sensation of warmth in a cold environment, but this sacrifices core heat to the skin, and thus cools the victim more quickly. The hypothalamic thermoregulator is chemically depressed in acute intoxication, and the chronic alcoholic with Wernicke's encephalopathy will have a primary hypothalamic dysfunction. Furthermore, the most efficient internal heat generator (shivering) is less likely to function with even low-grade intoxication. Barbiturates act in a similar fashion. They are known to suppress hypothalamic regulation, slow basal metabolic drive by inhibiting the release of thyroid-stimulating hormone (TSH) and adrenocorticotropic hormone (ACTH), and depress cellular enzymatic reactions. Phenothiazines, including several psychotherapeutic and antiemetic drugs, are well known to suppress the shivering response and may even induce hypothermia at therapeutic levels. Heroin and other narcotics have also been reported to be associated with hypothermia cases, although primarily on the basis of immobilization. Medical workers should also remember that in hypothermia states all metabolic processes are inhibited, so that *any* medication currently affecting the patient may have unusual or prolonged toxicities.

The *accident* victim must be expected to be hypothermic; all too often in the rush to evaluate and stabilize the patient's condition in acute trauma, a major, reversible source of morbidity will be overlooked if attention is not directed to the patient's temperature. At the accident scene, the patient may have been immobilized, trapped, and exposed for prolonged periods awaiting rescue or extrication. Even if unhurt, such a patient may not be able to protect himself or herself from the elements. With major traumatic insults, metabolic reserves will be taxed maximally and will be unavailable for thermoregulation, and frequently hypovolemia and acidosis will complicate attempted homeostasis. During resuscitation, the patient is routinely stripped of clothing without thought of warming, and large volumes of unheated solutions may be administered intravenously. Mild to moderate hypothermia, which otherwise could be easily overcome, can become a major component of the accident victim's demise. Prevention of this major complication falls directly on the triage nurse's identification of the problem and the primary care nurse's assessment and treatment.

The *adrenals* and other endocrine glands play a significant role in temperature homeostasis. Although rare as a direct cause of symptomatic hypothermia, malfunction of these glands may complicate recovery. The triage nurse should attempt to elicit a history of hypopituitarism, hypothyroidism, Addison's disease, diabetes, or chronic steroid use, and the primary physical assessment should also include consideration of signs suggestive of these problems. If such information is obtained, or if the patient is not responding to adequate treatment by rewarming by at least 1 °C per hour, patient evaluation should be directed toward these conditions. Whether or not the patient is diabetic, hypoglycemia is probable; intravenous dextrose (50 ml of 50%

dextrose in an adult) should be administered to supply a substrate for cellular metabolism.

The last category, *"and CNS,"* includes a diverse cluster of conditions that share two characteristics: immobility and possibly hypothalamic thermoregulatory malfunction. The acute stroke victim can have hypothalamic involvement or be unable to protect himself or herself from temperature extremes if not assisted by others; or the stroke itself may be secondary to an initial hypothermic insult. Hypercoagulation and intravascular sludging appear in significant hypothermia, and the resulting thrombus formation may precipitate the cerebrovascular accident. Some cerebral neoplasms, especially those that involve the third ventricle, and the injury associated with basilar skull fracture may affect the hypothalamus. Parkinsonian patients are also at risk, as their disease process may include centrally mediated vasodilation, excess sweating, and relative immobility. Similarly, patients with acute or chronic spinal cord injury may have lost much of their peripheral defense mechanisms.

Clinical Manifestations

The clinical picture of hypothermia is variable, roughly dependent on the patient's presenting core temperature. Although the disease process is a continuum, certain patterns are somewhat predictable within a given temperature range (Table 30–3). The patient presenting with a core temperature of less than 95° but more than 90°F has mild hypothermia. These patients may be shivering, although this reflex is abolished below 92°F, and they will usually be lethargic and confused or possibly combative. Confused behavior may include "paradoxical undressing" — such hypothermic patients may have a subjective sensation of heat, possibly owing to the failure of peripheral vasoconstriction as the syndrome develops. The nurse is unlikely to get much of a rational history from the patient and will need to depend upon his or her rescuers or companions for information about time and circumstances of exposure, past medical history, and similar data. Presenting vital signs (other than temperature) may be within normal limits, or there may be minor cardiac rate and rhythm disturbances, which will resolve with recovery. In the absence of other significant medical problems, these patients do well with simple, gradual passive rewarming, but will

---

TABLE 30–3
Clinical Presentation of Hypothermia
Based on Core Temperature

Core Temperature 95 to 90°F
  Shivering, lethargy, confusion
  Bradycardia or tachycardia (occasionally atrial fibrillation)
Core Temperature 90 to 87°F
  Generalized rigidity, coma
  Hypoventilation (respiratory acidosis)
  Bradycardia, increased myocardial irritability
  Hypovolemia, blood sludging (metabolic acidosis)
Core Temperature Less than 87°F
  Coma, areflexia, fixed and dilated pupils
  Apnea, cyanosis
  Bradycardia, ventricular fibrillation, asystole

require some monitoring to assure progressive recovery or will need to be investigated for underlying pathology.

Patients with a core temperature between 90° and 87°F can be classed as having "moderate" hypothermia, although these patients are profoundly ill and are at significant risk of death. They usually are in coma, with generalized rigidity, and will be both bradycardic and hypopneic. Blood pressure is usually obtainable only with Doppler augmentation but usually is present. The myocardium will be very irritable, and the risk of ventricular fibrillation is high. Both metabolic and respiratory acidosis may complicate the picture, and the patient will be hypovolemic and demonstrating signs of blood sludging secondary to the phenomenon of "cold diuresis." These patients can be killed by aggressive medical manipulation; refractory ventricular fibrillation is reported to be precipitated by moving the patient, placing an x-ray cassette behind the back, cardiopulmonary resuscitation (CPR), intubation, placement of central line catheters, or administration of intravenous drugs. This should not inhibit medically necessary manipulation, however; multihospital study of more than 400 patients (Danzl et al 1987) failed to find a single case of cardiovascular deterioration from intubation. The fibrillating or asystolic patient should be resuscitated aggressively, but the patient with a spontaneous cardiac rhythm, however slow, may be supplying his or her body's metabolic needs, and extreme caution is necessary. Consider the handling of this patient to be comparable to that of an acute spinal cord injury: "do no harm" should be the primary consideration.

The profoundly hypothermic patient will have a core temperature of less than 87°F, and usually will appear dead upon initial presentation. Comatose, cyanotic, apneic, areflexic, and with fixed and dilated pupils, these patients will be without obtainable vital signs. The cardiac monitor may show profound bradycardia, asystole, or ventricular fibrillation. If there is organized cardiac activity, Osbourne waves may be present (Fig. 30–2) on the monitor. Determination of death in the face of a low core temperature can only be made after aggressive core rewarming to at least 90°F without the return of a cardiac rhythm. To reiterate: *Nobody's dead till they're warm and dead!* Patients are reported to have recovered after 4 hours or more of CPR and core rewarming. The patient's age and underlying medical condition are the greatest determinants of overall recovery; chances for survival are better in hypothermia because markedly decreased metabolic demands lessen irreversible biochemical derangement. Every patient with a history even moderately suggestive of hypothermia who appears clinically dead and with low core temperature should receive a trial at rewarming therapy. No studies to date have correlated time from initial insult to resuscitation with recovery. Cause of death is usually refractory ventricular fibrillation.

As the process of core cooling proceeds, a number of physiologic changes occur than can result in complications on resuscitation. Shifts in intravascular volume to the core with peripheral constriction will stimulate a brisk volume correction, the so-called cold diuresis. Rapid cold challenges, such as immersion in water, can result in considerable loss of intravascular volume (while retaining blood elements), resulting in increased hematocrit, sludging of blood, and thus thrombotic complications: stroke, myocardial infarct, pulmonary edema, or acute tubular necrosis and renal failure. Decreased blood flow will allow lactate accumulation from anaerobic metabolism and metabolic acidosis. Pancreatitis and hyperamylasemia are also known to occur. Depressed laryngeal reflexes increase the risks of aspiration pneumonia, and increased bronchial secretions can complicate the picture.

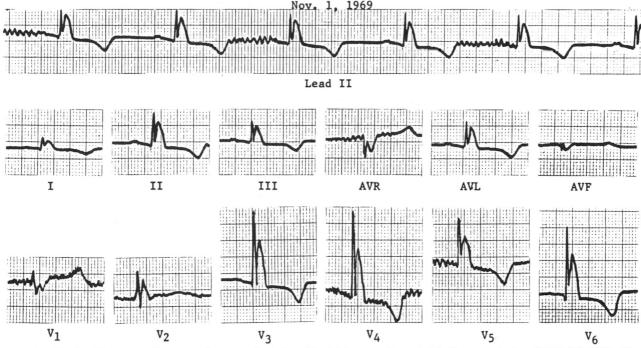

FIGURE 30-2. Electrocardiogram taken on admission. Rectal temperature at this time was below 90°F (32.2°C). The rhythm is sinus bradycardia at 40 beats/minute. The P-R, QRS, and Q-T intervals are prolonged and a prominent J wave is seen in most leads. Intermittent oscillations of the baseline are identified in lead II. (From Trevino, A. Archives of Internal Medicine, 1971, 127:470-473. Copyright 1971, American Medical Association.)

Treatment and Nursing Care

The patient with a core temperature of less than 90°F requires stage I nursing care, with special attention to serial monitoring and careful handling. A flow sheet should be created that will follow the patient through the first 48 hours, with hourly taking of vital signs, including temperature via rectal thermistor probe, blood pressure, central venous pressure (CVP), urinary output, cardiac rhythm, and serial arterial blood gases. This will require placement of a peripheral arterial line, a CVP monitor via the subclavian or internal jugular route, continuous cardiac monitoring with recording ability, an indwelling urinary catheter, intravenous (IV) access sites, and probable endotracheal intubation. It must be the responsibility of the primary nurse as well to protect the patient from inadvertent rough handling, especially during the critical temperature range of 87° to 90°F, at which cardiac irritability is a major problem.

During the initial rewarming period, a successful effort requires a gain of at least 1.5°F per hour in sustained temperature. This is best measured by a thermocouple probe placed at least 15 cm into the rectum. Although this is not a true core reading, it reflects changes in core temperature relatively accurately. Falsely low readings may be obtained in the presence of fecal impaction. Esophageal probes are also available but are more prone to falsely high readings when active core rewarming modalities are used (including aerosolized heated O_2). Most hypothermic patients are also hypovolemic and may require extensive fluid resuscitation. Fluid overload must be guarded against via serial CVP measurements; these patients are prone to pulmonary edema and to decreased cardiac and renal function. Arterial blood gas determinations will help assess adequate oxygenation and acid-base status, which can be particularly volatile during rewarming. Depressed body temperatures, however, may affect the results: pH may be falsely low and Po_2 and Pco_2 falsely elevated unless the laboratory is notified to correct for the patient's current temperature (although some authors suggest that more meaningful information is obtained by using the uncorrected test results). Initial laboratory tests are likely to include hemoglobin and hematocrit, serum glucose, electrolytes, blood urea nitrogen (BUN) and creatinine, and serum amylase. An initial chest radiograph should be obtained, as one third of major hypothermia victims will develop pulmonary edema or aspiration pneumonia. Review of the literature reveals that most authors agree that rewarming is the treatment of choice in accidental hypothermia. Unfortunately, at that point general agreement seems to end, as different modalities of treatment are championed mostly on the basis of case reports and retrospective studies.

Body Temperature, Altered, Hypothermia

There are three categories of rewarming methods, each with its own advantages and disadvantages. The simplest type is *passive rewarming*—essentially preventing further heat loss and allowing the body's endogenous heat to build back to normal. This is accomplished by removing the patient's clothes if wet, wrapping the patient in several layers of warm blankets (remember to cover the head and neck) and placing the patient in a warm, draft-free room. This method is suitable only for the mildest, most stable cases, as it relies on the body's internal reserves, but it has the advantage of being noninvasive, efficient, and non-labor-intensive.

Active external rewarming assumes that the internal reserves are not adequate for effective resuscitation and that heat must be added to complete rewarming. Heated Hubbard tanks, thermal blankets, hot water bottles, and microwave diathermy are all examples. Warming with these is more rapid yet noninvasive and can be done with relative ease by inexperienced personnel. Major drawbacks include loss of monitoring capability, lack of accessibility to the patient (especially with water baths), and the risk of rewarming afterdrop. This last problem is a well-recognized drop in core temperature of 0.5° to 3°F that occurs approximately 30 minutes into the rewarming phase. It is thought to be due to a return of blood flow to the extremities, which reopens perfusion beds previously shunted (with resulting hypotension) and allows a bolus of cold, acidotic blood to be released to the core, stimulating cardiac dysrhythmias, including asystole. Although this complication can be partially controlled by applying heat only to the trunk, or only to the areas of greatest fixed vascularity—the head and neck, axillae, and groin—this loss of heated surface area decreases efficiency and does not solve the accessibility problem.

Active core rewarming applies heat directly to the core, warming the heart and brain first. The techniques are, however, invasive and labor-intensive and require an experienced team. Modalities include heated, humidified O_2, heated intravenous fluids, heated gastric lavage, heated peritoneal dialysis, heated hemodialysis or extracorporeal circulation pumps, and post-thoracotomy mediastinal lavage.

Humidified oxygen, heated to 105° to 115°F and delivered by mask or endotracheal tube, is a relatively simple and useful adjunct in rewarming and can be used in all cases. Although a total of only 24 kcal/hour are delivered, the energy is delivered directly to the mediastinal area. (It requires 60 kcal to raise the temperature of a 70-kg person by 1.5°F.) Humidified oxygen cannot serve as a primary treatment, as by itself it is inadequate for active rewarming.

Heated intravenous fluid, primarily lactated Ringer's solution with 5% dextrose at a temperature of 115°F, is also a useful adjunct. Although the total heat delivered is low, only 17 kcal/L, warming the resuscitation fluids will add some heat and will avoid unnecessary temperature drop that would occur with room-temperature fluids. Heating can be performed by blood-warming coils, preheated water baths, or microwave warming (Box 30–1).

BOX 30–1 MICROWAVE WARMING OF INTRAVENOUS FLUIDS

Heated intravenous or dialysis fluids can be provided by using blood-warming coils or warm-water immersion of the fluids prior to use, but these methods entail significant delays either in the flow rate or in the time for warming. The common availability of microwave ovens now provides a rapid, simple means of obtaining heated fluids for such use. Intravenous solutions stored in flexible plastic containers may be heated with microwave radiation, although owing to variation in delivered energy with different models, some prior experimentation will be required to obtain the exact time and energy settings to heat the containers to 115°F. When attempting to standardize the technique for your hospital, remember to use a fixed number of containers for a given setting and to agitate the containers halfway through warming if the oven does not provide a rotating platform. Standardized procedures of this nature have been shown to provide consistent heating to plus or minus 1°C on repeat testing. Release of plasticizer from the containers during microwave heating has been studied and found not to be a problem. Fluid bags heated to 115°F in the oven should be wrapped in a towel prior to administration of the solution to prevent loss of heat.

Glass bottles have a potential risk of explosion from steam pressure generated with this procedure and thus should not be used. Containers that have metallic clips or attachments should never be placed in a microwave oven.

Gastric lavage, delivering and suctioning warmed fluids via a standard nasogastric tube, can be attempted only with caution. A patient whose condition is critical enough to require this therapy must be intubated prior to lavage, and large amounts of fluid should not be delivered by this route, as absorbed unrecovered fluid could result in electrolyte disturbance. The surface area of the stomach is not large; thus heat exchange will be relatively inefficient. The technique involves instilling 200 to 400 ml of warmed crystalloid via the nasogastric tube, clamping the tube for 5 minutes, and then suctioning to drain the stomach. This can be repeated throughout the resuscitation, but the volume of fluid not recovered from the tube should be limited.

Warmed peritoneal dialysis is a safe and effective technique when performed by trained personnel. With the insertion of two catheters, one in each peritoneal gutter, between 6 and 8 L of fluid can be exchanged in an hour, providing 102 kcal/hour to the core. The large surface area and extensive blood supply of the abdominal cavity provides an excellent heat transfer surface. Commercial dialysate solution can be used as the exchange fluid, or lactated Ringer's solution with 5% dextrose will work as well. Fluids can be preheated in a microwave oven to 115°F. The usual cautions and relative contraindications exist for this therapeutic lavage as for diagnostic lavage. Remember to always have a urinary catheter inserted prior to peritoneal catheter placement.

Other techniques available for use in severe hypothermia include heated hemodialysis or heated extracorporeal circulation (heart-lung bypass), although these usually require that a patient in unstable condition be removed from the acute care area and also need a standby technical team for operation and monitoring of the equipment. Emergency thoracotomy with open-heart massage and direct mediastinal lavage has been reported, but this is clearly a technique of last resort.

The use of these different rewarming devices will depend on the severity of the situation, the expertise of the emergency team, and the availability of equipment and personnel. As a general principle, patients can be divided into three categories for treatment: those with core temperatures greater than 90°F, those with core temperatures less than 90°F but cardiovascularly stable, and those with core temperatures less than 90° but cardiovascularly unstable (Fig. 30–3).

Summary

The patient with a core temperature greater than 90°F is medically the easiest category to manage. These mildly hypothermic patients are at little physical risk from their immediate condition and will do well with minor intervention. Initial triage and primary nursing assessment should include evaluation of the source of the hypothermia and a search for other, nonapparent problems, such as frostbite or unreported injury. The patient should have wet or frozen clothing removed and be wrapped in warm blankets and given heated, humidified O_2 by mask as adjunctive warming. Remember that the patient may be confused or otherwise uncooperative initially; protective observation and re-evaluation of the history after recovery may be needed. Core temperature readings should be taken hourly. If there is no temperature rise within 2 hours, evaluation of possible complicating factors such as hypothyroidism should be begun and active rewarming measures instituted. Recovered patients in this group do not need hospitalization and may be discharged from the ED, unless significant underlying disease is discovered or the cause of the hypothermia is unclear. Returning the patient to a situation of inadequate shelter, however, is tantamount to nursing malpractice. Investigation of the patient's social situation must be completed and provisions made for an appropriate discharge environment. The Social Service personnel may need to be consulted to arrange for housing or protective care.

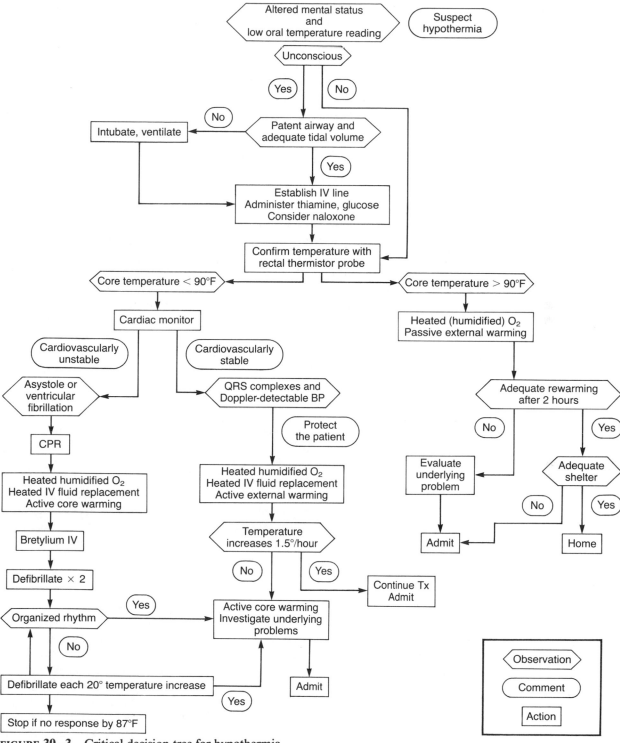

FIGURE 30–3. Critical decision tree for hypothermia.

The victim with a core temperature less than 90°F who has an effective cardiac rhythm, however slow, is a viable patient with an extremely high risk of iatrogenic death. These patients are usually in coma on arrival and will often have significant complicating diseases or concomitant injuries. Primary nursing assessment must be directed toward discovering these factors, and then the nursing plan must be directed toward intensive monitoring, protection against cardiovascular deterioration, and progressive rewarming. A flow sheet should be initiated upon arrival, including such parameters as core temperature, cardiac rhythm, pulse and blood pressure, CVP, IV intake and urinary output, level of responsiveness, and serial arterial blood gases, electrolytes, and hematocrit. Appropriate monitoring devices utilized should include rectal thermistor probe, continuous cardiac monitor with recording capability, arterial line, CVP catheter, and Foley catheter. The patient's airway must be protected and may need frequent suctioning. Extreme caution must be maintained in the handling of this patient, as cardiac deterioration to ventricular fibrillation or asystole may result from relatively minor stimulation. It is the primary nurse's responsibility to protect this patient: handle the victim with the level of care required for an acute spinal cord injury. As already noted, jostling, unnecessary movement, or overly aggressive instrumentation are all recognized to precipitate cardiac standstill that may not be convertible. Techniques of rewarming for this group of patients are the source of greatest controversy. All easily utilizable adjuncts should be employed, including heated O_2 and warmed IV fluids. Passive external rewarming or active external truncal rewarming are the methods most commonly advocated, as these patients are at the highest risk for afterdrop shock. Use of truncal microwave diathermy blankets seems to have significant advantages in this group of victims. Rewarming should proceed at a rate of at least 1.5°F per hour for optimal results; if this cannot be attained, then heated dialysis or other active core rewarming modalities will need to be employed.

Those patients with a core temperature of less than 90°F who are cardiovascularly unstable (i.e., do not have an organized cardiac rhythm) must be managed aggressively with full use of the resuscitation team, often for prolonged periods. Immediate intubation, all available monitoring capabilities, CPR, and any and all active core rewarming modalities should be started at once. Systemic acidosis should be corrected by controlled hyperventilation if possible, and adjusted by judicious use of sodium bicarbonate. Major effort should be directed toward core rewarming, with secondary concern for *initial* control of the cardiac rhythm. It is extremely difficult to defibrillate the heart below 85°F, and chronotropic and inotropic drugs do not work consistently at subnormal temperatures. Drugs administered during deep hypothermia will not be metabolized and may accumulate to toxic levels if given repeatedly during resuscitation. The resuscitation team recording nurse must be aware of this and keep all team members notified of total dosages employed during the hypothermic resuscitation. Lidocaine has not been shown to be of benefit for the cold, fibrillating heart, but several case reports support the use of a single bolus of bretylium to restore an organized rhythm. Electrical defibrillation can be used cautiously; recommendations are for two maximal-setting defibrillations at initiation of the resuscitation, followed by one further attempt with every 2 degrees of core temperature rise. Rewarming and CPR must be continued in asystole or ventricular fibrillation until the body is rewarmed to at least 87°F without conversion; there are recorded successful resuscitations after as long as 4 hours of continuous CPR. Again: *Nobody's dead till they're warm and dead.* Low core temperatures protect from metabolic derangement of vital organs during hypothermia; even full neurologic recovery has been reported.

Profoundly hypothermic patients will also be significantly hypovolemic from the previously described cold diuresis and will be in need of fluid resuscitation as well. Not only will aggressive heated fluid management supply extra kilocalories to raise the core temperature and help re-expand contracted vascular beds, but also supplemental crystalloid will help to lessen intravascular red blood cell (RBC) sludging with its associated hemolysis and thrombus formation. Fluid resuscitation must be guided by CVP monitoring and urinary output to guard against overload. Typical initial guidelines would include a 300-ml fluid challenge of lactated Ringer's solution with 5% dextrose, followed by 1 L/hour of continuous infusion. This should be modified by the patient's response, with the nurse keeping in mind that the dynamic process of rewarming with changing acid-base balance, variably recovering vascular beds, and suboptimal cardiac and renal function will require extremely close attention.

Steroids, thyroid extract, antibiotics, heparin, and other modalities have been advocated in hypothermia but have not been shown to have consistent benefit. They should only be given when specific indications are present to justify their use.

HEAT-RELATED EMERGENCIES

Failure of the heat-dissipation mechanisms is central to the development of heat-related emergencies. As discussed previously, the human body has more effective adaptive mechanisms for dealing with heat stress than with hypothermic conditions; however, these mechanisms can also be overwhelmed, with far more disastrous consequences. Damage done by excess heat causes greater morbidity and mortality and becomes irreversible at a much more rapid rate (Aphorism 30-6).

Aphorism 30-6 It doesn't take long to cook an egg or a neuron.

Etiology and Pathophysiology

The body's thermoregulatory system attempts to hold a core temperature of approximately 100°F in the face of continuously generated internal heat and widely variable environmental challenges. Basal heat production alone can result in a core temperature rise of 20°F per hour if dissipation mechanisms are paralyzed; even moderate work (300 kcal/hour) will cause an increase of 9°F per hour. The body also absorbs heat from a warm environment by radiation, convection, and conduction: sun exposure adds 150 kcal/hour, and significant quantities of heat will even be absorbed through the soles of the feet in a hot environment. Humans live and work in many settings where the ambient temperatures create major heat loads that must be continuously dispersed.

Temperature control is mediated by receptors in the hypothalamus that directly sense the warmth of the blood flowing to them. In response to this stimulus, blood is directed to the skin surface by relaxation of the vascular beds, and sweat gland (sudomotor) activity can also be enhanced. These responses are mediated by the endocrine glands and the autonomic nervous system. Dilation of the skin blood vessels improves radiation and convection losses when the ambient temperature is less than the skin surface temperature (about 92°F) but has only limited value in warmer weather. As the temperature increases, evaporative losses from sweating become the primary heat dissipation mechanism. Each 1.7 ml of sweat vaporized will release 1 kilocalorie of heat; sweating in the unacclimated, untrained individual can reach a maximum of 1.5 L/hour. Theoretically, then, heat loss from sweat can be as much as 882 kcal/hour, although the practical limit is about 650 kcal/hour owing to dripping and pooling of liquid. The body can tolerate sweat losses equal to about 5 per cent of body weight without difficulty, but physiologic derangement begins as losses approach 7% without replacement of fluid. Sodium and potassium losses can also be significantly high, especially in the unacclimated person. The body must adapt in other ways as well to meet the demands of cooling: Because dilation of the skin vascular beds can increase blood flow 20-fold, cardiac output must increase. Both rate and stroke volume are affected, and cardiac work (and oxygen utilization) can be maximal. The splanchnic bed contracts, shunting blood to the periphery, but this cannot match the dermal expansion. Salt and water are retained by the kidneys, owing to an increase in circulating aldosterone and growth hormone, saving fluid for evaporation. These mechanisms can maintain a reasonable core temperature for some period in any healthy person at rest; however, the stresses of excess generated heat of work, depressed physiologic adaptability, or simply prolonged exposure can cause the problems classed as heat-related emergencies.

With prolonged exposure to high ambient temperatures, the body develops accommodative responses that decrease internal stress and improve efficiency. This phenomenon, known as acclimation, takes about 2 weeks of heat or humidity or work exposure to develop fully. Several adaptive changes improve the body's ability to handle the heat stress until the effects of training increase efficiency (and thus decrease heat production) in muscular work. Chief among these is the ability to produce increased amounts of sweat, as much as 2.5 to 3 L/hour, with a marked reduction in excreted sodium. Plasma and extracellular fluid volume expand, and the heart's stroke volume and aerobic efficiency increase. Muscles develop increased glycogen stores and greater numbers of mitochondria, improving oxidative metabolism (Fig. 30–4). Such acclimation can occur at any age, but as cardiovascular reserve diminishes, maximal improvement levels will be lower. Until these changes occur, the person in a hot environment will be at risk. However, it should be noted also that exposure to this new heat and work environment should be gradual and must be continuous—brief nonexertional forays from within an air-conditioned enclosure will *not* create an acclimized ability to survive heat load stress.

Heat edema, heat cramps, heat exhaustion, and heat stroke, the four heat-related conditions, range from the trivial to the catastrophic. They are, however, all failures of the body to meet the physiologic needs of the adaptive responses to heat stress. Perceived in that manner, it becomes apparent that the correct medical approach must be to *enhance* the accommodation, rather than *attack* the problem as a "disease" brought about by external forces (Aphorism 30–7).

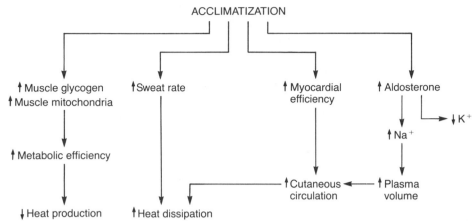

FIGURE 30–4. The metabolic effects of acclimatization are depicted schematically. (From Olson KR, Benowitz NL. 1984. Emerg Med Clin North Am 2:461.)

Aphorism 30–7 In heat, aikido is more effective than karate.

As in the case of hypothermia, only rarely will a patient come to the ED complaining of a heat related problem. To correctly serve these patients, the triage nurse must be aware of the risk factors for these conditions and stay alert to weather conditions and the population of the hospital's catchment area. Because heat-related emergencies are well recognized to be epidemic in nature, nursing supervisors should also consider these factors and make short-term staffing arrangements to handle an anticipated increased patient load in prolonged periods of unusually high heat and humidity. Factors that increase the likelihood of these problems include age, exertion, environment, drugs, and diseases (Table 30–4).

As with cold injuries, the patient's age is a significant factor, and for similar reasons. Infants, with their limited reserves and inability to protect themselves, are at risk in hot weather, especially if overdressed or bundled or if left in a hot, unventilated car. The young and healthy generally are at risk only when pushing themselves beyond the limits of their acclimation. This is a fairly common phenomenon and is the source of most of the cases of "exertional" heatstroke. It is the elderly, however, that fall victim to the majority of cases of so-called epidemic heatstroke, when prolonged high temperatures and humidity gradually overwhelm their limited reserves. Mortality in this group runs to 40 to 80% in various published series.

Muscular activity can produce impressive quantities of heat, as previously described, elevating core temperatures rapidly into the dangerous range unless there is proper dissipation of the heat. Acclimation can reduce the risks, but the majority of victims in this category succumb before full acclimation is reached. In the United States, the largest numbers of heat-related emergency cases are found among amateur athletes, especially high school football participants, and military recruits. Lack of conditioning, "macho" behavior or excessive zeal, and high ambient temperatures at

TABLE 30–4
Risk Factors Associated with
Heat-Related Conditions

Age
    Infants
    Young, healthy and unacclimated persons
    Elderly
Exertion
    Amateur athletes
    Military recruits
    Laborers
Environment
    High heat, high humidity
    Closed workspace
    Occlusive clothing
Drugs*
    Anticholinergic drugs
    Phenothiazines
    Tricyclic antidepressants
    Monoamine oxidase inhibitors
    Fat-soluble sedatives or hypnotics
    Lithium
    Diuretics
    Amphetamines
    LSD
    Phencyclidine
    Cocaine
    Beta blockers
    Sympatholytic antihypertensives
Diseases
    Alcoholism
    Parkinsonism
    Obesity
    Diabetes
    Spinal cord injury
    Hyperthyroidism
    Pheochromocytoma
    Status epilepticus
    Sudomotor Dysfunction
        Extensive prior burns
        Prior heat stroke
        Cystic fibrosis
        Ichthyosis
        Scleroderma
        Ectodermal dysplasia
        Miliaria
    Cardiovascular disease

*Excluded are drugs that cause nonenvironmental hyper-
thermia (e.g., malignant hyperthermia).

the beginning of training all contribute to the problem, as do the unfortunate practices of water deprivation, lack of warmup exercises, occlusive clothing (plasticized
sweatsuits, leather padding), and forced maximal participation. Persons in some
occupations are at risk, usually owing to the extreme temperature ranges in which
they must work. Roof-tarrers, blast-furnace workers, underground miners, and fire
fighters are typical high-risk groups.

Because the body's accommodative mechanisms to heat are so extensive, climatic conditions must generally be relatively extreme before they are overwhelmed. High temperatures (130°F or more) can be tolerated at rest with low humidity, but when humid conditions and still air make evaporation inefficient, effective cooling cannot be maintained. This is especially true when there is a prolonged heat wave, which gradually overtaxes the elderly's limited accommodative powers, or when these environmental extremes are coupled with major exertion. Mini- and microclimates must also be considered: victims in closed, unventilated spaces with high ambient temperatures or persons whose clothing does not allow adequate air circulation (joggers in occlusive suits, hazardous material (hazmat) workers in protective garments) are prone to difficulties.

Drugs can impair many portions of the accommodative reflexes to heat load or can be a source of heat generation in their own right. Malignant hyperthermia, a devastating drug reaction characterized by rapidly spiking core temperatures after the administration of succinylcholine or halothane, is not discussed here, nor are medications known to induce hypermetabolism. Some medications will impair hypothalamic function, such as the phenothiazines and possibly ethanol. Sudomotor activity is mediated by the cholinergic sympathetic nervous system; thus, drugs with anticholinergic properties (including antihistamines, benztropine, and tricyclic antidepressants) will dull the sweating response. Critical electrolyte imbalance can be a factor with lithium or the diuretics, diminishing reserve; cardiac response can be blunted by beta blockers or by sympatholytic antihypertensive agents. A wide variety of drugs are known to cause increased muscular activity, thus generating excess heat. These include amphetamines, cocaine, LSD, phencyclidine, and monoamine oxidase inhibitors (MAOIs)

Similarly, medical conditions that blunt the physiologic response to heat or diminish reserve will incline the victim to heat problems. Special mention should be made of diseases that impair sweat production, as this may not be obvious initially. Recovered victims of heatstroke may have no obvious physical stigmata, but they are known to frequently have nonfunctional, necrotic sweat glands. Many skin diseases, including miliaria (prickly heat) damage sweat glands, and patients with prior third degree burns over large surface areas will lack appropriate skin elements over those areas. Finally, the patient in status epilepticus will generate vast quantities of heat from the continual muscular tension, and as a result represents a special category of a double emergency, in which the complications of each problem have a multiplicative effect on the patient's morbidity.

Alertness to these risk factors will help the triage nurse to assess suspicious conditions for their acuteness and severity and may allow judicious initiation of treatment prior to the patient's entry into the care area. Certainly, in the milder conditions, knowledge of the self-limited nature of the problem can aid in appropriate triage when space is limited, and the patient can be reassured that this disease is not a harbinger of catastrophe. Initial assessment of these patients must include, then, time of onset of the complaint, the patient's local environment and level of activity at time of onset and immediately prior to it, current medications, and chronic medical conditions including skin diseases, as well as routine chief complaint, vital signs, and other routine features. The patient's temperature at time of arrival will be important, but less often is it diagnostic of the condition, and in fact, if environmental conditions are not kept in mind, moderate temperature elevations may lead the workup astray in pursuit of causes of a fever.

Minor Heat-Related Emergencies

These conditions generally occur early in the course of acclimation and are the result of attempts at physiologic adaptation to the heat stress. In such attempts, the body does successfully overcome the heat load, but with mild metabolic derangement, which produces symptoms. These disorders are self-limited and usually respond well to only minor intervention; recurrences can be prevented by proper patient education.

Heat Edema

Swelling of the hands, feet, and ankles is a common symptom seen during the first few days of heat exposure, even in the absence of any heart or kidney disease. It is especially seen in the elderly, unacclimated person, and may reach the point of pitting edema. The patient will generally have no other symptoms or significant physical findings. Most patients will not seek attention for this, although the uncomfortable tightness of the shoes or the fear of heart disease may prompt their decision to seek medical assistance. The condition is secondary to a heat-induced hyperaldosteronism and usually resolves in a few days.

Treatment and Nursing Care • Generally, no confirmatory testing is necessary; reassurance and simple elevation of the legs for comfort are all that is needed. The major complication is iatrogenic: initiation of diuretics on the basis of these symptoms increases the risk of later heat stroke.

Heat Cramps

This condition is usually seen in fully acclimated laborers or athletes and is characterized by extremely painful spasms in the exerted muscle groups, occurring some time after cessation of activity. Victims usually report good physical health and acclimation, adequate fluid replacement, but suboptimal salt intake during exertion. The patient will have few other symptoms (although occasionally nausea is reported) and will have essentially normal vital signs. The pathophysiology is thought to be systemic and local muscular hyponatremia, owing to loss of sodium in sweat. The acclimated worker, although relatively able to conserve salt, is capable of a 50% net increase in sodium excretion owing to higher volumes of sweat produced.

Treatment and Nursing Care • Although extremely painful, these cramps will resolve with administration of oral balanced salt solution (Gatorade or 1 teaspoon of salt in 500 ml water) or intravenous crystalloid if oral liquids are not tolerated. Although they are not at major risk, these patients should be brought immediately to the treatment area for purposes of pain control. Elevation, oral fluids, and gentle massage of the afflicted area will usually resolve the problem; narcotics are not necessary.

Two similar conditions that must be considered in this setting are tetanic cramps and rhabdomyolysis. Tetanic cramps will occur *during* rather than after the heat stress and are secondary to the hyperventilation response to heat load. Cooling and CO_2 rebreathing promptly resolve the problem. Rhabdomyolysis or muscle breakdown usually occurs secondary to direct injury or ischemia and can also be manifested by muscle pain. Myoglobin is released from damaged tissue and will precipitate in the kidney, causing renal failure. Screening for this condition should always be done, using a simple urine dipstick test for hemoglobin (which also becomes altered with myoglobin). Heme-positive urine in the absence of microscopic hematuria must be considered evidence of significant myoglobinemia and a risk for kidney damage. Occasionally, a patient has severe abdominal cramps and a boardlike abdomen due to spasm of the abdominal muscles. Relatively prompt resolution on treatment along with an appropriate history will help differentiate this from a surgical emergency (Box 30–2).

BOX 30–2 NOTES ON RHABDOMYOLYSIS

In exertional heat stroke, extreme muscular work from activity or seizures is a major source of heat load. When this muscular activity level is accompanied by the low blood flow states of frank heatstroke, lactic acidosis and muscular necrosis will commonly appear. These may also occur due to direct thermal effects, trauma, or pressure necrosis and thus may occasionally be seen in "classic" heat stroke cases as well. Muscular necrosis releases myoglobin, potassium, and muscle enzymes (CK and others) into the circulation. Cellular muscle damage itself is of little consequence, producing no recognized long-term effects; however, myoglobin, a complex iron-containing molecule, will precipitate in an acid urine and lead to profound renal failure.

Myoblobinuria is easily detected by frequent urine sampling with the orthotolidine dipstick (Heme Dipstix) test: If positive, in the absence of corresponding microscopic hematuria, this *must* be considered evidence of significant myoglobinuria and treated appropriately. Remember, however, that high or low urine flow states may not allow adequate concentration of myoglobin to permit detection with this qualitative test; in these settings, frequent assessment of blood CK levels must serve as a warning for the presence of myoglobin.

Aggressive osmotic diuresis with mannitol is the treatment of choice. Alkalinization of the urine is also recommended but may be difficult to manage in the face of concomitant electrolyte disturbances. Hypokalemia makes alkalinization especially difficult to maintain and should be cautiously corrected. Occasionally, temporary hemodialysis is necessary to support the patient over the acute renal injury.

Knowledge Deficit • After evaluation and resolution of acute heat cramps, the patient may be discharged home from the ED. Aftercare teaching should stress the need for adequate salt replacement to prevent a recurrence. Replacement is best accomplished by lightly salting food during times of high heat stress; the practice of using salt tablets should be discouraged, as they can cause vomiting and will cause an interluminal hyperosmotic state that will draw fluid from the circulation and contribute to volume depletion.

Heat Exhaustion and Heat Syncope

These conditions occur with some frequency, usually in unacclimated, older patients laboring under a mildly exertional, environmental heat load. When they occur in patient clusters, they can be a harbinger of an impending heat stroke epidemic, and hospital personnel should be prepared for an influx of extremely ill patients.

These two conditions are essentially the result of volume and electrolyte depletion, brought about by major activation of the heat dissipation mechanism. Heat dissipation succeeds, but the body is unable to control the physiologic stress. Some authors suggest that these disorders lie on a continuum with frank heat stroke; thus, they should be treated aggressively. Fluid and electrolyte losses occur via sweating, sequestering of fluid in interstitial muscle, and dilation of the dermal and muscular beds during work and heat stress. If adequate intake is not maintained (and it has been shown that response to the sensation of thirst does *not* provide enough fluid) and cardiac output cannot meet the continued demands, a hypotensive collapse is imminent.

Clinical Manifestations • The patient complains of a prodrome of fatigue, lightheadedness, nausea, vomiting, diarrhea, headache, and a feeling of impending doom; he or she may progress to hyperventilation, giddiness, or hysteria. Vital signs reveal hypotension, tachycardia, and tachypnea; temperature will usually be moderately elevated, occasionally as high as 104°F. Physical assessment will show an awake patient, possibly mildly confused, often complaining of headache, who has an ashen and profusely sweaty skin. Peripheral vascular contraction, lack of neurologic deficit, and lower body temperature help to differentiate this condition from full-blown hyperthermia.

Treatment and Nursing Care

Fluid Volume Deficit

Obviously, any hypotensive patient should immediately be brought into the patient care area, where the primary nurse should begin detailed assessment and stabilization. The patient should be undressed and allowed to cool. If hypotension continues, initial Trendelenburg position may be helpful. Most patients will require an IV line of normal saline solution and an assessment of status after a 300-ml fluid challenge. The severity of the patient's condition dictates the aggressiveness of care. Rapid, aggressive fluid resuscitation usually is not necessary; the majority of cases of hypovolemia relate to vascular dilation, not absolute fluid loss. Cooling and rest will constrict these beds, and large quantities of fluid may lead to overload. Occasionally such a patient will have a significant sodium deficit and may demonstrate signs of water intoxication, requiring treatment with hypertonic saline.

Further evaluation is required to rule out other potential causes of hypotension. In the absence of these, the otherwise healthy patient who returns to normal within a few hours of treatment may be discharged from the ED. Elderly or chronically debilitated patients, especially those with cardiovascular disease, should be admitted to the hospital for observation and cautious rehydration. Before discharge, careful inquiry should be made about the precipitant for this event; returning patients to settings in which they still will not be able to protect themselves from heat stress will place them again at risk. Instructions should be given to encourage fluid intake and increase dietary salt intake. Follow-up evaluation is necessary only in chronic medical conditions that may affect the handling of heat stress.

Heatstroke or Hyperthermia

The most catastrophic, but fortunately the rarest, of the environmental emergencies is heat stroke. Simply speaking, the syndrome is composed of (1) core temperature greater than 106°F, (2) neurologic impairment, and (3) lack of sweating. This is a true medical emergency, requiring immediate priority intervention (Aphorism 30–6). The syndrome is brought about by a failure of the heat dissipation mechanism, owing either to lack of physiologic reserve or to overwhelming heat load. Formally, the underlying mechanism serves to distinguish "classic" from "exertional" heat stroke, but initial treatment of the two entities is the same.

Prognosis is related to age and health of the patient and length of time at the hyperthermic extreme.

Clinical Manifestations • Classic heat stroke is seen in the elderly and physiologically impaired, as the result of a gradual depletion and deterioration of body reserves in the face of heat stress. It appears in epidemic form during periods of prolonged heat and humidity, usually after three or more days and nights of unrelieved oppressive weather. Fluid and electrolyte depletion brought about by copious uncompensated sweating causes an initial dehydration hypovolemia. This, when coupled with the relative hypovolemia of the expanded skin vascular beds, produces a significant cardiac stress, which will result in either peripheral vascular shutdown and sudomotor (sweat gland) collapse or frank cardiac decompensation. After initial dehydration, the patient develops progressive confusion and lethargy; when sweating ceases, the core temperature rises rapidly, and the patient exhibits hot, dry skin, a markedly elevated temperature, and a variable but abnormal neurologic picture. Alternatively, the victim may have an ashen, dehydrated complexion, but this is a grave prognostic sign associated with cardiac collapse.

Exertional heat stroke strikes the young, athletic, partially acclimatized person, usually after heavy exercise on a hot, humid day. Although dehydration is often a component of the problem, electrolyte disturbances, especially hypokalemia, seem to play a crucial role in the process. Collapse is often sudden, with little or no prodrome. As this can be a precipitous decompensation, the picture may be somewhat confused. Anhidrosis may not be apparent owing to residual sweat present as the heat load soared: do not assume that wet skin rules out hyperthermia. Occasionally these patients will have a core temperature less than the expected 106°F because the cessation of internally generated heat (as a result of loss of consciousness) will allow some cooling, which may be augmented by rescuer efforts by the time of arrival in the ED.

Treatment and Nursing Care • When a patient at risk arrives in the ED, initial assessment must be rapid and proceed concomitantly with aggressive treatment. If a history suggestive of heat stroke is obtained and a markedly elevated core temperature is confirmed, this is all that is needed to make a tentative diagnosis and begin cooling. *Treatment should never be delayed for confirmatory studies* (Table 30–5). A

TABLE 30–5
Treatment of Heatstroke

ABC
  Airway management and 100% oxygen
  Respiratory assistance
  Intravenous fluids (beware of overload)
Cooling
  Evaporative cooling: tepid water mist and fans
  Ice packs to head, neck, axillae, and groin
  Suppress shivering (intravenous diazepam)
  Core cooling only if no response
    (do not use ice baths, alcohol rubs, or
    antipyretics)
Monitor
  Core temperature (thermistor probe) continuously
  Vital signs every 5 minutes until stable
  Blood pressure via arterial line if hypotensive
  CVP or pulmonary capillary wedge pressure: fluids or cardiac failure
  Cardiac monitor for dysrhythmias
  Urine output (frequent checks for myoglobinuria)
  Arterial blood gases (corrected for core temperature)
  Electrolytes, clotting studies, liver function tests

patient with this suspected diagnosis must be treated with full resuscitation team efforts, with immediate physician attendance, two-to-one nursing care, and assistance from respiratory therapists until the initial cooling phase is completed.

Potential for Injury, Related to

• Hyperthermia

Although cooling is the mainstay of treatment, immediate attention should be directed, as always, to the ABCs of airway, breathing, and circulation. Because these patients are in a hypermetabolic state, oxygen supplementation is essential. A patent airway must be guaranteed, with intubation if necessary, and 100% oxygen is supplied until the patient reaches a near-normothermic level. Respiratory assistance may be necessary, depending upon the patient's alertness. Intravenous fluids are needed, but caution must be maintained; deficits may be variable and difficult to determine. Fluid overload is a definite hazard; high-output cardiac failure, vasomotor paralysis, and renal failure all reduce the margin of safety. CVP or Swan-Ganz monitoring may be required. All patients with an altered mental status should receive an intravenous bolus of 50% dextrose in water; hypoglycemia is a frequent complication of heat stroke and may be a primary precipitant in the debilitated patient.

Initial cooling efforts should have been begun in transit; on arrival, the victim should be taken immediately to the trauma or resuscitation room, where he or she should be stripped completely (with a quick assessment for occult injuries) and cooling begun while other stabilization maneuvers are in progress. Evaporative cooling is most efficient, removing 540 kcal/kg of water evaporated. Tepid water should be used as a mist spray over the victim, with a strong continual breeze from electric fans. This can be assisted by ice packs placed in areas of obligate blood flow: the scalp, neck, axillae, and groin. Alcohol sponging should not be used because toxicity from inhaled fumes is a reported complication, potentially affecting both the patient and the staff. Remember that evaporative cooling will be efficient only in a relatively low-humidity microclimate; air-conditioning and air circulation are required. If such conditions are unavailable, wrapping the patient in ice-soaked sheets will maintain close surface contact between ice and skin and provide adequate cooling. Fanning to enhance evaporation and frequent changing of sheets improve the temperature reduction effort. Skin massage and ice water baths are recommended by some authors, but have limitations of being too labor-intensive for too little gain (as well as being physically painful to the performer) and decreasing the monitoring capabilities during resuscitation (consider what would be involved in attempting defibrillation in an ice-water tub).

Other modalities, such as ice water lavage, cold water peritoneal dialysis, or temperature-controlled cardiopulmonary bypass, can also be considered but are rarely necessary. Aggressive temperature reduction should be continued until the core temperature is below 101°F, but care should be taken to prevent overshoot. Temperature reduction should be accomplished in 45 to 60 minutes. During initial temperature reduction, shivering may appear, especially if ice packs are used. Because the muscular work of shivering is an extremely efficient heat generator, it should be suppressed with intravenous diazepam or lorazepam. Chlorpromazine, which has been used in the past, is known to lower the seizure threshold and should be avoided if possible. Dystonias may be seen, but treatment should be directed toward rapid cooling or neuromuscular blockade, as the anticholinergic effects of diphenhydramine (Benadryl) or benztropine (Cogentin) may worsen the hyperthermia. Antipyretics such as aspirin or acetaminophen are of no use in heat-related emergencies, and in fact may contribute to complications of coagulopathy and hepatic damage.

Heat stroke patients are at high risk for morbidity and mortality. Intensive monitoring is absolutely imperative to reduce the severity of the complications, many of which may not be manifested until 12 to 24 hours later. Upon the patient's arrival, a flow sheet must be created that should remain in use for the first 24 hours of the patient's hospital course. It should include initial vital signs, with core temperature taken by rectal thermistor probe, repeat vital sign determinations every 5 minutes until stabilized, cardiac rhythm via continuous monitoring (with hard copy sampling of changes), CVP readings during fluid resuscitation or pulmonary artery wedge pressures if cardiac failure is impending, hourly urinary output and observation for myoglobinuria, arterial blood gases corrected for core temperature, electrolyte determinations, clotting studies, and liver function tests.

Appropriate instrumentation of the patient must therefore include rectal thermistor temperature probe; IV access routes, both peripheral and central, with capacity for CVP or Swan-Ganz catheter placement; endotracheal intubation; cardiac monitor; arterial line with blood pressure transducer; urinary catheter with hourly urinometer measurement; and nasogastric intubation with low continuous suction.

Although the diagnosis of heat stroke may in many cases be obvious, there are some conditions that must also be considered when a hot, neurologically impaired patient arrives in the ED (Table 30–6). Rapid cooling remains a priority, but if the hyperpyrexia is resistant or other factors appear, a different cause for the picture must be sought. Infections, including meningitis, encephalitis, and septic shock, may have a clinical picture very similar to that of heat stroke. Primary hypothalamic lesions (hemorrhage or tumor) may be associated with temperature disturbance and should

TABLE 30–6
Differential Diagnosis of
Heat Stroke

Meningitis (meningococcemia)
Encephalitis
Septic shock
Rocky Mountain spotted fever
Malaria
Typhus
Typhoid fever
Hypothalamic lesion (infarct or tumor)
Midbrain hemorrhage
Thyroid storm
Drug intoxications
   Anticholinergic poisoning
   Salicylism
   Amphetamine
   Phencyclidine
Drug withdrawal
   Alcohol
   Sedatives
Malignant hyperthermia
   Halothane
   Succinylcholine

be considered, especially when hyperthermia appears with unilateral anhidrosis or diabetes insipidus. If the diagnosis is unclear, computed tomography (CT) followed by diagnostic lumbar puncture may be necessary. Although the fever is seldom high enough to mimic heat stroke, fever spikes that occur with altered mental status may suggest hyperthermia in Rocky Mountain spotted fever, typhus, typhoid fever, or malaria. Thyroid storm may be initially confusing, although secondary markers for hyperthyroidism should make that diagnosis obvious. Anticholinergic poisoning or salicylate intoxication must be considered; acute intoxications with amphetamines or phencyclidine also produce an elevated temperature and a bizarre, combative state. Similarly, withdrawal from alcohol or other depressants produces a metabolic overdrive and confusion that can mimic, or when combined with recurrent seizures, can progress directly to heat stroke. The syndrome of malignant hyperthermia, which occurs during or shortly after administration of halothane anesthesia or succinylcholine, is indistinguishable from heat stroke, except, of course, for the setting in which it appears.

Recognized complications that must be anticipated include lactic acidosis, hyper- or hypokalemia, hypoglycemia, hyponatremia, hypocalcemia, and volume depletion; high-output cardiac failure, pulmonary edema, or myocardial necrosis or infarction; rhabdomyolysis and muscular necrosis; renal failure secondary to hypotension or myoglobinuria; intestinal paralytic ileus or gastrointestinal bleeding; disseminated intravascular coagulation (DIC) or thrombocytopenia; hepatocellular necrosis and liver failure. Each of these can be treated with standard medical therapies as they appear; however, the sooner they are detected and treatment is begun, the better the prognosis. Cardiac failure may respond to simple cooling or cautious fluid replacement; digitalis or pressor agents such as dopamine or dobutamine may be necessary, however. Pressor agents with peripheral constrictive alpha-adrenergic effects (e.g., norepinephrine) must be avoided — the peripheral constriction will impair critical heat dissipation and worsen the primary problem.

All patients with heat stroke will need to be admitted to an intensive care unit setting for at least 24 hours, as late complications can appear suddenly and require one-on-one management. Seizures or cerebral ischemia, rhabdomyolysis and renal failure, late cardiac decompensation, and gastrointestinal bleed are all relatively common occurrences. Long-term prognosis is variable, depending on prior state of health, length of time under heat stress, and adequate oxygenation. Survival is not necessarily related to initial core temperature, and recovery without neurologic impairment has been reported after an initial reading of 115.7°F.

Families can be counseled to expect a prolonged recovery and anticipate at least initial neurologic disability. Cardiac injury is usually limited to focal necrosis, possibly creating a hypodynamic wall segment, but coronary insufficiency and thus progressive damage or dysfunction is usually not significant. Most cases of renal failure are reversible, and patients do not require prolonged dialysis; hepatocellular necrosis, however, can be severe. On discharge from the hospital, patients must be advised to return to their previous level of function slowly; special caution should be advised in situations of subsequent heat stress, as sweat gland necrosis and thus sudomotor impairment is common in heat stroke survivors.

When the ambient temperature and humidity rise, these patients should be advised to avoid prolonged exposure to heat if possible, to increase fluid intake beyond levels of thirst control ("clear" urine is a good measure of appropriate intake), to add extra salt to foods, and to avoid salt tablets, alcohol, and optional anticholinergic medications (e.g., antihistamines for hayfever). Athletic persons can return to prior levels of function in the absence of other impairments, provided they are specifically counseled about slow, progressive acclimation to hot weather and adequate fluid intake during heavy work. This may be as much as 3 to 5 L/hour and should be accompanied by appropriate electrolyte supplementation.

CONCLUSION

The human body has limited defenses to control its microclimate under environmental stresses; when these are overwhelmed, a wide range of derangement syndromes can appear. In relative low-temperature situations, peripheral damage (frostbite) can cause superficial or deep tissue damage that can be hard to distinguish during initial presentation. Local rewarming, gentle handling, and pain control are the mainstays of emergency care. Careful attention must be paid to protecting the patient from refreezing the injured area.

Hypothermic patients have disruption of their core temperature, resulting in significant metabolic changes manifested most obviously by alteration in function of the heart and brain. Such patients may initially appear dead, but are resuscitatable with potential for full recovery. Careful handling, core rewarming, and fluid replacement enhance chances for survival. A high index of suspicion and confirmed initial temperatures on all patients will alert the medical team to this protean disease process.

Hyperthermic emergencies may produce symptoms along a continuum depending upon the extremes to which the patient is stressed, and the degree of acclimation established prior to the stress. Fluid and electrolyte disturbances are the hallmark of the lesser syndromes, but heat stroke is manifested as profound metabolic derangement and has a high mortality rate. Rapid cooling (evaporative is most efficient) and precise monitoring for complications of myocardial injury, renal or hepatic damage, electrolyte disturbance, DIC, or rhabdomyolysis improve chances for survival; mortality is high.

These patients are fragile, and the disease manifestations are easily confused with those of other processes or are easily overlooked. Awareness is the key; careful handling the mainstay of care.

REFERENCES

General Environmental

Auerbach PS, Geehr EC. 1980. Environmental medical emergencies. Topics Emerg Med 2:1–154.

Auerbach PS, ed. 1987. Proceedings of the 1987 UAEM/IRIEM Research Symposium on Environmental Emergencies. Ann Emerg Med 16:643–649.

Kizer KW, ed. 1984. Environmental emergencies. Emerg Med Clin North Am 2:457–698.

Kodet ER, Angier B. 1975. Being your own wilderness doctor. Harrisburg, PA, Stackpole Books.

Stewart EC, ed. 1987. Perspectives in rational management: Selected environmental emergencies. Cyberlog 2:1.

Wilkerson JA. 1975. Medicine for Mountaineering, 2nd ed. Seattle, Mountaineers Publishers.

Cold-Related Emergencies

Bangs CC. 1984. Hypothermia and frostbite. Emerg Med Clin North Am 2:475–488.

Danzl DF. 1981. Accidental Hypothermia (monograph). Philadelphia, Smith-Kline/ACEP.

Danzl DF, Sowers MB, Vicario SJ, et al. 1982. Chemical ventricular defibrillation in severe accidental hypothermia (letter). Ann Emerg Med 11:698–699.

Danzl DF, Pozos RS, Auerbach PS, et al. 1987. Multicenter hypothermia survey. Ann Emerg Med 16:1042–1055.

Fergusson NV. 1985. Urban hypothermia. Anaesthesia 40:651–654.

Gong V. 1984. Microwave warming of IV fluids in management of hyperthermia (letter). Ann Emerg Med 13:645.

Hansen JE, Sue DY. 1980. Should blood gas measurement be corrected for the patient's temperature? (letter) N Engl J Med 303:341.

Harnett RM, Pruitt JR, Sias FR. 1983. A review of the literature concerning resuscitation from hypothermia: Part II. Selected rewarming protocals. Aviat Space Environ Med 54:487–495.

Heggers JP, Robson MC, Manavalen K, et al. 1987. Experimental and clinical observations on frostbite. Ann Emerg Med 16:1056–1062.

Kochar G, Kahn SE, Kotler MN. 1986. Bretylium tosylate and ventricular fibrillation in hypothermia (letter). Ann Intern Med 105:624.

McCauley RL, Hing DN, Robson MC, et al. 1983. Frostbite injuries: A rational approach based on the pathophysiology. J Trauma 23:143–147.

Miller JW. 1980. Urban accidental hypothermia: 135 cases. Ann Emerg Med 9:456–461.

Mills WJ Jr. 1980. Accidental hypothermia: Management approach. Alaska Med 22:9–11.

Reuler JB. 1978. Hypothermia: Pathophysiology, clinical settings and management. Ann Intern Med 89:519–527.

Sarnaik AP, Vohra MP. 1986. Near-drowning: Fresh, salt, and cold water immersion. Clin Sports Med 5:33–46.

Trevino A. 1971. The characteristic electrocardiogram of accidental hypothermia. Arch Intern Med 127:470–473.

Zell SC, Kurtz KJ. 1985. Severe exposure hypothermia: A resuscitation protocol. Ann Emerg Med 14:339–345.

Heat-Related Emergencies

Abramowicz M, ed. 1985. Exertional heat injury. Med Lett 27:55.

Clowes GH, O'Donnell TF Jr. 1974. Heat stroke. N Engl J Med 291:564–567.

Graham BS, Lichtenstein MJ, Hinson JM, et al. 1986. Nonexertional heatstroke. Arch Intern Med 146:87–90.

Kilbourne EM, Choi K, Jones TS, et al. 1982. Risk factors for heatstroke. JAMA 247:3332–3336.

Knochel JP. 1975. Dog days and siriasis: How to kill a football player. JAMA 233:513–515.

Knochel JP. 1974. Environmental heat illness. Arch Intern Med 133:841–864.

Murphy RJ. 1984. Heat illness in the athlete. Am J Sports Med 12:258–261.

Olson KR, Benowitz NL. 1984. Environmental and drug induced hyperthermia. Emerg Med Clin North Am 2:3.

Shibolet S, Lancaster MC, Danon Y. 1976. Heat stroke: A review. Aviat Space Environ Med 47:280–301.

Slovis CM, Anderson GF, Casolaro A. 1982. Survival in a heatstroke victim with a core temperature in excess of 46.5°C. Ann Emerg Med 11:269–271.

Stewart CE. 1987. Preventing progression of heat injury. Emerg Med Rep 8:16.

Weiner JS, Khogali M. 1980. A physiologic body cooling unit for treatment of heat stroke. Lancet 1:507–509.

Susan Woolley, RN
Charles Drueck III, MD

Burn Injuries

Burn injuries are acute events, painful and sometimes dramatic in appearance. Two to three million burn injuries occur in the United States yearly. Of these cases, 300,000 result in hospitalization and ultimately 12,000 patients die of burn-related injuries. Most burn injuries can be treated on an outpatient basis after evaluation in the emergency department (ED). Recognition of those patients requiring hospitalization because of the extent of injury, the area burned, or potential complications from the type of burn is the role of the ED nurse. Fluid resuscitation, care of the burn wound, relief from pain, emotional care, and preparation for admission must progress in an orderly fashion and are coordinated by the ED nurse.

The nurse's approach to the patient will depend on the extent and depth of the burn injury and factors such as smoke inhalation, damage to internal organs, blunt trauma, or fractures. The age of the patient may contribute to potential mortality from a burn. Both infants less than 2 years of age and elderly patients over 60 years of age have less reserve available to survive a major burn (Fig. 31–1). The risk of elder or child abuse or foul play must also be considered if the burn wound distribution does not correspond to the history of the injury.

The skin is the body's largest organ system and protects the person by temperature regulation, prevention of bacterial or viral invasion, and conservation of body fluids and electrolytes. These functions of the skin are lost with a burn injury. The more extensive and deeper the burn injury, the more complications that are encountered and the greater the potential mortality.

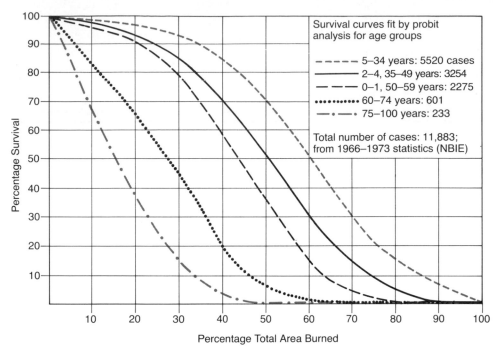

FIGURE 31-1. Burned patient survival: age group versus percentage of total area burned. The two severity factors (age and total area burned) greatly affect chance for survival. Keep in mind, however, that these averages improve with excellence in burn care. NBIE = National Burn Information Exchange. (Modified from Emergent Care of the Burn Victim, p 42, 1979, National Institute for Burn Medicine, with permission.)

PATHOPHYSIOLOGY OF BURN INJURIES

An insult to skin integrity affects not only the skin but also many other organ systems. Soon after a burn injury is sustained, a release of histamine occurs from the thermally injured cells. This causes a vasodilation and an increase in capillary permeability, permitting fluid and electrolytes to leak into the interstitial spaces beneath the burn and surrounding tissue. Colloid osmotic pressure decreases as protein is lost from the vascular space, causing an even greater shift of fluid into the interstitial space. This places the patient at great risk for hypovolemic shock. Platelets and leukocytes aggregate in the capillaries beneath the burn, resulting in thrombosis and further tissue damage.

Fluid is also lost directly through the burn wound. The rate of this fluid loss may be up to 15 times the normal insensible fluid loss. As the lost fluid evaporates, a decrease in body temperature occurs. This causes an increase in basal metabolic rate, an increase in caloric expenditure, and hypothermia.

Burn shock is a term applied to the cardiovascular status of the burned patient as a result of hypovolemia. Within the first several hours of an extensive burn injury, the loss of first local, then systemic capillary integrity results in massive intravascular fluid loss. If left untreated, this condition leads to rapid hypovolemia and circulatory collapse. Dysrhythmias secondary to electrolyte imbalances and hypovolemia can occur. Acute renal failure may ensue unless there is proper fluid replacement. Acute gastrointestinal ileus and even ulceration may develop owing to constriction of the splenic blood vessels.

CLINICAL MANIFESTATIONS

When the burn patient arrives in the ED, a rapid assessment is performed. Airway, respiratory status, and circulation are first priorities, followed by an assessment of other injuries and, last, an estimate of the extent, depth, and location of the burn injuries. The greatest and earliest threat to life in a major burn is inhalation injury. This results from inhaling superheated smoke, steam, gas, or toxic fumes. Clinical findings suggestive of pulmonary injury are history of the burn injury occurring in an enclosed space, burns of the face and neck, sooty mucous membranes, singed nasal hairs, circumoral burns, and restlessness. Later symptoms include hoarseness, wheezing, dyspnea, stridor, hemoptysis, or carbonaceous sputum. Nasal flaring with inspiratory retraction are signs of impending respiratory failure. Any of these suggest smoke inhalation and, if the patient is not already intubated, the ED nurse should be prepared to assist with prophylactic endotracheal intubation. Early control of the airway, when there has been significant smoke inhalation, avoids loss of the airway and respiratory arrest from edema of the supraglottic space.

Continuous assessment of respiratory status is essential in the burn patient. The rate, depth, and effort of respiration are observed every 15 to 30 minutes; auscultation of the lungs also is performed at these times. The stethoscope can be placed directly over a burn wound if necessary. Rales may indicate fluid overload secondary to overzealous fluid resuscitation or leaking of fluid into alveoli secondary to loss of capillary integrity. Absence of lung sounds may indicate pneumothorax or hemothorax secondary to related trauma.

Carbon monoxide poisoning must not be overlooked. Frequently the patient with carbon monoxide poisoning will be disoriented. Skin and mucous membranes will have a cherry-red appearance even in the burn wounds. Carbon monoxide has an affinity to hemoglobin 240 times greater than that of oxygen. Arterial blood gases of persons with carbon monoxide poisoning will show a normal plasma content of dissolved oxygen (PaO_2). The oxygen saturation (O_{2SAT}) will be abnormally low. Because carbon monoxide is preferentially bound to hemoglobin, the patient suffers a functional hypoxemia as a result of interference with hemoglobin-mediated oxygen transport and unloading at the tissues. The patient with a major burn injury loses a massive amount of fluid into the wound. Because the protective functions of the skin are lost, insensible water loss, which is normally 30 to 50 ml/hour, may increase up to 700 ml/hour in a severely burned person. The result of this fluid shift is a circulating volume depletion. Symptoms of hypovolemic shock will become clinically evident and can lead to cardiac arrest if left untreated.

The patient will develop edema and will continue to become more edematous as time passes, even in body parts not burned. Intravenous fluid therapy must be initiated as soon as possible to prevent hypovolemic shock. However, once therapy is initiated, careful monitoring must occur to maintain circulatory integrity as well as prevent a rebound hypervolemia owing to miscalculated volume requirements.

The patient will be hypotensive and tachycardic. Heart rates of up to 160 beats/minute are not unusual and may stay relatively high owing to the stress of the burn and the increased metabolic rate after the resuscitation.

The patient will need resuscitation with large volumes of lactated Ringer's solution to maintain cardiovascular stability. Level of consciousness and urine output are monitored frequently as they are indicators of adequacy of cardiac output.

In general, burn injuries do not bleed or cause unconsciousness. Therefore, presence of hypovolemic shock or decreased sensorium might suggest central nervous system injury, hypoxemia, or internal injuries.

The triage nurse ascertains as many facts about the patient and the mechanism of burn injury as possible. This information helps determine the severity of the burn injury and plan of care. The following information is obtained from prehospital care providers such as emergency medical teams (EMTs), allied medical personnel, or family: type of burn (thermal, chemical, electrical, inhalation) (if it is a chemical burn, the exact name of the chemical must be obtained); duration of exposure; presence of noxious fumes; exposure to smoke or burn in an enclosed space; bruises, lacerations, or fractures; related accidents—explosions, falls, motor vehicle accident; patient's age; and past medical problems and allergies.

A known history of other problems, especially cardiovascular or pulmonary, is important for selection of treatment and evaluation of the patient's response to treatment.

An in-depth history, including habits and family illnesses, is obtained when the patient is out of immediate danger.

SEVERITY OF BURN INJURY

The severity of the burn injury is determined by the extent of the burn (percentage of body surface area burned [%BSA]), the depth of the burn wounds, age of the patient, past medical history, and area of the body burned.

Extent

The extent of the burn is determined by calculation of the percentage of surface area burned. This calculation is very important because initial fluid resuscitation is based on this estimate. The Rule of Nines is a simple and common method where by the body is divided into areas of 9% or multiples of 9% with the perineum constituting 1% (Fig. 31–2). This method is not completely accurate, however, and must be modified for children. The Lund-Browder Chart, although more time consuming, allows for age differences and is more accurate (Table 31–1). The palm on the

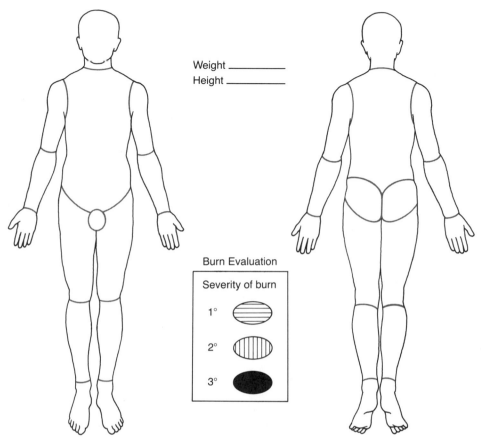

Weight _____
Height _____

Burn Evaluation

Severity of burn

1°

2°

3°

FIGURE 31–2. Rule of Nines. An estimation of the extent of the burn can be made by using the Rule of Nines. The total body surface is sectioned into the following percentages: head and neck, 9%; each upper extremity, 9%; chest and abdomen, 18%; upper back, 9%; lower back and buttocks, 9%; each leg and foot, 18%; and the genitals and perineum, 1%.

patient's hand is roughly equivalent to 1% of the body surface area and can be used as a ready ruler, especially to measure smaller burn wounds.

Depth

Assessment of the depth of the burn injury is not a factor in initial fluid resuscitation. It is, however, helpful for planning and implementing appropriate care. Many times the exact depth is difficult to determine until several days after injury (Fig. 31–3).

A *first-degree* burn involves only partial-thickness damage to the epidermal layer of the skin. It is like a sunburn. The skin is erythematous and painful. There is mild vasodilation and the patient feels chilled. Within 7 days, the damaged epithelium will slough as it is replaced by new healing cells. Usually the skin recovers without permanent scarring but may be bright pink for several weeks.

TABLE 31–1
Lund and Browder Chart

Area	Age–Years 0–1 (%)	1–4 (%)	5–9 (%)	10–15 (%)	Adult (%)	% 2°	% 3°	% Total
Head	19	17	13	10	7			
Neck	2	2	2	2	2			
Ant. Trunk	13	17	13	13	13			
Post. Trunk	13	13	13	13	13			
R. Buttock	2 1/2	2 1/2	2 1/2	2 1/2	2 1/2			
L. Buttock	2 1/2	2 1/2	2 1/2	2 1/2	2 1/2			
Genitalia	1	1	1	1	1			
R.U. Arm	4	4	4	4	4			
L.U. Arm	4	4	4	4	4			
R.L. Arm	3	3	3	3	3			
L.L. Arm	3	3	3	3	3			
R. Hand	2 1/2	2 1/2	2 1/2	2 1/2	2 1/2			
L. Hand	2 1/2	2 1/2	2 1/2	2 1/2	2 1/2			
R. Thigh	5 1/2	6 1/2	8 1/2	8 1/2	9 1/2			
L. Thigh	5 1/2	6 1/2	8 1/2	8 1/2	9 1/2			
R. Leg	5	5	5 1/2	6	7			
L. Leg	5	5	5 1/2	6	7			
R. Foot	3 1/2	3 1/2	3 1/2	3 1/2	3 1/2			
L. Foot	3 1/2	3 1/2	3 1/2	3 1/2	3 1/2			
					Total			

Source: Lund CC, Browder NC. 1944. Surg Gynecol Obstet 79:352–358, with permission.

Second-degree burns are also partial-thickness burns but injure only the upper portion of the dermis of the skin. These burns can be divided into superficial and deep partial-thickness injuries. The superficial partial-thickness burn extends beyond the epidermis and superficially into the dermis. The burn is characterized by blister formation and a very red and weepy appearance; in addition, it is very painful because of exposed nerve endings. A clean partial-thickness burn will heal in 7 to 10 days. Deep partial-thickness burns are more difficult to assess, in that their appearance is similar to that of a full-thickness injury. The wound is dry and pale. There may be a mottled or white appearance, but pinprick sensation is preserved. This injury extends deep into the dermis, leaving only a few of the regenerative epithelial elements, such as sweat glands and hair follicles. This burn may require up to 3 weeks to heal and has the potential to convert to full-thickness if the burn wound becomes infected. All first- and second-degree burn wounds are partial-thickness injuries.

The *third-degree* or full-thickness burn extends entirely through the epidermis and dermis into the subcutaneous tissues, leaving no regenerative epithelial elements. This injury is most common with flame burns, but can occur from other sources, depending on the temperature and duration of exposure. The burn is characterized by a dry, leathery appearance. It may be charred, mottled, white, or mahogany-colored. Thrombosed blood vessels may be visible through the burned skin, which is called eschar (devitalized tissue due to coagulation necrosis). The full-thickness burn destroys the nerve endings. Because of that, the wound generally is not sensitive to pinprick.

Most burn injuries are a mixture of full- and partial-thickness wounds.

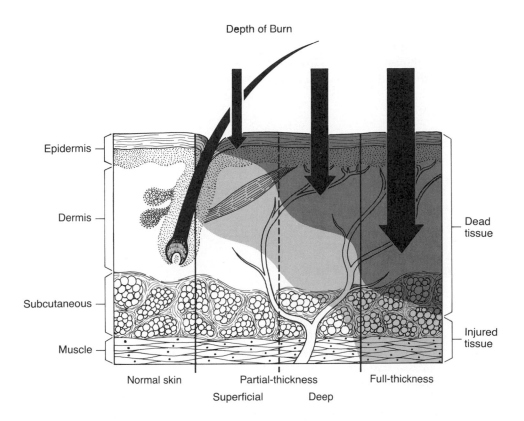

Partial-thickness Burn		Full-thickness Burn
Normal or increased sensitivity to pain and temperature	Sensation	Anesthetic to pain and temperaure
Large, thick-walled, will usually increase in size	Blisters	None, or if present, thin-walled and will not increase in size
Red, will blanch with pressure and refill	Color	White, brown, black or red; if red, will not blanch with pressure
Normal or firm	Texture	Firm or leathery

FIGURE 31–3. Depth of burn. The arrows represent degree of heat or intensity of burning agent and the time of contact with skin. The darker shaded area represents dead tissue; the lighter shaded area, damaged or injured tissue that will heal with good care. When all tissue (epidermis and dermis) has been destroyed, the burn is termed full-thickness. In partial-thickness burns, only part of the skin has been destroyed. (Redrawn from Emergent Care of the Burn Victim, p 41, 1979, National Institute for Burn Medicine, with permission.)

Age

Statistics have shown higher mortality rates in burn-injured patients who are under 2 or over 60 years old. Both infants and elderly patients have less reserve to survive a major burn injury.

It is also important to note that the skin of infants and older patients is thinner, requiring a shorter duration of exposure to produce as deep a burn as in a young adult.

Past Medical History

The patient's past history can greatly influence his or her ability to survive a burn injury. The stress caused by the burn can exacerbate pre-existing conditions such as diabetes mellitus or pulmonary disease. It is also important to note drug sensitivities and drug or alcohol abuse as these may affect the caregiver's ability to reduce pain.

Part of the Body Burned

The area of the body burned is important in determining severity. Burns of the head, neck, and chest may lead to pulmonary difficulties. Burns of the perineum are prone to early infection and, if the genitalia are burned, have a tremendous emotional impact on the patient. Burns of the hands pose a potentially serious loss of function.

Other factors that contribute to the severity of burns are smoke inhalation and multiple other injuries in addition to the burn.

Classification of the burn wound as major, moderate, or minor is based on assessment of not only the extent but also the depth and area of the body burned (Table 31–2).

TABLE 31–2
American Burn Association Burn Classification

Major Burn Injuries
   Second-degree burns over > 25% BSA adult or > 20% BSA child
   Third-degree burns involving ≥ 10% of BSA
   All burns of the hands, face, eyes, ears, feet, or perineum
   All inhalation injuries
   Electrical burns
   All burns with associated complications of fractures or other trauma
   All high-risk patients (e.g., those with pre-existing renal, pulmonary, or cardiovascular disease)
Moderate Burn Injuries
   Second-degree burns over 15 to 25% BSA adult or 10 to 20% BSA child
   Third-degree burns of 2 to 5% BSA
   Burns not involving eyes, ears, face, hands, feet, or perineum
Minor Burn Injuries
   Second-degree burns over < 15% BSA adult or < 10% BSA child
   Third-degree burns of 2% BSA or less

TREATMENT AND NURSING CARE FOR BURN WOUNDS

Once the patient's condition has been stabilized and the extent and depth of burn determined, care of the burn patient involves continued resuscitation with monitoring and wound care.

Diagnostic Data

The individual with a major burn injury (more than 20% BSA) should have a complete blood count, urinalysis, and serum electrolyte determination. Hemoconcentration will produce an increased hematocrit. Urine specific gravity will be high, and there may be evidence of protein and ketones in the urine. Serum electrolytes are monitored closely in the early phases of burn injury. Later sodium moves into the interstitial space, resulting in a decreased serum sodium level. Hyperkalemia secondary to hemolysis of red blood cells or tissue destruction can also occur.

The more extensive the burn injury, the greater the number of systemic effects encountered. Therefore, an electrocardiogram and chest radiograph are obtained as a baseline. The patient with smoke inhalation specifically needs a chest radiograph and determinations of arterial blood gases and carboxyhemoglobin level.

Medications

All patients should have tetanus immunization updated or Hypertet and tetanus-diphtheria vaccine given if not previously immunized.

Narcotic analgesics should be administered intravenously.

Antibiotic use is controversial in the emergent phase of burn injury. Some burn physicians administer intravenous penicillin to prevent group A beta-hemolytic streptococcal infections. Other physicians prefer not to use antibiotics until there is a documented infection.

Wound Care

Care of the burn wound is considered only after the stabilization of the patient's condition has taken place. The initial wound care is directed toward removing soot and debris from the burn wound and débridement of broken blisters, cleansing of the wounds, and prevention of infection.

It is important to note that many burn units have transfer protocols for burn patients. These generally include a description of wound care that should take place prior to transfer. In some instances, especially if the burn unit is nearby, it may be requested that the patient only be washed and wrapped in a sterile sheet. This will allow for immediate visualization of the patient's wounds on arrival at the burn unit.

Cleansing and Débriding

The initial care of the burn wound should be accomplished in a clean, low-traffic area of the ED. Mask, gloves, and gown should be worn. Supplies needed for wound care include gauze sponges, small sterile bowls, instrument pack (containing scissors and forceps), sterile towels, gauze rolls, a topical antimicrobial cream, and antiseptic liquid soap. Wound care can be expedited by having all supplies open and accessible before starting.

Evaluate the patient's need for analgesic medication prior to wound care. Carefully explain the procedure and its importance in prevention of infection.

Wash the wound with a gauze sponge soaked in a diluted solution of antibacterial soap and water or saline solution. All soot, clothing fragments, dirt, and debris should be washed away. Loose epidermis will slough and blisters will break with slight pressure. Rinse with water or saline solution. Blistered areas are excised with scissors and forceps (Fig. 31–4). Hair is shaved to a one inch border of unburned skin. Eyebrows are not shaved because they may not grow back. A baseline wound culture should be obtained during débridement of blistered areas.

Once cleansing and débridement are accomplished, the wound may need to be reassessed for depth and extent of the burn injury. For patients not being transferred, an appropriate topical agent is applied and the wounds are covered with a bulky gauze dressing.

Topical Antimicrobials

A variety of topical antimicrobials are currently in use for the care of the burned patient, among them silver sulfadiazine, mafenide acetate, povidone-iodine, bacitra-

FIGURE 31–4. Débridement.

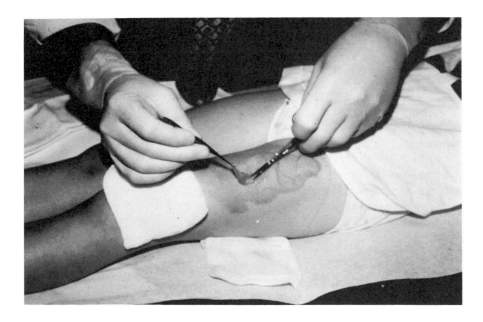

cin, and nitrofurazone. Topical antimicrobial therapy is aimed at controlling bacterial proliferation in the burn wound.

Silver sulfadiazine (Silvadene, SSD) is a mixture of a sulfa antibiotic and silver salt in a micronized water-soluble cream base. Its advantages are broad-spectrum coverage, low sensitivity, and painless application. The disadvantages are development of resistant strains of gram-negative bacteria, which proliferate after prolonged use on major burn wounds, and occasional leukopenia and hypersensitivity.

Mafenide acetate (Sulfamylon) is also a sulfa drug in a water-soluble cream base. The advantages of Sulfamylon are broad-spectrum coverage, especially against resistant gram-negative bacteria — specifically *Pseudomonas* species — and easy penetration into eschar. The disadvantages are pain or burning on application, occasional hypersensitivity, and a metabolic acidosis secondary to carbonic anhydrase inhibition. Fungus infection is not controlled by mafenide acetate. Sulfa-containing drugs should not be used in the last trimester of pregnancy because of adverse effects on the fetus.

Povidone-iodine (Betadine) is an iodine-containing antimicrobial solution or ointment. It has a broad spectrum against gram-negative and gram-positive organisms and is very effective against fungi. Serum iodine levels may rise, but no adverse effects are seen from this.

Silver nitrate solution, 0.5%, is applied as a wet dressing. It has antimicrobial properties against staphylococci, streptococci and *Pseudomonas* and is inexpensive. Problems include discoloration of everything that comes into contact with the solution, lack of eschar penetration, and severe electrolyte imbalances. Silver nitrate solution is used only in burn units and dressings must be constantly remoistened to keep them wet; the solution cannot be used for outpatient care.

Other agents, such as bacitracin (Baciguent) and nitrofurazone (Furacin), also are used, but not generally as the primary topical agent. Bacitracin ointment may be used on facial burns (especially on the lips and eyelids). It produces few allergic responses, and its appearance on the face (colorless) is better than white antibacterial creams.

Topical antimicrobial creams are generally applied 1/8-inch thick with sterile gloved hands or sterile tongue blades. Silvadene may be applied a little thicker, but Sulfamylon should be applied in a thin layer because it may be difficult to remove.

Dressings

Many burn units practice an open method of wound treatment (wounds are not dressed with gauze after the application of topical antimicrobial cream). It is best to check with the receiving hospital about its protocol before applying a dressing.

If dressings are to be placed, continue to observe sterile technique by using sterile gauze and gloves. Pure, coarse, cotton gauze is the best to use, because it is absorbent and it promotes mechanical débridement of the wound with its removal. Synthetic gauzes often are not absorbent and may cause maceration by leaving lint in the wound. Extremities are loosely wrapped with circular gauze rolls from distal to proximal direction in a figure-of-eight fashion to aid venous return (Fig. 31–5). Gauze should be placed between burned fingers and toes before wrapping. It may be necessary to leave a portion of the gauze open after wrapping to obtain blood pressure

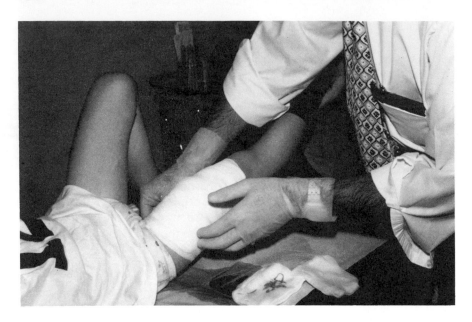

FIGURE 31–5. Figure-of-eight dressing.

readings or to monitor pulses. Large gauze sponges may be used to cover trunk burns. It may be helpful to hold gauze in place with tubular elastic netting, which is less irritating than tape. To allow for an adequate airway and facial muscle motion, dressings are not usually applied to the face.

If a patient has open lacerations or has had an escharotomy, it may be necessary to protect subcutaneous structures, such as muscle, tendon, or bone. The topical antimicrobial cream is applied directly to the area and covered with a saline-soaked gauze.

SPECIFIC THERMAL INJURIES

Flame Burns

Flame burns constitute over 50% of all burn injuries and are associated with smoke inhalation about 20% of the time. The added smoke inhalation increases morbidity and doubles the predicted mortality for the burn injury.

Clinical Manifestations

Most often flame burns are full-thickness injuries with only a narrow rim of partial-thickness injury. Frequently areas of the body covered by many layers of clothing (such as the belt line) are spared or are burned to a lesser extent. The burn wounds often are sooty and covered with carbonaceous debris. Loose skin and blisters may cover portions of the burn wound (Fig. 31–6).

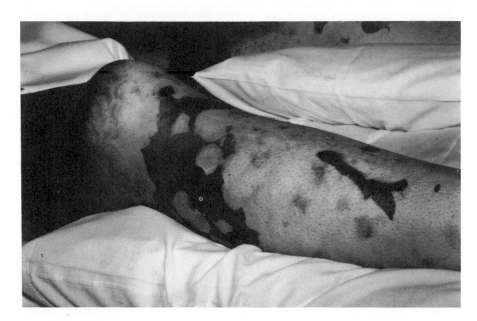

FIGURE 31–6. Burn wound covered with carbonaceous debris.

Scald Burns

One third of all injuries are scald burns. These injuries primarily occur in the bathtub or shower or from hot liquids and steam. Scald burns are very common in the pediatric age group and also are common in child abuse.

Clinical Manifestations

Scald burns are usually partial-thickness injuries. The liquid will produce an immersion, splash, or spill pattern with the central injury being the deepest. As the liquid flows away, it cools and the periphery has a more superficial burn. It takes 6 minutes in water at 130°F to produce a full-thickness burn but only seconds in water at 160°F (Fig. 31–7).

   Clothing may hold the heat and should be removed quickly at the scene.

   A child or noncommunicative adult with an immersion burn pattern (that is, an area of the body that looks as if it had been dipped into hot liquid, without areas of splash) should be evaluated for abuse.

Treatment and Nursing Care

The initial priority in care of the stable patient with flame or scald burns is cooling of the burn. This can be accomplished by applying dressing compresses moistened with cool distilled water. Frequent moistening and reapplication of the compresses is

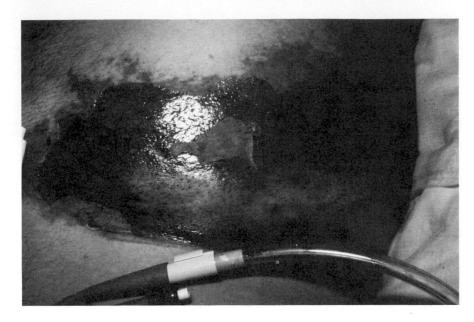

FIGURE 31–7. Scald burn.

necessary to assure continued cooling. A mild soap (e.g., Joy dishwashing soap) may be added to the distilled water.

Care of the patient with a burn injury of more than 20% BSA is best accomplished in a burn unit. The patient with a moderate burn injury (10 to 20% BSA) should be treated as an in-patient on a surgical service if the admitting physician is knowledgeable about caring for burn injuries. Minor burn wounds (10% BSA or less) can usually be treated on an outpatient basis.

The patient who has a minor burn and will be discharged from the hospital will require wound care, prescriptions, instructions, follow-up evaluation, and perhaps supportive services. It is the responsibility of the ED nurse to facilitate these plans for the patient.

With all burn injuries, tetanus immunization should be updated. Wound care of the minor burn is accomplished with clean (not sterile) technique. The patient or family is taught wound care while the nurse is carrying it out. Analgesic medication may be necessary prior to caring for the wound. The wound is cleansed and débrided. A topical antimicrobial is applied and covered with a fairly bulky gauze dressing. The patient will require both verbal and written instruction because his or her ability to retain information may be impaired owing to pain and anxiety.

Prescriptions for topical antimicrobial and pain medication should be given. Follow-up care is essential in most cases. A referral for follow-up in the ED, burn clinic, or private physician's office should be arranged prior to discharge from the ED.

A person with no family or assistance at home may require help with burn care. The Visiting Nurses' Association and other nursing agencies are easily contacted and can provide in-home nursing support for burn wound care. The patient without insurance and with limited financial resources may require assistance from the hospital social worker to obtain resources available to him or her.

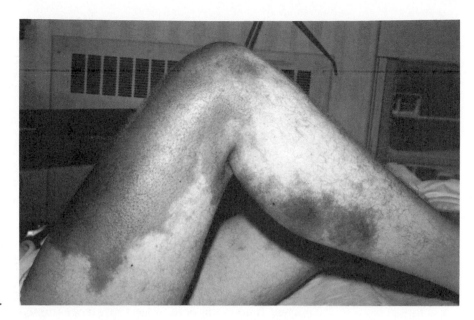

FIGURE 31–8. Alkali burn.

Chemical Burns

Chemical injuries account for a much smaller percentage of hospital admissions. Chemical agents are considered to be either acid or alkali. More than 25,000 products are available that are capable of producing a chemical burn.

Clinical Manifestations

Chemical agents are primarily liquid and produce burn injuries that may have a spill pattern to them. Most chemicals will produce a full-thickness burn by coagulating tissue protein, which results in cellular death. The depth of burn is related to type and concentration of chemical and duration of exposure. Alkali tends to penetrate deeper into the tissues, producing deep necrosis and placing the patient at risk for systemic absorption and toxicity. The burn wound often develops an eschar with or without blister. The eschar may be soft, appear depressed from the surrounding skin, and can range in color from white to yellow-green depending upon the causative agent (Fig. 31–8).

Treatment and Nursing Care

The treatment in the first hour following a chemical injury can greatly affect the depth of the burn. The most important action is to flush the area copiously with tap water for a minimum of 30 minutes. All clothing containing chemical must be removed. No effort should be made to neutralize an acid burn with an alkali or vice versa at the scene because the combination of the chemicals is exothermic and may further damage the skin. Dry powder should be brushed off first and then the area should be flushed with water. After adequate flushing, the chemical burn wound is treated as are all other burn wounds. The following special circumstances exist:

Hydrofluoric acid burn wounds are special in that they need to be flushed with water and then neutralized with an injection of calcium chloride into the burn wound. The calcium precipitates the fluoride ion, preventing penetration into deeper tissue. Without this, the chemical reaction would continue and the patient would note continued severe pain in the wound.

Chemical burns of the eyes need an ophthalmologist's evaluation as soon as possible. The initial flushing with saline solution or water should be carried out. An alkali burn of the cornea may lead to global perforation because of its continued chemical reaction with the eye tissues if it is not recognized and adequately flushed with water or saline solution.

Electrical Burns

Electrical burns involve less than 10% of the burn injured population. Electrical current follows the path of least resistance through the body. The severity of electrical injury depends on voltage, tissue resistance, pathways of current through the body, and length of exposure to the current. Current that passes through vital organs, such as the heart or brain, can produce serious internal damage. Fibrillation, dysrhythmias, and even evidence of a myocardial infarction may be present. The muscles and nerves in the arms or legs may be severely damaged. Respiratory arrest may occur if the current passes through the brain stem.

Clinical Manifestations

Electrical injury produces deep, well-circumscribed wounds at the points of entry and exit, with extensive underlying damage. The electrical arcing may cause further flame burns and can ignite the patient's clothes.

Entrance and exit sites may be charred and dry and painless. Often the exit site (or sites) is larger than the entrance site. Burns at these sites are usually full-thickness and often extend to muscle and bone. The areas have well-defined borders and become very edematous (Figs. 31–9 and 31–10).

Treatment and Nursing Care

Nursing assessment of the electrically injured patient must be performed in a thorough fashion because, even though the skin surface injury is small, the internal injuries may be major. Care must be taken to evaluate for other injuries. The patient may have fallen or have been thrown as a result of the electrical shock. A baseline electrocardiogram (EKG) and cardiographic monitoring for 24 hours (or until the patient's condition remains stable beyond that) are necessary as the electrical current can cause cardiac irritability. Cardiac arrest due to ventricular fibrillation is not unusual. Radiographs should be taken to determine the possibility of fractures from

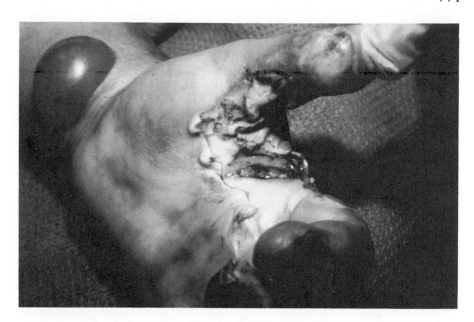

FIGURE 31–9. Full-thickness
electrical burn of the hand.

falls. Both entrance and exit sites should be determined. The scalp, which is covered
with a thick coat of hair, may hide an entrance or exit site. It will be necessary to shave
the head if there is a wound present.

The passage of the electrical current through the extremity will damage muscle
cells, leading to release of the muscle protein myoglobin, which enters the circulation
and is excreted by the kidney. The nurse must ensure adequate hydration to prevent
the myoglobin from precipitating in the kidney tubules, which will cause acute

FIGURE 31–10. Charred electrical burn of foot.

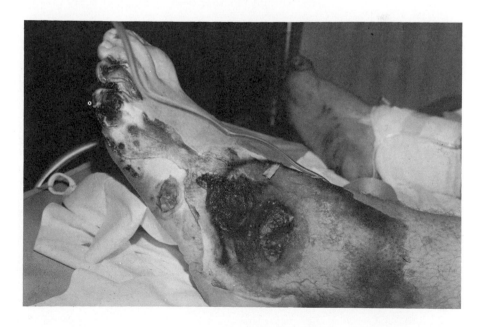

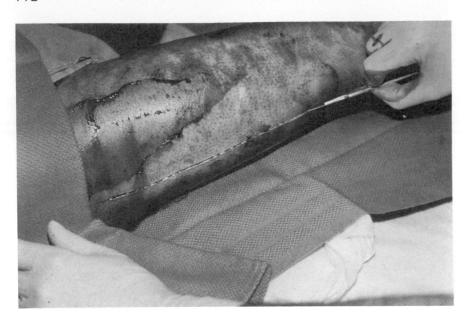

FIGURE 31–11.   Incision for fasciotomy.

tubular necrosis. Urine containing the excreted myoglobin protein may appear bloody, but it is not. Intravenous fluids (lactated Ringer's solution) must be given at a rate to maintain a urine output of 75 to 100 ml/hour. In addition, it is suggested that the use of mannitol (12.5 g) *or* sodium bicarbonate (44.5 mEq/L of lactated Ringer's solution) is beneficial. Mannitol initiates diuresis and sodium bicarbonate alkalinizes the urine. Both promote the excretion of the myoglobin. Internal muscle damage and swelling may necessitate fasciotomies in the first 24 hours to release the tension in the muscle compartments (Figs. 31–11 and 31–12). Arterial pulses in affected extremities should be monitored by Doppler every 30 minutes.

FIGURE 31–12.   Fasciotomy.

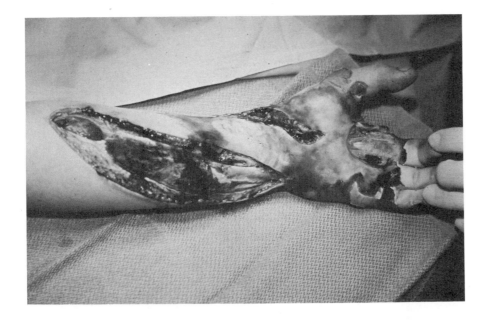

Laboratory evaluation of serum and urine myoglobin (because of potential muscle damage) and cardiac isoenzymes (because of potential cardiac and skeletal muscle damage) should be performed in addition to usual laboratory evaluation.

Sunburn

Patients with sunburn or sunlamp injuries are usually more in need of comfort measures or rehydration than they are of antibiotic therapy or hospitalization. Blistering may not develop for 24 to 36 hours after a sunburn because the partial-thickness damage is usually very superficial. Pain medication and a lanolin-containing lotion with a topical anesthetic will help relieve pain and add moisture to the skin for the first day or two. As with other partial-thickness burn injuries, significant blistering should be treated with a topical antimicrobial cream.

Hot Tar

Burns caused by hot tar or asphalt are particularly difficult to treat. The hot mass of tar adheres to the skin and continues to burn until cooled. Therefore, treatment includes immediate cooling of the tar at the scene and subsequent removal of the tar in the ED. This is a major undertaking for the nursing staff and often requires several nurses working tediously to remove the tar. A variety of methods can be used for tar removal. Bacitracin ointment softens the tar and, at the same time, provides antibiotic protection to the injured skin. Other solvents, such as mineral oil and nonirritating adhesive removers, can also be used. The tar often pulls off the outer layer of skin and hair shafts before coming loose. The larger the mass of tar and the hotter the tar on contact, the more likely it is that the burn injury will be full-thickness.

Hot Object

A hot object burn, such as from an iron, will leave an imprint of the object on the skin. The injury may be partial- or full-thickness depending on the temperature and length of contact.

TREATMENT AND NURSING CARE

Complications of major burn injury affect all organ systems. In the immediate hours after a burn injury, the major systems affected are respiratory, circulatory, and gastrointestinal. Stage I care focuses on stabilization of the burn patient's condition.

Ventilatory failure may progress rapidly in the patient with inhalation injury. Therefore, the nurse must anticipate and plan for a variety of treatments, including potential intubation, cricothyrotomy, or tracheostomy. All patients with smoke inhalation should receive high-flow humidified oxygen by mask. The clinical signs and symptoms and response to treatment will guide further therapy. Aggressive tracheobronchial toilet, use of bronchodilators, intubation, and mechanical ventilation may become necessary.

Serum carboxyhemoglobin levels should be determined; levels of 8 to 40% are not uncommon in persons involved in a fire. Levels of 50% or higher are generally accompanied by coma and brain damage from hypoxia. The patient with elevated carboxyhemoglobin levels should receive 100% oxygen until the level has returned to normal (less than 4%). Hyperbaric therapy (when available) provides the most rapid treatment by saturating the blood with oxygen at high pressures. Arterial blood gas determinations will provide more data as well as provide guidelines for treatment. An arterial pH of 7.35 or less, Po_2 of 60 mmHg or less, and Pco_2 of 40 mmHg or more paired with a respiratory rate of 40 or more breaths per minute suggests severe smoke inhalation and impending ventilatory failure.

The risk of loss of the airway is great in the patient with smoke inhalation. Therefore, early intubation to protect the airway is safest. The nurse should prepare for intubation by gathering necessary supplies, informing other caregivers (e.g., respiratory therapists), and explaining the procedure to the patient. If the patient is not in respiratory failure and can speak, the nurse can help to alleviate the patient's anxiety by prearranging a method of communication before intubation. This may include use of pad and paper if the patient is able to use them or simply eliciting yes and no responses from the patient.

Ideally, endotracheal intubation is performed because there is less risk of infection, but when heat damage to the upper airway has been severe or left untreated, airway edema or spasm might make endotracheal intubation difficult or impossible and cricothyrotomy or tracheostomy will be the alternative. The nurse must anticipate the need for sterile gowns and drapes because although this procedure is optimally performed in the operating room, it may need to be performed urgently in the ED.

The physician may wish to perform a bronchoscopy before intubation, although this usually occurs after the patient's condition is stable. The purpose for this might be strictly to obtain more information by visualizing the lower airway or to provide deep, thorough tracheobronchial toilet through a cleansing bronchoscopy. Soot, burns, and edema in the lower airway are demonstrative of the inhalation injury, and the patient should be intubated if this has not already been done to protect the airway.

The patient may become extremely anxious owing to hypoxia or the fear of unknown procedures. The nurse must ensure adequate pain relief with narcotic analgesics. In addition, the nurse can do much to relieve the patient's anxiety by careful explanation of procedures and by always providing an avenue of communication for the patient.

The nurse must continuously evaluate treatment by assessing the patient's behavior, obtaining and interpreting laboratory results and monitoring vital signs, auscultating lung fields, and observing chest expansion and use of accessory muscles.

Breathing Pattern, Ineffective, Related to

- *Constriction Interfering with the Mechanics of Breathing*

In addition to inhalation injury, circumferential burns of the upper abdomen, chest, or neck also compromise respiratory effort. As edema formation progresses, circumferential eschar becomes constricting. These burns, when on the chest or abdomen, interfere with the mechanics of breathing. When the burns are on the neck, actual mechanical obstruction may occur. Signs and symptoms include inability to handle secretions, hoarseness, stridor, air hunger, and extreme respiratory effort. Arterial blood gas determination will show a rising Pco_2 and a falling Po_2 with eventual respiratory arrest.

If the patient is not severely symptomatic, the tidal volume may be measured to determine the patient's ability to ventilate. This can be a useful periodic measurement to determine the patient's need for assistance.

Endotracheal intubation or tracheostomy may become necessary depending on the patient's condition. An escharotomy, which is an incision through the eschar into the underlying tissue, may be required to relieve constrictions of the extremities or chest (Fig. 31–13). This procedure is performed with a scalpel over the cleansed (antiseptically prepared) burn wound. The nurse's responsibility during this procedure is to provide patient comfort and to help control local bleeding, which may require application of pressure or suturing.

Stage II care involves evaluating effectiveness of treatment. Close patient observation and assessment of respiratory status for deterioration are essential. Monitoring of arterial blood gases contributes data indicating signs of respiratory compromise.

Fluid Volume Deficit, Intravascular, Related to

- ### Interstitial Fluid Sequestration Secondary to Leaky Capillary Syndrome

A major burn (greater than 20%) results in progressive hypovolemia owing to loss of vascular fluid into the burn wound. If an intravenous line has not been established previously, it is necessary to obtain at least one venous route with a large-bore catheter.

Peripheral line placement in an unburned area is preferred because of the risk of infection. However, central line placement or venous cutdown through a burn

FIGURE 31–13. Proper sites for escharotomy.

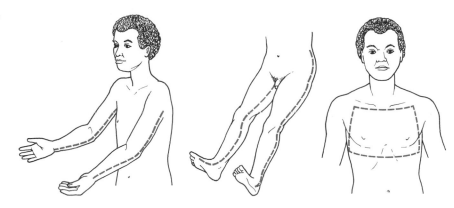

wound may be necessary if venous access is limited by the burn size. Multiple intravenous routes may be necessary if fluid replacement volumes are large. An indwelling Foley catheter is inserted and urine output is closely monitored. Large volumes of lactated Ringer's solution will be needed intravenously to maintain cardiovascular stability for the patient with a major burn wound. Colloids are not usually given in the first 24 hours because increased capillary permeability allows leaking of the protein into the interstitium, adding to edema formation.

A number of formulas may be used for fluid resuscitation of the burn patient (Table 31–3). The Parkland Formula is the most widely used and accepted guide for fluid requirements during the first 24 hours. The Parkland Formula supplies 4 ml of lactated Ringer's solution multiplied by the body weight (in kilograms) multiplied by the burn size (BSA). For example, a 70-kg person with a 50% burn will require 14,000 ml of lactated Ringer's solution in the first 24 hours. One half of this amount (7000 ml) is given in the first 8 hours, and one quarter (3500 ml) is given in the second and third 8-hour periods. It should be noted that the first 8-hour period begins at the time of burn, not at initiation of fluid therapy. Therefore, it is not uncommon to give a fluid bolus initially in the ED.

The goal of fluid therapy is to maintain an adequate vascular volume and prevent fluid overload. In a previously healthy individual, a urine output of 0.5 to 1.0 ml/kg/hour or 30 to 50 ml/hour for most adults can be used as a measure of adequate fluid replacement.

Cardiac monitoring of the patient with a major burn is important because electrolyte imbalances and hypovolemia may cause dysrhythmia. Measurement and recording of intake and output must be extremely accurate to evaluate effectiveness of fluid replacement. This also provides the receiving hospital or unit with much needed information.

Pediatric burn victims need closer observation during their fluid resuscitation because their normal requirements (i.e., unburned) are proportionally greater than an adult's. Lactated Ringer's solution given by the Parkland Formula of 4 ml/kg/% BSA for major burns should provide adequate resuscitation, but smaller burns, of less than 25% BSA, may require additional fluids over the amounts estimated by the Parkland Formula. The goal is an adequate blood pressure, pulse, and urine output in the child, which may require more fluid than the burn formula estimated.

Stage II care involves measurement of the urine output and vital signs every 30 to 60 minutes to evaluate the effectiveness of therapy. The urine will be dark, with a high specific gravity (1.035 to 1.040) if the vascular volume is inadequate. The volume of intravenous fluid is adjusted (or titrated) up or down to maintain a urine output of 0.5 to 1.0 ml/kg/hour, a heart rate between 60 and 140 beats/minute, and a systolic blood pressure between 100 and 140 mmHg. The central venous pressure (CVP) (if available) will be low or negative. It is not advisable to try to "catch up" with the formula calculations by speeding the intravenous rate or slowing down if excess volumes were given unless the blood pressure (less than 100 or greater than 140 systolic), pulse (less than 60 or greater than 140 beats/minute), urine output (less than 30 ml or greater than 70 ml/hour adult), and CVP (less than −1 or greater than +2) indicate a need for change. As fluid replacement progresses, the urine will clear and the specific gravity will decrease. If the response to fluid replacement is not favorable within 2 hours of its initiation, the burn size should be recalculated and intravenous catheter placement checked. A urine output of more than 70 ml/hour

TABLE 31-3
Fluid Therapy for Burn Victims

Evans Formula

    Dr. Everett Idris Evans introduced the first formula in 1952. He calculated the amount of fluid to be replaced by taking into consideration both the size of the wound and the weight of the patient. Evans recommended that the total estimated amount of colloids and crystalloids (electrolytes) be given during the first 24 hours and one half of this amount be given during the next 24 hours with an appropriate amount of glucose to cover insensible water loss. He was the first to caution that in a burn involving more than 50% of the body surface, to avoid overhydration the fluid requirements should be estimated as though only 50% of the body surface had been burned.

Brooke Formula

    The Brooke Formula was first published in 1953 and is a modification of the Evans Formula. This formula estimates the following requirements for the first 24 hours after a burn:

Colloids (blood, dextran, plasma): 0.5 ml/kg/% BSA burned.

Crystalloids (lactated Ringer's–Hartmann's solution): 1.5 ml/kg of body weight/% BSA.

Water (5% glucose in water): Dependent on age and size of patient to replace insensible fluid loss.

    One half of the estimated fluid requirements for the first 24 hours is given in the first 8 hours, one quarter of the total in the second 8 hours, and one quarter of the total in the third 8-hour period. The second 24-hour period requirements for colloids and lactated Ringer's–Hartmann's solution is about one half that for the first 24 hours. In applying this formula to burns of larger than 50%, requirements must be calculated as though only 50% of the body had been burned.

Parkland (Baxter) Formula

    The Baxter Formula recommends crystalloid replacement only in the first 24-hour period, given at a replacement rate of 4 ml of solution per kilogram of body weight times percentage of burn up to 50% total body area. Half of this amount is given in the first 8 hours. Colloids are not given in the first 24 hours because Baxter did not find a significant reduction in need for crystalloid when colloids were given in the first 24 hours. However, colloids are given in the second 24 hours after the burn and are effective in correcting residual plasma volume deficits.

EXAMPLE: 70-kg patient, 25 years of age, with 50% total area burned.

FIRST 24 HOURS:

Colloid Solutions (blood, plasma, plasma expander): None.

Electrolytes (lactated Ringer's–Hartmann's solution): 4 ml $\times$ 70 kg $\times$ 50% = 14,000 ml *in first 24 hours.*

Glucose in Water: None (2 L given in second 24-hour period).

TOTAL 24 HOUR INTAKE: 14,000 ml

RATE OF ADMINISTRATION:

1/2	1/4	1/4
First 8 hours after burn 7000 ml	Second 8 hours after burn 3500 ml	Third 8 hours after burn 3500 ml

    From Emergent Care of the Burn Victim, 1979, p 540 National Institute for Burn Medicine, with permission.

    Although fluid therapy should be individualized for each patient, it is useful to complete calculation of a formula as a guideline and make a 24-hour double check to prevent copious fluid replacement and overload.

along with an increased blood pressure and pulmonary rales are indications of fluid overload and should be treated immediately with restriction of infused fluids.

    The patient with a large burn injury or the elderly patient may need more invasive monitoring of cardiac status (such as pulmonary artery catheter monitoring) during resuscitation because of decreased myocardial reserve. The risk of catheter infection should be considered against the benefit of the information gained. Because of this risk, invasive monitoring of the burn patient should be done in a burn unit.

Tissue Perfusion, Altered (Peripheral), Related to

• *Vasoconstriction*

The release of vasoactive substances after a thermal injury causes an intense vasoconstriction. This, combined with the constricting effects of circumferential eschar over swelling tissue, can have a profound effect on the peripheral circulation.

Clinical presentation of compromised circulation includes numbness and decreased sensation, decreased capillary refill, cyanosis, and diminished or absent peripheral pulses. Monitoring of peripheral pulses on affected extremities is necessary at least every 1 to 2 hours during the first 24 hours. Pulses should be palpated from distal to proximal (e.g., radial artery, brachial artery). If pulses are not palpable, they should be obtained by Doppler ultrasound directly over the course of the artery even if over the burn wound. If pulses are absent or diminished, an escharotomy will need to be performed (Fig. 31 – 13). Preparation for an escharotomy includes explanation of the procedure to the patient, antibiotic preparation solution, scalpel, suturing instrument, and sterile towels. Bleeding (if any) is controlled with direct pressure or suturing with an absorbable type of suture material. Once the incision has been made, the eschar separates, thus relieving the underlying pressure with a return of a peripheral pulse. These areas are washed and dressed with the antibiotic cream as are the rest of the burn wounds during wound care.

Gastrointestinal Dysfunction,* Related to

• *Major Burns*

Patients with burns of 20% BSA or greater will develop gastric dilation and ileus of the small bowel. Hypovolemia causes constriction of the splenic blood vessels. Symptoms include nausea and vomiting, abdominal distention, pain, and an absence of bowel sounds.

The nurse should anticipate development of an ileus and prepare to insert a nasogastric tube or sump and connect to intermittent suction. This decreases the risk of vomiting and aspiration. The patient with a major burn should be given nothing by mouth during the first 24 hours. Antacid therapy may be initiated in the ED in an effort to prevent stress-related ulcerations of the stomach (Curling's ulcer), which have been shown to develop early.

Pain, Related to

• *Major Burn*

Many factors influence a patient's response to pain. These include cultural influences, previous experience with illness or hospitalization, severity of injury, and personal losses as a result of the injury.

---

* Non – NANDA-approved nursing diagnosis.

Narcotic analgesics should be administered as soon as the patient is hemodynamically stable and other injuries are ruled out. It is necessary to administer pain medication intravenously so that absorption and drug effects are reliable and observable. Generally morphine (2 to 25 mg) or meperidine (5 to 15 mg), administered in small increments to avoid hypotension and respiratory depression, is the drug of choice.

Stage II care involves careful assessment of effectiveness of medications in reducing pain and monitoring for hypotension and respiratory depression. Emotional support, calm explanations, and reassuring the patient that analgesics will be provided for pain will often reduce the quantity of analgesics needed.

Application of saline-soaked towels may cool and relieve pain in partial-thickness wounds but should be limited for the patient with major burn injury because of the potential of hypothermia. Avoid placing ice directly on the burn wounds because the cold can cause further thermal damage. Diversionary techniques, such as conversation or counting, and relaxation techniques, such as rhythmic breathing, in addition to analgesics may help the patient get through the pain of a difficult procedure or wound care.

Family Processes, Altered, Related to

• *Ill Family Member*

A major burn injury is one of the most devastating traumas a patient can endure. The burn-injured patient may be alert and talking on arrival to the emergency department. He or she may appear to have minimal discomfort, especially if the burns are full-thickness. For this reason it is imperative that health care givers remain as calm and as direct as possible. The burned person sustains many physiologic as well as psychologic stresses. In addition to causing pain, the injury itself produces many anxieties, including fear of the unknown, powerlessness, change in body image, and fear of death. The burned person's psychologic well-being and his or her social support greatly affect the outcome of the injury. The ED nurse promotes this well-being by providing simple explanations, comfort measures, and skillful, knowledgeable care.

When considering emotional response, the patient and family should be looked on as a unit. The ED nurse is often the first health care professional to have contact with the patient's family. They may have to wait a period of time before being allowed to see the patient. The nurse can allay much of their anxiety by giving short but frequent progress reports. The family must be prepared verbally prior to seeing the patient. A detailed description of edema formation, burn wound appearance, and tubes and machinery in place should be given. Family members often imagine much worse than the reality of what has happened.

It is equally important to include the family in anxiety-relieving efforts. Their support for the patient and cooperation with the health care team is crucial to the patient's participation in his or her care and even to the patient's survival. The intubated patient will have an increased anxiety owing to an inability to communicate. This person should not be left alone but given the opportunity to communicate either by written means or by responding with yes and no to questions.

Occasionally the burn injury is a result of a suicide attempt. This person may be violent and abusive, requiring restraints and sedation, or he or she may be withdrawn with no response to painful stimuli. In either case, it is best to involve a psychiatric professional as early as possible.

TRANSFER GUIDELINES

Many hospitals do not have the resources available for the patient with major burn injuries (more than 25% BSA). Once the patient's condition is stabilized — that is, the airway maintained and burn shock treatment begun — the patient can be safely transferred. There may or may not be a choice of burn facilities, depending on the geographic area. Metropolitan areas may have three or four burn units that are relatively equidistant, and rural areas may have only one possibility many miles away. In either case, it is important to have telephone contact with the nearest burn unit early on. This will establish bed availability as well as provide more information for the transfer plan and treatment protocols.

The following responsibilities must be agreed upon between the two physicians: who will arrange transport; whether transport will be ground or air; who will accompany the patient; and what additional medical support may be necessary during the transfer. The transport vehicle should be equipped as a Mobile Intensive Care Unit with trained staff. Generally, air transportation is used when the burn unit is more than 60 miles away, when the transport is occurring during heavy traffic hours, or when either the sending or the receiving hospital is equipped with their own air ambulance service.

Information about the following must be communicated between the ED nurse or physician and the burn unit nurse or physician: airway; fluid therapy (including intake and output); pertinent history; all medications given; wound care; escharotomy; patient's emotional response; and other treatment given, such as nasogastric tube, Foley catheter, or arterial line insertion. The receiving hospital will want to know the estimated time of arrival.

Many burn units have printed transfer protocols that they are willing to share with any ED in their region. The use of such a protocol helps expedite care for the patient at both facilities. A directory of burn facilities in the United States is available from the American Burn Association.

CONCLUSION

Emergent care of the burn victim in order of priority includes airway management, fluid resuscitation, emotional support, wound care, and pain relief. This is a challenge to all the caregivers, especially to the ED nurse who has only infrequent experience with patients with major burns. An understanding of the pathophysiologic changes that occur with the burn injury will help the nurse to provide skillful physical care to the patient. Anticipating and providing for the patient's and family's emotional needs will help pave the way for good communication, cooperation with care, and rapid healing.

REFERENCES

Artz C, Moncrief J, Pruitt B. 1979. Burns: A Team Approach. Philadelphia, WB Saunders Co.

Braen GP. Emergency Management of Major Thermal Burns. 1977. Kansas City, MO, Marion Laboratories.

Desai MH. Inhalation injuries in burn victims. 1984. CCQ 7(3):1–7.

Edlich RF, Haynes BW, Larkham V, et al. 1978. Emergency department treatment, triage and transfer protocols for the burn patient. J Am Coll Emerg Phys 7:152–158.

Feller I, Jones CA. 1973. Nursing the burned patient. Ann Arbor, MI, Institute for Burn Medicine.

Freeman JW. 1984. Nursing care of the patient with a burn injury. Crit Care Nurse 4(6):51–68.

Jacoby F. 1984. Care of the massive burn wound. CCQ 7(3):44–53.

Johnson C, O'Shaughnessy EJ, Fostergren G, et al.

1981. Burn management. New York, Raven Press.

Kenner C. Thermal injuries. 1984. In Beyers M, Dudas S, eds. The Clinical Practice of Medical-Surgical Nursing. Boston, Little, Brown and Company, 1411–1449.

Klein DG, O'Malley P. 1987. Topical injury from chemical agents: initial treatment. Heart Lung 16:49–54.

Richardson JD, Polk H, Flint L. 1987. Trauma: Clinical Care and Pathophysiology. Chicago, Year Book Medical Publishers.

Roberts ML, Pruitt B. 1979. Nursing care and psychological considerations. In Burns: A Team Approach. Philadelphia, WB Saunders Co., 370.

Wachtel T, Kahn V, Frank H. 1983. Current Topics in Burn Care. Rockville, MD, Aspen Publications.

Marianne Genge, RN MS

Surface Trauma

Surface trauma, or trauma to the skin, is a common cause for admission to the emergency department (ED). Skin trauma may be due to any one of the following: burns, falls, industrial accidents, motor vehicle accidents, gunshot wounds, and human or animal bites. These injuries often occur in conjunction with other life-threatening injuries and therefore are given minimal attention initially. However, quick astute nursing care can limit psychologic as well as physical scarring from such injuries.

The skin is the largest organ in the body and serves to protect the other body parts from injury, infection, and dehydration. It also helps to regulate body temperature. The skin is composed of two layers of tissue: the epidermis and the dermis (Odland 1983). Beneath this is a layer of subcutaneous fatty tissue (Fig. 32–1). The epidermis, or surface layer, is avascular, is composed primarily of epithelial cells, and is 10% water (Griepp 1988). This layer is thicker on the dorsal and extensor surfaces of the body. The epidermis is the layer responsible for the regeneration of the skin and can do so if the necessary elements are left intact. The dermis is composed of connective tissue and fibroblasts, microphages, and fat cells. The dermal layer is vascular, with lymph channels and nerves. The structures that form hair, nails, and sebaceous and sweat glands begin in the dermis and extend to the epidermis.

Beneath the dermis lies a group of structures collectively called the hypodermis or subcutaneous tissues. Included in this layer are fat, smooth muscle, the areolar bed, blood vessels, and nerves. This layer cushions, insulates, and provides energy, owing to the fat and areolar bed present here (Thompson et al 1986).

The skin serves the following functions: protection, control of body tempera-

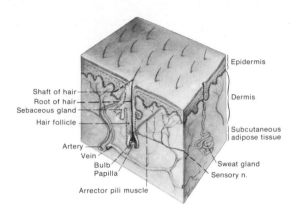

FIGURE 32–1. Cross section of the skin. (From Jacob SW, Francone CA. 1989. Elements of Anatomy and Physiology, 2nd ed. Philadelphia, W. B. Saunders.)

ture, primary sensation, excretion of water and salt as needed, preservation of body fluids, and production of vitamin D. Thus, injury to the skin can potentially have a profound effect on the rest of the body. Thorough nursing care can limit these effects.

INTEGUMENTARY ASSESSMENT

Surface trauma is not always a priority during the initial assessment of a patient. A thorough integumentary assessment is conducted only after airway, breathing, circulation, and life-threatening injuries have been stabilized.

Assessment of surface trauma should begin with a thorough history of the present injury. Where, when, and how did the injury occur? Timing of the injury is important. If surface injuries are more than 6 hours old, they should be considered contaminated and cared for differently than clean wounds (Knezevich 1986). For example, the area may need to be cleansed more thoroughly. Determining where the injury occurred can help establish how the wound may have been contaminated. What was the mechanism and force of the injury? Knowing the mechanism of injury can help determine what type of injury was sustained and what nursing care should be anticipated. What was the amount and type of bleeding (pulsating or oozing)? Did the patient experience pain? Is there any numbness or tingling distal to the injury? It should also be determined if any interventions had been done at the trauma scene. Who assisted the patient? Were any medications administered? How did the patient get to the ED?

A thorough medical history should also be obtained. The past medical history should include information regarding illnesses that may affect the integumentary system, such as diabetes or cardiovascular disease (with regard to healing), dermatologic problems, and bleeding disorders. The nurse should also note if the patient is presently taking any medications, such as aspirin, immunosuppressants, steroids, or anticoagulants; note also if the patient's tetanus immunization is current. A thorough medical history should provide the nurse with data that will enhance planning for care throughout the patient's ED stay.

After obtaining the past medical history, the nurse should obtain a complete psychosocial history. Surface trauma can often leave disfiguring scars. How has the patient coped with stress in the past? Does the patient have significant others who are supportive? The patient's body image and self-concept are areas that will need to be addressed in further depth after emergency care is given. The nurse needs to start obtaining information to set the groundwork for later nursing interventions.

Following the psychosocial history, the nurse should conduct a complete review of the systems with an emphasis on the skin. It should be determined if the patient has had any dermatologic problems prior to trauma. How quickly does the patient's skin normally heal? The nurse should gather sufficient data to anticipate which patients may develop complications in healing following trauma.

The age of the patient should be determined. The skin of the elderly is very friable, and the skin tears can be jagged. Peripheral vascular status is usually poorer in these patients also. Both factors can contribute to delayed healing and to infection. Nutritional status, which also contributes greatly to the healing process, should be assessed.

Inspection is the primary technique used in assessing the integument. The nurse should look for edema, location of foreign bodies, presence and location of necrotic tissue, color of the skin, and the extent of damage to the skin. The nurse should observe the patient flex, extend, abduct, adduct, and circumduct the affected limb. Because palpation might cause additional injury, infection, and pain, it is not used to a great degree with the integumentary system, although the nurse should palpate for tenderness and temperature. The nurse should evaluate the wound and describe the injury as completely as possible. Sensation should be tested by touch, pinprick, or two-point discrimination. Pulses distal to the wound should be assessed. In the case of facial wounds, the function of cranial nerves that innervate the face should be tested. Radiographs should be taken if the presence of a fracture or foreign body is suspected when surface trauma exists. Arteriograms can confirm loss of circulation.

ETIOLOGY AND PATHOPHYSIOLOGY

Surface trauma is basically a break in the continuity of the skin due to a stretching of the skin beyond its capacity, thus producing damage where the shear force is the greatest. As a result of such trauma, two physiologic responses occur: loss of the epithelial reactions and the inflammatory and vascular reactions. Loss of the integrity of the epithelial layer can lead to both fluid and electrolyte imbalances as well as an alteration in the body temperature. The severity of these consequences depends on how much epithelium is lost. Surface trauma includes open and closed wounds. An open wound involves a break in the skin with exposure of underlying tissue. Closed wounds, such as a contusion or bruise, have no breaks in the skin.

Surface trauma can be described according to the mechanism of injury: abrasions, avulsions, contusions, lacerations, and puncture wounds. An abrasion is a scrape in which either the skin or the mucous membrane is rubbed off. Usually both the epidermal and dermal layers are involved. An avulsion is a full-thickness skin loss whose edges cannot be approximated. A contusion does not break the skin and is caused by blunt trauma to superficial tissue. Blood extravasates into skin or mucous membranes. A laceration is a tear in the tissue. A puncture wound is usually caused by a pointed instrument that penetrates the tissue (Wolff et al 1983). Puncture wounds include human and animal bites. There is minimal blood loss with puncture wounds. Because they tend to seal off, they present the potential for infection.

The second response of the skin to trauma is its inflammatory and vascular reactions. Vasoactive elements released during the inflammatory response cause pain, edema, and vasodilation (redness). Because the scalp and face are very vascular, they tend to bleed profusely with lacerations and abrasions.

TREATMENT AND NURSING CARE

During stage I care the nurse addresses the most life-threatening patient needs, such as airway maintenance and circulation. Hemorrhage related to surface trauma needs to be controlled initially by direct pressure or elevation, or both. Supplemental oxygen may be administered.

General wound care is concerned with limiting the degree of scarring, preventing infection, decreasing the loss of mobility associated with such injuries, and basically closing the wound with the least amount of tissue damage possible (Stillman 1981). In the case of puncture wounds, the wound may be soaked for 15 to 20 minutes in an antiseptic soap solution to permit thorough débridement. Radiographs may be ordered to identify retained foreign bodies in the wound such as metal, stone, or wood. A xerogram is obtained to rule out retained glass fragments within the wound. At times, the puncture wound may need to be opened surgically to be examined and cleansed more thoroughly. Removal of foreign material is important not only to prevent infection but also to prevent significant scarring. It is suggested that the area not be shaved, as this tends to increase the risk for infection. Prophylactic intravenous antibiotics may be administered. Copious irrigation with normal saline is the preferred method of protection against infection. Débridement may be utilized for imbedded debris.

The method of wound closure depends on the degree of wound contamination and the extent of the injury. Primary closure is the approximation of wound edges within 6 to 8 hours of the time of trauma. Clean wounds are treated in this manner. Delayed primary closure is usually done for large, edematous, and infected wounds. In delayed primary closure, the wound is cleansed, debrided, and kept open for 3 to 5 days before suturing. This allows swelling and infection to run their course. A scar usually results following such a closure (Knezevich 1986). In some instances a sterile dressing may be sufficient wound care. A dressing is applied to a wound to absorb drainage and limit fluid loss and to protect the wound from further damage.

Infection, Potential for, Related to

- *Surface Trauma*
- *Foreign Matter in Wound*
- *Pre-existing Infection*

The nurse should inspect the wound thoroughly for foreign matter, which should be removed. The skin around the wound should be assessed for pre-existing infection, vascular compromise, and the severity of injury. A complete medical history and review of systems should be geared toward gaining an insight on potential risk factors for infection.

If the patient has diabetes, depending on how well it is controlled, there may be a poor vascular supply to the wound, contributing to delayed healing and a risk for infection. If the patient is immunosuppressed, this may also contribute to the risk of infection.

The wound should be thoroughly cleansed, and prophylactic antibiotics should be administered as ordered. The wound should be irrigated with normal saline solution under high pressure as needed. Current research does not support the use of iodine or surgical scrub solution. Cultures should be obtained from wound sites if the wound is an animal or human bite and if the object that caused the injury was contaminated with pathogenic organisms. Sterile technique should be followed during all dressing changes. Tetanus and rabies vaccinations should be administered as appropriate. (See Guidelines on TD and Tetanus Immunoglobin, Table 16–1.)

Skin Integrity, Impaired, Related to

- *Surface Trauma*

The nurse needs to assess the skin after admission to determine if the wound is increasing in severity. The skin is the patient's first line of defense against invading organisms. Assess the tissue surrounding a wound and attempt to salvage viable tissue. Thorough cleansing and dressing of the wound should foster these attempts.

Fluid Volume Deficit, Related to

- *Hemorrhaging Open Wounds*
- *Draining Wound*

If surface trauma reaches the dermis and below, bleeding will occur. If the trauma extends further, larger blood vessels may be injured and more bleeding can occur. Hemorrhaging is best stopped by direct pressure for a few minutes. Care should be taken to use sterile technique when pressure is applied to an open wound. If possible, clean wounds are closed within 6 hours. Dressings are applied to draining wounds in an attempt to limit drainage and contain fluid loss via evaporation.

Pain, Related to

- *Surface Trauma*

Nerve endings are not present in the epidermis but are present in the dermis and subcutaneous layers. Surface trauma pain can be managed well with mild oral analgesics.

Anxiety, Related to

- *Surface Trauma*
- *Potential for Disfigurement*

Surface trauma initially appears more severe than it actually is. Abrasions may bleed slightly, but they heal quickly without scarring, as do some lacerations. The nurse should explain to the patient the type of wound that has been sustained. The course of treatment and the probable outcome will probably be explained to the patient by the physician; however, the nurse can assist by clarifying and answering patient questions. The patient should be instructed on how to care for the wound appropriately to avoid infection. The patient should be allowed adequate time to ask questions to help alleviate anxiety.

EVALUATION

Ongoing evaluation of a patient with surface trauma includes assessing the severity of the injury and hemorrhage, and pain management. If the wound is minor, this is fairly simple. However, if the wound is associated with other trauma, it could be more challenging to manage.

Patients who are discharged from the ED with dressings on their wounds need to be taught wound care. They should be instructed regarding analgesic and possibly antibiotic therapy that has been prescribed. They should also be instructed to arrange a follow-up appointment with a physician.

CONCLUSION

Surface trauma may occur at any time over the lifespan. Although most such wounds are not life-threatening, emergency care is often needed to stop hemorrhage and at times prevent scarring. Emergency nursing care begins with stabilizing the patient and assessing which wounds need immediate attention, such as those with uncontrolled arterial hemorrhaging, scalp lacerations in which the patient has signs and symptoms of hypovolemia, and lacerations with neurovascular impairment. The nurse needs to determine in which cases treatment can be delayed, such as with many abrasions and contusions.

Discharge of the patient with surface trauma from the ED is usually to the home, if the wound is an isolated injury without complication. In the case of multiple trauma the patient is usually hospitalized. If the patient is discharged home, nursing care should include patient teaching regarding the basic process of wound healing and associated care of the wound, pain management, infection control, and follow-up care. The patient should also be cautioned to avoid direct sunlight to injured areas, which may now burn more easily.

Thus, the ED nurse's role is not limited only to treatment but extends to education of the patient.

REFERENCES

Griepp EB, Robbins ES. 1988. Epithelium. In Weiss, L, ed. Cell and Tissue Biology. Baltimore, Urban & Schwarzenberg, 115–148.

Knezevich BA. 1986. Trauma Nursing: Principles and Practice. Norwalk, CT, Appleton-Century-Crofts, 165–167.

Odland GF. 1983. Structure of the skin. In Goldsmith LA, ed. Biochemistry and Physiology of the Skin. New York, University Press, 3–63.

Peacock EE, VanWinkle W. 1976. Surgery and Biology of Wound Repair, 2nd ed. Philadelphia, WB Saunders Co, 271–366.

Stillman R. 1981. Wound closure: Choosing optional material and methods. Emergency Room Reports, 2(10).

Thompson JM, et al. 1986. Clinical Nursing. St. Louis, CV Mosby Co, 543–547.

Wolff LW, Weitzel MH, Zarnow RA, et al., eds. 1983. Fundamentals of Nursing. Philadelphia, JB Lippincott, 642–649.

Karen Blesch, RN MS

Oncologic Emergencies

Cancer patients may require emergency care for a wide variety of conditions that arise as a result of either their disease or its treatment. Many of the so-called oncologic emergencies are not unique to cancer patients; the same conditions may arise from a variety of nonmalignant causes (e.g., spinal cord compression related to severe rheumatoid arthritis, disseminated intravascular coagulation related to trauma, gastrointestinal bleeding related to gastric ulcers). However, when emergency conditions are associated with cancer, the underlying malignancy introduces special considerations for medical diagnosis and treatment as well as the patient's response to the emergency situation — the province of nursing.

The meaning of a trip to the emergency department (ED) may be very different for an individual with cancer as opposed to someone who is being treated for an acute, but nonetheless "curable," condition. To the person who has been living successfully with cancer for some time, the need for emergency care may be perceived as a setback in a long series of battles against the disease. Patients with advanced cancer whose conditions have deteriorated progressively may have thoughts of imminent death foremost in their minds. This may also preoccupy their significant others. And, for some persons with cancer, the ED may be "where it all started." Although this is not usually the case, it is not unheard of for a patient to come to the ED with superior vena cava syndrome, pain or shortness of breath, or symptoms of spinal cord compression, from widely disseminated but heretofore undiagnosed cancer. It is important, then, for the emergency nurse to be particularly sensitive, not only to the situational crisis normally precipitated by a need for emergency care, but also to the special emotional needs a person with cancer may have.

Almost all cancer patients require emergency care at some time during the course of their disease. The increasing ability to treat cancer successfully — for either cure or control — has increased the number of people living with cancer. Cancer is no longer considered an acute, immediately terminal disease. Rather, it becomes a chronic disease with remissions, relapses, and complications. It is usually for a complication of the disease or its treatment, or during a period of relapse, that an oncologic emergency arises.

This chapter identifies emergency situations that may be associated with cancer and proceeds to a discussion of the etiology, pathophysiology, clinical manifestations, treatment modalities, and nursing interventions for several specific oncologic emergencies.

ONCOLOGIC EMERGENCIES: AN OVERVIEW

Although most oncologic emergencies are not immediately life-threatening, many of them can lead to significant morbidity and mortality if not promptly and appropriately diagnosed and treated. Hospitalization is almost always required to stabilize and treat the problem. Table 33–1 provides a brief overview of potential oncologic emergencies as described by Arseneau and Rubin (1983). It should be remembered that many of these situations can arise outside of cancer. It is also important to be aware that cancer patients are just as likely to develop emergencies not related to their cancer as the rest of the population. Thus, although a history of cancer is useful in diagnosing an oncologic emergency, it should not be used to rule out the presence of other, "benign" pathophysiologic processes.

Determining if a patient has a history of cancer or cancer treatment is an essential part of the nurse's role when a patient has symptoms that could signal an oncologic emergency (Table 33–1). Some cancer patients, as do those with other chronic diseases, come to the ED frequently and become well known to emergency department personnel. This may be particularly true in a community setting. However, this familiarity with the patient's history should not bias the nurse and keep him or her from fully documenting the patient's presenting problem and considering other pathophysiologic processes that may be present. Therefore, while maintaining a high index of suspicion for oncologic emergencies, emergency department personnel also need to remain as objective as possible in their patient evaluations.

SPECIFIC DISORDERS

Spinal Cord Compression

Spinal cord compression is a true emergency in terms of morbidity, whose early symptoms may be misdiagnosed as benign musculoskeletal pain. Early cord com-

TABLE 33-1
Oncologic Emergencies

Condition	Etiology	Signs and Symptoms	Treatment
Cardiovascular System			
Pericardial tamponade	Pericardial metastases or radiation pericarditis causes fluid to accumulate in pericardial sac	Anxiety, oppressive chest discomfort, dyspnea, confusion, coma	Pericardiocentesis; pericardial radiation; surgical creation of "pericardial window"
Superior vena cava syndrome	Tumors in mediastinum (breast, lung, lymphoma) compress superior vena cava, resulting in fluid accumulation in upper body	Facial (periorbital), head, neck, upper extremity edema; cyanosis; clubbing of fingers	Immediate radiation therapy or chemotherapy (nitrogen mustard) to shrink mediastinal mass
Central Nervous System			
Increased intracranial pressure	Pressure from primary or metastatic brain or meningeal tumors	Headache, nausea, visual disturbances, personality changes, lethargy, coma	Prompt administration of corticosteroids (dexamethasone, 4 mg IV, q6 h); radiation therapy, intrathecal chemotherapy
Spinal cord compression	Lymphoma or tumors metastatic to vertebral bodies (lung, breast, prostate) or adjacent soft tissues puts pressure on spinal cord	Back pain, weakness of extremities, sensory changes, bowel or bladder dysfunction, overt paresis (advanced)	Corticosteroids (dexamethasone, 4 mg IV, q6 h); emergency decompression laminectomy; radiation therapy; chemotherapy
Gastrointestinal System			
Bowel obstruction	Primary (colon, lymphoma) or metastatic tumor (breast, ovary) compresses and ultimately occludes bowel lumen	Early satiety; cramping abdominal pain; constipation; nausea; vomiting (may be feculent)	IV fluids and electrolytes; nasogastric tube for decompression; surgery
Bowel perforation	Rupture of primary tumors of bowel or stomach or necrosis of gastrointestinal lymphomas induced by chemotherapy or radiation results in spillage of bowel contents into peritoneal cavity (peritonitis)	Sudden, severe abdominal pain; shock; fever; rigid abdomen	IV fluid and electrolyte support; antibiotic therapy to cover anaerobes; surgical exploration as soon as patient is stable
Esophageal obstruction or perforation	Primary esophageal tumor (occasionally lymphoma or metastatic lung tumor) compresses and obstructs esophagus (external) or ruptures it (internal)	Dysphagia, regurgitation, aspiration on swallowing	Nutritional support with total parenteral nutrition or gastrostomy feeding tube; surgery; radiation therapy; chemotherapy
Ascites	Portal hypertension secondary to metastatic liver disease (breast, colon), peritoneal carcinomatosus (ovary, breast, gastrointestinal malignancies), extensive gastric lymphoma cause accumulation of fluid in peritoneal cavity	Abdominal discomfort; difficulty eating; abdominal distention ("bloating"); dyspnea if severe	Diuretics (spironolactone, 25 mg qid); paracentesis; chemical sclerosis of peritoneal cavity; peritovenous shunt; control of underlying disease
Hematologic Emergencies			
Disseminated intravascular coagulation	Release of thromboplastin-like material from necrosing neoplastic cells after cytotoxic therapy (especially promyelocytic leukemia; prostate adenocarcinoma)	Internal or external hemorrhage	Transfuse fresh frozen plasma; intravenous heparin

TABLE 33-1
Oncologic Emergencies *(Continued)*

Condition	Etiology	Signs and Symptoms	Treatment
Leukostasis	In leukemias with peripheral blast cell count > 100,000/mm³, leukemic cells plug small capillaries, resulting in multiple microinfarctions and hemorrhage	Usually occurs in brain or lung with symptoms appropriate to affected organ; often fatal	Chemotherapy with hydroxyurea, 5000–6000 mg as a single dose
Thrombocytopenic hemorrhage	Bone marrow replacement with tumor (leukemia, lymphoma), intravascular coagulation, myelosuppression secondary to chemo- or radiation therapy results in thrombocytopenia	Circulating platelets < 20,000/mm³ places patient at risk; hemorrhage may be internal (intracranial, intraabdominal) or external	Platelet and blood and fluid replacement
Infectious Emergencies Leukopenic sepsis	Bone marrow suppression from chemo- or radiation therapy, or bone marrow replacement by neoplastic cells (leukemia, lymphoma, myeloma) severely compromises patient's ability to fight infection	WBC < 1000/mm³ places patient at high risk of developing sepsis; fever, septic shock may develop rapidly	Hospitalization; immediate initiation of broad-spectrum antibiotics intravenously
Disseminated viral infections	Immunosuppression related to disease or treatment allows normally trivial viral infections (e.g., influenza, upper respiratory tract infection) to become severe or systemic	Fever, flulike symptoms; rash or skin lesions with herpes zoster (shingles)	Hospitalization; intravenous antibiotics to prevent secondary infection; antiviral therapy (acyclovir), supportive care
Fungal infections	Immunosuppression secondary to disease or treatment allows growth and colonization of normally harmless fungi, which may become systemic	*Candida albicans:* sore throat, mouth with red mucosa and white patches that bleed with attempted removal; may become systemic	Oral nystatin; amphotericin or 5-fluorocytosine, or both, if systemic
		Aspergillus: sudden cough, pleuritic pain, appearance of lung infiltrates; may simulate pulmonary embolism; can also cause gastroenteritis, nephritis, esophagitis	Hospitalization for stabilization and lung biopsy for diagnosis; amphotericin
		Cryptococcus: meningitis symptoms (fever, headache, stiff neck)	Lumbar puncture for diagnosis, hospitalization; amphotericin
Parasitic diseases	Immunosuppression causes growth and colonization of normally harmless parasites	*Pneumocystis carinii pneumonia:* rapid appearance of bilateral interstitial pulmonary infiltrates associated with cough, fever, hypoxia	Hospitalization for lung biopsy, supportive care; intravenous sulfamethoxazole (Bactrim); pulmonary therapy
Metabolic Emergencies Hypercalcemia	Metastatic bone disease (breast, lung, kidney, myeloma) causes release of unbound calcium ions into serum; occasional ectopic	Nausea, vomiting, constipation, urinary frequency, lethargy, confusion; may progress to coma or death; should be suspected in any	Hospitalization; vigorous intravenous hydration with normal saline; diuresis with furosemide or ethacrynic acid; mithramycin

TABLE 33–1
Oncologic Emergencies *(Continued)*

Condition	Etiology	Signs and Symptoms	Treatment
	hormone production by tumor (thyroid, parathyroid)	confused or comatose cancer patient	
Hyperuricemia	Death of high number of malignant cells (leukemia, lymphoma) releases uric acid into blood stream	None—must be anticipated and prevented; major hazard is renal tubule damage and renal failure	Give allopurinol prophylactically; forced diuresis and alkalinization of urine; dialysis may be necessary on a temporary basis
Hypoglycemia	Excessive insulin production by islet cell carcinoma; excessive glucose consumption (with large retroperitoneal tumors)	Sweating, anxiety, dizziness, tachycardia, confusion, coma	Intravenous administration of 50% dextrose solution; long-term control of disease
Lactic acidosis	Anaerobic glycolysis in rapidly proliferating malignant cells (usually lymphoma) produces large amounts of lactic acid	Weakness, lethargy, tachypnea, coma, Kussmaul respirations	Intravenous sodium bicarbonate; long-term control of disease
Tumor lysis syndrome	Rapid necrosis of large numbers of malignant cells releases massive amounts of intracellular material into circulation—usually occurs during initial therapy of rapidly growing, bulky tumors (lymphoma)	Hyperkalemia, hyperphosphatemia, hypocalcemia, hyperuricemia, acidosis—can be very rapid in onset with development of lethal cardiac dysrhythmias	Immediate correction of metabolic imbalances; forced diuresis; cardiac monitoring by telemetry
Orthopedic Emergencies Pathologic fractures	Lytic bone metastases (breast, lung, renal cell, thyroid, myeloma) destroy and weaken bone	Chronic bone pain prior to fracture with slight increase in pain and possible "snapping" sensation when fracture occurs; may occur in spinal column, ribs, long bones, pelvis	Internal fixation if possible; radiation therapy; use *extreme* caution when lifting, transferring, or moving patient; pain control
Ophthalmic Emergencies Orbital and ocular tumors	Tumor infiltration or metastasis to orbit	Exophthalmos, pain, visual difficulties	Emergency radiation therapy
Herpes zoster involving trigeminal nerve	Trigeminal nerve innervates cornea	Corneal ulceration, blindness, trigeminal pain	Emergency ophthalmic consultation
Renal Emergencies Bilateral ureteral obstruction	Obstruction of ureters by pelvic or retroperitoneal tumors (bladder, cervix, prostate, ovary, colon, lymphoma)	Uremia, oliguria, anuria	Surgical intervention to relieve obstruction; possible hemodialysis if uremia is life threatening and underlying disease is not imminently terminal
Respiratory Emergencies Upper airway obstruction	Compression of trachea by upper mediastinal tumors (head and neck carcinomas; thyroid cancer)	Cough, respiratory distress, inspiratory stridor	Emergency radiation therapy; tracheostomy usually not possible or useful because of location of tumor
Pneumothorax	Complication of thoracentesis or erosion of tumor from bronchus into pleural space	Sudden chest pain, cough, dyspnea, tachycardia	Chest tube placement
Pleural effusion	Pleural metastases (breast, lung); obstruction of lymphatic drainage by	Progressive dyspnea with oppressive discomfort or pain on affected side	Thoracentesis with possible chest tube placement; control of underlying dis-

TABLE 33–1
Oncologic Emergencies *(Continued)*

Condition	Etiology	Signs and Symptoms	Treatment
	tumor involvement of mediastinal lymph nodes (lymphoma)		ease; chemical sclerosis of pleural space
Symptomatic Emergencies			
Pain	Bone (bone metastases); pleural (pleural metastases); abdominal (retroperitoneal tumors, enlarged liver, GI obstruction); nerve (nerve root obstruction or irritation—head and neck, retroperitoneal, pelvic tumors); headache (intracranial tumors)	Pain—site, severity, and quality variable, depending on cause	Variable according to cause and success of varying pain management approaches
Nausea, vomiting	Most often side effect of antitumor therapy; may be caused by GI obstruction	Variable degrees of nausea and vomiting	Determine cause, give antiemetics, possible need for fluids and electrolytes, nutritional support if severe
Mucositis	Side effect of chemotherapy, radiation therapy	Pain; erosions in mouth, other mucous membranes	Topical anesthetics, gentle but meticulous oral hygiene
Dyspnea	Pulmonary involvement with tumor; pneumonia; bronchospasm; effusions; edema; or emboli; can occur secondary to interstitial fibrosis from bleomycin, busulfan therapy; postirradiation pneumonitis	Subjective feeling of "not being able to breathe"	Administer oxygen and possibly parenteral morphine sulfate; diagnose and treat underlying cause

pression may follow an insidious course for weeks or months (Rodriguez and Dinapoli 1980; Zevallos et al 1987). It is often not diagnosed until the pain is severe or neurologic signs such as weakness, paralysis, or bladder and bowel dysfunction are present. From this point, however, progression of the cord compression may be rapid, resulting in permanent functional loss. It has been demonstrated that treatment of spinal cord compression is most effective when neurologic dysfunction is not present. Patients whose condition is allowed to progress to gross neurologic dysfunction (e.g., inability to walk) rarely regain function (Findlay 1987; Zevallos et al 1987). Spinal cord compression per se is not fatal, although it usually occurs in an advanced stage of cancer, and many patients do not live beyond 6 months to 1 year after the episode. Nevertheless, long-term survival does occur (Gilbert et al 1978), and early and aggressive treatment is warranted because the quality of life may be profoundly affected.

Etiology and Pathophysiology

Spinal cord compression is thought to occur in about 5% to 10% of all cases of cancer, most frequently breast and lung cancer. Other tumors that can cause cord compression include carcinomas of the prostate or kidney, carcinomas of unknown origin, lymphoma, and myeloma. Less commonly, carcinomas of the colon, stomach, thyroid, testes, and adrenal glands may compress the spinal cord (Rodriguez and Dinapoli 1980).

Spinal cord compression in cancer can occur by several mechanisms. Actual invasion of the spinal cord by tumor is rare; tumor involvement usually occurs in the epidural space. The tumor may invade the epidural space by a variety of mechanisms: direct extension from a vertebra affected by metastatic disease (from breast, lung, prostate); invasion through prevertebral lymph nodes (lymphoma); hematogenous spread through venous or arterial pathways (myeloma) (Rodriguez and Dinapoli 1980). Cord compression can also arise from a variety of "benign" disorders, including herniated disc, severe arthritis, or ankylosing spondylitis. Discussion of these disorders is beyond the scope of this chapter; however, a high index of suspicion should be maintained for any patient who comes to the ED with radicular back pain, with or without neurologic signs.

The symptoms of spinal cord compression arise from direct mechanical compression of the spinal cord by tumor, by interruption of the vascular supply to neural structures by tumor (resulting in edema or tissue ischemia), or by direct compression by vertebrae that have collapsed, been fractured, or been dislocated by tumor (Rodriguez and Dinapoli 1980). It is important to remember that localized, primary tumors seldom cause cord compression. Cord compression is most often caused by tumors that have invaded or metastasized to structures adjacent to the spinal cord. Cord compression, then, usually indicates advanced, systemic disease.

Clinical Manifestations

As noted earlier, pain is the earliest and most frequent symptom associated with spinal cord compression. The pain is usually gradual in onset and may have been progressing steadily for weeks or months before the patient comes to the emergency department. It is localized to a particular level of the spine, and may be felt at a location one or two vertebral bodies below the level of the actual compression (Glover and Glick 1985). Localized back pain may become radicular in nature (radiating through a specific dermatome) as nerve roots become compressed (Rodriguez and Dinapoli 1980). The pain may be aggravated by lying down, weight-bearing, sneezing, coughing, or the Valsalva maneuver, and it may be relieved by sitting (Glover and Glick 1985). Other symptoms may include sensory changes, extremity weakness, and changes in bladder and bowel function. Table 33-2 describes specific symptoms (other than pain) that may be present in spinal cord compression (Glover and Glick 1985; Rodriguez and Dinapoli 1980).

Treatment and Nursing Care

The focus of emergency nursing care in spinal cord compression is on facilitating rapid, appropriate diagnosis and treatment, preventing further injury, and caring for the patient and family's psychologic needs, such as for information and emotional support. To these ends, the nurse plays a critical role in taking a complete history and

TABLE 33–2
Specific Symptoms Associated with Spinal Cord Compression

Symptoms	Comments
Sensory Changes Numbness, tingling, loss of feeling, coldness, unsteadiness (sensory ataxia), loss of vaginal, rectal, or urethral sensation, decreased perineal sensation, decreased sensation in lumbosacral dermatomes	Loss of sensation in pelvic structures and saddle area may occur with metastases to the cauda equina
Weakness Stiffness, dragging of limb, unsteadiness	
Bladder or Bowel Dysfunction Bladder: Hesitancy, incomplete emptying, progressing to urinary retention with overflow Bowel: Constipation, obstipation; poor sphincter tone	

ordering initial diagnostic tests. The patient should not be kept waiting but should be placed in an examining or treatment area to be seen promptly. Stage I care focuses on the initiation of lifesaving measures and initial resuscitation. For the patient who has cervical pain, special attention to respiratory status is critical, because rapidly progressing cord compression in this area may lead to respiratory paralysis. Stage II care involves preparing the patient and family for admission to the hospital as well as conducting further diagnostic measures and treatment, which will be initiated on an urgent basis. Definitive diagnosis of spinal cord compression may be made by myelography, an invasive procedure involving special patient preparation and informed consent. Magnetic resonance imaging (MRI) is a highly accurate and sensitive, noninvasive diagnostic tool that is rapidly replacing myelography in the diagnosis of spinal cord compression. Treatment may involve chemotherapy, radiation therapy, surgery, or corticosteroids. The treatment modality used depends on several factors, including the tumor type, its location, and other treatments the patient has received. If the tumor is known to be highly sensitive to chemotherapy (for example, multiple myeloma or lymphoma), antineoplastic drug therapy may be initiated. Radiation therapy is considered the treatment of choice by some authors (Zevallos et al 1987) for radiosensitive tumors, such as breast cancer or certain lymphomas, or in situations in which surgery may not be feasible. Decompression laminectomy is a major operative procedure that requires that the person undergoing it be in fairly good health as well as to have a life expectancy of at least 4 to 6 months. Many cancer patients whose presenting feature is spinal cord compression have advanced disease and do not meet these criteria. In addition, the location of the tumor, its size, and its involvement with adjacent structures, such as nerves and blood vessels, may make it inoperable. On the other hand, surgery may be the treatment of choice if the patient has a longer life expectancy and is in overall good health; if the patient has already received the maximum radiation dose to the affected area; if the tumor is known to be radio- and chemotherapy resistant; or if the lesion is located high on the cervical spine and immediate decompression is necessary to prevent respiratory paralysis. Corticosteroids are given to reduce local edema and thus relieve pressure on the spinal cord. Intravenous dexamethasone therapy may be started in the emergency department.

Mobility, Impaired Physical, Related to

• Spinal Cord Compression

The initial history obtained by the nurse should be specific for cancer and cancer treatment. The patient should be asked specifically about his or her symptoms, including length of time present, and any changes or progress in the symptoms. Symptoms of back pain, weakness, sensory changes, or bowel or bladder dysfunction should be carefully and specifically explored. Radiographs of the involved area of the spine should be ordered. If the suspected compression is due to vertebral changes, such as dislocation, collapse, or structural defects, this will be revealed on radiographs.

Physical assessment includes a complete neurologic examination, which may be partially performed by the nurse. The examination should include tests for muscle strength and assessment of deep tendon reflexes and sensory perception, including pain and temperature sensations (Wilkowski 1986). Significant findings on physical assessment include worsening of pain with straight leg raising, neck flexion, and percussion near the level of the compression. Decreased rectal sphincter tone and loss of perineal sensation may be present. Deep tendon reflexes may be hyperactive or sluggish, depending on the location and type of compression. Muscle tone may be flaccid or spastic, again depending on the location and type of compression (Glover and Glick 1985; Rodriguez and Dinapoli 1980). In general, the symptoms reflect nerve compression and are not unique to spinal cord compression caused by malignant processes; instead they may be present in any pathologic condition causing neurologic compromise, such as disk protrusion or traumatic spinal cord injury. The patient should be made as comfortable as possible; however, analgesics may be withheld until after the initial physical assessment because they may mask the pain — a significant diagnostic indicator. Positioning of the patient for comfort and limiting his or her mobility are extremely important. The patient should be transported on a stretcher, lifted or log-rolled for transfers, and not be allowed to ambulate. In case of vertebral instability, traction may be instituted. Any change in the intensity, location, or character of the pain should be noted and reported to the health care team. Sensorineural changes should be noted, as should signs of bladder or bowel dysfunction (Wilkowski 1986). The symptoms of spinal cord compression may progress from pain to loss of neurologic function within hours. Careful monitoring, reporting, and documentation of patient status is critical.

As noted earlier, treatment of spinal cord compression requires admission to the hospital. Stage II care involves caring for the patient and family during the diagnostic and admission phase.

Knowledge Deficit, Related to

• **Disease Process and Treatment**

It is important for the nurse to keep the patient and family informed of the reasons for the various tests and of the seriousness of the situation. Test results and progress toward diagnosis and treatment should be communicated. The patient will probably be admitted to the hospital before treatment is begun, and the emergency nurse should help the family prepare for admission.

Coping, Ineffective Individual, Related to

• **Situational Crisis**

Spinal cord compression and the potential loss of function represent a true crisis for the patient and family. The nurse should provide reassurance that all appropriate tests and procedures are being completed and that the patient will be treated on a timely basis. Emotional support in the form of a calm, knowledgeable presence will be helpful in this stressful situation. Helping a family decide who should stay with the patient, explaining procedures and activities, and providing supportive services, such as information about telephones, appropriate waiting areas, and availability of food service and coffee or soft drinks, will assist families in coping.

Spinal cord compression is an emergency whose early symptoms may be overlooked or misdiagnosed by a patient and health care professionals. Treatment in the early stages of cord compression is essential to avoid permanent loss of function and maintain quality of life.

Superior Vena Cava Syndrome

Superior vena cava syndrome (SVCS) is another oncologic emergency that is insidious in onset and not immediately life-threatening, but that results in significant morbidity and possible mortality if allowed to progress to an acute stage. It occurs in approximately 3 to 5% of patients with carcinomas of the lung or lymphoma. Although over 95% of cases of SVCS are due to malignancy (primary or metastatic mediastinal tumors), the syndrome can also occur in benign conditions such as substernal goiter, mediastinal fibrosis, and aortic aneurysms (Carabell and Goodman 1985; Varricchio 1985). Lung cancer and lymphoma are by far the most common malignancies associated with SVCS, but intrathoracic metastases from other tumors can also cause this syndrome. Recently, a related entity, iatrogenic superior vena cava syndrome, has been reported in patients with long-term indwelling central venous catheters (e.g., Hickman, Broviac) (Bertrand et al 1984). Although these patients usually have cancer, they show no evidence of tumor involvement in the mediastinum.

Etiology and Pathophysiology

Superior vena cava syndrome occurs when venous return to the heart from the head, trunk, and upper extremities via the superior vena cava is compromised in some way.

The most common cause of the obstruction is extrinsic compression by mediastinal tumor or malignant intrathoracic lymph nodes. Intrinsic obstruction may be caused by thrombus formation with or without an indwelling central venous catheter. The superior vena cava and its tributaries are vulnerable to extrinsic obstruction because of the closeness of intrathoracic structures (allowing little room for tumor growth or lymph node enlargement), as well as the thinness of their walls and low intravascular pressure (Carabell and Goodman 1985; Glover and Glick 1985). Once the obstruction is severe enough, clinical symptoms begin to appear. These include edema of the face, neck, upper extremities, and trunk. Neck veins may be distended, and the patient may complain of dysphagia, chest pain, cough, or dyspnea. When the syndrome is slow in onset, collateral circulatory patterns develop in the chest to compensate for the compromised superior vena cava. This is evident by venous engorgement and distention in the chest area.

Clinical Manifestations

Superior vena cava syndrome has been classified as both an acute and a subacute emergency (Morse et al 1985). In its subacute phase, symptoms and findings may include subtle breathing changes (heaviness, dyspnea on exertion), weight gain, tight rings on fingers, and the appearance of venous patterns on the chest indicating the development of collateral circulation. As noted earlier, these events are subtle and insidious in onset, and it is not likely that a patient would come to the ED at this stage for this problem. The acute phase may present a true emergency, however, as the patient may complain of severe dyspnea, chest pain, and weakness. There may be tracheal edema in addition to the readily observable swelling of face, neck, upper extremities, and trunk. The face may be flushed and thoracic veins distended. The patient may complain of visual disturbances, proptosis, and periorbital edema. Funduscopic examination may reveal blurred disk margins and venous engorgement. The patient may be tachypneic (Morse et al 1985).

Patient assessment includes a history specific for cancer or cancer treatment, indwelling central venous catheter, and exploration of the symptoms and their development. Physical assessment includes observation of physical signs (e.g., edema, venous distention), vital signs, and funduscopic examination.

There are two schools of thought regarding the value and need for diagnostic tests. The diagnosis is traditionally a clinical one, based on the patient's history and physical findings. There are very few conditions that mimic SVCS (although congestion and edema due to cardiac tamponade, pericarditis, and allergic reactions are occasionally confused with SVCS) (Varricchio 1985), and the invasive measures necessary to definitively diagnose it and determine a cause may be dangerous in marked cardiovascular compromise. Another school of thought holds that a diagnostic work-up should be done unless the condition is immediately life-threatening. The minimal work-up may include a chest radiograph to determine the presence of a mediastinal mass. Other tests include sputum cytology, fiberoptic bronchoscopy, tomography, esophagoscopy, venous pressure manometry, surgical exploration, radionuclide venography, and mediastinoscopy (Varricchio 1985). The purpose of the more complete work-up is to determine the location and extent of the obstruction, to identify the precise cause, and to make a primary diagnosis if one has not been made.

Obviously, a complete work-up will take at least 24 to 48 hours, and the patient will be admitted to the hospital.

Treatment and Nursing Care

Treatment for SVCS is aimed at reducing the symptoms and eliminating the underlying cause (e.g., extrinsic pressure from intrathoracic tumor). Radiation therapy, chemotherapy, and possibly surgery are aimed at reducing the size of the compressing tumor. Diuretics, steroids, and anticoagulants are used to relieve the symptoms. The goal of therapy for SVCS caused by malignancy is palliation rather than cure (Varricchio 1985). Treatment for iatrogenic SVCS is not well determined. In this case, a diagnostic work-up has been recommended to rule out mediastinal mass and find a definitive cause. Treatment may include removal of the catheter, anticoagulants, or fibrinolytic drugs (Bertrand et al 1984). The level of diagnostic work-up for SVCS and treatment approaches will depend on the clinical experience and preferences of the treating physician, although radiation therapy is usually the primary treatment modality (Carabell and Goodman 1985).

Nursing care for the patient with SVCS will depend on the level of acuity of the syndrome. At triage, a careful history should be taken, with special attention to history of lung cancer or lymphoma, and the presence of an indwelling central venous catheter. The duration of the symptoms and a description of how they have progressed is important. If the patient is acutely dyspneic and in distress, he or she should be placed in an examining room immediately to be evaluated by a physician.

Stage I care focuses on further patient assessment and stabilizing his or her status. If the patient is profoundly dyspneic or cyanotic, the focus may be on maintaining an open airway and emergency measures to relieve symptoms (e.g., diuretics, positioning to promote maximal comfort) and promote tissue oxygenation. Stage II care involves monitoring the patient for changes in symptoms and preparing the patient and family for admission to the hospital, treatment, and diagnostic tests.

Tissue Perfusion, Altered, Related to

• **Decreased Cardiac Output, Obstructed Airway**

Nursing interventions include maintaining a high index of suspicion for the development of SVCS, particularly in patients with known lung cancer or lymphoma or in those indwelling central venous catheters (Morse et al 1985). In early SVCS the patient may only be symptomatic in the morning owing to the effects of gravity on hemodynamics. The history should track the presence of symptoms throughout the day. It is important to monitor vital signs continuously. The respiratory rate will probably be greater than 30 breaths per minute and the patient may be tachycardic (Varricchio 1985). Blood pressure readings may be inaccurate if upper extremity edema is present, and a large blood pressure cuff on the lower extremities should be used (Morse et al 1985). In acute SVCS the patency of the airway should be evaluated continuously, and the development of gurgling, rattling, stridor, cyanosis, and rib retractions, and the use of accessory muscles to breathe, should be noted and reported to the physician immediately. Maintenance of an open airway and tissue oxygenation are critical. Suctioning may be necessary. Cerebral edema may also develop, causing headache, increased intracranial pressure, and changes in mental status (Varricchio 1985). These symptoms should be observed, documented, and reported. Medications should not be given intravenously if upper extremity edema is present because sluggish blood flow may slow drug distribution and cause vascular wall irritation (Carabell and Goodman 1985). If possible, the lower extremities should be used for vascular access. If this is not possible, the left arm is preferred over the right (Morse et al 1985).

Electrolyte Balance, Altered, *Related to

- **Hypoxia**

In the event of airway obstruction or respiratory embarrassment, hypoxemia may occur, leading to a multiplicity of electrolyte and acid-base imbalances. Arterial blood gas values should be obtained and monitored. Carbon dioxide retention with respiratory acidosis will result in a compensatory metabolic alkalosis. Mental status changes may occur with electrolyte and acid-base imbalances and should be considered a significant indication for the evaluation of these parameters (Varricchio 1985).

Coping, Ineffective Individual, Related to

- **Situational Crisis, Fear of Impending Death**

The symptoms of acute SVCS may cause feelings of anxiety and suffocation, and fear of impending death in the patient. Family members accompanying the patient will also be anxious and may not be able to cope with the situation. Nursing interventions include comfort measures (e.g., positioning, administration of oxygen), and the administration of analgesics or tranquilizers to relieve anxiety. The patient and family should be kept informed of the patient's status, and calm, accurate explanations about medical and nursing treatments should be provided (Varricchio 1985).

In its early stages, SVCS is not immediately life-threatening and can be treated successfully. Allowed to progress, the symptoms may become acute and life-threatening, necessitating emergency treatment. Early detection of SVCS by knowing risk factors and recognizing early symptoms, along with patient education regarding the potential for developing this complication, are important nursing interventions. In acute SVCS the nursing focus is on maintenance of tissue perfusion, patient comfort, and reversal of symptoms. Survival in SVCS is most closely related to the underlying malignancy.

Infection and Septicemia

Infection is a frequent cause of morbidity and mortality in cancer patients. Many cancer patients die, not from the disease itself, but from overwhelming infection. A

---

* Non–NANDA-approved nursing diagnosis.

localized infection can rapidly become systemic, and septicemia and septic shock can ensue. An oral temperature of greater than 100°F in a neutropenic cancer patient constitutes an oncologic emergency.

Etiology and Pathophysiology

It is well known that cancer patients are extremely susceptible to developing fulminant, life-threatening infections as a result of both their disease and its treatment. Severely compromised host defenses (from either the disease or its treatment), coupled with exposure to multiple sources of infection, jeopardize the cancer patient's safety in this area (Table 33–3). Multiple, interrelated etiologic and pathophysiologic processes contribute to this problem, and a complete discussion of these mechanisms is beyond the scope of this chapter. Pizzo and Young (1985) have reviewed the cause and pathophysiology of infection in cancer patients in some detail, and the reader is referred to this source for a more in-depth overview of the problem. It is important for the emergency nurse to be aware of the problem of infection in cancer patients and to understand that a localized infection in these persons may become systemic and progress to septicemia within hours. A fever of 100°F coupled with neutropenia (less than 1000 neutrophils/mm^3) (see Box 33–1), or a known history of cancer, or cancer treatment, or use of an indwelling central venous catheter, or any combination of these, should arouse the suspicions of the emergency nurse. It is important to remember that the source of the infection may be bacterial, fungal, viral, parasitic, or any combination; that the microorganism(s) may not be considered pathogenic under "normal" circumstances (over 80% of the infections that occur in cancer patients arise from endogenous flora); and that any body system may have been the original site of infection. Mortality from septicemia ranges from 10 to 40% but may be as high as 70%, depending on the site of the primary infection (e.g., lungs) and the number of microorganisms involved. Septicemia is the cause of fever in approximately 20% of neutropenic cancer patients (Pizzo and Young 1985).

TABLE 33–3
Factors Contributing to Infectious Complications in Cancer Patients

Disruption of the physical integrity of skin and mucous membranes by surgery, radiation therapy, chemotherapy (stomatitis), and indwelling vascular access devices (e.g., Hickman, Broviac, and other types of catheters)

Alteration of microorganism receptors on epithelial and mucosal cells by disease or treatment permits colonization by potential pathogens

Bone marrow suppression by chemotherapy or radiation therapy depletes numbers of neutrophils and alters their function

Bone marrow involvement with disease (leukemia) produces dysfunctional neutrophils

Disruption of cellular and humoral immunity by disease (lymphoma, myeloma) or treatment

Malnutrition contributes to body's inability to maintain normal defenses

Multiple invasive procedures and therapies increase transmission of microorganisms (e.g., total parenteral nutrition, parenteral antibiotics and analgesics)

Use of multiple antibiotics alters normal flora, permitting colonization by fungi and other pathogens

Frequent hospitalizations increase risk of nosocomial infections

Indwelling catheters and pumps provide a source of colonization

Source: Pizzo PA, Young RC. 1985. In DeVita VT, Hellman S, Rosenberg SA, eds. Cancer: Principles and Practice of Oncology, 2nd ed. JB Lippincott, 1963–1988.

BOX 33-1 DETERMINING NEUTROPENIA

The terms *neutropenia* and *granulocytopenia* are often used interchangeably when discussing clinical features in cancer patients. Neutrophils (or granulocytes) are the "fighters"—the white blood cells that are responsible for defending the host against infection by most bacteria and fungi. The bone marrow reserves of these cells must be replenished on a continual basis. When bone marrow function is compromised by cancer or its treatment, granulocytopenia occurs, and the patient is at great risk for infection. To determine the presence of granulocytopenia it is essential to calculate the absolute granulocyte count (AGC). This is done by taking the total percentage of polymorphonuclear leukocytes, bands, and segmental leukocytes from the differential white blood cell (WBC) count and multiplying that percentage by the total WBC count. The product of these numbers is the absolute number of neutrophils (or granulocytes) per cubic millimeter of blood, and is the basis for determining neutropenia. Generally an AGC between 500 and 1000/mm^3 is considered to place a patient at risk for developing serious infection. The normal values for the differential WBC count are shown below (see note):

WBC (leukocytes) 5000-10,000/mm^3
   neutrophils (polymorphonuclear, bands, segmental) 50-70%
   lymphocytes 20-30%
   monocytes 3-7%
   eosinophils 1-3%
   basophils 0-0.75%

     The following is an example of the WBC differential count in a neutropenic individual:

WBC (total) 3200
   polymorphonuclear 1%
   bands 2%
   segmental 2%
   lymphocytes 82%
   monocytes 10%
   eosinophils 2%
   basophils 1%

Only 5% of the total WBC count of 3200 are granulocytes, or an AGC of 160. This patient is severely neutropenic and at extremely high risk of developing overwhelming, life-threatening infection.

Note: Laboratories vary in what they establish as normal ranges for blood values. They also vary as to how the differential is reported. Some laboratories report polymorphonuclear leukocytes, bands, and segmental cells. Others only report bands and segmental leukocytes. The three terms describe varying stages of maturity of granulocytes (polymorphonuclear cells being least mature and segmental forms most mature); however, all are considered capable of fighting infection. It is important to remember that the differential count is always reported as a percentage of the total WBC count.

Clinical Manifestations

The only manifestation of infection in a cancer patient may be fever. Patients who are neutropenic frequently do not exhibit "normal" inflammatory responses at infection sites, because these reactions depend on a functional immune system. Thus, body fluids such as sputum, urine, or wound drainage may not be purulent. Redness and swelling may be absent. Nonetheless, all potential sites of infection should be examined and material taken for cultures. Chills and rigors may be present in bacteremia. Any history of cancer, recent cancer treatment, or recent hospitalization should be elicited. Laboratory tests should include a complete blood count with special attention to the differential count, culture and sensitivity testing of blood, urine, sputum, and wounds (including central venous catheter exit sites), and a chest radiograph. In patients with indwelling venous access catheters, the catheter may or may not be used in the emergency department for drawing blood for cultures and administering fluids and medications, depending on the preference and experience of the physician. If the catheter is the source of the infection, drawing blood for cultures through it may mask the presence of other microorganisms in the blood. Using an infected catheter to administer fluids may introduce more bacteria into the circulation. Catheters suspected of being infected are usually not removed unless aggressive treatment fails to clear the infection. A decision to remove the catheter will not usually be made in the ED. For more detailed information on the management of vascular access devices in the ED, refer to Chapter 34.

Treatment and Nursing Care

A cancer patient arriving in the ED with a fever and neutropenia should be promptly started on intravenous antibiotic therapy and admitted to the hospital for further diagnosis and treatment. It is not considered wise to wait for the infectious organism to be identified before beginning treatment. Thus, empiric antibiotic therapy, perhaps using a combination of two or three broad-spectrum antibiotics, is usually begun immediately. The antibiotics will be "fine-tuned" to the specific organism(s) causing the infection when culture and sensitivity test results are available. Stages I and II care may overlap and focus on monitoring and stabilizing the patient's condition, obtaining specimens for laboratory tests, and initiating treatment. Antibiotics should be started as soon as culture and sensitivity specimens are obtained, in the ED. The febrile, neutropenic cancer patient should not be considered "stable," as sepsis and septic shock can develop rapidly and without warning. The need to initiate resuscitation and other life-saving measures should be anticipated for the duration of the patient's stay in the ED.

Potential for Injury, Related to

- **Infection**

It is again extremely important for the nurse to obtain a history for cancer, cancer treatment, recent hospitalization, and duration of the presenting symptom (fever). In this instance, it is also critical to determine if the patient has had allergic reactions to any antibiotics. The patient should be placed in an examining room and evaluated promptly by the physician, especially if a high temperature (over 102°F) or rigors or chills are present. Specimens for cultures and sensitivity testing should be obtained, as should a chest radiograph. Nursing care involves monitoring the patient's vital signs and general condition, including level of consciousness, color, temperature, condition of skin, and the patient's overall feeling of well-being. If shock develops, resuscitative and other life-support measures will be necessary. Under ordinary circumstances, antipyretics and antibiotics generally are started as soon as blood cultures are obtained.

Septic shock may develop rapidly and without warning. An increase in body temperature, tachycardia, a drop in blood pressure, cool, clammy skin, and a decrease in level of consciousness may be apparent. Nursing care involves notifying the physician and beginning treatment for shock. Administration of oxygen and intravenous fluids and measures to reduce the fever should be carried out (e.g., acetaminophen, hypothermia blanket). Samples for measuring arterial blood gases will be needed, and a venous blood sample should also be obtained for a coagulation profile. Medication to stabilize blood pressure (e.g., dopamine) and cardiac function may be administered. Septic shock may stabilize with initial treatment, or it may progress to disseminated intravascular coagulation, or cardiorespiratory arrest, or both (Pizzo and Young 1985; Sumner 1987). When treating septicemia in the neutropenic cancer patient, it is important to remember that the patient may also be thrombocytopenic, and bleeding complications could occur. The nurse should also remember that this patient is severely immunocompromised, and careful handwashing and scrupulous aseptic technique for invasive procedures should be followed.

As with other oncologic emergencies, the patient with septicemia will be admitted to the hospital for inpatient care. The patient and family will need emotional support in the form of explanations, reassurance, and information about supportive services. Infection and septicemia are truly life-threatening oncologic emergencies.

Hypercalcemia

Hypercalcemia is one of many metabolic emergencies that can occur with malignancy. It is undoubtedly one of the most common metabolic emergencies, affecting approximately 10 to 20% of all cancer patients at some time (Fields et al 1985). It occurs most often in carcinomas of the breast, lung, and kidney and in multiple myeloma, but it has been associated with primary tumors in various other sites (Levine and Kleeman 1987). Treatment is aimed at restoring a normal calcium balance; however, the underlying malignancy must be controlled to resolve the problem completely.

Etiology and Pathophysiology

Hypercalcemia of malignancy is due to multiple disruptions of extremely well-balanced and tightly controlled mechanisms that maintain calcium homeostasis. Normal calcium metabolism involves a complex series of interactions between various hormones and other substances and the bones, kidneys, and gut. These mechanisms are not completely understood, nor are the pathophysiologic mechanisms underlying the hypercalcemia of malignancy. Both processes have been reviewed (Levine and Kleeman 1987; Mundy 1987), and the reader is referred to these articles for a more in-depth explanation than can be provided within the scope of this chapter.

Hypercalcemia of malignancy occurs in three conditions: solid tumor without bony metastases, solid tumor with bony metastases, and multiple myeloma (Fields et al 1985). Hypercalcemia in malignancy results from resorption of calcium from bone and the inability of the kidneys to excrete the higher calcium load. It is believed that the tumor itself produces various substances that cause this problem, affecting both bone metabolism and renal function. It is not simply a matter of calcium leaching from lytic bone lesions into the serum and kidney function compromised by the disease, its treatment, or other causes, although these factors certainly seem to play a role (Mundy 1987). It is important for the ED nurse to know that hypercalcemia can occur in almost any malignancy, with or without bony metastasis, and that it results from a complicated interplay of multiple and, as yet, not fully understood factors. Hypercalcemia can have nonmalignant causes (most commonly primary hyperparathyroidism), although it is rare that "benign" hypercalcemia would be diagnosed in the ED, as these syndromes are usually chronic and less severe and do not rapidly produce symptoms.

Clinical Manifestations

The clinical manifestations of hypercalcemia in malignancy are vague and nonspecific. They may include neurologic changes, such as fatigue, muscle weakness, mental status changes, stupor, and coma. Polyuria and polydipsia may be present. Gastroin-

---

BOX 33-2 INTERPRETING SERUM CALCIUM LEVELS

When interpreting the serum calcium level, it is important to remember that calcium is present in the serum in three forms: free calcium ions (about 45%); calcium bound to albumin (about 40%); calcium bound to multiple organic and inorganic anions (e.g., phosphate, sulfate) (about 15%). Only the free calcium ions are physiologically active, yet routine serum calcium measurements usually reflect the *total* amount of calcium. Therefore, the serum calcium level may not accurately reflect the level of circulating free calcium ions or the presence of "true" hypercalcemia (Levine and Kleeman 1987). It may be necessary to calculate an adjusted serum calcium level to compensate for changes in serum albumin concentration. The following formula may be used:

corrected calcium (mg/dl) = measured calcium + [4 − albumin (g/dl)] × 0.8*

Ionized serum calcium measurements may be available. It is important to know how the laboratory used by the ED calculates and reports serum calcium levels.

---

* Fields ALA, et al. 1985. In DeVita VT, et al. Cancer: Principles and Practice of Oncology. JB Lippincott.

testinal disturbances are common and include anorexia, nausea, vomiting, weight loss, and severe constipation, unrelieved by laxatives. The myocardium is very sensitive to calcium balance, and there may be changes in the EKG. Bone pain and headache may also occur (Fields et al 1985; Mahon 1987).

Assessment of the patient begins with a blood chemistry profile and proceeds to more complex and specific analyses of blood, urine, bones, and endocrine function. The serum calcium level should be interpreted carefully (Box 33–2) and should be considered along with the patient's history, presenting symptoms, and other serum values. Any ionized calcium value higher than the normal parameters (about 8.8 to 10.4 mg/dl for men and 8.5 to 10.1 mg/dl for women) should be considered significant. The higher the serum calcium value, the more severe the hypercalcemia is considered to be. Further assessment of the patient includes obtaining a history of cancer or cancer treatment, exploration of the presenting symptoms, and further diagnostic testing.

Treatment and Nursing Interventions

Emergency treatment for hypercalcemia focuses on restoring fluid volume (these patients are often dehydrated) and enhancing renal excretion of calcium. The patient will be admitted to the hospital for further treatment of the hypercalcemia (aimed at reducing calcium resorption from bone), further diagnostic testing, and possible treatment of the underlying malignancy. Treatment of hypercalcemia involves intravenous fluids (2 L of normal saline solution over 2 to 3 hours) followed by intravenous furosemide, bumetanide, or ethacrynic acid every 2 to 4 hours to enhance urinary excretion of calcium. Sodium, potassium, and magnesium will also be lost, and these electrolytes need to be monitored and replaced. Longer-term treatment includes continued hydration and diuresis, plus the possible use of a number of agents to reduce bone resorption (e.g., mithramycin, calcitonin, glucocorticoids, etidronate disodium, and others) (Levine and Kleeman 1987). Hypercalcemia will recur unless the underlying malignancy is controlled.

Hypercalcemia

The patient's overall condition should be assessed by the nurse, including mental status and history of any symptoms. If the patient is a woman with a history of metastatic breast cancer treated with estrogen or the antiestrogen tamoxifen (Nolvadex), this should be noted. A transient episode of hypercalcemia may occur when this therapy is initiated. Known as a "flare" reaction, it may be symptomatic and require treatment, but it does not persist for a long period of time. The flare reaction is thought to be a temporary episode of bone resorption activated indirectly by changes in the hormone level. History of use of other drugs known to aggravate hypercalcemia, such as vitamins A and D, calcium supplements, thiazide diuretics, and lithium, should also be obtained. Use of digitalis should be ascertained, as hypercalcemia can augment its effect, leading to digitalis toxicity (Levine and Kleeman 1987). A full serum chemistry panel should be ordered and the patient evaluated as soon as possible. Stage I care involves initiating intravenous fluid therapy and perhaps diuretics and electrolytes. A Foley catheter should be inserted and intake and output monitored closely. A 12-lead EKG should be obtained. Stage II care involves monitoring the patient, especially for mental status changes, relief of other symptoms (e.g., pain), and preparing the patient and family for the hospitalization. It is always important to provide explanations and reassurances to the patient and invariably anxious family members.

Hypercalcemia of malignancy is potentially life threatening. It is usually diagnosed by measurement of serum calcium level, as the clinical presentation is vague and nonspecific. Specific treatment modalities used depend on the severity and duration of the calcium imbalance, but include hydration and diuresis.

Malignant Effusions

Cancer is frequently complicated by the development of pleural, peritoneal, and pericardial effusions. Although effusions are usually not acutely life threatening (with the exception of pericardial effusion, which can develop rapidly, leading to cardiac tamponade), they can cause considerable discomfort to the patient, precipitating a visit to the ED.

Pleural Effusion

Etiology and Pathophysiology • A pleural effusion is the accumulation of fluid in the pleural space, between the visceral and parietal pleurae. Normally, a small amount of fluid circulates through this potential space, allowing the two surfaces to move freely against one another during the movements of respiration. Fluid accumulates when the normal turnover of pleural fluid is disrupted. In cancer this can happen in several ways: malignant cells find their way to the pleura, causing irritation of the pleural surfaces and accumulation of fluid in the pleural space; lymphatic involvement with tumor obstructs normal lymphatic drainage from the pleural space; malignant cells are shed from the pleurae into the pleural fluid, causing a "tumor cell suspension" in the pleural space; finally, vascular invasion by tumor cells may obstruct capillary flow within the pleurae, causing changes in hydrostatic pressure gradients and accumulation of fluid in the pleural space (Gobel and Lawler 1985). Pleural effusions may be localized or loculated (small pockets of fluid throughout the pleural space) and occur most frequently in breast cancer, lung cancer, ovarian cancer, and lymphoma.

Clinical Manifestations • The symptoms of pleural effusion may include dyspnea, cough, or chest pain, or the patient may not be symptomatic at all. The cough is usually dry and nonproductive. Dyspnea may be described as breathlessness or difficulty breathing either at rest or with activity. The chest pain may be vague and uncomfortable. Pleuritic pain is usually not present unless the pleura are inflamed simultaneously. Diagnosis is made by physical examination of the chest, chest radiograph, and analysis of pleural fluid (Wegmann and Forshee 1983). Significant findings on physical assessment include intercostal prominence, dullness to percussion, reduced or absent breath sounds over the affected area, and possibly tracheal deviation if the effusion is large. A posteroanterior chest radiograph, taken with the patient in the lateral decubitus position (lying on his or her side) will reveal even a small effusion. Wegmann and Forshee (1983) suggest that the x-ray technician should be told that the area of interest is the dependent hemithorax, as this may influence the technique used. The patient should lie on the affected side for at least 5 minutes before the film is taken to allow the fluid to drain to the dependent side. A thoracentesis will be required to obtain pleural fluid for analysis. This procedure may or may not be done in the ED.

Treatment and Nursing Care • The only treatment for a malignant pleural effusion that would be performed in the emergency department would be a thoracentesis to drain the infusion, and possibly the insertion of a thoracostomy tube for continued drainage. Other treatments for malignant pleural effusion include the instillation of various chemical agents to sclerose the pleural space (after the original effusion has drained), pleurectomy, radiation therapy, and the use of intrapleural radioisotopes, all beyond the scope of emergency care (Gobel and Lawler 1985). Nursing interventions focus on facilitating the diagnosis and maintaining patient and family comfort during the diagnostic tests and process of admission to the hospital.

Comfort, Altered, Related to

• *Dyspnea, anxiety*

Tissue Perfusion, Altered (Cardiopulmonary), Related to

• *Hypoxemia*

The nurse should obtain information about history of malignancy or cancer treatment. The patient's symptoms should be explored. A history of weight fluctuation may be significant: weight loss is frequently seen with pleural effusion, and recent weight gain may indicate fluid retention. The patient's respiratory and mental status should be determined. Pleural effusion can lead to hypoxemia. Vital signs should be taken, with special attention to respiratory and heart rates. The patient should be asked directly about dyspnea, chest pain, and cough. Wegmann and Forshee (1983) have described the nursing assessment for pleural effusion in detail. Unless there is severe respiratory distress and need for immediate intervention, stage I care involves primarily monitoring the patient's respiratory and mental status for sudden deterioration and taking appropriate action should the patient's condition deteriorate. Stage II care involves preparing the patient for chest radiograph and ensuring his or her comfort. While waiting, the patient should be allowed to assume the position that allows him or her to breathe most comfortably. If a thoracentesis for either diagnostic or therapeutic purposes is to be performed in the ED, the patient and family will require explanations and emotional support. The nurse may be requested to assist with the thoracentesis and chest tube insertion.

Peritoneal Effusions (Ascites)

Etiology and Pathophysiology • A peritoneal effusion is the accumulation of fluid in the potential space formed by the visceral and parietal peritoneum. It occurs most frequently in ovarian, endometrial, gastric, pancreatic, mammary, and colonic cancer, usually at an advanced stage of the disease. Several factors may contribute to the development of malignant ascites. Seeding of malignant cells within the peritoneum may cause capillary damage, resulting in increased capillary permeability. Obstruction of the vasculature by tumor may interfere with venous drainage, allowing fluid to accumulate in the peritoneal space. Lymphatic obstruction interferes with lymphatic drainage. Hypoalbuminemia, commonly seen in advanced cancer, may cause a fluid shift from intravascular to extravascular spaces within the peritoneum (Zehner and Hoogstraten 1985).

Clinical Manifestations • Symptoms of ascites may include loss of appetite, indigestion, weight gain, enlargement of abdominal girth, dyspnea, orthopnea, and generalized discomfort. There may also be constipation, nausea, and vomiting. These symptoms are caused by increased pressure of fluid within the abdomen. On physical assessment, the abdomen may be obviously distended and tense. A "fluid wave" may be elicited by gentle ballottement of the abdomen. Obvious respiratory effort may be present, particularly if the diaphragm has been displaced upward by the effusion. Bowel sounds may be diminished. Occasionally, a coexistent pleural effusion is present, thought to be caused by leakage of ascitic fluid through diaphragmatic lymphatic channels into the pleural space. Abdominal radiographs, ultrasound, and computed tomographic (CT) scanning will help identify potential bowel obstruction, presence of tumor, and full extent of the effusion (Zehner and Hoogstraten 1985).

Treatment and Nursing Care • The immediate aim of treatment is to remove the fluid from the intraperitoneal space. This is done with paracentesis to drain the fluid. Peritoneal effusions may be massive (over 12 L) and may require repeated drainage. A catheter may be left in place for several days with intermittent clamping until the ascitic fluid is drained. Generally, no more than 1 to 2 L of fluid should be drained at any given time, to avoid massive shifts in fluid volume and possible hypovolemic shock. Peritoneal effusions tend to recur, and the ultimate aim of treatment is control of the underlying disease with chemotherapy. A LeVeen peritoneal venous shunt may be placed as a longer-term palliative approach. This shunt drains fluid from the abdomen into the superior vena cava, allowing it to be dispersed into the systemic circulation (Zehner and Hoogstraten 1985).

Coping, Ineffective Individual, Related to

• *Advanced disease, situational crisis*

As noted earlier, malignant ascites usually occurs in advanced stages of cancer. Nursing care focuses on patient comfort and safety and on patient and family education and support. The patient history should be specific for cancer and should explore the development of signs and symptoms. It should be determined whether this problem has occurred in the past, and history of paracentesis or insertion of a LeVeen shunt should be obtained. The patient should be positioned comfortably (usually the upright position is more comfortable as it relieves pressure on the diaphragm). The patient and family should be offered emotional support, and explanations of any diagnostic procedures or physical findings. If a paracentesis is to be performed in the ED, the nurse should be prepared to assist with the procedure and monitor fluid drainage.

Pericardial Effusion

Etiology and Pathophysiology • Although pericardial effusion can result from a variety of nonmalignant causes, cancer and radiation therapy are the most common etiologic factors. In cancer, pericardial effusion may develop when tumor invades the pericardium. This may be a direct extension of a primary thoracic tumor (lung and breast cancer) or a metastasis from a tumor at a more distant site (lymphoma, leukemia, melanoma) (Concilus and Bohachick 1984). Pericardial effusion may also occur as a result of pericarditis secondary to mediastinal radiation therapy. The pathophysiology of pericardial effusion is similar to that of the other malignant effusions. Fluid accumulates in a potential space, this time formed by the two surfaces of the pericardium. The mechanisms of inhibition of lymphatic drainage, venous flow obstruction, and changes in capillary flow are similar. The problem is that pericardial effusion can lead to the development of pericardial tamponade, a life-threatening emergency. The diagnosis and management of pericardial tamponade are described elsewhere in this text; here only the management of pericardial effusion is discussed.

Clinical Manifestations

It is important to know that malignant pericardial effusions can progress slowly or rapidly. If the accumulation of fluid in the pericardium is slow and gradual, the normally inelastic pericardial membrane may stretch to accommodate the increased fluid volume, causing minimal symptoms. However, if the effusion develops rapidly, even a small amount of fluid will cause sufficient pressure on the myocardium to initiate tamponade. Ultimately, a slow-growing effusion will also result in cardiac tamponade. Symptoms of pericardial effusion include cough and dyspnea and the symptoms of acute pericardial tamponade. Physical findings may be insignificant, unless a tamponade is developing. A chest radiograph, CT scan, cardiac fluoroscopy, and echocardiogram may detect a more slowly developing pericardial effusion (Zehner and Hoogstraten 1985).

Treatment and Nursing Care • If a patient is asymptomatic with a slowly developing or stable effusion and is responding to therapy for the underlying malignancy, the pericardial effusion may not be treated. Treatments for pericardial effusion may include pericardiocentesis, creation of a pericardial window (allows fluid to drain into the pleural space), instillation of chemical sclerosing agents, and radiation therapy (Zehner and Hoogstraten 1985). None of these procedures would be conducted in an ED unless acute pericardial tamponade were in progress, in which case an emergency pericardiocentesis would be performed to relieve pressure on the myocardium.

Decreased Cardiac Output, Related to

• *Cardiac tamponade*

   The nurse should maintain a high index of suspicion for any cancer patient with cardiovascular symptoms. If pericardial effusion is suspected, the patient should be monitored very closely and the emergency department staff prepared to begin emergency pericardiocentesis and resuscitative efforts. As with all other emergencies, the patient and family will require a great deal of emotional support, particularly if cardiac tamponade ensues. When pericardial effusion and cardiac tamponade are appropriately treated, the patient's survival will depend on the underlying malignancy. As with other oncologic emergencies, the disease is usually in a more advanced stage, and the patient may not survive longer than a few months to a year. Nonetheless, successful intervention in this and all other oncologic emergencies may improve the quality of life remaining, allowing the patient and family to settle their affairs.

CONCLUSION

Cancer patients are likely to be seen in the emergency department for a variety of situations. Although many of the oncologic emergencies are not immediately life-threatening, several are, and these require prompt medical and nursing intervention. The emergency nurse can have a significant impact on the quality of life the cancer patient has remaining by maintaining a high index of suspicion for oncologic emergencies when a cancer patient enters the ED.

REFERENCES

Arseneau JC, Rubin P. 1983. Oncologic emergencies. In Rubin P, ed. Clinical Oncology for Medical Students and Physicians. New York, American Cancer Society, 516–533.

Bertrand M, Presant C, Klein L, et al. 1984. Iatrogenic superior vena cava syndrome. Cancer 54:376–378.

Carabell S, Goodman RL. 1985. Superior vena cava syndrome. In DeVita VT, Hellman S, Rosenberg SA, eds. Cancer: Principles and Practice of Oncology, 2nd ed. Philadelphia, JB Lippincott, 1855–1860.

Concilus EM, Bohachick PA. 1984. Cancer: Pericardial effusion and tamponade. Cancer Nurs 7:391–398.

Fields ALA, Josse RG, Bergsagel DE. 1985. Metabolic emergencies. In DeVita VT, Hellman S, Rosenberg SA, eds. Cancer: Principles and Practice of Oncology, 2nd ed. Philadelphia, JB Lippincott, 1866–1881.

Findlay GFG. 1987. The role of vertebral body collapse in the management of malignant spinal cord compression. J Neurol Neurosurg Psychiatry 50:151–154.

Gilbert R, Kim J, Posner J. 1978. Epidural spinal cord compression from metastatic tumor: Diagnosis and treatment. Ann Neurol 3:40–51.

Glover DJ, Glick JH. 1985. Managing oncologic emergencies involving structural dysfunction. CA—A Cancer Journal for Clinicians 35:238–251.

Gobel BH, Lawler PE. 1985. Malignant pleural effusions. Oncol Nurs Forum 12(4):49–54.

Levine MM, Kleeman CR. 1987. Hypercalcemia: Pathophysiology and treatment. Hosp Pract 22(7):93–110.

Mahon SM. 1987. Symptoms as clues to calcium levels. Am J Nurs 87:354–356.

Morse L, Heery M, Flynn K. 1985. Early detection to avoid the crisis of superior vena cava syndrome. Cancer Nurs 8:228–232.

Mundy GR. 1987. The hypercalcemia of malignancy. Nephrol Forum 31:142–145.

Pizzo PA, Young RC. 1985. Infections in the cancer patient. In DeVita VT, Hellman S, Rosenberg SA, eds. Cancer: Principles and Practice of Oncology, 2nd ed. Philadelphia, JB Lippincott, 1963–1998.

Rodriguez M, Dinapoli R. 1980. Spinal cord compression. Mayo Clin Proc 55:442–448.

Sumner SM. 1987. Septic shock. Nursing 76(2):33.

Varricchio C. 1985. Clinical management of superior vena cava syndrome. Heart Lung 14:411–416.

Wegmann J, Forshee T. 1983. Malignant pleural effusions: Pertinent issues. Heart Lung 12:533–543.

Wilkowski J. 1986. Spinal cord compression: An oncologic emergency. Emerg Nurs 12(1):9–12.

Zehner LC, Hoogstraten B. 1985. Malignant effu-sions and their management. Semin Oncol Nurs 1:259–268.

Zevallos M, Chan PY, Munoz L, et al. 1987. Epi-dural spinal cord compression from meta-static tumor. Int J Radiat Biol Phys 13:875–878.

Rita Wickham, RN MS

Long-Term Venous Access Devices

Intravenous (IV) therapy has become widely used during the last 50 years, with nurses having increased primary involvement for only about 30 years. Intravenous catheter technology has paralleled the availability and growing need for IV therapy, along with other sophisticated diagnostic and therapeutic measures. From the early days of stainless steel needles that were used, resharpened, sterilized, and reused, we have seen the advent of various disposable plastic and stainless steel peripheral devices, polyethylene subclavian catheters, and silicone central venous catheters. Plastic and polyethylene catheters are suited only for short-term central catheterization because they tend to become brittle over time and are more highly thrombogenic than silicone catheters.

Broviac and colleagues (1973) developed a silicone central venous catheter more suited to long-term placement because of lower risks for thrombogenicity, infection, dislodgment, air embolism, or hemorrhage. Many variations of the silicone central venous catheter have subsequently been developed. These include nontunneled catheters, tunneled catheters, and totally implanted venous access ports. Although these devices are used most frequently for cancer patients, patients with other short- or long-term medical problems requiring prolonged IV therapy or access may also benefit from long-term catheter placement. Examples of such patients include those with debilitating cardiac disease, Crohn's disease (requiring total parenteral nutrition), sickle cell anemia, acquired immunodeficiency syndrome (AIDS), and cystic fibrosis. Patients with extensive burns and those with severe infections such as osteomyelitis who require an extended course of IV antibiotics may also benefit from long-term venous access devices. It is likely that these catheters will continue to have a growing use for many more persons in this era of decreasing hospital stays and increasing outpatient care. Therefore, it is imperative that emergency department (ED) nurses, in particular, be knowledgeable and skilled in the care of these catheters that are a virtual lifeline for many individuals. This chapter focuses on the three major types of long-term venous access devices (VADs), their assessment and access, and the management of common catheter-related problems.

OVERVIEW

VADs are similar in many respects, but they differ in how and if they exit the body. Nontunneled and tunneled catheters exit the body, whereas implanted ports lie completely beneath the skin and must be accessed with special needles. Nontunneled catheters are inserted peripherally into the basilic or cephalic vein at the antecubital space or centrally into the subclavian vein. The device enters the vein a short distance from the exit site. A short extension tubing, such as a T-connector, is secured to the catheter hub, and this may extend beyond the dressing to provide access to the system. Tunneled catheters, on the other hand, extend for several inches in a subcutaneous tunnel between the exit site and the point where the catheter enters the vein. Tunneled catheters have a Dacron cuff that lies about 5 cm from the exit site and serves to anchor the catheter and to minimize the risk of infection. Nontunneled and tunneled catheter systems are closed with Luer-Lok injection caps (Fig. 34–1).

Virtually all catheters are constructed of silicone, which to date has been identified as the most biocompatible material. Two implanted ports, the titanium Port-A-Cath (Pharmacia Deltec, Inc.) and the Implantofix (Burron Medical, Inc.) have polyurethane catheters. Polyurethane not only has similar biocompatibility to silicone but also is stiffer than silicone, allowing for easier placement (Linder et al 1984). Once the polyurethane catheter comes into contact with the blood vessel, it softens, thereby decreasing thrombogenicity.

Catheters are placed in a generally similar fashion (Fig. 34–1). One of the major veins of the upper chest, such as the subclavian, jugular, or cephalic, is cannulated. The tip of the catheter is advanced until it lies in the superior vena cava at or above the junction of the right atrium. Nontunneled central catheters exit at the neck or antecubital space, close to where they enter the vein. Tunneled catheters usually exit midway between the nipple and sternum, at a site distal from venous insertion. A similar placement technique is used for implanted venous access ports. A small excision on the upper chest exposes the vein selected for cannulation. The catheter is inserted and advanced so that the tip lies in the superior vena cava. A subcutaneous pocket is then formed nearby, into which the portal body is sutured. Finally the incision is closed. In cases of superior vena cava obstruction, the saphenous vein is cannulated and the catheter tip is advanced to the inferior vena cava. In this case, the catheter exits or the portal body is implanted in the lower abdomen or groin and should not be mistaken for a jejunostomy, gastrostomy, or peritoneal dialysis catheter.

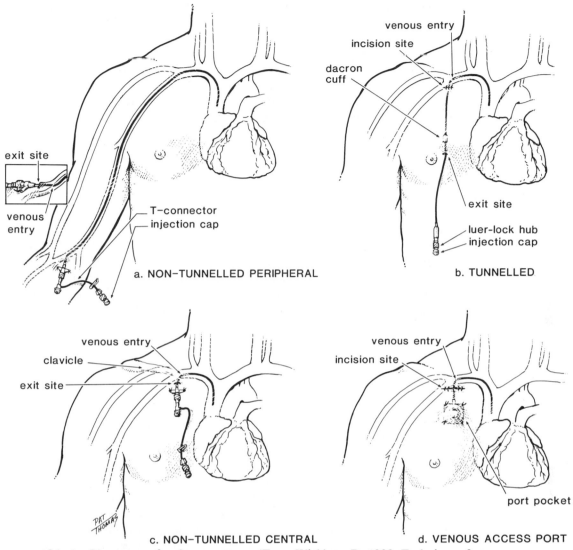

FIGURE 34-1. Placement of catheter systems. (From Wickham R. 1988. Techniques for venous access. Proceedings of the 5th National Conference on Cancer Nursing. American Cancer Society, Atlanta, GA.)

Nontunneled Catheters

Nontunneled silicone catheters are small-gauge catheters (19-to 23-gauge). Although central catheters are always inserted by a physician, peripheral catheters may be inserted by physicians or specially trained nurses (Chathas 1986; Lawson et al 1979). Peripheral catheters include those that are sutured at the exit site (e.g., the Intrasil, Baxter Healthcare Corp.) and those that are not sutured (e.g., the Per-Q-Cath, Gesco International).

Although nontunneled catheters have the smallest internal lumen, they are quite versatile and can be used for many months for IV boluses or continuous infusions of medications, fluids, blood and blood products, and total parenteral nutrition; they can also be used to obtain blood samples (Goodman and Wickham 1984; Slater et al 1985). Double-lumen central catheters are available from some manufacturers, which further increases the versatility of the catheter.

Although no comparative studies have been done, the rate of infection or other serious complications for nontunneled catheters does not appear to be greater than with other catheters (Lawson et al 1979). This may be related to the skill and experience of those persons caring for and teaching patients with this type of catheter. Another advantage is the ability to replace the catheter by an over-the-wire technique if a catheter-related infection or sepsis is suspected or if the catheter becomes damaged.

Major disadvantages of nontunneled catheters include high care requirements, restrictions on activity, and changes in body image. An occlusive dressing must be worn over the exit site at all times. Because the catheter exits the body an inch or less from where it enters the vein, sterile technique is usually recommended for dressing changes. These factors, plus the need for daily flushing with heparinized saline solution, make the care costs for this type of catheter high. In addition, because the catheter exits at the neck or antecubital space, it limits activities such as swimming and is difficult to "hide," affecting body image.

Tunneled Catheters

Many brands of silicone tunneled catheters (e.g., Hickman, Leonard, Raaf, Corcath, Groshong) are available. These thick-walled, large-bore, highly versatile catheters are available in models with single, double, and even triple lumens. A dressing over the exit site is required until the site has healed and the Dacron cuff has become enmeshed with fibroblasts, which takes about 3 to 4 weeks. After healing has occurred, many practitioners do not require the nonimmunocompromised patient to wear an occlusive dressing over the exit site. Some persons choose to keep a Band-Aid or other dressing over the exit site. Dressing changes need not be as meticulous as for nontunneled catheters, but the patient must keep the exit site clean and assess it regularly, particularly for signs and symptoms of infection, catheter dislodgment, or catheter damage. Tunneled catheters should always be looped back and secured to the patient to minimize the risk of traction, accidental removal, and catheter damage.

The Groshong catheter (Catheter Technology Corp.) is one of the newer tunneled silicone catheters. The Groshong is constructed of thin-walled silicone and is available in several sizes, from 3.5 to 8 French. It is also available in a double-lumen model. The 8 French is of comparable lumen to the Hickman gauge catheter (1.06-mm internal diameter), whereas the 7 French is comparable to the Broviac catheter (1.0-mm internal diameter). Another difference between the Groshong catheter and other tunneled catheters is that the Groshong catheter is blind-ended, with a patented two-way slit valve at the end of the catheter (Fig. 34–2). The valve remains closed unless fluids are being infused or blood is being withdrawn. The catheter is flushed once weekly with sterile saline solution when not used, after blood is withdrawn or

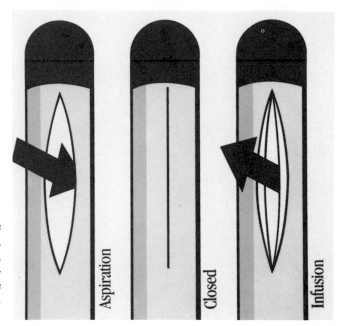

FIGURE 34–2. The patented two-way slit valve of the Groshong catheter (patent nos. 4,431,426, 4,549,879, 4,559,046, 4,547,194, 4,327,722, 4,671,796, 4,701,166, 4,753,600, 4,772,276, and 4,529,399) remains closed unless positive pressure opens it to allow infusion or negative pressure closes it to permit withdrawal of blood samples. (Courtesy of Catheter Technology Corporation.)

fluids infused. The risks of air embolism, hemorrhage, and clotted catheter are reduced with this design.

Tunneled catheters are the most versatile long-term catheter. It is generally easy to draw blood from them because of their large gauge, which is not always true with smaller-gauge nontunneled catheters. In addition, a double or triple lumen allows for multiple infusates (although it also increases the care requirements of the catheter). Fewer patients have double-lumen nontunneled catheters or ports. Furthermore, tunneled catheters can be repaired if damaged distally to the exit site.

Disadvantages of tunneled catheters include care requirements and cosmesis. Costs of catheter supplies (heparin flush, syringes and needles, alcohol wipes, injection caps, cleansing materials, antiseptic ointment, and dressing supplies) can be considerable, especially if a dressing over the exit site is always prescribed. Some persons have difficulty accepting tubes exiting from their bodies, whereas others may lack the mental or physical ability to care for such a device.

Venous Access Ports

Several brands of single- and double-lumen implanted venous access ports are available. The components include the portal body and attached catheter (Fig. 34–3). The portal is constructed of plastic, stainless steel, or titanium and contains a dense silicone septum overlying a reservoir. The septum lies approximately parallel to the skin when implanted. If correctly accessed, the septum will withstand 1000 to 2000 needle sticks. The silicone (or polyurethane) catheter is either permanently attached to the portal (one-piece design) or attached at time of placement (two-piece design).

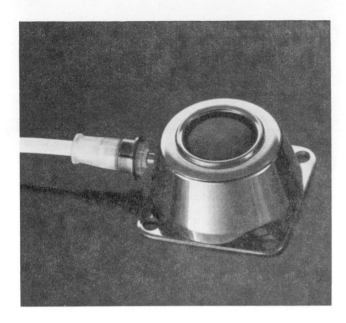

FIGURE 34-3. Venous access port. (Courtesy of Phar-
maciDeltec, Inc., St. Paul, MN.)

Since no part of the system exits the body, the portal must be accessed with a
Huber point needle (Fig. 34-4). This specially designed needle has a deflected tip
that tears rather than cores the septum. This allows the portal to reseal when the
needle is withdrawn. Huber point needles are available in several sizes ($\frac{3}{4}$ inch to $1\frac{1}{2}$

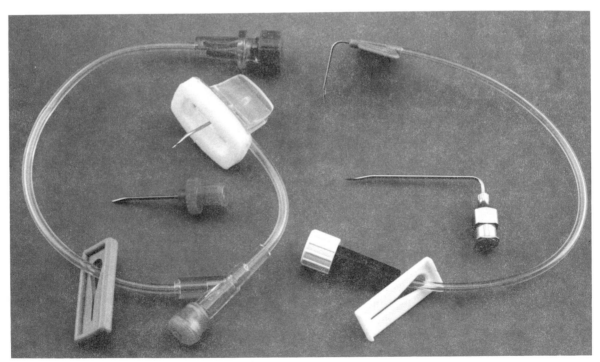

FIGURE 34-4. Huber-point needles.

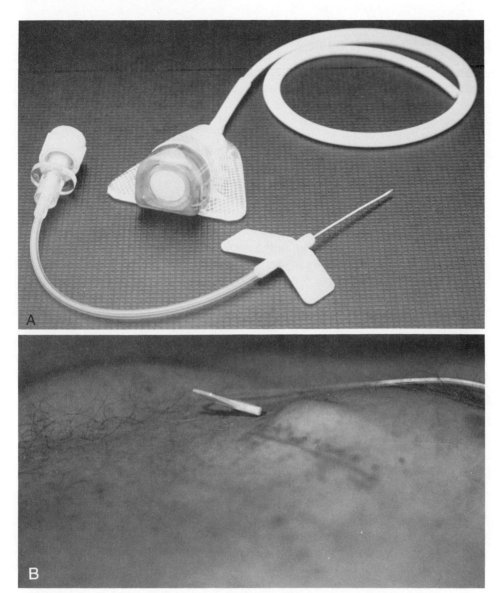

FIGURE 34–5. *A*, Norport SP 5. requires cannulation with straight Huber needle, *B*, which ultimately lies parallel to the skin. (Courtesy of Norport Medical Products, Inc.)

inches or longer), in straight or 90-degree forms, and in several gauges (19-, 20-, and 22-gauge).

Recently a new port, the Norfolk SR (Norfolk Medical) has become available. This port differs greatly from all ports in that the portal body is rotated 90 degrees, requiring a different cannulation procedure (Fig. 34–5). The manufacturer believes this design facilitates safe and reliable continuous infusions because of a thick septum and because a straight Huber point needle is used to cannulate the port. Once cannulated, the needle lies parallel to the skin, decreasing the risk of needle dislodgment and subsequent extravasation of infusate.

Ports are not quite as versatile as tunneled catheters because two incompatible infusates cannot be infused simultaneously into a single-lumen device, and few patients have double-lumen ports placed. However, ports can be used for blood sampling as well as bolus and continuous IV infusions. Because the entire system is enclosed under the skin, there are little or no care requirements for the patient. Some patients are taught to discontinue infusions, flush and heparinize the system, and decannulate their ports on completion of ambulatory infusions. Ports are flushed with heparinized saline solution after use or once every 4 to 8 weeks when not in use.

Although care requirements are minimal, the patient needs to assess the portal site for signs and symptoms of port pocket infection. A port may be less objectionable in terms of body image, but the patient may object to the pain of the needle stick. Some surgeons denervate the area over the portal at time of insertion to decrease the discomfort associated with cannulation.

Insertion costs for ports are higher than for nontunneled or tunneled catheters. These include the cost of the device ($250 to $400 plus hospital fee), the surgeon's fee, and hospital costs (surgery and postanesthesia recovery). Although the procedure is usually done in outpatient surgery, these costs can be considerable. Ports, then, generally are most suitable for the person who will require venous access for more than 2 to 3 months or who is not a suitable candidate for an external catheter because of inability to care for catheter, previous catheter sepsis, repeated external catheter damage, or dislodgment.

EVALUATING LONG-TERM CENTRAL VENOUS CATHETERS

It may not initially be known whether a patient who comes to the ED has a long-term venous catheter. Thus, the nursing history should elicit this information from the patient or significant others. If the patient is not conscious, physical examination easily provides evidence of external catheters, although it may not be clear that these are intravenous catheters as opposed to intra-arterial or peritoneal catheters. Radiographic confirmation of the catheter tip above or at the right atrium may be necessary. Totally implanted ports may also be difficult to assess. Catheter manufacturers generally supply a wallet-sized identification card along with the catheter, which the surgeon may give to the patient. In addition, some health care providers give the patient additional written information about their catheters. Therefore, the patient should be asked or his or her physical effects examined for any identifying information about the type of catheter and how to use it, or at what hospital it was inserted.

The catheter exit site or port pocket should be carefully examined before the catheter is accessed. The nurse should look for evidence of catheter damage or slippage; swelling or pain in the ipsilateral shoulder, arm, or neck; and signs and symptoms of local infection, including erythema, swelling, discomfort, or purulence. Consultation with a physician is necessary before accessing any catheter with these findings.

ACCESSING LONG-TERM CENTRAL VENOUS CATHETERS

If the nurse is unfamiliar with a particular catheter, it is important to find an experienced colleague from the ED or another part of the hospital (e.g., an oncology nurse) to assist with catheter access and use. At the very least it is distressing for the patient who has gone through catheter placement to have nurses or physicians start peripheral IVs because they are unfamiliar with access procedures. On the other extreme, the catheter may provide the only reliable access in a critically ill or injured person.

Patients may come to the ED with a catheter-related problem or with a non-catheter-related problem but require venous catheterization. Therefore, procedures for access for infusion and blood sampling along with general information regarding the three major types of long-term VADs are discussed in this section.

GENERAL INFORMATION: NONTUNNELED AND TUNNELED CATHETERS

Information	Rationale
1. Nontunneled and tunneled catheter systems are closed with a Luer-Lok injection cap.	1. A Luer-Lok decreases the risk of accidental dislodgment of the cap from the catheter. The injection cap allows for bolus injections or short-term infusions without opening the catheter system.
2. If accessing a catheter through the injection cap use $\frac{5}{8}$-inch to 1-inch needle of smallest gauge feasible (20- to 25-gauge).	2. One inch is the longest needle that can be inserted through the injection cap without risking damage to the catheter.
3. Routine clamping of nontunneled and tunneled catheters is not recommended; if clamping is preferred, metal clamps (bulldog) should not be used.	3. Routine clamping, especially with metal bulldog clamps, increases the risk of catheter damage.
4. Clamp (with nonmetal clamp) when the cap is removed.	4. Clamping closes the system, minimizing the risks for air embolism, hemorrhage, or clotted catheter.
5. Incompatible solutions should never be infused simultaneously through a single catheter lumen.	5. Incompatible solutions may cause irreversible catheter occlusion.
6. External catheters or IV tubing should always be secured to the chest or abdomen, as with a "stress loop."	6. A stress loop minimizes the risk of needle dislodgment from an implanted port or accidental catheter dislodgment from direct traction.

Continued

GENERAL INFORMATION:
NONTUNNELED AND TUNNELED CATHETERS *Continued*

Information	Rationale
7. Always wash hands before accessing any catheter even if sterile gloves are worn.	7. The most frequently cultured organisms in documented catheter-related infections are bacteria commonly found on skin (Hansell et al 1986; Peterson et al 1986).
8. Always inspect catheter exit site daily and before use.	8. Local infections are easily detectable and require treatment.

IMPLANTED VENOUS ACCESS PORT

1. It is important to select an appropriate needle:	
a. A ¾- to 1-inch long 90-degree Huber point needle is sufficient for most persons; for those patients whose ports are deeply implanted (e.g., under adipose tissue or breast tissue), a longer needle may be necessary.	a. Ideally the port is not implanted so deeply that it is difficult to palpate or cannulate and to stabilize the needle; the needle tip should reach the backstop of the portal without a great amount of the needle protruding beyond the skin.
b. The needle gauge selected is dependent on the rate of infusion and the infusate(s); potential IV needs should be anticipated before cannulating the port.	b. A 22-gauge needle is used if less than 250 ml IV fluid/hour is infused; a 19- to 20-gauge needle is used if more than 250 ml IV fluid/hour is infused, if blood is infused, if IV riders are administered in addition to continuous IV infusion, or if total parenteral nutrition (TPN) is infused.
2. Adequate assessment of the portal is imperative before cannulation. This includes locating the borders of the port with two fingers or three fingers (triangulation) as well as assessing how the top of the portal lies in relationship to the skin.	2. The septum is not always parallel to the skin surface; for instance, surgical placement or contracture of scar tissue may result in a tilted port, the patient may have a side access port, or the portal may have turned over because of "twiddling" by the patient (Gebarski and Gebarski 1984); a clear idea of where the septum is and how it lies in relationship to the overlying skin will result in the most suc-

GENERAL INFORMATION:
IMPLANTED VENOUS ACCESS PORT *Continued*

Information	Rationale
	cessful and relatively painless cannulation.
3. The needle is inserted perpendicularly into the port (not necessarily the skin) until the back of the portal reservoir is felt.	3. Perpendicular cannulation minimizes the chance of coring rather than tearing the portal septum; repeated coring decreases life and effectiveness of septum and may result in extravasation (leakage) of infusate from the portal.
4. The needle should never be rocked or rotated once the septum has been cannulated.	4. Movement of the needle in the septum may damage the septum, allowing extravasation of infusate. Therefore, during cannulation the needle should be held over the point at which it will ultimately be stabilized.
5. The hub of the needle in the septum should point away from large muscle masses involved with significant movement (e.g., the pectoral muscle).	5. Placement of the hub of the Huber point needle toward a muscle may increase rocking of the needle and increase the risk of needle dislodgment and extravasation of infusate.
6. When a port is cannulated for intermittent bolus or continuous IV infusion, the needle and short extension tubing are generally changed once weekly.	6. This interval is recommended by most manufacturers; there should be no increased rate of port pocket or systemic infection if asepsis is maintained when opening the system.
7. Incompatible solutions should never be infused concurrently through a single-lumen port.	7. Incompatible solutions may cause irreversible occlusion of the catheter; always flush with 10 to 20 ml of sterile normal saline solution between incompatible infusates.
8. Always wash hands before accessing a port, even though sterile gloves are worn.	8. The most commonly cultured organisms in documented catheter-related infections are bacteria commonly found on the skin (Lokich et al 1985; May and Davis 1988).
9. Always inspect for erythema, increased temperature, swelling, or tenderness of the port pocket site before access.	9. Port pocket infections preclude cannulating the port without physician approval.

PROCEDURES FOR CATHETER USE:
IV INFUSIONS, NONTUNNELED CATHETER

Administering Infusion:
Supplies

IV solution with IV tubing attached
Alcohol wipes
Tape
10-ml syringe of normal saline

Procedure	Rationale
1. Connect IV tubing to IV solution and flush tubing.	
2. Close clamp on microbore tubing attached to catheter.	2. Prevent air embolism, hemorrhage, or obstruction of catheter when system is opened.
3. Remove injection cap and discard, maintaining sterility of microbore tubing hub.	3. Minimize risk of contamination and catheter-related infection.
4. Cleanse hub with alcohol wipe.	4. Minimize risk of contamination and catheter-related infection.
5. Connect IV tubing to microbore hub, taping connection.	5. Minimize risk of accidental dislodgment of IV tubing.
6. Unclamp microbore tubing and start IV at ordered rate of infusion.	
7. Tape microbore catheter or IV tubing to chest or arm.	7. Minimize risk of traction and accidental catheter removal.

Discontinuing Infusion:
Supplies

Injection cap
10 ml of sterile normal saline solution (unless infusate is normal saline solution or 5% dextrose in water)
3-ml syringe (with needle attached) containing 1 ml heparinized saline solution (100 U/ml)

Procedure	Rationale
1. Turn off IV fluid and clamp microbore tubing.	1. Prevent air embolism, hemorrhage, or obstruction of catheter when system is opened.

PROCEDURES FOR CATHETER USE:
IV INFUSIONS, NONTUNNELED CATHETER *Continued*

Discontinuing Infusion:

Procedure	Rationale
2. Disconnect IV tubing and attach 10-ml syringe of normal saline to microbore tubing.	
3. Unclamp microbore tubing and flush with saline.	3. Prevent precipitation of incompatible solutions within catheter.
4. Clamp tubing and disconnect syringe.	
5. Connect injection cap to microbore tubing and unclamp.	
6. Flush with heparinized saline solution through injection cap.	6. Prevent clotting within catheter.

IV INFUSIONS, TUNNELED CATHETER

Administering Infusion:
Supplies

IV solution with IV tubing attached
Alcohol wipes
Catheter clamp
Tape

Procedure	Rationale
1. Connect IV tubing to IV solution container and flush tubing.	
2. Clamp catheter.	2. Prevent air embolism, hemorrhage, or obstruction of catheter when system is opened.
3. Remove injection cap and discard, maintaining sterility of catheter hub.	3. Minimize risk of contamination and catheter-related infection.
4. Cleanse catheter hub with alcohol wipe.	4. Minimize risk of contamination and catheter-related infection.
5. Connect IV tubing to catheter hub, taping connection.	5. Minimize risk of accidental dislodgment.
6. Unclamp catheter and start IV at ordered rate of infusion.	

Continued

IV INFUSIONS, TUNNELED CATHETER *Continued*

Administering Infusion:

Procedure	Rationale
7. Secure catheter to chest with safety loop.	7. Minimize risk of traction or accidental catheter damage or removal.

Discontinuing Infusion:
Supplies

Injection cap
10-ml syringe of sterile normal saline solution
3-ml syringe of heparinized saline solution (10 U/ml)* (if patient has other than a Groshong catheter)
22-gauge ⅝-inch to 1-inch needles

Procedure	Rationale
1. Turn off IV and clamp IV tubing.	
2. Clamp catheter (unless Groshong type) and remove tape from connection site.	
3. Wipe connection site with alcohol wipe.	3. Minimize risk of contamination and catheter-related infection.
4. Disconnect catheter from IV tubing and secure a new injection cap on catheter.	
5. Tape connection.	
6. Unclamp catheter and flush with 10 ml of normal saline if	
a. infusing solution incompatible with heparin or	a. Prevent precipitation within catheter.
b. patient has Groshong catheter.	b. Flush needed only with Groshong catheter.
7. If non-Groshong catheter, follow with 3-ml heparinized saline flush.	7. Prevent clotting within the catheter.

* Concentration of heparin flush is generally selected empirically and may differ from institution to institution. Concentrations of 10 U/ml to 100 U/ml are adequate to create a heparin lock and prevent clotting within the catheter.

IV INFUSIONS, IMPLANTED VENOUS ACCESS PORT

Cannulation for Continuous IV Infusion:
Supplies

Sterile 90-degree Huber point needle, 19- to 22-gauge, attached tubing or short extension set
10-ml syringe
10 ml of sterile normal saline solution
18-gauge needle
Sterile gloves
Steri Strips or 1-inch tape
3 povidone-iodine swabs
Antimicrobial ointment
Sterile 2 × 2 inch gauge squares
Occlusive dressing: 2 × 2 inch or 4 × 4 inch gauze squares and tape, or transparent dressing

Procedure	Rationale
1. Palpate site to locate port and septum (Fig. 34–6).	1. Adequate assessment is crucial to optimal cannulation.

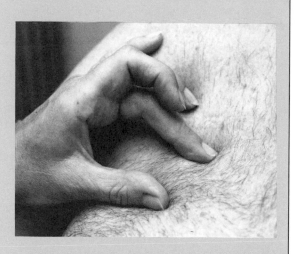

FIGURE 34–6. Palpate site to locate port and septum.

2. Examine site for redness, heat, swelling, or discomfort; notify	2. These signs and symptoms may be present until the port pocket

Continued

IMPLANTED VENOUS ACCESS PORT *Continued*

Procedure	Rationale
physician of any such occurrence before cannulation if beyond normal healing time.	is well healed, about 2 to 3 weeks; beyond this time such symptoms may indicate a port pocket infection.
3. Cleanse 3 to 4 inches of surrounding area about the port with a povidone-iodine swab.* Using a circular motion, start at center of port and work outward (Fig. 34–7). Repeat with two more povidone-iodine swabs. Allow to dry before cannulation.	3. A widely prepared area will allow for palpation and stabilization of the port, preventing contamination of the sterile gloved hand. Povidone-iodine is the recommended skin preparation for IV cannulation. It must be allowed to dry on the skin.

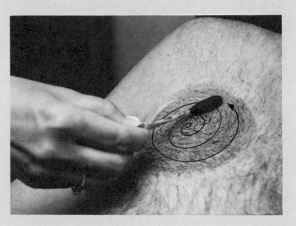

FIGURE 34–7. Cleanse area over port with povidone-iodine swabs, using a circular motion.

Procedure	Rationale
4. Open and place on sterile field: 10-ml syringe 18-gauge needle Huber point needle Extension tubing (if not attached to Huber needle) Sterile gloves	4. Sterility of these items is maintained until the port is cannulated.
5. To side, place Opened ampule of sterile normal saline solution Unopened antimicrobial ointment Tape Dressing	
6. Don sterile gloves.	6. Maintain sterile technique.

*Use alcohol wipes if patient is allergic or sensitive to iodine.

IMPLANTED VENOUS ACCESS PORT *Continued*

Procedure	Rationale
7. Connect extension tubing to Huber point needle, if necessary.	
8. Maintaining sterility, attach 18-gauge needle to 10-ml syringe, drawing up 10 ml of sterile normal saline solution.	
9. Disconnect 18-gauge needle from syringe.	
10. Connect syringe containing saline solution to tubing attached to Huber point needle.	
11. Prime tubing and needle with saline solution, leaving syringe attached.	11. Ensure patency of needle and clear the system of air.
12. Cannulate the port while stabilizing it between two or three fingers (Fig. 34–8). Use a sure, swift technique to push the needle through the skin and portal septum until the bottom of the port is felt.	12. A sure technique is more likely to result in correct needle placement as well as decreased patient discomfort.

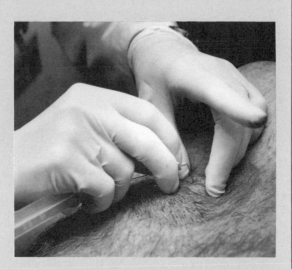

FIGURE 34–8. Cannulate the port while stabilizing it between two or three fingers.

13. Check for correct placement by flushing with the remaining saline solution in the syringe.	13. A correctly cannulated port will flush easily with no objective (swelling) or subjective (pain)

Continued

IMPLANTED VENOUS ACCESS PORT *Continued*

Procedure	Rationale
a. If unable to flush, recheck needle position by pushing the needle further against the backstop or recannulating.	signs of extravasation of sterile normal saline.
b. If swelling and pain occur about port, recheck needle position.	Inability to flush may indicate the needle has not been advanced through the septum or that the catheter is occluded.
c. Notify physician if pain or swelling occurs or if unable to flush once correct placement is ascertained.	
14. Apply antimicrobial ointment to needle site.	14. Minimize bacterial growth at needle insertion site.
15. Stabilize needle by placing 1 or 2 folded sterile 2 × 2 gauze squares under hub of needle, if necessary, and taping across needle hub about it in chevron fashion (Fig. 34–9).	15. Help to minimize risk of accidental needle dislodgment.

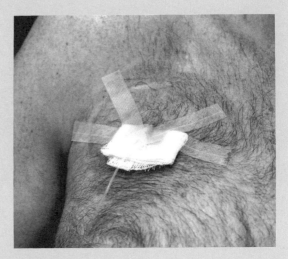

FIGURE 34–9. Stabilize needle by applying tape across hub and around it in a chevron pattern and by placing folded 2 × 2s beneath it if necessary.

16. Apply occlusive gauze and tape or transparent dressing over site.
17. Clamp tubing and remove syringe.
18. Connect to IV tubing and start infusion.
19. Tape connections.

IMPLANTED VENOUS ACCESS PORT *Continued*

Procedure	Rationale
20. Secure stress loop by taping back over chest or dressing.	20. Minimize risk of accidental needle dislodgment.

Discontinuing Infusion: Supplies

10-ml syringe
Sterile normal saline solution
3-ml syringe
Heparinized saline solution (100 U/ml)
18-gauge needles (2)
Alcohol wipes

Procedure	Rationale
1. Draw up 10 ml of normal saline solution.	
2. Draw up 3 ml of heparinized saline solution.	2. Heparinized saline solution (100 U/ml) is recommended by port manufacturer to prevent clotting within the catheter.
3. Remove dressing, taking care not to dislodge needle from port.	
4. Close clamp on short extension tubing.	4. Minimize risk of air embolism, hemorrhage, or obstruction of catheter.
5. Remove tape from connection and cleanse with alcohol wipe.	5. Minimize risk of contamination and catheter-related infection.
6. Disconnect from IV tubing if port had been used for continuous infusion.	
7. Connect normal saline syringe to Huber tubing.	
8. Open clamp; flush vigorously.	
9. Close clamp.	
10. Connect heparin syringe.	
11. Open clamp and flush.	
12. Close clamp.	
13. Stabilize port between two fingers; pull needle straight out.	
14. Examine site for redness or heat, swelling, purulent exudate, and discomfort.	14. Signs and symptoms of local infection should be reported to the physician.
15. Apply Band-Aid if desired.	

OBTAINING BLOOD SAMPLES, NONTUNNELED CATHETER

Note: Some institutions do not recommend the routine use of nontunneled catheters to obtain blood samples. The rationale for this policy is that opening the system places the patient at greater risk for infection (M.D. Anderson Hospital and Tumor Institute, Houston, Texas). Therefore, when it is necessary to draw blood from the catheter, meticulous sterile technique is advised.

Supplies

Laboratory tube(s)   Alcohol wipes
Requisitions for tests   Syringes for blood samples
Heparinized saline solution   3-ml syringe with needle
(100 U/ml)   2 10-ml syringes
Sterile normal saline solution   Injection cap

Procedure	Rationale
1. Draw up 10 ml of normal saline solution.	
2. Draw up 1 ml of heparinized saline solution.	
3. Clamp short extension tubing attached to catheter.	3. Prevent air embolism, hemorrhage, or obstruction of catheter.
4. Remove injection cap and discard.	
5. Connect empty 10-ml syringe.	
6. Open clamp and withdraw 7 ml of blood.	6. Heparinized saline solution remaining in catheter will dilute sample and may otherwise affect laboratory results.
7. Close clamp, detach, and discard this sample.	
8. Connect syringe for blood sample.	
9. Open clamp and withdraw blood slowly and steadily.	9. Exerting high negative pressure when attempting to withdraw blood rapidly may cause the catheter to collapse.
a. Blood samples for activated partial thromboplastin time (APTT) should not be drawn from heparinized silicone catheters.	a. APPTs of samples drawn from heparinized silicone central catheters and peripheral veins differ significantly (Almadrones et al 1987).
b. Blood for complete blood count should be placed immediately into a heparinized tube (before flushing catheter).	b. Clotting precludes analysis of complete blood count.

OBTAINING BLOOD SAMPLES, NONTUNNELED CATHETER *Continued*

Procedure	Rationale
10. Close clamp, detach syringe and attach 10-ml syringe of normal saline solution.	
11. Open clamp and flush catheter.	11. A new injection cap is used each time the system is opened to minimize the risk of infection.
12. Close clamp and attach new injection cap.	
13. Open clamp, cleanse injection cap, and flush with heparinized saline solution.	
14. Attach needles to syringes of blood and fill collection tubes.	
15. Label specimens and send to laboratory.	

OBTAINING BLOOD SAMPLES TUNNELED CATHETER

Supplies

Laboratory tube(s)
Requisitions for tests
Catheter clamp
Heparinized saline (10 U/ml)
Sterile normal saline
Syringes large enough for blood samples

Alcohol wipes (4)
3-ml syringe with needle
10-ml syringe with needle
18-gauge needles (2)
Vacutainer and Vacutainer needle*

Procedure	Rationale
1. Prepare sterile barrier.	1. Maintain the sterility of open syringes and needles.
2. Draw up 10 ml of sterile normal saline solution if catheter is connected to IV for continuous infusion; draw up additional 3 ml of heparinized saline solution if catheter is capped.	2. Catheters that are reconnected to continuous infusions will only need to be cleared of blood, whereas the capped catheter (except the Groshong type) will need to be heparinized.
3. Remove needles from both and place all on sterile barrier; place	3. Maintain sterility of all components that will touch catheter

Continued

**OBTAINING BLOOD SAMPLES
TUNNELED CATHETER** *Continued*

Procedure	Rationale
all other syringes on the sterile barrier.	hub and IV connectors.
4. Turn off infusion if indicated, clamping IV tubing.	
5. Clamp catheter, remove tape, and cleanse connection with alcohol wipe.	5. Minimize risk for introducing bacteria into catheter or IV tubing.
6. Disconnect IV tubing or cap.	6. Maintain sterility of all connecting sites.
7. Attach empty 10-ml syringe to catheter and cover IV tubing or injection cap with sterile needle securing Luer-Lok.	
8. Unclamp and withdraw 6 ml of fluid for discard.	8. Heparinized saline solution remaining in catheter will dilute sample and may otherwise affect laboratory results.
9. Clamp catheter and disconnect syringe.	
10. Connect collection syringe(s) and unclamp, withdrawing blood specimens slowly.	10. Negative pressure exerted to obtain blood return must not be so great as to collapse catheter wall, nor so slight as to allow clotting of blood within the catheter.
a. Draw blood for cultures first if drawing several specimens.	
b. Blood samples for activated partial thromboplastin time (APTT) should not be drawn from heparinized silicone catheters.	b. APPTs of samples drawn from heparinized silicone central catheters and peripheral veins differ significantly (Almadrones et al 1987).
c. Blood for complete blood count should be placed into heparinized collection tube immediately (before flushing catheter).	c. Clotting of the blood sample prevents analysis of complete blood count.
11. Clamp catheter and remove collection syringes.	
12. Vigorously irrigate catheter with 10 ml of saline solution, followed by 3 ml of heparinized saline solution (if catheter is capped). (Only Groshong catheter does not require heparin flush.)	12. Catheters that are reconnected to continuous infusion will only need to be cleared of blood, whereas the capped catheter (except the Groshong) will need to be heparinized.

OBTAINING BLOOD SAMPLES
TUNNELED CATHETER *Continued*

Procedure	Rationale
13. Clamp catheter and disconnect syringe.	
14. Wipe catheter hub with alcohol wipe.	
15. Remove needle cover from IV tubing or injection cap.	
16. Reconnect IV tubing or injection cap, taping connection.	
17. Attach needles to collection syringes and fill collection tubes.	
18. Label specimens and send to laboratory.	

---

* This procedure may be accomplished with Vacutainer if the catheter is capped: Repeat steps 1 to 5.

Procedure	Rationale
6. Attach Vacutainer needle to Vacutainer, placing 7-ml specimen tube into Vacutainer without puncturing rubber stopper.	
7. Wipe injection cap with alcohol wipe.	
8. Insert Vacutainer needle into injection cap.	
9. Making certain catheter is unclamped, push specimen tube all the way into the Vacutainer, puncturing the rubber stopper.	9. Negative pressure within specimen tube will draw fluid or blood from catheter.
10. Remove first Vacutainer specimen tube and discard.	10. First specimen will be diluted with heparinized saline solution.
11. Repeat with all specimen tubes.	
12. Withdraw Vacutainer needle and discard.	
13. Flush capped catheter with saline solution or heparinized saline solution or both, as appropriate.	
14. Label specimen tubes and send to laboratory.	

OBTAINING BLOOD SAMPLES
VENOUS ACCESS PORT

Blood samples may be drawn from a line established for blood sample or when the port is cannulated for IV infusion.

Supplies

Blood collection tubes
Requisitions for tests

Syringes of appropriate size to draw blood specimens

Continued

OBTAINING BLOOD SAMPLES
VENOUS ACCESS PORT *Continued*

Supplies

10-ml syringe
20-ml syringe
Sterile normal saline solution

18-gauge needles
Alcohol wipes

Procedure	Rationale
1. Place syringes, needles, and other equipment on a clean surface.	1. Although sterile gloves are not necessary, sterility of connections (catheter hub, ends of syringes, needles, IV tubing) must be maintained.
2. Draw up 20 ml of sterile saline solution and remove needle from syringe.	
3. Clamp the short extension tubing attached to Huber point needle. a. Cannulate the port if necessary (see Cannulation for Continuous IV Infusion, steps 1 to 13), or b. Clamp IV tubing if port was previously cannulated for infusion.	
4. Untape connection and cleanse with alcohol wipe if port was previously cannulated for infusion.	4. Minimize the risk of introducing bacteria into the catheter or IV tubing.
5. a. Connect empty 10-ml syringe to Huber tubing, or b. Disconnect IV tubing from Huber tubing, connecting empty 10-ml syringe to Huber tubing and 18-gauge needle to IV tubing.	5. Maintain sterility of all connecting sites.
6. Unclamp Huber tubing and withdraw 6 ml of blood.	
7. Clamp tubing, disconnect this syringe, and discard specimen.	7. Heparinized saline solution will dilute the sample and may otherwise affect laboratory results.
8. Connect collection syringe.	
9. Unclamp tubing and steadily withdraw the blood specimens.	9. The negative pressure exerted to obtain blood return must not be

OBTAINING BLOOD SAMPLES
VENOUS ACCESS PORT *Continued*

Procedure	Rationale
	so great as to collapse the catheter wall, nor so slight as to allow clotting of blood within the catheter or Huber needle.
a. Blood samples for activated partial thromboplastin time (APTT) should not be drawn from heparinized silicone catheters.	a. APPTs of blood drawn from heparinized silicone central catheters and peripheral veins differ significantly (Almadrones et al 1987).
b. Blood for complete blood count should be placed into a heparinized collection tube immediately (before flushing catheter).	b. Clotting of the blood prevents analysis of these parameters.
10. Clamp Huber tubing and disconnect collection syringe.	
11. Connect 20-ml syringe of normal saline solution immediately.	
12. Unclamp Huber tubing and flush briskly with 20 ml of sterile normal saline solution.	12. Residual blood within the needle, portal body, or catheter may clot within a short time.
13. Clamp Huber tubing and disconnect 20-ml syringe.	
14. a. Reconnect Huber tubing to IV tubing, taping connection, or	
b. Prepare to heparinize and discontinue the Huber point needle (see Discontinuing Infusion, Procedure, under Implanted Venous Port), or	
c. Attach injection cap to maintain cannulated and heplocked port.	
15. a. Restart IV infusion, or	
b. Flush system with 3 ml of heparinized saline solution (100 U/ml) if discontinuing the Huber needle or heplocking port.	
16. Fill collection tubes, label, and send to laboratory.	

CATHETER COMPLICATIONS

A risk of several complications exists for all catheters. These are summarized in Table 34–1. Major complications that may lead to the patient's coming to the ED are discussed. These include infection, extraluminal venous obstruction, intraluminal catheter obstruction, extravasation, and catheter damage. First, however, a general overview of the assessment of patients coming to the ED with catheter-related problems is given.

Assessment of Catheter-Related Complications

When a person comes to the ED with a catheter-related complication, initial assessment must determine his or her level of illness acuity. Triage assessment must focus on the patient's chief complaint, examination of the catheter site, and vital signs. Most patients will be considered stable and will thus be able to wait for further assessment and intervention. In a few instances, most likely catheter-related sepsis, the patient may be in a life-threatening situation and therefore must be treated as quickly as possible.

In the treatment area, the chief complaint of the patient is investigated more fully. Information elicited should include what type of catheter the patient has, where

TABLE 34–1
Catheter-Related Complications

Complication	Nontunneled Catheter (NT)	Tunneled Catheter (TN)	Venous Access Port (VAP)	Sources
Catheter-related infection or sepsis	X	X	X	Chathas 1986; Fuchs et al 1984; Hansell et al 1986; Lawson et al 1979; Lokich et al 1985; May and Davis 1988; Press et al 1984; Slater et al 1985; Verghese et al 1985
Catheter occlusion: Withdrawal Mural thrombus Intraluminal clot	X	X	X	Bertrand et al 1984; Chathas 1986; Lawson et al 1979; Lokich et al 1985; Peterson et al 1986
Extravasation*		X	X	Lokich et al 1985; Rubenstein et al 1985
Catheter damage with or without migration	X	X	X	Lokich et al 1985; Reed et al 1983; Rubenstein et al 1985; Slater et al 1985
Other (rare or less serious): Phlebitis†	X			Chathas 1986; Lawson et al 1979
Pneumothorax‡	X	X	X	Lawson et al 1979; Slater et al 1985
Twiddler's syndrome			X	Gebarski and Gebarski 1984
Accidental removal, hemorrhage, air embolism	X	X		Ostrow 1981; Peterson et al 1986; Reed et al 1983
Cardiac perforation§ or tamponade	X	X		Peterson et al 1986

* Most common with VAP, although reported with other catheters.
† Occurs with peripherally placed catheters.
‡ Occurs shortly after insertion when catheter is placed by the direct subclavian approach.
§ Use of stiff catheters (polyvinylchloride or polyethylene) and advancement of the catheter tip into the atrium increase risk.

it exits the body, how long he or she has had it, what the catheter is used for, and when it was last used for therapeutic purposes. Other questions to ask the patient relate to the specific catheter-related problem.

Examination of the catheter site follows the history-taking. Because most catheters are placed in one of the large veins of the upper chest or neck, it is important to examine the entire upper chest, arms, neck, and face using good lighting. Comparison of the ipsilateral and contralateral (to the catheter) sides may yield important clues. The nurse should look for any subtle or obvious swelling over the chest wall, neck, shoulder, or arm on the side of the catheter, increased venous pattern over the chest or shoulder, tenderness or pain at the exit site or over a port pocket, tenderness or pain along a catheter tunnel, erythema over any part of the catheter, and purulence or crusting at the exit side. The catheter should also be examined for signs of slippage from the exit site (a length of catheter just distal to the exit may appear cleaner or the catheter cuff may be visible) or for frank signs of catheter damage. The most common laboratory test ordered for this patient is the complete blood count with differential count.

INFECTION

Catheter-related infection is a most serious complication and may occur at several sites: at the exit site of a nontunneled or tunneled catheter, in a port pocket, along the catheter tunnel, within a mural thrombus surrounding the intravenous segment of catheter, or as a septicemia seeded from the colonized catheter tip. The majority of infections occur at the exit site and in the tunnel (Press et al 1984). It is suggested that venous access ports are associated with a lower risk of catheter-related infection (May and Davis 1988).

Etiology and Pathophysiology

Risk factors for catheter infection include the indications for catheter placement, duration of placement, and catheter-related thrombosis. Catheters used primarily for TPN have the highest rate of infection (22.9%), followed by those used mainly for antibiotic therapy (12.7%) or chemotherapy (4.4%) (Fuchs et al 1984). Fuchs and coworkers also indicated that increasing duration of the catheter placement might also be a risk factor. On the other hand, Press and colleagues (1984) found only catheter thrombosis strongly associated with the onset of a catheter infection. Other factors, such as the patient's immune status, nutritional status, and underlying disease process, as well as the adequacy of teaching, the nursing and medical support available, and the mental and physical ability of the patient and significant others to care for the catheter may also influence the risk of infection. The relative importance of these factors, however, has not been established.

Clinical Manifestations

The chief complaint of the patient may or may not indicate the severity of the infection. Local signs may not be present in the most serious infections (septicemia and septic thrombosis). Patients with septicemia may progress to septic shock.

Exit site infections are manifest by erythema, induration, tenderness, or purulence within 2 cm of the exit site (Press et al 1984). Tunnel infections are accompanied by pain, erythema, and induration along the subcutaneous tunnel more than 2 cm from the exit, with or without signs of inflammation and purulent exudate at the exit site. Definite catheter-related bacteremia alone occurred in 18.8% of patients in the series of Press and colleagues, although 75% of patients with exit infections and 38% of those with tunnel infections had associated bacteremia as well.

Bacteremia is confirmed by fever with or without chills and by positive blood cultures. *Staphylococcus epidermidis* is the most commonly cultured organism in documented catheter-related bacteremia (Hansell et al 1986; Peterson et al 1986; Press et al 1984). The complete blood count is essential and may reveal leukocytosis or, in patients with bone marrow suppression following chemotherapy, a decreased total white blood cell count along with a decrease in the relative percentage of neutrophils.

Septic thrombosis occurs infrequently, but is potentially the most serious catheter-related infection. Injury to the venous endothelium along the catheter or at its tip, irritating intravenous solutions, or irregular blood flow or stasis about the catheter may contribute to thrombus formation (Slagle and Gates 1986). The thrombus may be colonized from contaminated IV fluids or TPN, bacterial migration from the external site, or a bacteremia related to a distant infection (Verghese et al 1985).

Patients with septic thrombosis have symptoms of bacteremia, and some may have evidence of venous obstruction (e.g., swelling of neck or arm and increased venous pattern over chest and shoulder). The presence of a thrombus may be confirmed radiologically with a venogram through a peripheral vein on the affected side (Verghese et al 1985).

Port pocket infection is manifested as erythema, tenderness, and induration over or about the port pocket. If a port pocket infection is suspected, the nurse should not cannulate the device before medical consultation because of the risk of tracking the infection through the septum, into the catheter, and into the circulatory system. If the port is already cannulated, the needle may be left in place to draw blood for cultures and to infuse antibiotics (Moore 1987).

Treatment and Nursing Care

Infection, Related to

- ### *Presence of Long-Term Venous Access Device*

It is imperative to determine the severity of the infection, particularly if impending septic shock is suspected. Assessment of vital signs, particularly temperature and blood pressure, mental status, and indications of altered cardiac output (flushing or pallor, warm or cool skin, decreased urinary output) is essential. Cultures of all likely

TABLE 34–2
Catheter-Related Infections

Site	Manifestations	Treatment
Exit	Erythema, tenderness, induration with or without purulence within 2 cm of exit	Resolve with adequate neutrophils; possible oral or IV antibiotics
Tunnel	Erythema, tenderness, induration along subcutaneous catheter tract 2 cm from exit, with or without purulence at exit site	IV antibiotics, possible catheter removal*
Septicemia	Fever and bacteremia or fungemia; uninflamed catheter tunnel; fever resolves upon catheter removal	IV antibiotics; remove catheter if fever does not resolve in 48 hrs*
Septic thrombosis	Venous occlusion about catheter; bacteremia and fever	IV antibiotics; catheter removal,* with or without surgical resection of thrombus or affected vein
Port pocket	Erythema, tenderness, induration, with or without fever; purulence at pocket	IV antibiotics; if cannulated, draw blood for cultures from port and from peripheral vein; administer IV antibiotics through port If port not cannulated, do not cannulate; administer antibiotics through peripheral IV line, with or without catheter removal*

* Do not remove for fever of unknown origin.
Source: Adapted from Moore CL, 1987. Precept Press, pp 74–99; Press OW. 1984. Medicine 63:189–200.

sources of infection, including blood cultures from the catheter and a peripheral vein, urine, and wound, need to be done before antibiotic therapy is initiated. Although catheter removal is indicated in some cases, more commonly a more conservative approach, including ruling out other sites of infection and a course of intravenous or oral antibiotics, is used initially (Table 34–2). The patient with a serious infection will be hospitalized. Cancer patients experiencing profound leukopenia (fewer than 1000 WBCs/mm^3) and symptoms of infection, particularly fever, will also be hospitalized. IV antibiotics may be initiated in the ED, and the catheter may generally be used for this purpose unless a port pocket infection is suspected. Persons with less severe infections (e.g., exit infection in the absence of significant leukocytosis) may return home with a prescription for oral antibiotics.

Every person who has a long-term venous access device must be considered at risk for infection, not only because of the catheter, but also because of the factors that necessitate the placement of the catheter. Thus, the ED nurse should ascertain whether the patient knows how to care for the catheter and whether he or she has the ability to care for it. This includes not only conceptual ability, but physical ability and financial resources to purchase catheter supplies. In addition, availability of supplies (e.g., heparinized saline solution) may be a problem in some communities. Follow-up by the nurse may take care of these difficulties.

EXTRALUMINAL OBSTRUCTION

The nurse may suspect an obstructed catheter when he or she is unable to draw a blood sample from it (withdrawal occlusion). However, it must be recognized that the inability to draw blood may not necessarily indicate actual intraluminal catheter occlusion. Several extraluminal factors may cause withdrawal occlusion. These include catheter placement, fibrin sheath formation, and mural thrombus. Catheter placement and fibrin sheath formation are associated with withdrawal occlusion whereas mural thrombus may or may not be associated with withdrawal or infusion occlusion, or with both. Fluids can generally be infused unless there is intraluminal occlusion of the catheter.

Etiology and Pathophysiology

Catheter Placement

Some physicians insert the catheter so that the tip is in the right atrium. However, catheters that extend too far into the atrium may impinge on the endocardium and cause withdrawal occlusion (Reed et al 1983). Optimal placement of the catheter tip is in the superior vena cava at or above the junction of the right atrium.

Fibrin Sheath Formation

Fibrin sheath formation is common to all catheter materials but occurs earlier and more frequently with short-term central venous catheters. A fibrin "sleeve" starts to form at the point where the catheter enters the vein and may eventually propagate along the entire length of the catheter. In time, the sleeve may become so extensive as to extend beyond the tip of the catheter (Brismar et al 1981). Withdrawal occlusion results. Fibrin sleeves are not seen on routine chest radiographs and usually are confirmed by infusing contrast material while withdrawing the catheter.

Mural Thrombus

In a few instances a mural thrombus may form about a catheter, which may or may not be associated with withdrawal occlusion or infusion occlusion, or both. This type of clot originates at some point along the catheter, where it contacts the intima of the vein. The coagulation cascade is initiated at this site, with platelet aggregation and fibrin deposition. The resultant clot may eventually propagate to completely occlude the vein or catheter (Borrow and Crowley 1985).

Clinical Manifestations

Symptoms of venous occlusion include pain in the neck, shoulder, chest wall, or scapula; swelling of the ipsilateral arm, neck, or upper chest; and collateral venous dilation (Bertrand et al 1984; Smith et al 1985). Careful history and examination, comparing one side of the neck, chest, and arm to the other, is mandatory as findings may be subtle.

Treatment and Nursing Care

Anxiety, Related to

• *Inability to Draw Blood Sample from Catheter*

An obvious benefit of most catheters is the ability to obtain venous access for blood sampling and infusion without painful needle sticks. Understandably, the patient may become anxious or angry when blood sampling is not possible. The nurse needs to reassure the patient that symptoms reflective of the withdrawal occlusion do not necessarily mean that the catheter cannot be used and must be removed.

If the nurse suspects either catheter impingement or a fibrin sleeve is causing withdrawal occlusion, repositioning the patient may eliminate the problem. The nurse should instruct the patient to alternately raise and lower the arms, sit up, or lie down on the back or side while trying to draw the blood sample. Another measure is to have the patient perform the Valsalva maneuver or to place him or her in the Trendelenburg position if not contraindicated. These measures to change the position of the catheter tip are sometimes successful.

If these measures are not successful, a chest radiograph may be helpful. Because all catheters are radiopaque, correct placement can be confirmed by chest radiograph. If it is correctly placed, the physician may order a trial of low-dose fibrinolytic medication to be administered through the catheter (see Declotting a Catheter Appendix 34–1), which may restore the ability to draw blood from it (Peterson et al 1986).

Injury, Related to

• *Iatrogenic Obstruction of Major Veins Secondary to Mural Thrombus Resulting from Central Venous Catheter*

Medical management of mural thrombus may include continuous infusion of a thrombolytic agent (urokinase or streptokinase) in an attempt to lyse the clot, or continuous infusion of heparin followed by low-dose coumadin to minimize clot extension. In some instances the catheter will be removed to prevent further propagation of the clot (Lokich et al 1985). This is not done hastily because of the expense related to inserting catheters and because of the further limited venous access for the patient. The patient may be hospitalized to confirm whether or not symptoms are related to the catheter. This is usually done by venography through a peripheral vein. If the patient has minimal symptoms and the catheter is patent, the physician may adopt a wait-and-see attitude.

Patients with extensive mural thrombus may be admitted for large-dose continuous-infusion urokinase. Monitoring of these patients' coagulation parameters demonstrates that prothrombin time (PT), partial thromboplastin time (PTT), and fibrin split products remain normal while abnormal fibrinogen levels may signify toxicity (Fraschini et al 1987).

Evaluation

In some instances the measures to change the position of the catheter tip, as well as those to lyse a fibrin sleeve, will eliminate withdrawal occlusion. Similarly, the patient who has a thrombus about the catheter may experience a return of blood sampling capability. On the other hand, it is never possible to draw blood from some catheters. Furthermore, if conservative management has been used, the patient must understand the importance of promptly reporting worsening signs and symptoms.

INTRALUMINAL CATHETER OBSTRUCTION

Blood cannot be withdrawn, nor can fluids be infused, if a catheter is occluded. This may occur as the result of several factors but most commonly is due to precipitation of drugs or clot formation within the catheter.

Etiology and Pathophysiology

Drug precipitation occurs infrequently, usually when incompatible drugs (e.g., heparin and doxorubicin) are infused simultaneously through a single catheter lumen. Other drugs, including diazepam and phenytoin, interact with silicone to precipitate. It is seldom possible to clear the catheter in this case, which leads to catheter removal.

Clot formation within the catheter can occur if the catheter is not flushed properly, if positive pressure is not maintained within the catheter (e.g., when blood is drawn back into a syringe or the injection cap is removed from unclamped catheter), or perhaps because of other catheter- or disease-related factors (e.g., hypercoagulability secondary to malignancy).

Clinical Manifestations

The chief complaint of persons coming to the ED with catheter occlusion is that they are unable to flush their catheters. Because the source of catheter occlusion is intraluminal, blood is still able to flow around the catheter. As such, the patient may not exhibit any of the previously mentioned signs and symptoms related to extraluminal causes of catheter obstruction.

Treatment and Nursing Care

In all cases of catheter occlusion, the nurse should question the patient about catheter care. Any knowledge deficits which the patient may have related to catheter care or techniques must be identified. In addition, any problems that the patient may have that impede his or her ability to care for the catheter must also be identified (e.g., financial problems, mental or physical limitations, poor psychologic acceptance of catheter). If any of these factors appear causally related to the obstructed catheter, reinforcement of teaching and arrangement for follow-up care from a community care nursing agency or outpatient clinic is appropriate.

Potential for Injury, Related to

- ### *Catheter Occlusion Secondary to Precipitation of Drugs or Clot Formation with Catheter*

An occluded catheter should never be irrigated forcefully. The foremost reason is not the risk of pushing a clot into the pulmonary circulation but that forceful irrigation will expand the catheter and it will rupture at its weakest point. The ruptured catheter must then be removed.

If a clot is suspected, gentle instillation of a thrombolytic agent will usually restore patency in 30 to 60 minutes (see Declotting a Catheter, Appendix 34–1) (Lawson et al 1982). Urokinase is generally used for this purpose. Although it is more expensive than streptokinase, urokinase is less pyrogenic and allergenic (Fraschini et al 1987). It is available in single doses for declotting catheters (Abbokinase Open-Cath, Abbott Laboratories). This product is easy to reconstitute and to administer in the correct dose. Sometimes it is necessary to instill a second dose to completely lyse the clot and restore catheter patency. The instilled urokinase should be aspirated from the catheter if possible. Although 5000 units is a very small dose and urokinase has a half-life of 14 minutes, caution should be used in patients with active internal bleeding or increased risk of bleeding.

EXTRAVASATION

Extravasation, or leakage of caustic infusate from a vein or about a catheter into subcutaneous tissue, is associated with local discomfort (pain or burning, or both), erythema, and swelling. Certain drugs, particularly some antineoplastic agents, can cause soft tissue necrosis, resulting in chronic pain and functional loss if they extravasate. Known vesicant drugs and recommended management of extravasation from peripheral veins are listed in Table 34-3. As there are few documented instances of management of extravasation from central catheters, it would be prudent to apply the same management principles to extravasation from central veins.

Etiology and Pathophysiology

The risk of extravasation is greatest with implanted ports, but it can occur with other catheters as well. Accidental dislodgment of the Huber needle from the port is implicated most frequently (Lokich et al 1985). Other causes include damage to the catheter during or after placement that allows infusate to leak from the catheter, or clot formation at the catheter that causes the infusing drug to backtrack along the catheter (Lokich et al 1985; Rubenstein et al 1985).

TABLE 34-3
Management of Extravasation of Vesicant Drugs

Antineoplastic Agents	Antidote	Other	Source
Doxorubicin (Adriamycin) Daunorubicin (Cerubidine)	—	Cold: qid for 15 min for 48 hrs Elevate extremity Consult plastic surgeon for pain persisting beyond a few days	Rudolph and Larson 1987 Cancer Chemotherapy Guidelines 1988
Mitomycin C (Mutamycin)	Topical DMSO, 50–100%, 1–2 ml of 1 mMol, apply one time	Consult plastic surgeon for pain persisting beyond a few days	
Vinblastine (Velban) Vincristine (Oncovin)	Hyaluronidase, 150 U/ml;, reconstitute with 1 ml normal saline solution and inject 150–900 U SQ around site of extravasation	Apply warm compresses	Cancer Chemotherapy Guidelines 1988
Mechlorethamine (Nitrogen mustard)	Sodium thiosulfate, 1 g/10 ml; inject 5–6 ml into IV line or subcutaneously around site of extravasation		Cancer Chemotherapy Guidelines 1988
Other Agents Calcium salts (calcium chloride, calcium gluconate)	Hyaluronidase 150 U/ml (? amount)		Jameson and O'Donnell 1982
Vasopressors (epinephrine, dopamine, aramine, dobutamine, norepinephrine)	Phentolamine (Regitine), 2.5 mg, plus hyaluronidase, 300 U in 5–10-ml syringe; draw up together and inject subcutaneously		Jameson and O'Donnell 1982

DMSO, dimethylsulfoxide; SQ, subcutaneously.

Clinical Manifestations

The patient with an implanted port or other catheter who comes to the emergency room with signs and symptoms of extravasation requires careful management. The history should elicit information about what drug was being infused and when the infusion was started. Attention to the nature and duration of symptoms is essential. The possibility of extravasation should be considered if the patient complains of pain or burning in the port pocket or the ipsilateral chest, chest wall, or neck that began after commencement of the infusion.

Treatment and Nursing Care

Comfort, Altered, Related to

- *Infiltration of Soft Tissues with Locally Damaging Drug*

    Continuous infusion of cancer chemotherapy agents in particular is done in many instances, and patients can receive their treatment at home using ambulatory infusion devices. These persons will always have a central venous catheter if they are receiving vesicants. Extravasation is a rare occurrence, but it must be recognized immediately if it occurs. If the infusion device is still on, it should be turned off. If the patient has an implanted port, the dressing over the port site should be removed, taking care not to dislodge the needle if it is still in place. The attending physician will need to be consulted, as management may differ depending on the drug being infused and the extent of the extravasation. A plastic surgeon may also see the patient, as some cases of extravasation require surgical intervention (Rudolph and Larson 1987).

DAMAGED CATHETERS

An advantage of tunneled catheters is that they can be repaired if damaged in the external portion. This is not so with totally implantable catheters, which would require a surgical procedure to repair or replace the device. Similarly, damaged nontunneled catheters may be replaced by the physician using an over-the-wire technique. Damage to external catheters is discussed here.

Etiology and Pathophysiology

About 12 inches of the nontunneled catheter extends from the exit site, and it may become damaged if not properly secured to the patient's chest. External catheters may sustain damage if patients use a needle longer than $\frac{5}{8}$ inch to flush the catheter, if they inadvertently forget to remove the catheter clamp when flushing the catheter, if they attempt to vigorously flush a clotted catheter, if they continuously use a high-tension clamp over an unprotected catheter, or if they inadvertently cut the catheter with a scissors.

Clinical Manifestations

A patient is most likely to come to the ED if he or she accidently severs the catheter or notices that it is leaking at some point distal to the exit site. The history should elicit information on how long it has been since the damage was noticed and how it occurred, as well as signs and symptoms of complications that could arise as a result of catheter damage. These include infection, obstructed catheter, and less commonly hemorrhage or air embolism. Examination of the catheter may reveal frank damage. On the other hand, a pinpoint hole may not be evident until the catheter is flushed.

Treatment and Nursing Care

Injury, Related to

• *Damaged Catheter*

The nurse should clamp the catheter between the exit site and the point of damage. If the catheter has been severed, a sterile 4 × 4 inch gauze square should be secured about its end. In most instances a physician will repair or replace the catheter, although repair of a tunneled catheter can be done by the nurse. Supplies for this include the repair kit, a sterile field, sterile scissors, sterile gloves, and povidone-iodine preparation. If immediate use of the catheter is indicated, the nurse may repair it with an intracatheter for short-term use (see Emergency Repair of Tunneled Catheter, Appendix 34–2) (Ford 1985). If damage to the catheter is related to a lack of knowledge or noncompliance, reinforcement of teaching and referral for follow-up are indicated.

CONCLUSION

Rapid advances in long-term central catheter technology present a challenge to patients and caregivers. All must gain an immense amount of knowledge and skills to adequately care for and use these devices. The ultimate benefit is that the presence of a catheter may allow a patient to safely receive complex treatment in a variety of settings, which may have a positive impact on the patient's quality of life.

REFERENCES

Almadrones L, Godbold J, Raaf J, et al. 1987. Accuracy of activated partial thromboplastin time drawn through central venous catheters. Oncol Nurs Forum 14(2):15–18.

Bertrand M, Presant, CA, Klein L, et al. 1984. Iatrogenic superior vena cava syndrome. A new entity. Cancer 54:376–378.

Borrow M, Crowley JG. 1985. Evaluation of central venous catheter thrombogenicity. Acta Anaesthesiol Scand Suppl 81:59–64.

Brismar B, Hardstet C, Jacobson S. 1981. Diagnosis of thrombosis by catheter phlebography after prolonged central venous catheterization. Ann Surg 194:779–783.

Broviac JW, Cole JJ, Schribner BH. 1973. A silicone rubber atrial catheter for prolonged parenteral alimentation. Surg Gynecol Obstet 136:602–606.

Cancer Chemotherapy Guidelines. 1988. Module 5: Recommendations for the Management of Extravasation and Anaphylaxis. Pittsburgh, Oncology Nursing Society, 2–20.

Chathas NK. 1986. Percutaneous central venous catheters in neonates. J Obstet Gynecol Neonatal Nurs 15:324–332.

Ford R. 1985. History and organization of the Seattle-area Hickman catheter committee. NITA 8:123–135.

Fraschini G, Jadeja J, Lawson M, et al. 1987. Local infusion of urokinase for the lysis of thrombosis associated with permanent central venous catheters in cancer patients. J Clin Oncol 5:672–678.

Fuchs PC, Gustafson ME, King JT, et al. 1984.

Assessment of catheter-associated infection risk with the Hickman right atrial catheter. Infect Control 5:226–230.

Gebarski SS, Gebarski KS. 1984. Chemotherapy port "Twiddler's syndrome." Cancer 54:38–39.

Goodman MS, Wickham R. 1984. Venous access devices: An overview. Oncol Nurs Forum 11(5):16–23.

Hansell DT, Park R, Jensen R, et al. 1986. Clinical significance and etiology of infected catheters used for total parenteral nutrition. Surg Gynecol Obstet 163:469–474.

Jameson J, O'Donnell J. 1982. Guidelines for extravasation of intravenous drugs. Infusion 7:157–161.

Lawson M, Bottino JC, Hurtubise MR, et al. 1982. The use of urokinase to restore the patency of occluded central venous catheters. Amer J Intravenous Ther Clin Nutr 9(9):29–32.

Lawson M, Bottino JC, McCredie KB. 1979. Long-term IV therapy: A new approach. Am J Nurs 79:1100–1103.

Linder LE, Curelaru I, Gustavson B, et al. 1984. Material thrombogenicity in central venous catheterization: A comparison between soft, antebrachial catheters of silicone elastomer and polyurethane. J Parenter Enter Nutr 8:399–406.

Lokich JJ, Bothe A, Benotti P, et al. 1985. Complications and management of implanted venous access catheters. J Clin Oncol 3:710–717.

May GS, Davis C. 1988. Percutaneous catheters

and totally implantable access systems. A review of reported infection rates. J Intravenous Nurs 11:97–103.

Moore CL. 1987. Nursing management of infusion catheters. In Lokich JJ, ed. Cancer Chemotherapy by Infusion. Chicago, Precept Press, 74–99.

Ostrow LS. 1981. Air embolism and central venous lines. Am J Nurs 81:2036–2038.

Peterson FB, Clift RA, Hickman RO, et al. 1986. Hickman catheter complications in marrow transplant recipients. J Parenter Enter Nutr 10:58–62.

Press OW, Ramsey PG, Larson EB, et al. 1984. Hickman catheter infections in patients with malignancies. Medicine 63:189–200.

Reed WP, Newman KA, deJongh C, et al. 1983. Prolonged venous access for chemotherapy by means of the Hickman catheter. Cancer 52:185–192.

Rubenstein RB, Alberty RE, Michels LG, et al. 1985. Hickman catheter separation. J Parenter Enter Nutr 9:754–757.

Rudolph R, Larson DL. 1987. Etiology and treatment of chemotherapeutic agent extravasation injuries: A review. J Clin Oncol 5:1116–1126.

Slagle DC, Gates RH. 1986. Unusual case of central vein thrombosis and sepsis. Am J Med 81:351–354.

Slater H, Goldfarb IW, Jacob HE, et al. 1985. Experience with long-term outpatient venous access utilizing percutaneously placed silicone elastomer catheters. Cancer 56:2074–2077.

Smith NL, Ravo B, Soroff HS, et al. 1985. Successful fibrinolytic therapy for superior vena cava thrombosis secondary to long-term total parenteral nutrition. J Parenter Enter Nutr 9:55–57.

Verghese A, Widrich WC, Arbeit RD. 1985. Central venous septic thrombophlebitis—the role of medical therapy. Medicine 64:394–400.

Emergency Procedures

DECLOTTING A CATHETER

Supplies

1-ml tuberculin syringe or 3-ml syringe
Urokinase (Abbokinase Open-Cath), 5000 U/ml
3-ml syringe
2 10-ml syringes filled with sterile normal saline solution
Alcohol wipes
Injection cap
Heparin flush: Port, 3 ml, 100 U/ml
               Tunneled catheter, 2.5 ml, 10 U/ml
               Nontunneled catheter, 1 ml, 100 U/ml
Note: Use urokinase, 5000 U/ml: 0.5 ml to declot nontunneled catheter, 1 ml to declot tunneled catheter or implanted port. If double-lumen catheter is being declotted, both lumens must be instilled with the appropriate volume of urokinase.

Procedure	Rationale
1. Wash hands.	
2. Clamp tunneled catheter or extension tubing of nontunneled catheter or extension tubing of Huber needle in implanted port.	2. Prevent air embolism when system is opened.
3. Wipe connection site between the catheter or extension tubing hub and injection cap.	
4. Remove injection cap and attach 10-ml syringe of saline solution.	
5. Open clamp and *gently* try to irrigate catheter.	5. Forceful irrigation may rupture catheter.
6. If unable to irrigate, close clamp and attach empty 3-ml syringe. *Note:* If patient has an implanted	

Procedure	**Rationale**
port, recannulate at this point and repeat attempts to irrigate.	
7. Reconstitute urokinase according to manufacturer's directions and draw up appropriate amount into a tuberculin syringe or 3-ml syringe.	7. Preceding procedures may have established catheter patency. Reconstitution before this point results in an unnecessary cost.
8. Open clamp and try to withdraw any residual fluid from the catheter.	
9. Reclamp and detach this syringe.	
10. Attach syringe of urokinase and open clamp.	
11. Gently instill urokinase. This may take a few moments, exerting a back-and-forth action on the syringe plunger.	11. The total volume of catheters varies from less than 1 ml to about 1.5 ml. The catheter will accept this volume and the urokinase will diffuse through the remaining fluid to reach the clot.
12. When total volume is instilled into catheter, clamp, leaving the syringe attached.	
13. Allow urokinase to remain in catheter for 30 minutes.	13. Some practitioners advise checking every 5 minutes, for the first 30 minutes (Lawson et al 1982), but it is often more practical to wait a longer period.
14. Attempt to withdraw urokinase. If unsuccessful, try again in 30 minutes.	
15. If unsuccessful at 60 minutes, repeat the procedure.	
16. If unsuccessful in two attempts, consult physician.	16. Catheter may be occluded with precipitate.
17. If successful, follow with appropriate heparin flush.	

EMERGENCY REPAIR OF A TUNNELED CATHETER

Supplies

Povidone-iodine swabs
Sterile drape
Sterile gloves

Angiocatheters: 14-gauge for 1.06-mm internal diameter (ID) catheter
18-gauge for 1.0-mm ID catheter

Supplies

Tongue blade
Sterile scissors
Syringe with 10 ml of sterile saline solution
3-ml syringe

Sterile 4 × 4 inch gauze squares
Injection cap
1-inch tape
3-ml syringe with heparin flush (10 U/ml)

Procedure

1. Clamp catheter between exit site and site of damage.
2. Wash hands.
3. Open sterile equipment on sterile drape: gloves, angiocatheter, tongue blade, 4 × 4 gauze squares, injection cap, sterile scissors.
4. Cleanse area of catheter proximal to damage with povidone-iodine swabs, placing catheter on sterile drape or gauze, allowing to dry.
5. Don sterile gloves.
6. Cut catheter with sterile scissors close to site of damage, replacing trimmed catheter exiting from patient on sterile field.
7. Remove stylet from angiocatheter and insert the angiocatheter to its hub into the trimmed catheter.
8. Tape connection between catheter and the hub of the angiocatheter.
9. Attach the empty syringe to the hub of the angiocatheter.
10. Unclamp and aspirate 2 to 3 ml of blood.
11. Clamp catheter, detach syringe, and discard.
12. Attach syringe of saline solution, unclamping to flush.
13. Flush with heparinized saline solution.
14. Clamp and close system with injection cap.

Rationale

1. Prevent hemorrhage, obstruction of catheter, or air embolism.

6. At least a few inches of undamaged catheter needs to extend from the exit site to repair it permanently.

10. Remove air from catheter and establish patency.

Procedure	**Rationale**
15. Break tongue blade in half and cover with 4 × 4 gauze square.	15. Cover sharp edges to prevent further catheter damage.
16. Secure catheter with angiocatheter to tongue blade.	16. Stabilize catheter until permanent repair is accomplished.
17. Notify physician or specially trained nurse for permanent catheter repair.	

Management Issues Affecting Emergency Nursing

Donna Young, RN MS
Barbara White, RN MS

Fiscal Considerations in a Competitive Environment

Changes in the health care industry resulting from aggressive efforts to control costs have created a new and challenging environment for the hospital emergency department (ED). Traditionally, the ED has been an important gateway for patient admissions and utilization of hospital services (Vestal 1984). Admissions generated through the ED have provided substantial revenue for the hospital. In this day of prospective payment, however, ED admissions may not be as financially appealing as in the cost-based reimbursement environment (Munoz et al 1985).

In this rapidly changing industry, hospital-based EDs face competition for patients from physician offices and free-standing emergency centers. The successful ED will position itself to meet the needs of today's consumer. In addition, human and material resources must be managed effectively to remain financially successful.

The nurse plays a vital role in the success of the ED. The nurse must be cognizant of the changes in this competitive environment, including attributes of today's consumer, the demand for or utilization of services, and the financial performance of the ED.

This chapter provides an overview of factors that affect the financial viability of hospital EDs. Attributes of today's consumer are discussed, and strategies for increasing revenue and decreasing operational costs are presented. Information that is required to monitor and positively affect the financial success of the ED is identified.

FACTORS AFFECTING FINANCIAL VIABILITY OF EMERGENCY DEPARTMENTS

Systems of Reimbursement

Many factors have influenced health care delivery and reimbursement systems. However, the most dramatic effect on hospital reimbursement was the implementation of the prospective payment system (PPS) by the federal government in 1983. The PPS was implemented to decrease the rising cost of inpatient hospital services through the use of diagnostic related groups (DRGs). Under this system, the hospital is reimbursed a fixed payment based on the patient's discharge diagnosis or diagnoses.

The result of prospective payment has been a decrease in length of hospital stay, reduction of inpatient admissions, and a dramatic increase in the utilization of outpatient services. The PPS has given hospitals the incentive to treat patients in outpatient settings rather than utilizing expensive inpatient services. As a result of this increased use of outpatient services, the costs of outpatient services are escalating, and the federal government is examining strategies to reduce outpatient care costs.

The ED remains under a cost-based reimbursement system. However, since ED services constitute the largest portion of hospital-based outpatient services (Sabin 1986), future efforts to reduce ED use and reimbursement will affect the financial viability of hospital-based EDs.

Competition

The number of visits to hospital EDs increased dramatically until 1980. In the United States, there was a gradual decrease in patient visits from 82.4 million in 1980 to 78.8 million in 1984 (Powills and Matson 1985). What are the factors that have caused this decrease in ED visits?

Beginning in the 1970s, free-standing emergency centers (FECs) were developed and competed with hospital EDs for patients who required minor emergency care (Ferber and Becker 1983). In 1985 there were 1697 walk-in ambulatory care centers in the United States according to the American College of Emergency Physicians (Powills 1985). Orkand Corporation estimates that there will be an increase to over 5000 centers in the 1990s (Magill and Hartzke 1984). Although the hospital ED remains the predominant provider of emergency care, FECs are a competing force.

The proliferation of health maintenance organizations (HMOs), preferred provider organizations (PPOs), and other employee benefit plans have also affected the use of emergency services (Powills and Matson 1985). Enrollees in these programs are often required to seek prior approval for emergency services at specified emergency centers in order to ensure payment for these services. These requirements are aimed at discouraging inappropriate use of emergency services in an effort to decrease health care costs.

The third competitive factor affecting ED use is the physician's office. Physicians have become more sensitive to consumers' requests for more convenient hours. Office hours have been extended into evening hours and weekends. As a result, patients often seek minor emergency care in the physician office rather than in the ED.

In today's changing and competitive health care environment, everyone associated with the hospital ED, including nurses, must be sensitive to those factors affecting use of EDs. The financial viability of EDs depends on the ability to sustain the patient population and to maintain or increase revenue. One strategy that may prove beneficial in sustaining hospital-based ED populations is to provide ED patients referrals for follow-up care to physicians who are affiliated with that institution.

UNDERSTANDING CONSUMERS

The patient's first impression of a hospital is often made at the source of first contact. Hospital and ED personnel must be aware that the ED is the hospital's front door for many patients. Munoz and colleagues (1985) demonstrated that 18% of all hospital admissions in a large teaching hospital were from the ED. It is imperative that this first judgment be based on an impression inspired by an attractive facility providing effective, efficient, and humane treatment.

The astute emergency nurse must understand the attributes of consumers. Operations of the ED may require alteration in order to be responsive to both consumers seeking minor emergency care and those requiring acute emergency services.

Numerous studies have investigated preferences and utilization practices of the consumer of emergency care services (Inguanzo and Harju 1985a; Magill and Frommelt 1985; Inguanzo and Harju 1985b). Consumers today are better educated than ever before and seek episodic health care based on a number of predictable variables. Convenience — ease of accessibility, convenient hours, and short waiting times — is important. The perception of having received high-quality, sensitive care is also important. Women often select the health care facility for their families, and many working women find the convenience of FECs' evening hours attractive. Positive or negative experience in terms of the criteria previously described is likely to affect selection of a facility for future health care.

The media abounds with marketing efforts to inform consumers of facilities providing emergency services. Persons most likely to seek treatment at FECs include people who live in metropolitan suburbs or medium-sized cities, graduated from college, and live in households with an annual income of $40,000 or more (Inguanzo and Harju 1985b). Individuals who are least likely to go to FECs and most frequently go to hospital EDs for minor care are between 18 and 24 years old, have less than a high school education, are unmarried, and live in small towns or rural areas. The challenge for an ED is to become visible within the community and provide convenient, affordable emergency care.

Convenience

Convenience is a major factor in selecting emergency care providers. In one study, 79% of persons who used an FEC regarded convenience as a factor in their decision to use the center (Magill and Frommelt 1985). The hospital-based ED must be as accessible to the consumer as are the FECs. Hospitals located near shopping areas or dense residential populations are ideal. However, accessibility can be achieved by placing signs in locations that easily lead the consumer to the ED. Adequate parking in close proximity to the ED entrance increases convenience.

Consumers are busy and have competing demands upon their time. Increasing numbers of Americans move each year, thus breaking ties with their family physicians. This population may select EDs for their episodic care. The ED is available to meet consumers' health care needs on a 24-hour basis.

Health care consumers do not like to wait for service. Consumers using the hospital ED for minor care will not be satisfied to wait for extended periods while life-threatening emergencies and other acute care needs are met. The ED that can successfully operate an efficient and effective minor care service has a competitive advantage. Strategies for delivering minor care in the ED are discussed later in this chapter.

Cost Consciousness

The American public is increasingly aware of health care costs. As consumers become more directly accountable for a portion of the bill for ED services, they become more selective in seeking care. In view of this, many hospitals have changed or will change their ED pricing structure to respond to local competition. This is particularly important because charges at FECs are typically 35% to 50% of the charge at a hospital ED for comparable care (Magill and Hartzke 1984).

Humane Services

Compassionate treatment by staff is important to consumers seeking emergency care (Magill and Frommelt 1985). The patient and the family expect to be treated with respect and courteousness. The nurse at the bedside (or stretcher-side) can best identify the patient's needs and hear complaints. The manner in which the nurse responds to these consumer needs dramatically affects the overall impression of the care received.

STRATEGIES FOR MAXIMIZING ED REVENUE

Nursing staff in collaboration with hospital administration must determine consumer needs and implement strategies to maximize ED revenue. Marketing, competitive charge structures, documentation, effective delivery systems for minor emergency care, and implementation of cost-effective practices are strategies that are discussed in the following sections.

Marketing the ED

Marketing is one component of a strategy for success. The literature abounds with marketing strategies and campaigns used in the health care field. The nursing staff must understand basic marketing principles. Kaplan (1985) stated that successful marketing depends upon addressing the four Ps: product, place, price and promotion. Product is the service provided—in this case health care in the emergency setting. Products that may be provided in the ED include minor care and pre-employment physicals for industry. Place is the location and environment. Price relates to competitive pricing structures and is described later in this chapter. The fourth P, promotion, is advertising. Kaplan emphasizes that the sequence is essential. The first three (product, place, and price) should be addressed before promoting the facility.

Knowing the consumer using the ED allows the staff to respond to consumer needs. Patient information from medical records can be analyzed to identify the market segment served by the hospital ED. Do not assume that you know what consumers want or what they should have.

The ED nursing staff must work closely with the hospital marketing department. The nurses must continually assess the needs and preferences of consumers utilizing services and identify those the ED can provide. The nursing staff must be oriented to the hospital's marketing goals to provide emergency services efficiently and responsively.

Implementation of a Variable Charge System

A traditional cost-based reimbursement system is currently used for emergency services by Medicare, Medicaid, and insurance carriers. Emergency services are reimbursed based on "reasonable" charges (Baptist and Feller 1985). However, restrictions on ED reimbursement have been instituted to discourage ED use and to reduce costs to third-party payers. Studies are being funded to identify a capitated reimbursement system for ambulatory care services (Riffer 1986). A capitated system would reimburse hospitals at a fixed price for providing emergency care, similar to DRG payments for inpatient hospital care.

The most frequent complaint from patients who use ED services is that the charge may be higher than the intensity of service and time spent in the emergency room may seem to warrant (Buckley 1983). The price has traditionally been set by what the market will bear as opposed to the actual cost of services. An American Hospital Association (AHA) survey shows that nearly 70% of responding hospitals have changed or will change the ED pricing structure to meet local competition (Howard 1986). Sabin (1986) recommends bundling services that have similar resource consumption and applying a price that reflects the actual cost of service. Lower fees for less emergent visits will keep the ED competitive for minor emergency treatment.

Buckley (1983) describes a variable pricing structure for a hospital ED. Four charge categories were developed based on patient diagnosis, level of illness, type of injury, treatment and procedures involved. The nursing time, supplies utilized, and equipment required were also considered. Table 35 – 1 identifies each of these charge

TABLE 35-1
Criteria for Levels of ED Service

I. Brief	**III. Intermediate**

I. Brief

Requires no or minimal treatment
Brief history and physical examination with negative or minimal findings and treatment
Treatment refused
Immunizations associated with minimal first aid or no wound care
Examination, advice, and minimal treatment prescribed
Advice only
Cast removal/cast repair
Private M.D. check, no nursing care other than vital signs
Throat culture

II. Limited

Requires routine treatment
Phlebotomy requiring no observation
Suturing, minor; no nurse required
Requires radiography/laboratory tests
Anterior nasal packing
Initial limited history and physical; care, including advice and administered medications
Vaginal and rectal examinations
Treatment of sprains or fractures with or without premolded splints including plastic splints
Evaluation of sprains and fractures with referral for treatment
Minor burns with minimal physician and nursing time required
Evaluation of medical or surgical problems with referral for definitive treatment
Foreign body removal, nonoperative (eye, ear, nose, etc., with or without fluorescein staining for eye)
Allergic reaction, with generalized hives and edema
Application of dressings when no sutures required
Treatment of local allergic reactions
Evaluation and treatment of poisoning without induced emesis or gastric lavage

III. Intermediate

Requires moderate care or definitive therapy (medical or surgical)
Rape, with routine laboratory tests and follow-up
Emotional disturbances, patient not requiring constant attendance
Extended history and physical with diagnosis and treatment
Treatment of moderate burns with or without dressing application
Incision and drainage with or without local anesthesia
Evaluation and treatment of poisoning with induced emesis and/or gastric lavage
Application of extensive dressings
Treatment of sprains or fractures requiring casting or plaster splinting
Complicated allergic reaction
Diagnostic invasive procedures (e.g., thoracentesis)
Posterior nasal pack
Acute myocardial infarction, uncomplicated or suspected

IV. Comprehensive

Requires extensive therapy
Rape, requiring significant emotional support
Psychiatric patient requiring constant attendance or holding room
Life support assistance required or imminent
Acute myocardial infarction with complications
Vascular collapse
Acute respiratory failure
Severe multisystem disease
Severe trauma
Severe allergic reactions with anaphylaxis
Severe poisoning
Extensive burns

Source: Buckley DS. Unpublished. Submitted in partial fulfillment of the requirements for advancement to Fellowship in the American College of Healthcare Executives, all rights reserved by the American College of Healthcare Executives. Reproduced with permission.

categories—brief, limited, intermediate, and comprehensive—with guidelines for each.

Prior to implementing a variable charge system, an analysis of personnel time and ancillary services and supplies is advisable. A comprehensive management engineering study may be indicated to provide the data needed to develop a patient classification system. In the absence of a detailed study, a random selection of patient records can be reviewed to analyze intensity of services rendered and personnel resources required per visit. A pilot study will demonstrate the percentage of visits for various levels of service. Revenue projections can be developed from this data. Charges for the less acute services must be competitive with local FECs. In order to improve department profitability, charges for high-volume procedures and more intense services, such as multiple trauma and extensive burns, may exceed the actual cost (Currie and Howard 1985).

Following implementation, revenue generated by the variable pricing system should be compared with revenue generated under the previous charge system. Since a primary concern of the finance department is the potential loss of revenue, adjustments to the charges may be necessary to maintain profitability.

Documentation of Services

Complete and accurate documentation of patient information and treatments provided will maximize reimbursement from third-party payers. Nurses must document the care they give in detail, always with one eye toward its economic implications (McClain and Sehhat 1984). In the current cost-containment environment, insurance audits may result in lost revenue for services that are not recorded.

In the busy environment of an ED, time for documentation is limited. Documentation forms must be easy to use and must avoid duplication of information. A sample of ED records can be evaluated monthly to assure accuracy of patient charges and completeness of documentation.

Effective Delivery Systems for Minor Emergency Care

It has been reported that up to 80% of the patients who use hospital-based EDs do not require true emergency medical care (Magill and Hartzke 1984). Consumers are seeking quality-oriented, cost-effective care in a convenient and caring environment. Therefore, the emergency nurse must be sensitive to consumer issues and proactive in order to sustain the minor care population.

Lengthy waiting periods are cited as one reason consumers are reluctant to use the hospital ED for minor care. The waiting time for treatment in an FEC is 15 to 20 minutes. (Magill and Hartzke 1984). Waiting creates a high probability that the consumer will seek another source of care for the next minor care incident.

In order to reduce waiting times in the hospital ED, Sabin suggests setting up separate processing systems for minor care and emergency care (Punch 1985). One strategy is to completely separate the minor care area from the acute care area. This arrangement may include a separate entrance and separate registration and treatment areas for minor care patients. Staff could be rotated through both areas or could be assigned to the minor care area based upon desire to work with this specific population. Creative uses of other health care professionals such as nurse practitioners can be considered in striving to provide more cost-effective and efficient emergency services.

When it is impractical to provide separate areas, separate processing systems may be developed. For example, specific nurses and physicians may be assigned to the minor care population. Whether the hospital-based ED provides care to acute and minor emergency care patients in the same or separate areas, the ED staff must switch from the life-threatening situations to minor care with equal commitment.

Implementing Cost-Effective Practices

In an environment in which cost containment is a major priority, decreasing operational costs is essential. The ED nurse-manager must monitor expenses monthly to evaluate effectiveness of cost-containment strategies. Nursing staff must work collaboratively with the nurse-manager to identify and implement strategies to enhance productivity and decrease operational costs.

Managing Personnel Resources

The largest cost in the hospital and ED budget is nursing personnel salaries and benefits. Therefore, the effective use of personnel resources is essential to control costs in the ED.

The Joint Commission on Accreditation of Hospitals (JCAH) requires that the nursing department "shall define, implement, and maintain a system for determining patient care requirements for nursing care on the basis of demonstrated need, appropriate nursing intervention, and priority for care" (Accreditation Manual for Hospitals 1987). The patient classification system designed for ED use is an important tool to forecast staffing needs.

Although patient classification systems are not widely used in EDs, a few have been developed and are gaining more widespread use (Schulmerich 1984; Stevenson et al 1978). The patient classification system is a valuable tool to justify staffing needs, redistribute nursing staff, and adjust the skill-mix the better to meet patient needs (Schulmerich 1984). The nurse-manager can control personnel costs by using alternative scheduling options, such as 8-, 10-, or 12-hour shifts. Flexible scheduling also allows the appropriate personnel resources to be available to meet projected patient needs. The use of volunteers to assist with non-nursing tasks in EDs to supplement ED personnel should be considered.

In hospital EDs using variable charging, the system of patient classification can be the basis for the charge system. This would reduce documentation by avoiding two separate classifications of patients — for the charge system and for the staffing system. The patient classification system identifies, defines, and measures the nursing services delivered to the patient; it can be based on documentation of individual nursing services or nursing diagnoses for the individual patient (VanSlyck 1985). Financial data based on patient care needs and nursing resources used are valuable in negotiating contracts with HMOs and PPOs. Such data can also be utilized to charge for nursing services.

Managing Material Resources

Nursing staff must be well informed about supply and product costs and must participate in product decisions. Supply cost can be contained or even decreased by using supplies efficiently and decreasing supply and equipment loss.

Products and supplies that reduce labor or the cost of outpatient procedures decrease operational cost. New products being considered for ED use should be evaluated according to specific selection criteria. These criteria should address both clinical usefulness and financial impact. The criteria can be developed by the hospital products committee or the materials manager in collaboration with the ED nurses and physicians.

Although some equipment and supplies used in the ED may be unique, most products can be standardized throughout the facility. Product standardization increases volume use of each product. This allows the materials manager to negotiate substantial savings with vendors, especially if the hospital participates in a group purchasing program. In addition, costs of training personnel to use new equipment and supplies are reduced when products are standardized throughout the hospital.

MONITORING EMERGENCY DEPARTMENT PERFORMANCE

In the current competitive environment, data are required to evaluate the financial status of an ED. Data are used to assess the feasibility of expanding or eliminating services and contracts with HMOs, PPOs, and local employers. Data collection and storage are also essential if any new payment system, especially one that is prospective, is anticipated (Sabin 1986).

Generally, the ED manager receives revenue and expense data. Monthly financial reports include the projected budget, personnel, and material expenditures for the month and year-to-date and revenues generated for the month and year-to-date. Data evaluation allows the nurse-manager to determine whether or not controls have been effective in matching costs to use of resources.

However, additional information is needed by the ED manager to evaluate departmental performance and productivity. Table 35-2 lists some critical data that can be used by the nurse-manager (Ranseen and Thorton 1985).

Some institutions suffer from too many reports, making the evaluation of departmental performance difficult. The nurse-manager must determine what information is needed to evaluate ED performance, decide if the data are available on hospital and departmental reports, and identify what data is needed but not currently available. Information can be collected by the hour, day, month, or year, and evaluated by the nurse manager on at least a monthly basis.

TABLE 35-2
ED Data Elements

Total ED visits
ED visits by intensity level
ED length of stay by department, intensity level, and medical diagnosis
ED procedures
ED visits by age, sex, race, marital status
Total AMA
Transfers from ED by facility destination
Admissions to hospital: total, to ICU, OR, Pediatrics, and so forth
ED revenue by department, MD, ancillary tests
Visits by payer category
Average charge by department, MD
Average MD charge by procedure

The ED log can provide a substantial amount of necessary data. An automated log allows data manipulation for generating required reports. Data can be stored on the hospital mainframe computer. ED reports are generated from the mainframe or down-loaded to a microcomputer to allow data manipulation. If a hospital information system is not available, a microcomputer can be used to store data and generate reports.

Product Line Management

An effective strategy for responding to the competitive environment is managing emergency services as a hospital product line. Product line management (PLM) is a system that organizes products according to specific services, such as women's health, cardiac care, or geriatric care (Nackel and Kues 1986).

The manager for a product line such as emergency services is responsible for financial, operational, and marketing aspects of the service. The product manager has the authority and responsibility for the financial profitability of the service (Bruhn and Howes 1986).

Product line management is relatively new in the hospital industry. It provides interesting management opportunities for nurses and may be a critical element in the success of hospital EDs.

CONCLUSION

The implementation of prospective payment for inpatient hospital services has resulted in competition for limited health care dollars. Health care providers are marketing services to attract and increase customer use of their services. EDs are responding to competition by modifying traditional services the better to meet the needs of consumers. The goal is to provide courteous, convenient, and cost-effective emergency services.

A major factor affecting use of EDs is the proliferation of FECs. In an effort to be more responsive to patients who need minor care, EDs can develop variable charge systems to lower the price of minor emergency care. EDs should consider geographically separating minor care from emergency care patients to decrease the waiting time for the former. In addition, marketing efforts may promote increased use of hospital EDs by consumers.

Nurses play a significant role in the financial success of the ED. Efficient and humane nursing care delivery will attract patients to the ED. Nursing can effectively manage the use of personnel and material resources to enhance departmental profitability.

The emergency nurse must be aware of the changing health care environment and consumers' needs for emergency services. The ED that is responsive and efficient will continue to be successful.

REFERENCES

Accreditation Manual for Hospitals. 1987. Chicago, Joint Commission on Accreditation of Hospitals.

Baptist A, Feller J. 1985. Reimbursement of emergency centers. In Friend PM, Shiver JM, eds. Freestanding Emergency Centers: A Guide to Planning, Organization, and Management. Rockville, Md, Aspen Systems Corporation, 107–118. 1985.

Bruhn PS, Howes DH. 1986. Service line management. New opportunities for nursing executives. J Nurs Admin 16:13–18.

Buckley DS. 1983. The development and implementation of a variable charge structure in an ED. Unpublished. Submitted in partial fulfillment of the requirement for advancement to Fellowship in the American College of Healthcare Executives. All rights reserved by the American College of Healthcare Executives.

Currie D, Howard DM. 1985. Microcosting an emergency department. Top Health Care Financ 11:78–88.

Ferber MS, Becker LJ. 1983. Impact of freestanding emergency centers on hospital ED use. Ann Emerg Med 12:429–433.

Howard D. 1986. Ambulatory care hospitals. Prices Evolve 60:75–76.

Inguanzo JM, Harju M. 1985a. What's the market for emergency care? Hospitals 59:53–54.

Inguanzo JM, Harju M. 1985b. Hospitals still dominate emergency care market. Hospitals 59:84–85.

Kaplan A. 1985. Using the components of the marketing mix to market emergency services. In Winston WJ, ed. Marketing Ambulatory Care Services. New York, The Haworth Press, 53–62.

Magill JR, Frommelt JJ. 1985. Consumer satisfaction in FECs. In Friend PM, Shiver JM, eds. Freestanding Emergency Centers: A Guide to Planning, Organization and Management. Rockville, Md, Aspen Systems Corporation, 237–240.

Magill G, Hartzke L. 1984. Immediate care centers fast medicine for the 80s (DHHS Publication No. HRP-0905987). Springfield, Va, National Technical Information Service, US Department of Commerce, 3.

McCLain JR, Sehat MS. 1984. Twenty cases: what nursing costs per DRG. Nurs Manage 15:26–34.

Munoz E, Laughlin A, Regan DM, Teicher et al. 1985. The financial effects of ED-generated admissions under prospective payment systems. JAMA, 254:1763–1771.

Nackel JG, Kues IW. 1986. Product-line management: systems and strategies. Hosp Health Serv Admin 31:109–123.

Powills S. 1985. No wait service. Hospitals 59:54–56.

Powills S, Matson T. 1985. Hospital emergency departments learn how to make money. Hospitals 59:122–124.

Punch L. 1985. Hospitals must restructure emergency charges to retain patient base. Mod Health 16:122.

Ranseen TA, Thorton TL. The ED: a financial winner for hospitals in the 1980s? Healthcare Financ Manage 39:30–48.

Riffer J. 1986. Study paves way for outpatient revamp. Hospitals 60:87.

Sabin MD. April 1986. Strategic positioning for optimal response to proposed outpatient financing systems. Paper presented at meeting of The Virginia Organization of Nurse Executives, Richmond.

Schulmerich SC. 1984. Developing a patient classification system for the emergency department. J Emerg Nurs 10:298–305.

Stevenson JS, Brunner NA, Larabee J. 1978. A Plan for Nurse Staffing in Hospital Emergency Services (Publication No. 20–1696). New York, National League for Nursing.

VanSlyck A. 1985. Nursing services: costing, pricing, and variable billing. In Shaffer FA, ed. Costing Out Nursing: Pricing Our Product. New York, National League for Nursing, 39–53.

Vestal KW. 1984. Marketing concepts for the ED. J Emerg Nurs 10:274–276.

Rose Lach, RN MS

Quality Assurance in an Emergency Department

Why do people return to their favorite restaurant; book reservations on the same airline; have their cars repaired by the same mechanic; or return to the same health care institution? The answer is "quality."

Quality is evident when a particular place of business consistently provides excellent service. Meals are served warm with little delay. Flights are on time. Cars operate efficiently after repair. Health care is delivered immediately and efficiently.

Why is there an emphasis on quality in the United States, especially in health service? First, currently, the emphasis or need for quality is a result of several driving forces:

1. consumerism
2. government reimbursement of health care
3. increased costs of medical care
4. rapid advances in medical sciences
5. documented poor quality of care (Graham 1982).

Because consumers have become more educated and sophisticated about health care, quality is a primary concern for them. Consumers are beginning to recognize that there are differences in how health care personnel deliver services (e.g., whether they give discharge instructions and whether they are concerned about follow-up care). This emphasis on quality by consumers is evident by the increase in consumer participation in all aspects of health care and in the rise in malpractice suits in recent years.

873

Second, quality became of primary importance as the government became involved in the reimbursement for health care services through Medicaid and Medicare. The government became a third party purchaser of services for the poor and elderly. Because government representatives realized we were spending large amounts of funds on health care, they demanded that hospitals provide quality services. In 1972, the Bennet Amendment (PL 92-603) established Professional Standards Review Organizations (PSROs) to monitor quality of care in hospitals. PSROs became responsible for monitoring and evaluating the care of persons in federally financed programs (Graham 1982).

Third, quality of care became important as the government implemented a program to help curb the rise in medical care costs. This program is a prospective (as opposed to what was formerly a retrospective) system in which the government reimburses hospitals for care they administer to Medicare patients categorized under Diagnostic Related Groups (DRGs). This program has sorted illnesses and diagnoses under certain categories (DRGs) and has determined the cost of care and length of stay typically required within each category. According to the category a person is placed in under DRGs, the hospital is paid a predetermined amount, regardless of the patient's length of stay or acuity of illness. Because under the DRG system costs and length of stay are predetermined, this program is an incentive for hospitals to discharge patients quickly to remain profitable (Bull 1985).

Because of the DRG system, one of the challenges for hospitals is to provide cost-effective services without sacrificing quality of care. Quality of care is questioned when a patient remains acutely ill yet is discharged within the length of stay required by DRGs. As a result of this issue, hospitals expanded their quality monitoring departments to determine if hospital personnel delivered the appropriate services required and if they recommend needed follow-up care (Graham 1982).

Fourth, quality standards need to be developed in an age in which rapid advances in medical science and technology occurs. Heart, liver, and kidney transplants have been accelerated in the last decade, yet standards have not been developed by which to measure quality of care. Criteria must be formulated which determine if pre-, intra-, and postoperative care was adequate (Graham 1982).

Fifth, and last, quality is an issue because there has been documented evidence of poor quality of care. In 1984, Levy and coworkers reported the results of a medical records review in an emergency department (ED). At the end of 1 year, approximately 74,000 ED medical records were audited to determine if ED personnel administered care according to pre-established audit standards. Of these charts reviewed, 744 did not meet audit criteria. Because of this quality review, 79 patients were called back for necessary follow-up, and 665 patients were called back to recommend further extension of services that involved additional diagnostic studies and referrals to appropriate clinics.

In summary, quality of care has become a primary issue in response to social, political, economic, technical, and legal pressures. These pressures include consumers' concern over health care, government involvement in Medicare and Medicaid reimbursement and the establishment of DRGs, rapid advancement in technology, and concern about documented poor quality of care. Because of these driving forces, the development of programs to measure the quality of care is a priority in health care today.

This chapter identifies and discusses the components of a quality assurance program. First, however, the definition of quality is discussed. This chapter then closes with the highlights of requirements of the Joint Commission on the Accreditation of Hospital Organizations (JCAHO) for a quality assurance program.

DEFINING QUALITY

Granted that quality is necessary today, what *is* quality?

The following definitions describe not only quality but also quality assurance. Quality assurance is the name given to most programs that define, measure, and identify components of quality.

Definitions of quality or quality assurance include the following:

- A degree of excellence; superiority of kind (Mish 1985, 963).
- In essence, quality assurance consists of the establishment of standards, evaluation of these standards, and finally, implementation of actions that assure adherence to these standards (Lieske 1985, 45–46).
- Quality is the degree of adherence to generally recognized contemporary standards of good practice and achievement of anticipated outcomes for a particular service, procedure, diagnosis, or clinical problem (Rowland and Rowland 1987, 6).

These definitions imply that a quality assurance program encompasses a process and an application. The *process* of quality assurance includes establishment, measurement, and evaluation of standards as well as actions to improve attainment of 100 per cent compliance with these standards. The *application* of a quality assurance program can be broad or narrow. It can involve an institution or individual departments or services, and the clinical problems those services address.

Because the focus of this chapter is on ED quality assurance programs, the remaining sections deal with a departmental program. A departmental program establishes, measures, and evaluates standards and implements actions to achieve attainment of these standards.

DEVELOPING A QUALITY ASSURANCE PROGRAM

This section on developing a quality assurance program has a dual purpose. One purpose is to identify the steps involved; the second purpose is to recognize the essential components of a quality assurance program, which are often referred to as the "monitoring and evaluating process."

Following are 10 essential steps that are necessary to develop a quality assurance program:

1. Assign responsibility.
2. Delineate the scope of care or service.
3. Identify the important aspects of care.

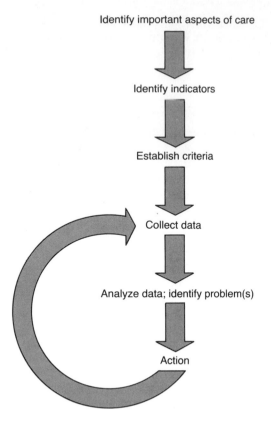

Identify important aspects of care

Identify indicators

Establish criteria

Collect data

Analyze data; identify problem(s)

Action

FIGURE 36-1. The monitoring and evaluation process, steps 3 through 9. (Adapted from *Monitoring and Evaluating Nursing Service,* 28. Copyright 1988 by the Joint Commission on Accreditation of Health Care Organizations, Chicago. Reprinted with permission.)

4. Identify indicators.
5. Establish criteria.
6. Collect data.
7. Analyze data.
8. Take actions to resolve identified problems.
9. Assess actions and document improvements.
10. Communicate relevant information (JCAH 1986).

The most essential components of the monitoring and evaluating process are steps 3 through 9 (Fig. 36 – 1). These components are interrelated. Successful completion of one step is essential before the nurse can proceed to the next step. The remainder of this section explains each step and how to implement it.

Step 1. Assign Responsibility

The director of a department is directly responsible for monitoring and evaluating activities of the ED. Although he or she is ultimately accountable, the director often delegates responsibility to other assistants, physicians, or nurses in the department. The director must identify who performs what activities (e.g., establish standards, collect data, and evaluate results) and determine if the duties are being performed (JCAH 1986).

Before the director delegates responsibilities, he or she must have formulated a quality assurance plan. Although JCAHO does not require it be written, a concise written plan provides a formal record of

1. the type of monitoring activities for review, such as diagnostic, therapeutic, or clinical components of care, and

2. assignment of responsibility for the monitoring and evaluation process.

Because the written quality assurance plan provides a formal record of the scope and organization of activities, it can be reviewed and revised annually, as necessary (Rowland and Rowland 1987).

Step 2. Delineate the Scope of Care or Service

"Delineating the scope of the care or service is defining what a department/service does" (Rowland and Rowland 1987, 8). In this step the department or service determines the functions and levels of health care, the diagnostic and therapeutic modalities it will monitor, and the type of patient it serves.

Rhee and coworkers (1987) formulated a framework that identifies the functions and levels of health care provided in an ED (Fig. 36–2).

These researchers stated that the scope of services for an ED include three functions and several levels of health care. The functions encompass providers of care, aspects of care, and those served. Levels of providers of care range from individ-

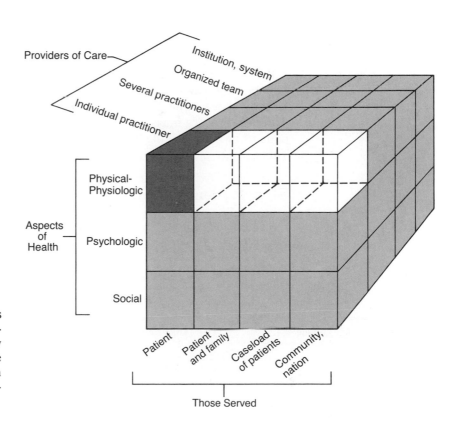

FIGURE 36–2. Functions and levels of health care. (From Rhee J, Donabedian A, Burney R. 1987. Qual Rev Bull, 13:5. Copyright 1988 by The Joint Commission on Accreditation of Health Care Organizations, Chicago. Modified with permission.)

ual practitioners to institutions or systems, and levels of care of persons served range from individual patients to nations. Aspects of health care have been identified as physical, psychologic, and social.

In an ED, quality monitoring activities are usually limited to the performance of individual practitioners in meeting the physical needs of an individual patient. These activities are represented by the shaded corner in Figure 36–2 (Rhee et al 1987).

An ED does not have to limit its quality monitoring to these levels of health care alone. It may expand monitoring from care rendered by an individual practitioner to that rendered by several practitioners (e.g., a code blue team) and from individual patients to families and communities (e.g., family teaching, participating in a community disaster). The director or his or her designates must choose the function and level of health care to be monitored.

In addition to determining functions and levels of health care, delineating the scope of care or service includes identification of major diagnostic and therapeutic modalities it performs. Examples of these modalities include performing electrocardiography (EKG), obtaining laboratory specimens, and administering medications.

Lastly, delineating the scope of service includes identifying the type of patients an ED serves. What are the major age or disability groups or disease entities it treats? Are the patients typically elderly cardiac, young pediatric, or young or middle aged trauma victims? The patient population will depend on the location (city or suburbs) and type (trauma or community) of ED (Rowland and Rowland 1987).

Thus, the scope of service should be defined. This includes major functions and levels of care, diagnostic and therapeutic modalities, and patients served.

Step 3. Identify Important Aspects of Care

After the director or designee defines the scope of services, he or she must choose therapies and modalities that are considered the *most* important aspects of care and monitor them. Important aspects of care are those that include a high volume of patients, involve a high degree of risk for patients, or usually cause problems for the patients or nursing staff (Rowland and Rowland 1987). Examples can be found in Table 36–1.

Step 4. Identify Indicators

Indicators identify specific populations related to an identified aspect of health care. For example, if fever is an aspect of health care to be monitored, a specific indicator

TABLE 36–1
Important Aspects of Care for an Emergency Department to Monitor

High Volume	High Risk	Problem Areas
Angina	Central venous access catheter insertion	Transport availability
Myocardial infarction	Nitroglycerin administration	Efficiency of obtaining laboratory results
Fever	Chest tube insertion	Bed availability
Trauma	Blood administration	Disaster drills

might be all infants (less than 1.0 year old) with a temperature greater than 103°F. Then standards are used to determine if appropriate care was rendered in relation to the identified indicator.

But what are the standards of quality to be measured? Standards are statements of expected care or behavior that are predetermined by experts or authorities. Standards of quality are predetermined by regulating agencies such as JCAHO or professional organizations such as the Emergency Nurses' Association (ENA) and the American Nurses' Association (ANA). An institution's policies and procedures and current literature may also be used to determine standards (Rowland and Rowland 1987).

Three types of standards to establish when monitoring an indicator are structure, process, and outcome standards.

Structure Standards

Structure standards define the required conditions for quality of care. Structure standards include number, mix, and qualifications of staff; the organization and management of staff; the policies and procedures; the appropriate physical facilities; and equipment (Donabedian 1982). In Table 36–2 there are examples of structure standards identified for a patient arriving in the ED with an injury related to a laceration with a moderate amount of bleeding.

Process Standards

Process standards are the actual direct care activities. "It is the action rather than the structure in which the action takes place that constitutes process" (Rowland and Rowland 1987, 31). Table 36–2 again lists examples of process standards.

Outcome Standards

Outcome standards measure the results of the nurse's actions. They are the end goals of action. In essence, these standards measure the effectiveness of previous actions (Lieske 1985). Table 36–2 also gives examples of outcome standards.

A point to note is that outcome standards must be established for different time frames. In this example, there are various stages of injury from acute bleeding at the initiation of treatment to elimination of bleeding at the end of treatment. Outcome standards usually indicate a time frame and stage of illness. This example is monitoring the end stage of treatment: bleeding has stopped by discharge and there is no evidence of infection 1 week post treatment.

In summary, step 3 requires the director to choose important aspects of care and step 4 requires him or her to identify indicators of this aspect of care. Standards are

TABLE 36-2

Standards and Criteria for Monitoring Injury Related to Laceration with Moderate Amount
of Bleeding Secondary to a Fall

Category	Standard	Criteria
Structure	Triage protocol present	The orientation manual has triage protocol present
	The ED is prepared to treat all patients it serves	A treatment room is available
		The necessary supplies are available
	Staff members are adequately prepared to care for all patients requiring ED services	All personnel receive an orientation to ED triage
Process	Measures are taken to control bleeding	Direct pressure is applied to the wound
		The wound is sutured
	Measures are taken to prevent infection	The wound is cleaned and irrigated for 5 minutes with povidone-iodine (Betadine) and saline solution
		The wound is covered with a sterile dressing
		Tetanus toxoid and antibiotics are administered according to physician order
		The nurse gives the patient wound care instructions
		The nurse explains wound care instructions
Outcome	The patient has no active bleeding on discharge 100% of the time.	The dressing is dry
		The patient has no orthostatic changes in blood pressure or pulse (no change greater than 10 mm Hg systolic from a lying to a standing position)
	The patient has no wound infection on follow-up 1 week post treatment 100% of the time	The patient has no fever (temperature of 98.6°F or less)
		The patient has no purulent drainage from the wound
		The patient has no cellulitis
	The patient has knowledge of wound care instructions on discharge 100% of the time	The patient has signed the form indicating he or she has received instructions
		The patient verbalizes understanding of instructions

then used to determine if appropriate care was rendered in relation to those identified indicators.

Step 5. Establish Criteria

After identifying indicators and standards of care, a director must establish criteria by which to measure standards. Criteria are the actual statements by which a person can *measure* standards (Rowland and Rowland 1987).

Criteria and standards are often confused, and one word is substituted for the other. However, standards are broad statements whereas criteria are very specific and precise measures of standards. In fact, several criteria are often established to measure one standard. A good example can be seen in Table 36-2. In this table, two criteria are listed that measure the process standard "Measures are Taken to Control Bleeding": apply pressure and suture the wound.

Criteria must be predetermined, reflect practice, and be measurable. Criteria must be established before data are collected. They must reflect practice and be in accordance with published criteria by professional associations and in the literature and be in agreement with the institution's policies and procedures. They are measurable if the data collector can easily distinguish between acceptable and unacceptable care (Rowland and Rowland 1987).

Step 6. Collect Data

In order to collect and analyze data, the following must be decided for each standard or criteria:

- data sources
- data collection method
- sample size
- time frame for data collection (Rowland and Rowland 1987)

Data Sources

Potential sources include patient records (nursing and medical notes, medication sheets, pathology and laboratory reports), incident reports, departmental records, minutes or reports of committees, patient interviews, direct observations of staff or patients, patient satisfaction questionnaires, and utilization review findings. One or several sources may be used to collect data for each standard or criterion.

Data Collection

Two methods of collection are *concurrent* and *retrospective* review. Concurrent review means data are collected while care is provided. Retrospective review means data are collected after care is provided or after discharge. Concurrent review is preferred since it is more pertinent to patient care and clinical performance.

In addition, the director must decide who the data collectors will be. They can be either those providing care or a chosen group outside the department or hospital.

Sample Size

There is no ideal number for sample size; but it must be adequate (usually at least 10 per cent of the population) and be representative of the population to be studied.

Time Frame

The persons responsible for the quality assurance program must determine the time frame for data collection. The time frame is based on the number of patients involved in the aspect of care to be monitored, degree of risk of the aspect of care, and how often the care is performed. The average time frame is quarterly data collection for a relatively small population with an aspect of care of average risk.

In conclusion, the director must make several essential decisions to accomplish this step. He or she must decide the data sources, data collection methods, sample size, and time frame.

Step 7. Analyze Data

Quality assurance personnel should tabulate the data collected and the director and delegates should analyze the results. The personnel can use charts, checklists, graphs, and computer printouts to tabulate and break down data. The director must then decide the number of criteria that will be met, the frequency in which criteria will be met, and which particular criteria must absolutely be accomplished for care, service, or performance to be acceptable (JCAH 1986).

Step 8. Take Actions to Resolve Identified Problems

Once a problem or deviation from a standard has been identified, the director must formulate a plan to resolve the problem. The plan must identify:

• who or what needs to change
• what actions are appropriate for the cause, scope, and severity of the problem
• who is responsible for implementing action
• when change is expected to occur (JCAH 1986).

This plan must be documented to establish a record for use in evaluating the effectiveness of actions taken. Table 36–3 provides an example of a plan.

There are three common causes of problems: lack of knowledge, defects in departments or hospital systems, and faulty behavior or performance of staff members. These problems can be corrected. Knowledge deficits can be corrected with education programs such as in-services, an orientation program, or patient or family classes. System defects might include altering policies and procedures, use of new or other supplies or equipment, or redistribution of staff. Behavior and attitude problems are more difficult to correct but can include counseling, changing responsibilities or duties, or transferring to another department or service (Brown 1986). Table 36–3 identifies wound infection as a problem and recommends in-services to correct the knowledge deficit and a review of protocol to correct any system defect.

Thus, an appropriate plan includes what, who, and when: what the problem is; who is responsible for change and implementing actions; and when will the actions be completed.

Step 9. Assess the Effectiveness of Actions

The entire quality assurance plan can be destroyed if there is lack of planning for follow-up for data collection to determine if the problem was resolved. A date for collection of data to reassess the problem must be set immediately after actions and a target date for completion has been identified. The director must ensure that the problem was resolved or that the standard was achieved (Wilbert 1985).

The data that are re-collected may reveal that the problem is reduced or eliminated or that the problem still exists. If the problem is reduced or eliminated, the corrective actions have been successful. However, if the problem still exists, the director must determine if the problem had not been correctly identified or if the corrective actions were inappropriate (Brown 1986).

TABLE 36–3
Quality Assurance Corrective Plan

Problem or Concern	Corrective Action	Responsible Person
Upon return visit for suture removal, 5 patients have had wound infections over a 1-month period	Review sterile technique with all ED staff Review protocol for indications for wound cultures, tetanus immunization, and antibiotics with ED director	ED clinical specialist Head nurse

Completion Date	Follow-up findings
1-1-89	Problem resolved; no wound infections detected
1-1-89	during last month's monitoring

Remember, monitoring and evaluating activities are ongoing. Problems, resolutions, and follow-up must be documented (Table 36–3) and continuous. Without this continuous reassessment, the director cannot determine if standards have been met.

Step 10. Communicate Information

The organization-wide quality assurance plan identifies who will receive reports and the type and frequency of reports required for departmental reporting of activities. Quality assurance reports are usually shared with members of other departments, who can contribute to the identification and resolution of problems monitored. Usually the type of reports include problems, corrective actions, and results of follow-up as seen in Table 36–3, as well as minutes of quality assurance meetings or staff meetings in which quality assurance was discussed. These reports are usually submitted to the hospital-wide quality assurance committee quarterly (JCAH 1986).

In summary of this second section, a quality assurance program is established by completing the 10 steps identified from assignment of responsibility through and including communication of information. The most crucial part of the process are steps 3 through 8, which are the monitoring and evaluation activities.

One step must be completed before the next can be accomplished. By using these guidelines, a quality assurance program will be established and the nurse will see an improvement in quality care service.

JCAHO REQUIREMENTS

Lastly, the ED director should be knowledgeable of JCAHO's requirements for a quality assurance program. These requirements are not discussed in detail here as they are accomplished by following the previously described steps. The requirements are that the quality assurance program be

- planned, systematic, and ongoing
- comprehensive (activities include all those providing care and encompass major diagnostic, therapeutic, and preventive functions)

- based on indicators and criteria agreed on by the department or service and acceptable to the organization
- of a nature that will result in appropriate actions to resolve identified problems
- continuous
- integrated with other departments or services and merged with information through the department (JCAH 1986).

CONCLUSION

Quality assurance is a primary concern in health care today. Because it is a primary issue, it is essential that a health care facility develop a sound quality assurance program. The 10 steps outlined are crucial to accomplish this task. Once this program is in progress, there will be *quality*—excellence in service and care.

REFERENCES

Brown, ML. 1986. Quality Assurance in Long-term Care. Chicago, IL, JCAH.

Bull MJ. 1985. Quality assurance: Its origins, transformations, and prospects. In Meisenheimer CG. Quality Assurance: A Complete Guide to Effective Programs. Rockville, MD, Aspen Publishers, 1–129.

Donabedian A. 1982. The quality of medical care. In Graham N, ed. Quality Assurance in Hospitals. Rockville, MD, Aspen Publishers, 15–26.

Graham N. 1982. Historical perspective and regulations regarding quality assessment. In Graham N. Quality Assurance in Hospitals. Rockville, MD, Aspen Publishers, 3–9.

JCAH. 1986. Monitoring and Evaluation in Nursing Services. Chicago, IL, JCAH.

Levy R, Goldstein B, Frott A. 1984. Approach to quality assurance in an emergency department: A one year review. Ann Emerg Med 13:166–169.

Lieske A. 1985. Standards: The basis of a quality assurance program. In Meisenheimer C. Quality Assurance. A Complete Guide to Effective Programs. Rockville, MD, Aspen Publishers, 1–129.

Mish F. 1985. Webster's Ninth New Collegiate Dictionary. Springfield, MA, Merriam-Webster.

Rhee K, Donabedian A, Burney R. 1987. Assessing the quality of care in a hospital emergency unit: A framework and its application. Qual Rev Bull 13:4–16.

Rowland H, Rowland B, 1987. The Manual of Nursing Quality Assurance. Rockville, MD, Aspen Publishers.

Wilbert C. 1985. Selecting topics/methodologies. In Meisenheimer C. Quality Assurance: A Complete Guide to Effective Programs. Rockville, MD, Aspen Publishers, 103–109.

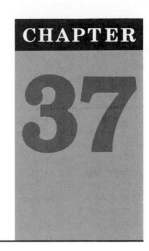
Ruth E. Rea, RN PhD CEN, LTC, US Army Nurse Corps

Emergency Nursing Productivity Issues

Confronted with increased pressure to contain costs, hospitals are now critically evaluating their cost effectiveness. Under the past system of cost-plus reimbursement, hospitals actually faced economic incentives to increase costs (Curtin 1984) to generate additional revenue. In contrast, in today's cost-containment environment, hospitals are struggling to employ effective methods to remain financially solvent. With this increased emphasis on cost containment, nurse administrators are challenged to describe nursing's contributions to the overall hospital's revenue and to define nursing productivity quantitatively. Most of these efforts to define nursing productivity have concentrated on the in-patient setting. However, as lengths of stay within hospitals shorten owing to prospective payment constraints, the acuity of illness in patients seen in emergency care settings has increased. It is anticipated that the issue of nursing productivity within the emergency care setting will become increasingly important as a means of justifying staffing and budget. Thus, the purpose of this chapter is to provide the reader with a basic understanding of productivity measurement issues with special focus on the evaluation and use of patient classification systems within emergency care settings. To foster this understanding, a review of generic productivity definitions is included, current in-patient classification systems are discussed, and current methods to document emergency nursing productivity are

---

The opinions or assertions contained herein are the private views of the author and are not to be construed as official or as reflecting the view of the Department of the Army or the Department of Defense.

analyzed. Additionally, problems with patient classification systems and methods to manage staffing shortfalls are presented.

PRODUCTIVITY DEFINITIONS

A measurement of productivity involves comparing output with input, simplistically formulated as follows:

$$\text{Productivity} = \frac{\text{Total Output}}{\text{Total Input}}$$

The critical issue in productivity measurement relates to the definition of the unit of analysis, specifically deciding what constitutes output and input. Within some health care settings, very basic formulas define output as clinic visits and describe input in terms of staffing hours or dollars. Thus, productivity is reflected in cost per clinic visit or required staff numbers per clinic visit. Although the calculations are fairly simple, productivity defined by this measurement method has limited applicability. The major limitation is that required nursing care as related to specific clinic visits cannot be determined accurately. It is well known that not all clinic or emergency visits require the same amount of nursing care time (e.g., a patient requiring major trauma resuscitation versus a patient with complaints of a urinary tract infection). It is impossible to determine, by using emergency visit as the output unit of measurement, the contribution of nursing to the emergency facility workload or the nursing staff's productivity.

A much more sensitive measure of nursing productivity compares the hours of required nursing care of patients seen in the emergency care facility with the hours of available nursing care. This productivity formula may be written as follows:

$$\text{Nursing Productivity} = \frac{\text{Hours of Available Nursing Time}}{\text{Hours of Required Nursing Time}}$$

The resulting index provides a basis by which the productivity of nursing can be evaluated. If the index is less than 1.0, the actual hours provided were less than the hours required by types of patients seen. This may mean that the staff was "more" productive, or it may mean that less than adequate nursing staff was available to provide professional nursing care to patients seen during the measured time period. An index greater than 1.0 indicates that actual hours of available nursing care exceeded those required by patients. Within the emergency care setting, this may not be uncommon owing to variations in patient arrival as well as seasonal and monthly fluctuations. It may also mean that staffing levels are higher than required for patient needs. In any case, a measurement of nursing care as required by specific types of patients is necessary if nursing productivity and the cost of nursing care are to be determined. A patient classification system that defines the required nursing care of specific patients is becoming increasingly necessary in emergency care settings.

IN-PATIENT CLASSIFICATION SYSTEMS

As the development of patient classification systems in the emergency care area has lagged behind that for the in-patient area, a brief review of the development of in-patient illness acuity measures may be helpful in understanding issues that influence measurement of productivity and acuity of illness within the emergency care facility. Driven by the cost-containment environment, in-patient classification systems have become increasingly complex. These systems can be divided into three basic designs, which represent a progression in the sophistication of measurement and data collection systems. These in-patient classification systems are as follows: (1) descriptive, (2) checklist, and (3) engineered unit standard (Lewis and Carini 1984).

A descriptive classification system groups patients into a certain category on the basis of a previously defined narrative description. For example, a patient on a mechanical ventilator might be categorized as a Level I patient whereas a self-care patient might be categorized as a Level IV patient. The major advantage of this system is that it provides a time-efficient method by which to categorize patients. Additionally, it does provide some guidelines by which to match direct patient care needs to required nurse staffing.

However, this system has several major limitations. First, it requires subjective interpretation by the nursing staff in that the same patient might be categorized into different levels by different nurses. Secondly, this system does not provide a mechanism by which to match the amount of nursing care hours quantitatively with specific categories of patients. Using the example already given, it can only be said that the Level I patient requires more nursing care than the Level IV patient. The exact or even the average amount of nursing care required by both patients is unknown. Thus, although this system is time efficient, it does not provide the data needed to measure productivity or to make budgetary decisions.

A checklist design is the second major form of in-patient classification system. In this method, various descriptions of patient activities or cooperative abilities are assigned point values on the basis of an estimation of time required to perform these tasks. Patients are then assigned to specific categories of care according to the total number of points.

Although this checklist design offers several improvements over the descriptive system, problems still exist. First, different nurses can still categorize the same patient differently. In addition, only direct nursing care is measured and the checklist frequently is not comprehensive. Finally, most often points are assigned to various activities only on the basis of an estimation of the time required to complete a given task.

The engineered-unit standard design represents the most complex patient classification system and provides the most objective data. However, the development of an engineered-based patient classification system is arduous and involves many complex steps. A tasking document must be developed that identifies both direct and indirect patient care activities. Each of the identified tasks needs to be defined to establish the specifications for measurement. After determining and defining these activities, timed observations must be conducted and obtained across all shifts and all days of the week. From an analysis of these measurements, nursing activities can be grouped into various patient care indicators and ultimately collapsed into three to five larger patient care categories. Each of these categories can be correlated with a specific amount of required nursing time.

Use of a patient classification system based on an engineered unit standard has several important advantages over the descriptive and checklist systems. It does provide an objective, quantitative method that relates patient care needs to required nurse staffing. It also provides a means to determine nursing budget on the basis of patient care needs. Finally, the information derived from engineered unit standards tends to have high credibility with hospital administrators because of their familiarity with industrial productivity models and engineering methodology.

However, use of an engineered patient classification system is not a total panacea as this method has some major limitations when used to measure nursing productivity.

First, the development of a patient classification system based on engineered standards requires a great deal of time. Additionally, these standards are finite and must be reviewed at least annually to ensure that they continue to reflect the current status of nursing practice and appropriate care categories for the current patient population (Alward 1983).

Second, engineered standards are facility specific. Although many institutions borrow engineered standards developed in other facilities, the nurse manager needs to be aware that differences in facility design, nursing philosophy, patient population, and categorization of direct and indirect patient care activities may invalidate the patient care categories and nursing staff requirements within a specific institution.

An additional problem with engineered standards is that these systems measure nursing as it is actually practiced. An engineered standard is not required to determine appropriateness of staffing levels or appropriateness of activities prior to determining time standards. For example, if a nursing unit is understaffed, it will be difficult to demonstrate a need to increase nursing staff as an engineered standard will reflect only the actual time associated with measured activities.

In a similar vein, engineered standards measure both direct and indirect patient care activities without analysis of the impact of staffing on both categories. For example, the absence of a unit clerk will increase the indirect care activities of professional nurses. Yet, most engineered standards do not calculate the time that could be spent in direct nursing care by the professional nurse if a unit clerk was present.

Perhaps the greatest weakness of engineered standards is that they do not reflect the discretionary aspects of professional nursing practice. Patient classification systems derived from these types of standards do not measure the timeliness of nursing interventions, analyze the required judgments, or evaluate the prioritizing of nursing activities (Curtin 1984).

EMERGENCY PATIENT CLASSIFICATION SYSTEMS

Although lagging behind the in-patient setting, the development of patient classification systems in the emergency care environment has paralleled the development of in-patient classification systems. Similar to the in-patient settings, emergency care

TABLE 37-1
PCS Evaluation Guidelines

1. Examine definitions of direct nursing care activities.
2. Review completeness of measured activities.
3. Review definitions of indirect care activities
4. Analyze unique issues of facility
5. Review reliability and validity information

systems are responsive to governmental and consumer concerns regarding the cost of health care and are attempting to control costs with productive use of staff (Federa and Bilodeau 1984). Managers in these settings are attempting to define productivity in the emergency care environment to determine appropriate staffing levels, to forecast future patient care needs, and to verify budgetary proposals.

Akin to occupied bed measurements, clinic visits have initially been used to determine staffing levels and to monitor productivity in the emergency care area. However, clinic visits are an inadequate measurement of acuity of illness or nursing productivity as this unit of analysis presumes that all emergency patients require similar levels of nursing care.

Within the past several years, quantitative patient classification systems have been developed for the emergency patient that purport to measure the required nursing care for specific categories of patients. Several factors must be considered when evaluating a quantitative patient classification for the emergency care setting (Table 37-1).

First, the listing that guided the measurement of direct nursing care activities should be examined. This direct care listing should allow the full range of professional nurse functioning as practiced in that facility. Many times, patient classification systems measure only the technical tasks (e.g., dressing changes, vital signs) associated with emergency care. Measures of discretionary professional nursing activities, to include assessment, prioritizing, evaluation, and patient teaching, should be recognized and timed by a patient classification system if the resultant staffing guidelines are to reflect appropriate nursing functions. In most cases, a tasking document with operational definitions of activities as originally developed and that guided the industrial engineer is available for examination by the nurse administrator.

Second, the listing of direct nursing care activities should be reviewed for comprehensiveness related to a specific practice setting. Several nursing functions may vary among emergency facilities to include triage, observation of patients within a holding area, and degree of patient teaching. Also, the presence of a medical residency program may either increase or decrease the amount of required nursing time.

Third, the category of indirect nursing activities also needs to be examined. Whether using an outside consultant or adapting a previously developed patient classification system, the definition of indirect care should be evaluated. In most cases, indirect nursing activities reflect the amount of time spent in activities not directly involved in patient care (e.g., meals, breaks, personal time, or wait time). Some patient classification systems define indirect care activities as all activities that do not occur directly with the patient. Using this definition, important emergency nursing functions such as family teaching and communication with other health care professionals would be considered indirect care. Additionally, some systems do not separate the direct care activities performed by the head nurse. Instead, all the nurse manager's time is considered indirect time. In both examples, the indirect care percentage is inflated. As indirect care ratios are closely monitored by most hospital administrators, it is important that the indirect time be determined accurately and be reflective of the nursing philosophy within the institution.

Fourth, several unique facility-specific factors must be considered. Unlike most in-patient areas, emergency patients tend to demonstrate great variation in arrival to the emergency care facility as indicated by fluctuations in patients seen per shift, day, month, or season of the year. It is also difficult to predict a patient's length of stay within an emergency environment as this length of stay may depend on factors beyond a patient's direct care needs (e.g., in-patient bed availability or medical staff requirements). Finally, transport distances to laboratory, radiology departments, and in-patient units influence the required number of nursing staff members to provide patient care. Thus, any patient classification system must be evaluated in relation to these areas when determining acceptability for use within a specific institution.

Finally, psychometric properties of a patient classification system should be reviewed. Although much can be discussed within this area, the nurse administrator should minimally evaluate reliability and validity. Reliability refers to the consistency with which the classification tools determines acuity of illness. The most common form of reliability for acuity instruments is interrater reliability. If the reliability coefficient is less than 0.85, developers of the patient classification should be questioned regarding the probable reasons why this has occurred. Validity refers to the accuracy of measurement and is more difficult to evaluate than reliability. As a minimum, the illness acuity tool developers should provide information related to content and criterion validity.

STAFFING DERIVED FROM PATIENT CLASSIFICATION SYSTEMS

Once acuity of illness is determined, translation of patient needs into nursing staff requirements can be accomplished. This involves the following steps:

- Categorization of patients on the basis of acuity points
- Determination of required direct nursing care hours on the basis of illness acuity
- Calculation of indirect nursing care hours
- Calculation of total required nursing care hours
- Determination of full-time equivalents (FTE) on the basis of total required nursing care hours.

Using Table 37–2 to illustrate the foregoing steps, four categories of patients have been developed according to the summation of illness acuity points for the patient. (Generally categories are determined statistically by the developers of the instrument.) Each category reflects an increase in nursing care needs, with a category I patient requiring an average of 0.5 nursing care hours and a category IV patient requiring 2.5 nursing care hours. Within each category, the number of patients is multiplied by the average required nursing care times. In the cited example, a total of

TABLE 37–2
Staffing Derived From PCS Data

	Category				
	I	II	III	IV	Total
Monthly Patient Illness Acuity Data—December					
Number of Patients	950	1500	400	50	2900
Average Nursing Hours per Patient	0.5	1.0	1.5	2.5	—
Total Nursing Hours	475	1500	600	125	2700
Staffing Calculation					
Step 1:	Direct time $= (950 \cdot 0.5) + (1500 \cdot 1.0) + (400 \cdot 1.5) + (50 \cdot 2.5) = 2700$ hours				
Step 2:	Indirect time $= 2700$ direct hours $\cdot 60\% = 1620$ hours				
Step 3:	Total nursing care hours $= 2700$ direct hours $+ 1620$ indirect hours $= 4320$ hours				
Step 4	Full-time equivalents (FTEs) $= 4320$ total nursing care hours $\div 168$ average available hours/person $= 25.7$ or 26 FTEs				

2700 direct nursing care hours was required for the 2900 patients seen during the month of December (step 1).

The indirect care time generally is calculated as a percentage of direct time, which is derived from actual work sampling measurements. This percentage may range from 50 to 75 per cent, depending on the exact definition of indirect nursing care. Using a 60 per cent factor in the cited example, the total number of indirect care hours is 1620.

After determination of direct and indirect care hours, the required number of full-time equivalents can be determined. An average of 168 hours is used as the divisor because this figure represents the average number of hours available on a monthly basis, accounting for the various holidays that occur throughout the year. In the example cited, 26 full-time equivalents are required on the basis of illness acuity and indirect time.

Once the full-time equivalents have been determined, scheduling of staff members will need to reflect the required seven days per week, 24 hours per day coverage. With more sensitive classification systems, information can be collected that reflects the average acuity of illness of patients per shift or per days of the week. This information is especially useful in matching required staffing with required patient care needs.

PATIENT CLASSIFICATION SYSTEM LIMITATIONS

Similar to the limitations identified with in-patient classification systems, methods used to describe emergency patient illness acuity and associated required nursing care also have some restrictions.

The first major limitation associated with emergency patient classification systems is that the recommended staffing may not reflect safe staffing when patient volume is low. Within the emergency care setting, a certain minimal number of staff members or "critical mass" needs to be available in spite of low volume. Thus, a patient classification system may recommend only one nurse on the night shift on the basis of patient volume; however, the minimum number of staff members will need to be two to three to safely respond to patients with a major emergency.

A second major problem area associated with emergency patient classification is the method by which activities are measured or timed. The preferred method by which to measure activities associated with emergency patient care is direct observation and timing. Many patient classification systems developed by specific institutions have used time estimates or self-reports of time required to accomplish certain activities (Genovich-Richards and Tracy 1984; Henninger and Dailey 1983). Although the use of time estimates or self-reports simplifies the development of a patient classification system, concerns are raised regarding the validity and reliability of the patient care measurements and associated staffing requirements.

Finally, the development of an emergency patient classification system needs to be tied to a professional standard of care as opposed to measuring activities only as currently performed (Simms et al 1985). For example, patient education might not be performed currently within a specific emergency care setting owing to staffing shortages. Thus, if time and motion studies are conducted, time for patient education might not be measured or included in the derivation of required patient care. Thus, it seems important to measure required nursing care on the basis of standards of care as developed by a specific institution to reflect types of patients seen, consumer expectations, nursing philosophy, nursing practice acts, and institutional policy.

The inclusion of standards as a means to develop an emergency patient classification system offers several advantages to the nurse manager. Standards of care clearly identify for the industrial engineer the activities that must be measured. Standards would ensure the incorporation of the discretionary aspects of professional nursing into the measurement approaches.

Moreover, the nurse manager can analyze the appropriate staffing level for each category of patient care. Use of standards of care can assist in determining appropriate qualifications of staff members as well as the total number of full-time equivalences.

Using standards as a basis for patient classification systems also identifies various courses of action for the nurse manager. When confronted with budgetary reductions, the nurse manager can specifically indicate resources needed to accomplish care. For example, when faced with a reduction in professional staff, the nurse manager could demonstrate that the function of patient discharge instructions requires specific resources. Jointly, the hospital administrator and nurse executive would need to develop a plan for selection or retention of staff members that realistically could provide the required service (Mason and Daugherty 1984). This may mean a re-evaluation of the decision to decrease staff, or it may mean the relocation of the function to other health care professionals (e.g., physicians).

MANAGEMENT OF PATIENT CLASSIFICATION SYSTEM SHORTFALLS

Patient classification systems provide information by which the required hours of nursing care can be compared with the available nursing hours. These systems do not

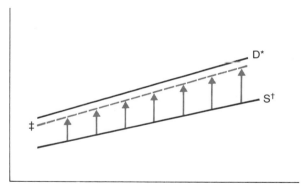

*D (Demand) = Required patient care hours
†S (Supply) = Available nursing care hours
‡ = New supply line

FIGURE 37–1. Supply line shift.

identify how to manage staffing shortfalls; this remains within the purview of the nurse manager to implement strategies to narrow this gap between required and actual hours of nursing care. Although most managerial efforts concentrate on increasing the supply of nurses, the prudent nurse manager should evaluate both methods to increase the supply of nurses and methods to alter patient flow into the emergency care facility.

In shortfalls, adjustment in the supply of nursing staff is often the first response (Fig. 37–1). Several strategies should be evaluated as a means to increase the number of available nursing hours. First, the nurse manager needs to evaluate patient flow and to match staffing with peaks in the demands. Frequently, the early evening shift has a higher patient illness acuity and volume than the later evening hours. By staggering or extending shifts (e.g., 10- or 12-hour shifts), nursing staff members can overlap at appropriate times to match the higher patient volume or illness acuity. Additionally, if certain days of the week have increased patient care requirements (e.g., weekends), per diem staff can be used to provide the extra required nursing hours.

Second, the nurse manager needs to evaluate the current staffing mix. The nurse manager may consider increasing the number of professional nurses on the staff. Professional nurses tend to be more productive as they do not need supervision, and they are able to perform the full range of nursing activities. Allied health professionals may need supervision in certain activities. In addition, they may be "available" (not performing other activities), but the required task may be beyond the scope of their practice. For example, an allied health professional may not be busy at the time someone is needed to start an intravenous line. However, because the task may not be within this staff member's job description, the allied health professional must wait for the professional nurse to start the intravenous line. Thus, the professional nurse with the broader scope of practice tends to be more productive and incurs less indirect time (specifically, waiting time).

To optimize the staffing mix, the nurse manager might also evaluate job descriptions and reorganize job content to reflect more productive use of staffing. This reorganization might result in consolidation of nonpatient care activities to the appropriate allied health professional level. It might also result in the development of

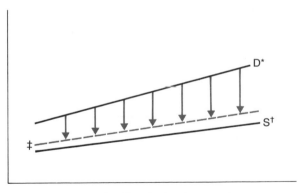

*D (Demand) = Required patient care hours
†S (Supply) = Available nursing care hours
  ‡ = New demand line

FIGURE 37–2. Demand line shift.

more flexible job descriptions, which encourage cross-training and cross-utilization of professional nursing staff (e.g., rotation between emergency care settings and adjunct clinics).

Although patient flow is evaluated infrequently by the nurse manager, strategies aimed at adjusting the patient flow or demand into the emergency care facility can reduce the gap between actual and required nursing care hours (Fig. 37–2).

Patient flow needs to be evaluated to determine appropriateness of emergency visits and to analyze if other facilities within the institution are more appropriate sources of care. Clinical hours might be evaluated in relationship to demand. For example, it might be noted that an increase in pediatric patients occurs regularly between 3:00 and 5:00 P.M., after the pediatric clinic closes. Cost analysis should be conducted to determine if it is more beneficial to extend pediatric clinic hours or to hire additional emergency nursing staff as a means of closing the gap between required and actual nursing care hours.

CONCLUSION

As a result of the recent emphasis on cost containment, emergency nurse managers are increasingly focusing on productivity issues. Initially, it seemed that the development of patient classification systems would be a panacea for determining required nurse staffing levels. However, a closer examination of patient classification instruments indicates that the nurse managers must carefully evaluate the use of these instruments within a given facility. It should be recognized that the use of a patient classification system is only the initial step in the analysis of productivity. Many variables influence productivity. The prudent nurse manager will need to identify the critical variables as well as ensure the development and use of a patient classification system that measures professional nursing practice.

REFERENCES

Alward RR. 1983. Patient classification systems: The ideal vs. reality. J Nurs Adm 13:14–19.

Anderson J, McCall P. 1983. Productivity and staffing: Cost-effective issues of the 1980s. J Emerg Nurs 9:172–173.

Channon B. 1983. Dispelling productivity myths. Hospitals 57:103–104, 106.

Curtin LL. 1984. Reconciling pay with productivity. Nurs Management 15(2):7–8.

Danis DM. 1987. Management. In Rea R E, Bourg P, Parker JG et al, eds. Emergency Nursing Core Curriculum Philadelphia, WB Saunders, 865–900.

Federa RD, Bilodeau TW. 1984. The productivity quest. J Ambulatory Care Management 7(3):5–11.

Genovich-Richards J, Tracy RL. 1984. An assessment process for nursing staff patterns in ambulatory care. J Ambulatory Care Management 7(2):69–78.

Hanson RL. 1982. Managing human resources. J Nurs Adm 12(12):17–23.

Henninger D, Dailey C. 1983. Measuring nursing workload in an outpatient department. J Nurs Adm 13(9):20–23.

Herzog T. 1985. Productivity: Fighting the battle of the budget. Nurs Management 16(1):30–34.

Jarrard JK. 1983. Engineered standards in hospital nursing. Nurs Management 14(4):29–32.

Johnson EA. 1981. Thinking conceptually about hospital efficiency. Hospital Health Serv Adm 26:12–26.

Lewis EN, Carini PV. 1984. Nurse, Staffing and Patient Classification. Rockville, MD, Aspen Systems.

Mason EJ, Daugherty JK. 1984. Nursing standards should determine nursing's price. Nurs Management 15(9):34–48.

Prescott RA, Phillips CY. 1988. Gauging nursing intensity to bring costs to light. Nurs Health Care 9(1):17–22.

Schulmerich SC. 1984. Developing a patient classification system for the emergency department. J Emerg Nurs 10:298–305.

Simms LM, Price SA, Ervin NE. 1985. The Professional Practice of Nursing Administration. New York, John Wiley and Sons.

Topf M. 1986. Three estimates of interrater reliability for nominal data. Nurs Res 35:253–255.

Vestal KW. 1983. Promoting excellence in the emergency department. J Emerg Nurs 9:290–293.

Wenke PC. 1983. 13 steps toward enhancing productivity. Hospitals 57(19):109–110, 112.

Wilson Haas SA. 1984. Sorting out nursing productivity. Nurs Management 15(4):37–40.

Organ and Tissue Donation: What Emergency Department Nurses Should Know

Michael Schroyer, RN MSN CCRN CNA

Organ and tissue transplantations have become so commonplace that more than 100 transplants are performed daily in the United States.[1] Organs and tissues currently used for transplantation are heart, liver, pancreas, kidney, bowel, lung, cornea, bone and connective tissue, bone marrow, heart for heart valves, saphenous vein, and skin. With current advances in technique and immunosuppression, the concept and practice of organ and tissue transplantation into health-impaired or terminally ill patients has become a modern fact of life.

Even with an increase in the number of transplants per year, there are still thousands of people with end-stage organ and tissue disease waiting for a transplant, as shown in Table 1. Efforts to increase the number of available donor organs and tissues are under way to meet the increasing demand.

REQUIRED REQUEST

With the demand for donor organs and tissues for transplantation increasing, the federal government has taken steps to resolve some of the issues surrounding transplantation. In 1986, Congress passed the Omnibus Budget Reconciliation Act (OBRA), which became effective on October 1, 1987. The provisions of this bill, which apply to all hospitals receiving Medicare or Medicaid reimbursement, are as follows:

1. Hospitals must have written protocol for donor identification.
2. The family must be informed of the option of organ or tissue donation.
3. Discretion and sensitivity must be observed.
4. Organ procurement organization must be notified of potential organ or tissue donors.

The federal government also enacted the Organ Donation Request Act in January 1987. This act, better known as "Required Request," was developed in response

TABLE 1
Organ and Tissue Transplantation in the U.S.

Organ or Tissue	Transplants in 1987	One-Year Survival Rate (Per Cent)	Number Waiting (August 1988)
Kidney	9094	92–95	13,233
Heart	1438	75–85	919
Liver	1199	70	512
Pancreas	142	90	151
Heart-lung	49	50	184
Cornea	35,000	90–95	7500

Statistics obtained from Regional Organ Bank of Illinois, Chicago, Illinois.

to the reluctance of health care professionals to ask families for organ or tissue donation. Provisions of Required Request are as follows:

• Next of kin must be asked for consent.
• Consent can be secured by the attending physician.
• Deference should be paid to donor's religious beliefs.
• Notification must be made to the Organ Procurement Organization.
• No sanctions for hospital noncompliance.

According to both acts, hospitals must comply with the provisions in each act, or Medicare and Medicaid reimbursement may be withheld. To date, 44 states have written and adopted Required Request legislation in conjunction with the federal guidelines.

WHAT IS POSSIBLE FOR PROCUREMENT

The emergency department (ED) has a major role in identification of potential organ and tissue donors. Organ donation requires that respiratory (artifically maintained) and circulatory functions remain intact. Tissue donors can be either respiratory and circulatory maintained brain-dead patients or patients who have expired from cardiorespiratory arrest.

The ED is rarely involved in the procurement process of visceral organs. Organ donors usually are maintained in the intensive care unit until brain death can be declared and consent obtained from the family. However, the ED has a vital function in identifying and stabilizing the condition of patients fitting the donor criteria. Ideal organ donors are previously healthy individuals who have suffered irreversible catastrophic brain injury, often resulting from acute head or neurologic trauma, subarachnoid hemorrhage or stroke, primary brain tumor, drug overdose or smoke inhalation (in some cases), or hepatic coma.

Criteria for organ donation are as follows:[2]

• Under 65 years of age
• Arrived at the hospital with respirations and heartbeat intact

- Unconscious with fixed dilated pupils and no reflexes
- Ultimately requires a ventilator
- Functioning kidneys and no history of kidney disease, chronic hypertension, or long-standing diabetes
- No systemic infection, communicable disease, or malignancy (except for primary brain tumor)
- Reasonable expectation of cardiovascular stability

Many tissue donors are identified and maintained in the ED. Because no ventilatory and cardiovascular support is necessary for tissue donation, any patient who dies in the ED can be a potential donor.* Tissues that can be procured are eyes or corneas, bone, and tissue (tendons, dura mater, fascia), heart for heart valves, saphenous vein, and skin.† Criteria for tissue donation are as follows:

Eye Donation[3]

- Age 1 to 75 years
- Absence of
    Acquired immunodeficiency syndrome (AIDS)
    Encephalopathies (Creutzfeldt-Jakob disease, rabies)
    Hepatitis
    Leukemia
    Lymphoma

Skin Donation

- Age 12 to 60 years
- Absence of
    Cancer
    Leukemia
    Skin infection
    Extensive dermatitis
    History of hepatitis, AIDS

Bone and Tissue Donation[4]

- Age 16 to 60 (may go to 65) years
- Absence of
    Hepatitis, AIDS, syphilis, tuberculosis
    Malignancy (other than primary brain tumor)
    Systemic infection

---

* Routine testing of all donors is done to detect antibodies for HIV and HB_sAg (hepatitis B surface antigen).

† Donors 40 to 60 (or 65) years old require a chest and abdominal autopsy to rule out malignancy. Donors for any transplantable tissue must not be in a high-risk category for AIDS, as defined by the Centers for Disease Control (e.g., homosexual men, intravenous drug abusers, prostitutes, hemophiliacs, or sex partners of the foregoing).

Autoimmune process
Intravenous substance abuse
Bone pathology
Musculoskeletal disease
Human growth hormone administration
Slow viral disease

Heart (for Heart Valves) Donation[5]

- Age birth to 55 years
- Cardiac asystole up to 12 hours acceptable
- Absence of
  Significant hypertension
  Insulin-dependent diabetes mellitus
  Communicable disease
  Injections of human pituitary–derived growth hormone
  Tumors (other than primary brain tumor)
  Progressive neurologic disorder (e.g., Creutzfeldt-Jakob syndrome)
  Neoplastic disease
  History of valvular heart disease
   No history of rheumatic disease
   No bacterial endocarditis
   No significant murmurs
  Cardiac trauma (chest compressions acceptable if length of time under 60 minutes)
  Sepsis
  AIDS, hepatitis, syphilis, cytomegalovirus disease
  Leukemia

Saphenous Vein Donation[5]

- Age 5 to 55 years
- Cardiac asystole up to 10 hours acceptable
- Absence of
  Vascular disease (arteriosclerosis, atherosclerosis, phlebosclerosis, varicosities in the area to be recovered)
  Trauma to area of potential vessel recovery
  Significant hypertension
  Sepsis
  Communicable disease
  AIDS, hepatitis, syphilis
  Leukemia
  Malignancy (except for primary skin and central nervous system lesions)
  Insulin-dependent diabetes mellitus
  Progressive neurologic disorder (e.g., Creutzfeldt-Jakob disease)
  Injections of human pituitary–derived growth hormone.

Body Donation

• Contact your local organ procurement organization

It is extremely important for the ED nurse or physician to obtain a complete past medical and surgical history on potential organ and tissue donors when they are admitted to the department. This will prevent disturbing the family for this information during a time of grief. Families of potential tissue donors between the ages of 40 and 60 (or 65) should be asked for consent for autopsy when consent for donation is obtained.

For tissue donors, several tubes of blood should be obtained so that the organ procurement organization and tissue banks can run serology tests to rule out human immunodeficiency virus, hepatitis, and syphilis. Blood cultures from three (minimum of one) different sites and a tube of blood for a white blood cell count and differential count should be obtained and sent to the laboratory in order to rule out any systemic infection.

When patients who fit the criteria for organ or tissue donation have been identified, the ED should notify the local organ procurement organization as soon as possible. A procurement coordinator will assist you in (1) determining if the patient is a suitable organ or tissue donor, (2) discussing organ and tissue donation with the patient's family, (3) obtaining permission from the medical examiner or coroner, (4) assisting with donor management, and (5) coordinating the recovery of all donated organs and tissues.

MEDICAL EXAMINER'S OR CORONER'S CASES

The ED staff often deals with Medical Examiner's or Coroner's cases. Cases seen in the ED that fall under the jurisdiction of the Medical Examiner or Coroner include the following:[2]

1. Deaths by homicide or suspicion of homicide
2. Deaths by suicide or suspicion of suicide
3. Deaths from accidental, traumatic injury
4. All deaths from poisoning or suspected poisoning
5. All deaths resulting from abortion
6. Deaths during or immediately following diagnostic, therapeutic, surgical or anesthetic procedures

Permission for organ and tissue donation must be obtained by the Medical Examiner or Coroner if the donor is a Coroner's case. The following information should be readily available when contacting the Medical Examiner or Coroner:

• Donor's name and address
• Time and type of accident
• Police report and badge number of officer at the scene
• Ambulance attendant's or allied health professional's report of the patient's condition at the scene of the accident and at arrival to the ED
• Most important, the time brain death was declared and by whom

DETERMINATION OF BRAIN DEATH

It is important for the nurse to check if his or her hospital has set criteria for determining brain death consistent with applicable state law. The state legal requirements determine the criteria for determination of brain death and the way they may be applied.

A neurologic or neurosurgical consultation should be obtained whenever possible. Brain death should not be determined by the surgeon(s) performing the organ removal.[6]

At present, 38 states and the District of Columbia have legislation recognizing the legality of brain death pronouncements. In those states that do not have brain death legislation, court decisions and institutional policies frequently permit the use of neurologic criteria to determine brain death.[7]

APPROACHING THE FAMILY

According to the Illinois Uniform Anatomical Gift Act, any person has, prior to death, the right to legally consent to donate all or part of his or her body after death for medical research, education, or transplantation. However, by common practice consent for organ or tissue donation is obtained from the donor's next of kin. The following is the order of priority of individuals from whom consent can be obtained:

1. Spouse
2. Adult son or daughter
3. Either parent
4. Adult brother or sister
5. Guardian of the decedent at time of death
6. Any other person authorized or under obligation to dispose of the body

Before anyone approaches the next of kin requesting organ donation, the local organ procurement organization should be consulted to determine the patient's suitability for organ donation.[8]

Approaching the family should be done in a dignified and professional manner by a designated professional determined by the hospital's required request policy. This person should have a positive attitude toward organ and tissue donation and should have knowledge about the donation process. If the professional designated to approach the family has a negative and nonprofessional attitude and approach toward organ and tissue donation, the family will likely decline.

Family members need emotional support during this time of bereavement. It is helpful for the nursing staff to comfort the family and allow them to express their feelings and doubts about organ and tissue donation. The ED nurse should notify clergy to help the family cope with their grief during this time.

The ED nurse must be empathetic and support whatever decision the family has made. The family should not be pressured to donate. If assistance in approaching the family is needed, contact the local organ procurement organization or tissue bank and ask for assistance from a procurement coordinator.

Following is a list of facts that are important to know when approaching a family for donation.

- No cost incurred during organ or tissue retrieval will be billed to the family or donor's insurance company.
- There is no disfigurement of the body during the procurement of organs and tissues. Wake and funeral arrangements may still be carried out in the usual manner.
- Organ and tissue retrieval is a dignified, sterile surgical procedure.
- Confidentiality of the donor and recipients is ensured.
- Organ and tissue donation may take several hours.
- A follow-up letter may be sent to the donor family by the organ and tissue procurement coordinator if requested.
- Donated organs are always given to those in greatest need.
- Religious leaders worldwide support organ donation.
- There often exist three options:
  1. Discontinue ventilation
  2. Continue ventilation until cardiopulmonary death occurs
  3. Organ and tissue donation is possible
- Organ and tissue donation often helps families cope with the loss of a loved one.[2]

ORGAN DONOR MANAGEMENT

The major goal in organ donor management is to maintain optimal hydration, oxygenation, and hemodynamic stability to ensure organ viability. The following guidelines should be utilized to promote optimal organ viability:

1. Maintain adequate fluid hydration, central venous pressure of 8 to 12 cm water.
2. Maintain minimal urine output of 80 to 100 ml/hour.
3. Maintain systolic blood pressure stability at a minimum of 100 mmHg.
4. Maintain adequate oxygenation.
5. Maintain electrolyte balance and blood sugar level.
6. Maintain normal body temperature.
7. Prevent infection; obtain blood, urine, and sputum cultures.

To maintain fluid volume, rapidly infuse normal saline solution or lactated Ringer's solution intravenously. Albumin may be used to increase the circulating volume. If the donor has hypovolemia owing to blood loss, transfuse with packed red blood cells.

Vasopressors may be used to maintain a systolic blood pressure of greater than 100 mmHg only after adequate fluid replacement has been attempted. Dopamine (Intropin) is the vasopressor of choice. Dosages of greater than 10 μg/kg/minute should be avoided. If dopamine does not correct hypotension, isoproterenol (Isuprel) may be used. The use of norepinephrine (Levophed) or metaraminol bitartrate (Aramine) should be avoided.

A urine output of 100 ml/hour should be maintained. If urine output is less than 100 ml/hour and does not increase with adequate blood pressure and optimal hydration with intravenous fluids, 12.5 to 25 g of mannitol should be administered and can be repeated every 6 hours until the organs are removed. If the patient has a high urine output, or has diabetes insipidus, the urine output should be replaced milliliter for milliliter plus 100 ml for insensible loss. Vasopressin (Pitressin) should be used only if necessary if the patient has diabetes insipidus.[2]

TISSUE DONOR MANAGEMENT

If both organs and tissues are being donated, use the organ donor management guidelines. Three blood cultures (minimum of 1) should be obtained from three different sites to rule out sepsis.

If only tissues are being donated, use the following guidelines.[5]

1. Tissue donors do not have to have cardiac activity.

2. Four to six red-top tubes of blood should be obtained. The tissue banks will use the tubes to run serology tests.

3. Three blood cultures (minimum of 1) should be performed.

4. A WBC count with differential should be obtained to detect infectious processes.

5. The donor should be kept in a refrigerated morgue until procurement of tissues can take place.

CONCLUSION

With the increase of organ and tissue transplants, many more patients wait for availability of an organ or tissue. This is due, in large part, to the lack of suitable organ and tissue donors. A contributing factor, however, is the lack of awareness of health care professionals with regard to organ and tissue donation.

The ED nurse is a vital link in the identification and management of potential organ and tissue donors. With increased awareness, the ED nurse can institute guidelines to identify organ and tissue donors, obtain consent, provide emotional support for the family, and provide proper medical management.

REFERENCES

1. Facts About Tissue Donation. Aug 1, 1988. Chicago, Regional Organ Bank of Illinois.
2. The Health Professional's Role in Organ and Tissue Donation. Oct 1, 1987. Chicago, Regional Organ Bank of Illinois.
3. Criteria for Eye Donation. 1988. Chicago, Illinois Eye Bank, p 2.
4. Rush-Presbyterian-St. Luke's Medical Center Tissue Bank. September 1988. Bone and Tissue Donor Criteria.
5. Donor Criteria for Heart (for Heart Valves) and Saphenous Vein Donation, established December 1, 1988. Marietta, GA. Cryolife, Inc.
6. American Hospital Association. 1986. Hospital Responsibilities in Requesting Organ Donations. Technical Advisory Bulletin, p 1.
7. Goldsmith J, Montefusco CM. 1985. Nursing care of the potential organ donor. Crit Care Nurse 5:22–29.
8. Illinois Uniform Anatomical Gift Act, PA 76–1209, Section 1, October 1, 1969.

Index

Note: Page numbers in italics *refer to figures; page numbers followed by (t) refer to tables.*

ISBN 0-7216-2374-3